DEDICATION

Andy, Matthew, and Katy –

May you provide encouragement, empower those you come into contact with,
work for justice, practice forgiveness, be self-aware, and celebrate life without caution.

S-

      Night, night

         Love you

            See you tomorrow

               Have a nice time sleeping

May the adventures continue

CONTENTS

16   Miscellaneous Wounds   397

17   Basic Dermatology   410

Heather Hettrick, PT, PhD, CWS, MLT, FACCWS

APPENDICES   437

INTRODUCTION

There are several distinguishing characteristics of this textbook that make it a superior learning tool for clinicians and students. First, each chapter begins with a list of key terms and chapter objectives to prepare the reader for the material that follows. Readers are encouraged to use these features as a self-study guide to check their understanding of the information provided. Second, the chapters include numerous tables, figures, and photographs to assist in highlighting information for readers and creating a link between the written text and actual patients in the clinic. Third, checkpoint questions within each chapter pose clinically relevant questions to promote reader comprehension. Fourth, review questions, located at the end of each chapter, provide an opportunity for readers to master chapter information. Answers to checkpoint and review questions are located in Appendix C to be used as a self-check. Fifth, the text models complete, concise documentation and provides readers with frequent opportunities to practice this vital skill. Sixth, a series of three case studies, located in Appendix B, encourage readers to apply their knowledge of basic science, examination, and interventions into a holistic plan of care for patients with open wounds. Readers are directed through a series of questions to describe photographs of patients with open wounds, hypothesize wound etiology, determine appropriate local wound care, and consider what additional interventions might be appropriate. Readers are encouraged to check their responses with the notes provided. Finally, www.myhealthprofessionskit.com **myhealthprofessionskit** is a supplement to the text, providing readers with additional full-color images, case studies, video clips of procedural interventions, and descriptions of various wounds, procedures, and products.

The text is organized into three major sections. Section I sets the stage for understanding wound care by reviewing basic science. Chapter 1 describes the normal anatomy of the integument and subcutaneous tissues. Chapter 2 reviews wound healing, including the phases of wound healing, wound healing processes, and abnormal wound healing. Chapter 3 presents factors known to adversely affect wound healing, including wound characteristics, local and systemic factors, as well as inappropriate wound care. The third edition includes expanded information on the normal phases of wound healing as well as the pathophysiology of chronic wounds to assist readers in clinical decision making.

Section II provides an overview of the examination of and interventions for patients with open wounds. Chapters cover examination, debridement, management of infection, dressing selection and bandaging, and modalities and physical agents. The section concludes with a chapter on the holistic management of patients with open wounds that provides detailed information on nutrition, adherence, and interdisciplinary wound management. By incorporating the most recent research available, the third edition provides increased depth on physical therapy tests and measures, biofilms, the use of silver, newer research-supported modalities and physical agents, and nutritional screening.

Section III builds upon the general patient and wound care information of Section II and applies this information to specific wound types, including arterial insufficiency ulcers, venous insufficiency ulcers, pressure ulcers, and neuropathic ulcers, as well as burns. Complete case studies have been incorporated into each of these chapters to allow the reader to integrate all aspects of anatomy, physiology, pathophysiology, and the five elements of patient management. A separate chapter addresses miscellaneous wounds such as abrasions, skin tears, surgical wounds, traumatic wounds, different types of bite wounds, wounds due to lymphedema, radiation fibrosis, and pyoderma gangrenosum. Each chapter describes the etiology, risk factors, classification, and characteristics for each wound type. The chapters provide detailed information on physical therapy tests and measures, as well as interventions for the successful management of patients with open wounds due to specific etiologies. Medical and surgical interventions that may apply to patients with open wounds are also discussed to provide the clinician with a better understanding of the valuable role these disciplines play in the management of patients with open wounds. Section III concludes with a chapter on basic dermatology to assist the clinician with screening intact skin.

Finally, the appendices include a wealth of information, including a glossary of terms, case studies, answers to chapter questions, total contact casting procedure, and a list of Internet wound care resources.

myhealthprofessionskit includes an image library, containing all of the photographs within the text as well as an electronic catalog of wounds of various etiologies such as trauma, burns, frostbite, and abuse. A separate section contains images and descriptions of various wound etiologies along with potential physical therapy interventions. Next, a separate section contains images and descriptions of various wound management procedures, modalities, and products. To further challenge the reader's understanding of wound management principles and practice, additional case studies, along with suggested answers, are provided. Documentation templates, following the framework within the text, are included to assist readers with incorporating didactic material into the clinic. Finally, the site contains video clips of many wound management procedures to enhance reader mastery of these skilled interventions.

The third edition contains many features for wound management course instructors. First, a PowerPoint™ presentation of each chapter, including tables and images, highlights key information. Second, sample laboratory activities and competencies for wound management interventions such as debridement, bandaging, and the use of modalities and physical agents are available to enhance student psychomotor skill development. Third, a bank of test questions for each chapter is provided to assess student cognitive integration of the information provided.

KEY UPDATES IN THE THIRD EDITION

Several key changes have been made in the third edition of this textbook to continue to provide a superior, holistic learning tool for students and clinicians. First, the landscape of medicine continues to change and all information and references have been updated to reflect current research and practice. Second, new sections including a chapter on lymphedema and an appendix on billing and documentation have been added. Third, the CD-ROM has been greatly expanded and reformatted into a website. MyHealthProfessionsKit **myhealthprofessionskit** includes access to images of most pathologies covered within the text, including open wounds, lymphedema, and dermatological conditions. In addition, the website contains chapter-by-chapter video clips including key information as well as demonstrations of proper procedural performance, such as debridement, modality use, dressing, and compression therapy.

ACKNOWLEDGMENTS

I would like to thank the following individuals who were key to the completion of this third edition:

- Stacy Takacs, whose problem solving, adaptability, and, dare I say, tact, have allowed me to continue to learn, grow, succeed, and enjoy.
- Melissa Kerian, whose patience and frequent reminders allowed this project to be completed (mostly) on schedule. Congratulations!
- Dr. Lam Le, for sharing her expertise and patients.
- Heather Hettrick, my safety plan and dermatology expert.
- My team of dedicated health care workers who cross state lines to keep me in the game.
- Arlene Dent and Myka, whose joy in life is just that.

REVIEWERS

Basic Science

1

Integumentary Anatomy

Chapter Objectives

After reading this chapter, learners will be able to:

1. Describe the normal structure and function of the epidermis.
2. Describe the normal structure and function of the dermis.
3. Describe the normal structure and function of the subcutaneous tissue.
4. State the main cells located within each layer of the integument and describe their functions.
5. Describe the normal structure of deeper tissues that may be exposed in open wounds including muscle, tendon, ligament, joint capsule, and bone.
6. Differentiate between viable and nonviable tissues that may be present in an open wound.
7. Differentiate between superficial, partial-thickness, and full-thickness wounds.

Key Terms

Adipose tissue	Keratin	Rete pegs
Basement membrane	Keratinocytes	Reticular dermis
Blisters	Langerhans' cells	Sebaceous gland
Callus	Macrophages	Sebum
Collagen	Mast cells	Stratum basale
Dermal papillae	Melanin	Stratum corneum
Elastin	Melanocytes	Stratum granulosum
Epidermis	Merkel cells	Stratum lucidum
Fascia	Nails	Stratum spinosum
Fibroblasts	Open wound	Subcutaneous tissue
Full-thickness wound	Papillary dermis	Sudoriferous glands
Hair	Partial-thickness wound	Superficial wound
Histamine	Phagocytizing	White blood cells

INTRODUCTION

This chapter describes the normal structure and function of the epidermis, dermis, subcutaneous tissue, and deeper tissues that may be involved in open wounds. In the average person, the skin weighs more than 4–5 kg, covers an area nearly 1.2 m^2–2.2 m^2, and ranges in thickness from 0.5 to 6.0 mm.[1–5] The thinnest skin is located on the eyelids and eardrums, while the thickest skin is located on the palms of the hands and the soles of the feet.[4,5] The integument is the largest organ system of the body,[1] and receives roughly one-third of resting cardiac output.[6,7] The skin is connective tissue that consists of cells, fibers, and an extracellular matrix organized into an outer epidermis and an inner dermis (see Figure 1–1). Beneath the dermis is a supportive subcutaneous connective tissue layer. Deeper tissues, including muscle, tendon, ligament, joint capsule, and bone, lie beneath the subcutaneous tissue layer. **Open wounds** involve a break in skin integrity, such as an abrasion, laceration, or ulcer. Open wounds may involve only the epidermis or may extend into deeper tissue layers. While the phases of wound healing apply to both open and closed wounds, the remainder of this text describes only open wounds.

Clinicians must be able to identify the extent of tissue involvement in order to classify open wounds and assess wound healing. Clinicians must also be able to differentiate normal, healthy, viable tissues from necrotic tissue and foreign materials that may be present in open wounds. In addition, clinicians must understand the impact tissue damage or loss can have both at the tissue level and for the patient as a whole. Chapter 17 provides detailed information on changes with aging skin.

EPIDERMIS

Epidermal Layers

The **epidermis** is the tough, leathery outer surface of the skin ranging in thickness from 0.06 to 0.6 mm, with the thickest portions located on the palms of the hands and the soles of the feet.[8] The epidermis is arranged into five layers that represent different stages of cellular differentiation. As new cells are formed, older cells elongate and their membranes thicken as they are pushed upward into the next epidermal layer. The deepest layer, the stratum basale, is attached to the dermis below by a thin, acellular **basement membrane.**

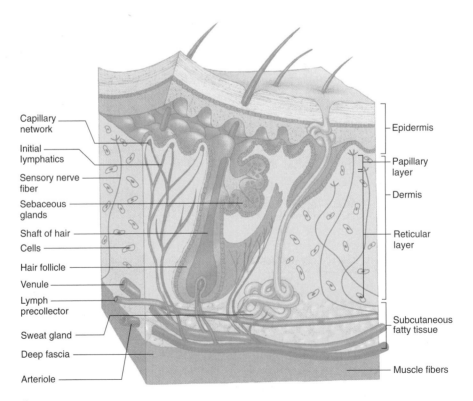

FIGURE 1–1   Skin structure.
Source: Emergency Care 10/e by Limmer/O'Keefe/Grant/Murray/Bergeron.

The basement membrane acts as a scaffolding for the epidermis and a selective filter for substances moving between the epidermis and the dermis.[8] The epidermis is avascular,[8] receiving its blood supply through the diffusion of nutrients from the dermis across the semipermeable basement membrane. The **stratum basale,** sometimes called the stratum germanitivum, is a single row of **keratinocytes,** continuously dividing cells that produce the protective protein **keratin.**[2] The **stratum spinosum** is the next layer. It consists of several rows of more mature keratinocytes, which appear "spiny" under a light microscope because of the keratin filaments.[4] Just above the stratum spinosum is the **stratum granulosum.** This layer contains three to five flattened cell rows with increasing concentrations of keratin.[2] As keratinocytes are pushed farther up and away from their dermal blood supply, they slowly die. The **stratum lucidum** contains a few layers of flattened, dead keratinocytes,[4] which appear clear through a light microscope. The outermost epidermal layer, the **stratum corneum,** or "horny" layer, consists entirely of dead keratinocytes.[2] The stratum corneum can be 20–30 cells thick and accounts for up to three-quarters of the thickness of the entire epidermis.[2]

The many layers of the stratum corneum serve as a physical barrier,[4,9] protecting the body from trauma and infection. The tight junctions between cells waterproof the skin, thereby helping regulate the body's fluid content. Dead cells of the stratum corneum are constantly abraded and replaced by cells from below. A cell's journey from the stratum basale up through the stratum corneum takes 14–21 days.[10] Occasionally, there is a localized buildup of cells of the stratum corneum due to pressure or friction. This is known as a **callus.**[2]

Epidermal Cell Types

Ninety percent of the epidermal cells are keratinocytes.[4] The epidermis contains three other main cell types: melanocytes, Merkel cells, and Langerhans' cells. **Melanocytes,** located in the stratum basale,[4] produce the pigment melanin.[2] **Melanin** protects the skin from the harmful effects of ultraviolet radiation from the sun and gives the skin its color.[4] Skin containing higher quantities of melanin appears darker in color, whereas skin with less melanin appears lighter.[2] Normally, the epidermis ranges in color from pale white to dark brown because of the presence of melanin. **Merkel cells** are specialized mechanoreceptors attached to keratinocytes by desmosomes[2,4] that provide information on light touch sensation.[8] **Langerhans' cells** present in the deeper layers of the epidermis help fight infection by attacking and engulfing foreign material.[4]

Epidermal Appendages

The epidermis has three appendages located within the dermis: hair, glands, and nails.[2] Hair follicles are present everywhere except in the palms and soles. **Hair,** composed of soft keratin, helps regulate body temperature by trapping air between the hair and the skin's surface.[2] Each hair follicle contains a **sebaceous gland** that secretes sebum.[2] If the more superficial epidermis is damaged, as with an abrasion, the deeper epidermal cells that line hair follicles serve as a source of epidermal regeneration (Chapter 2 provides a detailed description of wound healing). **Sebum** is an oily substance that lubricates the skin and hair.[1] **Sudoriferous glands,** present everywhere except the lips and ears, secrete sweat into ducts that lead to the skin's surface. Sweat is 99% water mixed with some salts and metabolic waste products.[2] The evaporation of sweat from the skin's surface helps cool the body. In addition, the oily sebum secreted by these glands may slow the growth of bacteria, thus helping reduce infection. **Nails,** located at the dorsal tips of the digits, consist of hard keratin.[1] Nails arise from cells within the stratum germinativum, protect the terminal digits, and assist with function.[2]

Additional Functions of the Epidermis

The epidermis has many important functions (see Box 1–1).[2] In addition to those described previously, the skin plays an important role in vitamin D synthesis by converting 7-dehydrocholesterol to cholecalciferol when exposed to ultraviolet light.[8] Vitamin D is essential for bone formation and the regulation of calcium levels within the body. For example, without Vitamin D, calcium cannot be absorbed from the gastrointestinal system. The epidermis is integral to cosmesis. The outer surface of the skin, hair, and nails adds to each individual's sense of self.

BOX 1–1   Functions of the Epidermis

- Provides a physical and chemical barrier
- Regulates fluid
- Provides light touch sensation
- Assists with thermoregulation
- Assists with excretion
- Critical to endogenous vitamin D production
- Contributes to cosmesis/appearance

☑ *Checkpoint Question #1*

If a wound extends only into the epidermis, will it bleed profusely? Explain your answer.

DERMIS

Dermal Layers

The dermis is 2–4 mm thick.[3] Although its layers are much less defined than those of the epidermis, the dermis can be described as consisting of two layers. The thin, superficial **papillary dermis** consists of loosely woven fibers embedded in a gelatinous matrix called ground substance.[2] The ridges and valleys of this layer (**dermal papillae**) conform to the contours of the stratum basale (**rete pegs**). This structural design, and the basement membrane, helps anchor the dermis to the overlying epidermis and protects the epidermal appendages. **Blisters** occur at this junction if there is friction between the epidermis and dermis. The deeper, **reticular dermis** makes up 80% of the dermal thickness[4] and consists of dense, irregularly arranged connective tissue.[2] The many thick fibers of the reticular dermis provide increased structural support to the skin.[2]

The dermis is highly vascular with many capillary beds providing nutrition to both the dermis and the overlying avascular epidermis.[4] The dermal capillaries provide the dermis with its characteristic color, ranging from pale pink to rosy red. Superficial lymphatics are also located within the dermis.[10] The lymphatic system helps return water, proteins, and other substances from the body's tissues to the blood vessels.[11] Healthy dermal tissue should have a shiny or moist appearance because of its high water content and a pink or rosy color due to its high vascularity. Collagen, elastin, and moisture make the dermis elastic and pliable.

Dermal Cell Types

Fibroblasts are the main cells found within the dermis. These cells produce the **collagen** and **elastin** fibers that give the dermis its characteristic strength and flexibility, respectively. **Macrophages** and **white blood cells** within the dermis help fight infection by engulfing harmful substances and releasing destructive enzymes.[2] **Mast cells** are specialized secretory cells throughout the dermis. They produce chemical mediators of inflammation, such as **histamine.**[4] These substances cause vasodilation and attract other cells to the area to help fight infection or repair injury. The dermis also contains several types of sensory receptors that provide information on touch, pressure, vibration, and temperature.[2]

Functions

The dermis has five main functions (see Box 1–2).[2] First, its vasculature provides nutritional support for itself and the epidermis. Second, if the outer epidermal layer is traumatized, the epidermal appendages housed within the dermis will multiply to help restore normal skin integrity. Third, many of the cells within the dermis help protect the body from infection by **phagocytizing** (engulfing and destroying) dead and foreign materials and initiating inflammation. Fourth, the dermis can play a role in thermoregulation by dilating the superficial vasculature to help dissipate body heat or by constricting these vessels to help conserve body heat. In fact, cutaneous blood flow is ten- to twentyfold more than is needed for tissue oxygenation and metabolism to help with thermoregulation.[4] Fifth, the neural supply adds to the epidermis's ability to provide information about the external environment.

Because the skin has so many important functions, loss of skin integrity can lead to serious and wide-ranging problems. For example, an individual with a deep burn covering the trunk and face would have an

BOX 1–2   **Functions of the Dermis**
• Supports and nourishes epidermis
• Houses epidermal appendages
• Assists with infection control
• Assists with thermoregulation
• Provides sensation

increased risk of infection and would lose massive amounts of fluid without intravenous fluid replacement. Once skin integrity is restored, the patient would be unable to sweat in the involved area, leading to skin that is easily abraded and traumatized. Loss of skin over such a large surface area would also decrease the patient's ability to dissipate heat by the evaporation of sweat from the skin's surface. Loss of melanocytes would increase the risk of sunburn and make the new skin pale in color, and loss of nerve endings would decrease the ability to perceive light touch. The resultant scars would alter the patient's physical appearance, potentially affecting self-esteem. The astute clinician remembers the link between skin structure and function when working with patients with integumentary injuries such as this. Holistic care should address not only the short-term problems associated with the loss of skin integrity, but also the long-term issues such as scar management and skin care to prevent secondary complications.

SUBCUTANEOUS TISSUE

Subcutaneous tissue, sometimes called the hypodermis, supports the skin.[2] It consists of adipose tissue and fascia. **Adipose tissue** is highly vascular, loose connective tissue that stores fat, which provides energy, cushioning, and insulation.[2] Fat-soluble vitamins, A, D, E, and K are stored in adipose tissue.[12] Healthy adipose tissue has a glistening white to pale yellow appearance, but may appear darker if dehydrated. **Fascia** is highly fibrous connective tissue that may be regularly or haphazardly arranged (see color image 1). Fascia separates and surrounds structures and facilitates movement between adjacent structures, including muscle, tendon, and bone.[13] Deeper lymphatic vessels are located within the subcutaneous tissue as well.[11] Subcutaneous tissue provides cushioning over bony prominences, such as the greater trochanter of the femur, thus decreasing the risk of pressure ulcers.[14]

DEEPER TISSUES

Because some wounds may extend beyond the subcutaneous tissue layer, it is important to understand the normal structure and appearance of deeper tissues. Muscles consist of regularly arranged fibers surrounded by fascia.[2] Muscle has a rich vascular supply, making it appear dark red in color and bleed readily if traumatized. In contrast, nonviable muscle will appear gray or black in color. Tendons are regularly arranged collagen fibers that may be enclosed in a fibrous sheath.[2] Ligaments and joint capsules consist of dense connective tissue. Ligamentous fibers are regularly arranged, whereas joint capsules have fibers running in varied directions.[2] When healthy, these tissues are glistening white in appearance. If nonviable, these tissues will appear dry or leathery, will be dark in color, and/or may no longer be continuous. Healthy bone will have a shiny, smooth, and milky white appearance and will feel hard when probed. Abnormal appearances include a moth-eaten, irregular surface or a bruised or dark discoloration. Severe pressure ulcers, diabetic ulcers, or burns, such as electrical burns, are likely to involve deeper tissues.

 Checkpoint Question #2

Your patient presents with an open blister on the posterior heel secondary to poor-fitting shoes. What tissues are involved with this type of injury?

DEPTH OF TISSUE INVOLVEMENT

By knowing the normal structure of the integument, subcutaneous, and deeper tissues, the clinician is able to determine the extent of tissue involvement in an open wound. Two examples will help clarify this point. First, consider a patient with a wound on the plantar aspect of the midfoot. The clinician would expect to find relatively thick integument that is free of hair follicles. If the wound extends beyond the integument, the clinician would expect to find the plantar fascia, fibrous tissue that appears pale yellow in color. If the wound penetrates through the fascia, the clinician may notice muscle, tendon, or bone within the wound bed. Alternatively, consider a patient with a wound over the superior, lateral thigh. The clinician would expect to find thinner skin than on the plantar aspect of the foot and evidence of hair growth. If the wound extends beyond the integument, the clinician may expect to find a variable amount of adipose tissue, pending wound location and the patient's percent body fat. If the wound extends farther toward the greater trochanter, there may be regularly arranged fascia from the tensor fascia lata or tendon from the attachments of the lateral rotators of the hip at the greater trochanter. If the clinician notes the presence of bone in the wound bed, it is likely the greater trochanter of the femur.

The extent of tissue involvement is typically categorized as superficial, partial-thickness, or full-thickness (see Table 1–1 and Figure 1–2). **Superficial wounds** affect only the epidermis.[15] An example of a superficial wound would be an abrasion[16] where the top layer of the integument has been removed, revealing the top layer of the dermis. **Partial-thickness wounds** involve the epidermis and part of the underlying dermis.[16,17] A second-degree burn such as a deep sunburn that results in blistering and peeling (described in Section III of the text) is an example of a partial-thickness wound.[9] In **full-thickness wounds,** tissue injury extends through both the epidermis and dermis to the subcutaneous tissue layer.[18] Full-thickness wounds may be further categorized as subcutaneous or subdermal tissue wounds if deeper tissues such as tendon, muscle, and/or bone are involved. A category/stage IV pressure ulcer with exposed bone in the wound bed (described in Section III of the text) is an example of a full-thickness wound. The classification of open wounds in the *Guide to Physical Therapist Practice*,[16] which is used throughout this text, is based on this categorization of the extent of tissue injury.

TABLE 1–1   Depth of Tissue Involvement in Open Wounds

Extent of Wound	Tissues Involved	Examples
Superficial	• Epidermis	Abrasion
		Superficial (first-degree) burn
Partial-thickness	• Epidermis	Blister
	• Dermis	Superficial and deep partial-thickness (second-degree) burn
		Stage II pressure ulcer
		Wagner grade 1 ulcer
Full-thickness	• Epidermis	Full-thickness burn
	• Dermis	Category/stage III pressure ulcer
		Wagner grade 1 ulcer
	• Subcutaneous tissue	Subdermal (fourth-degree) burn
	• May extend into deeper tissue layers (also called subdermal)	Wagner grade 2–5 ulcer

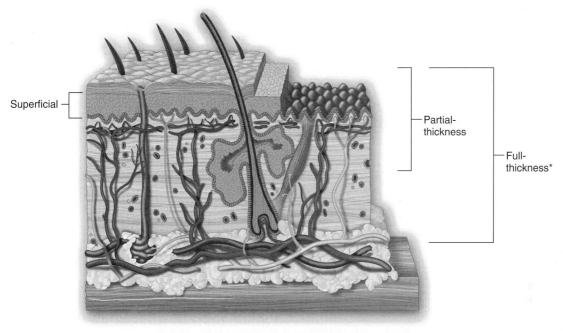

Superficial —

Partial-
thickness

Full-
thickness*

*Depth of injury extends *at least* to this layer.

FIGURE 1–2   Depth of tissue injury.
Source: Emergency Care 10/e by Limmer/O'Keefe/Grant/Murray/Bergeron.

 Checkpoint Question #3

Your patient's foot ulcer measures 5.0 cm length × 3.6 cm width × 0.8 cm depth. You conclude the ulcer involves what tissues?

CHAPTER SUMMARY

The skin consists of an outer epidermis and an inner dermis. The epidermis consists of five morphologically distinct layers of keratinocytes. The epidermis provides a physical and chemical barrier, helps regulate fluid and temperature, provides sensation, assists with vitamin D production, plays a role in excretion, and contributes to self-image. Open wounds with damage only to the epidermis are called superficial wounds. The dermis supplies the epidermis with nutrition and support, houses the epidermal appendages, assists with infection control and thermoregulation, and provides sensation. Open wounds involving the epidermis and dermis are called partial-thickness wounds. The subcutaneous tissue, consisting of fat and fascia, lies beneath the dermis. The subcutaneous tissue provides cushioning, insulation, and support to the overlying tissues, is an energy storehouse, and facilitates movement between structures. Wounds that extend into or beyond the subcutaneous tissue layer are called full-thickness wounds. Clinically, it is important to correctly identify structures within a wound to know the depth of tissue injury and to provide appropriate interventions.

REVIEW QUESTIONS

1. Label the left-hand side of Figure 1–3 (see on next page).
2. State the depth of tissue injury if a wound extends to level A, B, or C as noted on the right-hand side of Figure 1–3 (see on next page).

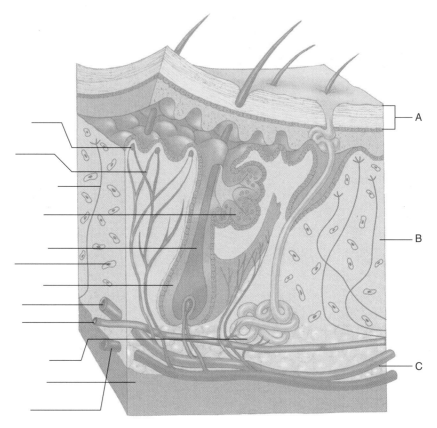

FIGURE 1–3 Skin structure.

3. How does the dermis assist with temperature regulation?

4. Your patient presents with a burn on his right arm after accidentally submerging his arm in a deep fat fryer. Based on the normal functions of the integument, describe the implications this injury will have acutely.

5. What is the extent of tissue loss shown in color image 1?

6. What is the extent of tissue loss shown in color image 2?

myhealthprofessionskit™

Use this address to access the Companion Website created for this textbook. Simply select "Physical Therapy" from the choice of disciplines. Find this book and log in using your username and password to access images, video clips, and additional learning tools.

REFERENCES

Go to myhealthprofessionskit.com to view this chapter's references.

Wound Healing

Chapter Objectives

After reading this chapter, learners will be able to:

1. Describe the vascular response of inflammation.
2. State the cells involved in the inflammatory phase and describe their functions.
3. Describe the proliferative phase of wound healing.
4. State the cells involved in the proliferative phase and describe their functions.
5. Describe the maturation and remodeling phase of wound healing.
6. Differentiate between wound closure by primary, secondary, and delayed primary wound closure.
7. Compare and contrast absence of inflammation and chronic inflammation.
8. Explain why absence of inflammation and chronic inflammation occur and interventions that may improve wound healing.
9. Compare and contrast hypogranulation and hypergranulation.
10. Explain why hypogranulation and hypergranulation occur and interventions that may improve wound healing.
11. Compare and contrast hypertrophic scarring, keloids, contractures, and wound dehiscence.
12. Explain why hypertrophic scarring, keloids, contractures, and wound dehiscence may occur and interventions that may improve wound healing.

Key Terms

Abrasion	Cytokines	Granulation tissue
Angioblasts	Cytotoxic agents	Growth factors
Angiogenesis	Dehiscence	Healed wound
Chemotactic agents	Delayed primary closure	Histamine
Chemotaxis	Diapedesis	Hypergranulation
Closed wound	Epibole	Hypertrophic scarring
Collagenases	Epithelialization	Hypogranular
Contracture	Exudate	Inflammation
Current of injury	Fibroblast	Integrins

Key Terms (*continued*)

Keloids
Macrophages
Margination
Mast cells
Matrix metalloproteases (MMPs)
Maturation/remodeling
Myofibroblasts

Platelets
Polymorphonuclear neutrophils
    (PMNs)
Primary closure
Proliferation
Prostaglandins
Scab

Secondary closure
Tissue inhibitors of matrix
    metalloproteases (TIMPs)
Transudate
Wound contraction

INTRODUCTION

This chapter reviews the body's response to injury. Normally, the epidermis is electronegative with respect to the dermis, creating a bioelectric field or "skin battery."[1,2] A break in skin continuity not only lowers the skin's electrical resistance, but also disrupts this skin battery, making the wound electropositive compared to the surrounding tissues.[2] It is thought that this local change in polarity, or endogenous **current of injury,** triggers the wound healing cascade.[3] Superficial wounds heal without scar tissue formation by simply regenerating the damaged epithelium.[1] However, the healing of deeper wounds consists of three phases: inflammation, proliferation, and maturation and remodeling. The key cells and events of each phase are described, followed by a discussion of three types of wound closures: primary, secondary, and delayed primary. The signs of abnormal wound healing are presented last. Common problems seen in each phase of wound healing are identified, and interventions are suggested.

PHASES OF WOUND HEALING

Normal wound healing is an organized and predictable process consisting of three overlapping phases: **inflammation, proliferation,** and **maturation/remodeling** (see Figure 2–1). Together, these three phases are sometimes called the inflammatory process. The body's first response to injury is inflammation. Inflammation allows the body to control blood loss and fend off bacterial invasion. It also signals the cells needed to restore the integument to the injured area. During the second phase of healing, the proliferative phase, new tissues are built to fill the gap left by damaged and debrided tissues. In addition, epithelial integrity is restored, and the wound is considered **closed.** The final phase of healing, maturation and remodeling, lasts up to 2 years after wound closure. During this time scar tissue is reorganized according to Wolff's law from a haphazard fiber arrangement to being oriented along the lines of tissue stress, until reaching maximum strength and function. Unfortunately, even after remodeling, scar tissue is less elastic than the original tissue and may only achieve a maximum of about 80% of the original tissue strength.[4] A wound is considered **healed** after it is resurfaced, and maximal attainable tissue strength is achieved. Scar tissue healing becomes of increased concern when a wound recurs in the same location, as is common with wounds due to venous insufficiency and neuropathic wounds. If this "second-generation" wound heals, its maximal strength will be 64% (80% of 80%) of the original tissue strength.

Inflammation

Inflammation involves both a vascular and a cellular response of living tissue;[5] therefore, inflammation does not occur in dead tissues or in tissues without adequate blood flow. The inflammatory phase assists with controlling bleeding and combating infectious agents that may be present.[5] Inflammation also sets the stage for further healing by signaling the cells necessary for repair and regeneration to come to the site of injury.[5,6] In an acute wound, the inflammatory phase begins at the time of injury and lasts a few days.[7]

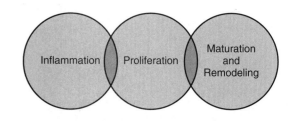

FIGURE 2–1   Overlapping phases of wound healing.

Color image 3 is an example of a wound in the inflammatory phase of wound healing.

Vascular Response

Tissue injury causes changes in local circulation. Immediately upon injury, the body responds in three ways to try to control blood loss. First, injured blood vessel walls allow fluid, called transudate, to leak out of the vessels and into the interstitial space, causing localized edema.[5] **Transudate** is a clear watery fluid made up of water, salts, and a small amount of protein. The resulting decrease in vessel pressure and increase in interstitial pressure help slow continued fluid leakage. Second, local blood vessels reflexively constrict for several minutes after injury to further reduce blood loss.[5] Third, **platelets** aggregate at the site of injury and are activated by contact with damaged endothelial cells lining vessel walls and exposed collagen.[5] Activated platelets become sticky, adhering to each other and the injured endothelium.[8] Activated platelets and fibrin form a plug that walls off the affected area.[5] Platelet plugs also close off lymphatic channels in the zone of injury, further increasing edema.[9] Activated platelets release numerous chemical mediators, including cytokines, growth factors, and chemotactic agents. **Cytokines,** such as interleukin-1 and tumor necrosis factor-α, are signaling proteins during the inflammatory phase.[5] **Growth factors** are endogenously produced hormone-like substances that control cell growth, differentiation, and metabolism.[5,10] **Chemotactic agents** are substances that attract cells necessary for wound repair to the area.[5,10]

Within 30 minutes of vasoconstriction, blood vessels then vasodilate, pushing still more fluid into the interstitial space and allowing more growth factors and inflammatory cells to reach the injured area.[11] This mixture of water, proteins, electrolytes, inflammatory mediators, waste products, and growth factors within the interstitial space is now called an **exudate.**[12,13] Because of the greater concentration of protein, exudate is more viscous than transudate and has a yellow or cream color. **Histamine** released by mast cells causes increased vessel wall permeability and short-term vasodilation, whereas **prostaglandins** released by injured cells induce a longer lasting vasodilation.[5] Vasodilation results in the localized redness, warmth, and swelling characteristic of inflammation. Pain, another sign of inflammation, is caused by swelling and chemicals within the injured area activating chemoreceptors and free nerve endings in the

area. Pain and swelling lead to decreased function of the affected area. These five signs—swelling, redness, warmth, pain, and decreased function—are known as the cardinal signs of inflammation.[5] They are commonly referred to by their Latin names—tumor, rubor, calor, dolor, and functio laesa.

As an example of the inflammatory response, consider what happens when a child falls on the sidewalk and "skins his knee." First, there is a break in skin integrity, an **abrasion,** causing bleeding. Soon, the bleeding begins to slow and a scab is formed. A **scab** is a collection of necrotic cells, fibrin, collagen, and platelets that serves as a biological Band-Aid™. If you examine the abrasion later that same day, you will notice a small amount of edema in the wound region and erythema around the wound margins. At that time, if you touch the area around the wound, you will notice it is slightly warmer than the skin farther away from the wound. The child may report that it is somewhat painful to bend or straighten the knee fully and may even walk slightly differently in an attempt to decrease the discomfort. Even in this commonplace example, the cardinal signs of inflammation are recognizable.

Cellular Response

In addition to the vascular response described previously, inflammation also involves a cellular response. Increased vessel wall leakiness causes a decrease in local blood volume. This slows the flow of circulating white blood cells, specifically **polymorphonuclear neutrophils (PMNs),** traveling within the capillaries and arterioles. Slower moving PMNs are then pushed to the sides of the vessel walls, a process known as **margination.**[5] As the process progresses, the PMNs begin to adhere to the endothelium paving the vessel walls. Next, the PMNs force their way into the interstitial space by extending small footlike projections, known as pseudopods, through the narrow openings within the vessel walls.[5] The migration of PMNs through capillary walls is known as **diapedesis.**[5] Using amoeboid-like movements, PMNs migrate toward the zone of injury. A chemical gradient formed by bacterial toxins, dead or dying cells, and changes in local pH guide the PMNs to the injured area. This process of active movement toward the area of highest concentration of a chemical signal is known as **chemotaxis.**[5]

PMNs are highly mobile scavengers, making them the first cells to reach the site of injury, usually within

12 to 24 hours.[14, 15] Once present, PMNs secrete chemotactic agents and mediators of inflammation, such as interleukin-1.[14] These substances attract more PMNs and inflammatory cells to the injured area, stimulate **fibroblast** migration, and induce new vascular growth. PMNs also secrete enzymes capable of breaking down damaged tissues and killing bacteria.[8] In addition to direct cellular killing of bacteria enzymatically, PMNs can also phagocytize bacteria and debris.[16] After capturing bacteria within its cell membrane, cellular lysosomes merge with the phagosome, releasing enzymes that destroy the bacteria.[5]

Circulating monocytes are the next cells to arrive on the scene. Once in the interstitium, these cells are called macrophages. **Macrophages** secrete nitrous oxide and bactericidal enzymes, which kill pathogens.[5, 6, 12] Macrophages are capable of phagocytosis,[5] but not as effectively as PMNs. Although larger and slower than PMNs, macrophages are essential to wound healing because they direct the repair process. Macrophages signal the extent of the injury, attracting more inflammatory cells to the area as needed.[14] Macrophages also produce numerous growth factors.[5, 17] Unlike the phagocytic macrophage, natural killer (NK) cells are a group of cells that kill bacteria, viruses, or infected host cells by directly contacting these items and inducing apoptosis (programmed cell death). NK cells also secrete inflammatory mediators to enhance the inflammatory response.[5] **Mast cells** from the dermis and local circulation help early in the inflammatory process by producing histamine and enzymes that accelerate the demise of damaged cells.[5] Mast cells produce chemical mediators that attract and activate inflammatory cells. See Table 2–1 for a summary of the key cells of the inflammatory phase.

Inflammation is essential to the healing process. Too often laypersons consider inflammation an undesired, and even unnecessary, consequence of wounding. It appears as if the results of inflammation, such as pain and swelling, are only negative. Clinicians direct patients to use ice and compression to decrease the inflammation associated with orthopedic injuries, such as a sprained ankle. Physicians may prescribe anti-inflammatory medications to control patients' aches and pains. Clinicians must remember, however, that inflammation is a normal and necessary series of events without which healing cannot occur. It is only when inflammation is excessive or prolonged that negative consequences may be encountered.

TABLE 2–1 Key Cells of the Inflammatory Phase

Cell	Functions
Platelet	• Forms platelet plug to control bleeding • Secretes growth factors and chemotactic agents
PMN	• First cells to the site of injury • Scavenger • Kills bacteria • Cleans wound • Secretes inflammatory mediators and MMPs
Macrophage	• Directs repair process • Assists with killing bacteria and cleaning wound • Secretes growth factors and MMPs
Mast cell	• Secretes enzymes • Secretes inflammatory mediators

Proliferation

As the inflammatory phase progresses, and the cells necessary for repair and regeneration reach the site of injury, the proliferative phase of healing begins. The phases of healing overlap and there is no one defining characteristic for progression between stages. In healthy individuals, it is possible for proliferation to begin within 48 hours of injury.[7, 18] The proliferative phase consists of four crucial events: angiogenesis, granulation tissue formation, wound contraction, and epithelialization.[16, 17] In general terms, this phase consists of rapid cell growth and replication, production of an extracellular matrix to fill the wound defect, and resurfacing of the wound bed. Color images 4 and 5 provide examples of wounds in the proliferative phase of wound healing.

Angiogenesis

Angiogenesis is the formation of new blood vessels. **Angioblasts**, endothelial cells that make up blood vessel walls adjacent to the zone of injury, bud and grow into the affected area.[19] These cells are directed by local tissue ischemia, vascular endothelial growth factor (VEGF), and by chemical mediators that are probably produced by macrophages.[19,20] Eventually these buds connect with other ingrowing buds to form new capillary loops.[19,21] Functioning capillary beds improve the nutrition to the injured area and the removal of waste products and cellular debris. Clinically, endothelial buds can be identified early on within the wound bed as tiny red dots. As angiogenesis progresses, these dots increase in number and size, and entire capillary networks are formed,[15] giving the wound bed a pink or rosy appearance.[22] Concomitantly, lymphatic channels begin to function again.[19] Open lymphatics and functioning capillary networks help reduce local edema created during the inflammatory phase.

Granulation Tissue Formation

Matrix metalloproteases (MMPs) are proteases produced by various cells, including neutrophils, macrophages, fibroblasts, and keratinocytes, during the wound healing process.[6] During normal wound healing, MMPs degrade the debris formed during the inflammatory phase,[23] leaving a defect that must be filled in order for healing to progress.[6,14] **Granulation tissue** is a temporary latticework of vascularized connective tissue that fills this void.[17,22,24] Fibroblasts from the general circulation and resting within the interstitium proliferate in the zone of injury and lay down an extracellular matrix.[5] This matrix is composed of water and proteoglycans that fill the spaces between collagen and elastin fibers.[9,14] The extracellular matrix allows fibroblasts and other cells to advance across the wound bed by providing a scaffolding on which they may migrate.[21] Surface cell receptors, called **integrins,** help cells recognize and reversibly bind to the extracellular matrix allowing this migration.[14] Fibroblasts are guided by chemotactic agents and low oxygen tension within the wound bed. Therefore, as new vessels are formed within the matrix, the stimulus for fibroblast proliferation decreases. Eventually, granulation tissue is replaced by scar tissue.

Wound Contraction

The extracellular matrix mediates **wound contraction.** Some fibroblasts within the wound bed are transformed into **myofibroblasts.**[25] Possessing properties similar to both smooth muscle cells and fibroblasts, myofibroblasts are the driving force of wound contraction.[26] The actin-rich myofibroblasts pull the wound margins together, decreasing the size of the defect.[27,28] The amount of wound contraction is affected by the shape, depth, and size of the wound. Linear wounds contract faster than square or rectangular wounds. Circular-shaped wounds contract the slowest.[9,27] Wound contraction is greater in full-thickness wounds than in partial-thickness wounds because of the increased amount of granulation tissue formation required for deeper wounds.[21] Because wound contraction involves stretching of the entire dermis without cellular proliferation, there is a limit to how much contraction can occur. Eventually, however, the thinned dermal layer is remodeled to near its full thickness.[9]

Epithelialization

As the wound defect is filled with granulation tissue, epithelial cells (keratinocytes) at the wound margins and epidermal appendages begin to multiply and migrate across the wound bed.[21,26,29,30] Keratinocytes elongate, extend pseudopods across the extracellular matrix, and then pull their parent cells with them as they advance, thus re**epithelializing** the wound.[9] Numerous growth factors within the wound milieu facilitate epithelial cell proliferation and migration.[21] Chemotactic agents guide keratinocytes toward the wound center.[30]

Epithelial cells cannot migrate over nonviable tissue; they must reach the oxygen-rich scaffolding of the granulation tissue. Therefore, keratinocytes must secrete enzymes to break down any debris in their path to reach down into the granulation tissue matrix. This is a slow, energy-consuming process. Thus, epithelialization is slowed by low oxygen tension and thick debris. Conversely, a moist, clean wound bed that is protected from further trauma facilitates movement.[9] The proliferative phase is complete when the wound is completely resurfaced with epithelial tissue, and the functional barrier of the skin has been restored. See Table 2–2 for a summary of the key cells of the proliferative phase.

Maturation and Remodeling

Wound healing is not finished once the wound bed has been resurfaced. The granulation tissue matrix laid down during the proliferative phase must be strengthened and reorganized to fit the surrounding tissue. Collagen synthesis continues at a rapid rate after

TABLE 2–2   Key Cells of the Proliferative Phase

Cell	Function
Angioblast	Forms new blood vessels
Fibroblast	Builds granulation tissue
Myofibroblast	Causes wound contraction
Keratinocyte	Reepithelializes wound surface

wound closure. Despite this, no increase in scar mass results because as new collagen is formed, old collagen is being broken down by endogenously produced **collagenases.** This synthesis and lysis balance is evident in the scar's appearance. A rosy, pink scar is still in the remodeling process, whereas a scar that is pale or more closely approximates the surrounding tissue color is fully remodeled.[9] Figure 14–1 provides an example of a burn wound in the maturation and remodeling phase of wound healing.

Collagen fibers transform from immature Type III collagen to mature Type I collagen and reorient along the lines of stress.[11,21] Two theories exist to explain the forces behind this reorientation.[9] The induction theory postulates that scar tissue tries to mimic the tissue surrounding it. Thus, if the scar occurs in dense, fibrous connective tissue, the scar will be made of dense, fibrous connective tissue. In contrast, the tension theory hypothesizes that internal and external stresses force collagen fibers to realign. When physical therapists and physical therapist assistants apply forces to scar tissue to attempt to change its qualities, they are following the tension theory. Range of motion exercises and scar tissue mobilization techniques such as cross-friction massage are grounded within the tension theory. Both the induction and the tension theory are supported by research.[9,11] It is likely, therefore, that scar maturation results from both internal *and* external influences.[9]

Remodeling continues up to 2 years following wound closure,[4,29] with the greatest amount of change occurring within the first 6–12 months.[9] Unfortunately, even once fully remodeled, scar tissue is at most only 80% of the original tissue's strength and elasticity.[5,12,31] In addition, the repaired tissue cannot function the same as the tissue it has replaced.[5] For example, the scar that appears after a full-thickness burn is unable to sweat due to a loss of sweat glands, is less sensitive to touch and temperature, and may have a different skin tone due to lack of melanin. Therefore, clinicians must consider that closed wounds may need continued protection and a gradual increase in stress to prevent future problems such as dehiscence and recidivism.[4] Table 2–3 lists the key growth factors involved in wound healing.[5,6,10,14,19,29,32–34]

TABLE 2–3   Key Growth Factors and Cytokines for Wound Healing

Name	Function	Effect on Wound Healing
Epidermal growth factor (EGF)	Growth factor	• Stimulates angioblast, fibroblast, and keratinocyte proliferation • Is a chemotactic factor for fibroblasts and keratinocytes
Keratinocyte growth factor (KGF)	Growth factor	• Stimulates keratinocyte proliferation
Fibroblast growth factor (FGF)	Growth factor	• Family of growth factors that stimulate all cell growth • Stimulates angiogenesis and epithelialization • Stimulates fibroblast growth and collagen production
Platelet-derived growth factor (PDGF)	Growth factor	• Is a chemotactic factor for macrophages and PMNs • Stimulates angioblasts, fibroblasts, keratinocytes, and macrophages • Stimulates matrix production and angiogenesis • Is the first growth factor approved for use in the United States and Canada

TABLE 2–3   Continued

Granulocyte-macrophage colony-stimulating factor (GM-CSF)	Cytokine	• Enhances wound contraction • Stimulates keratinocyte proliferation and migration • Stimulates angiogenesis • Is a chemotactic factor for macrophages and other inflammatory mediators
Transforming growth factor β (TGF-β)	Growth factor	• Family of growth factors made by fibroblasts, macrophages, keratinocytes, and platelets • Reverses steroid-impaired wound healing • Regulates matrix formation and collagen synthesis • Stimulates angiogenesis • Stimulates epithelialization • Inhibits MMPs and promotes TIMPs • Involved in scar formation • Stimulates cell growth
Tumor necrosis factor α (TNF-α)	Cytokine	• Stimulates fibroblasts • Activates neutrophils • Stimulates inflammatory mediators • Stimulates angiogenesis • Levels are increased in chronic wounds • Stimulates MMP and suppresses TIMPs
Interleukin-1 (IL-1)	Cytokine	• Stimulates fibroblasts and epithelial cells • Stimulates collagen synthesis • Stimulates angiogenesis • Is a chemotactic factor for inflammatory mediators
Vascular endothelial growth factor (VEGF)	Growth factor	• Very powerful stimulator of angiogenesis • Stimluates granulation tissue formation and epithelialization • Promotes collagen deposition • Increases secretion of MMPs and TIMPs for balanced extracellular matrix repair
Insulin-like growth factor I	Growth factor	• Reverses steroid-impaired wound healing

 Checkpoint Question #1

Your patient sustains a partial-thickness chemical burn. How do you think the body will reepithelialize the defect?

TYPES OF WOUND CLOSURES

Wound closure is accomplished one of three ways. **Primary closure** is generally the simplest and fastest type of wound closure as this occurs when the wound edges are able to be approximated with little or no granulation tissue formation. Typically, patients with wounds treated by primary closure are not seen by physical therapists *primarily* for wound care. Secondary closure requires the body to build a matrix of granulation tissue and, therefore, requires more time to reach wound closure. Most patients seen for wound care by physical therapists will go on to close by secondary closure. Delayed primary closure involves a combination of closure by primary and secondary closure. This type of wound closure may be preferable in patients with large wounds that are initially infected or that fail to successfully close by secondary closure. Physical therapists may work with patients to prepare their wounds for delayed primary closure.

Primary Closure

The simplest and fastest type of wound closure is referred to as healing by primary closure, also called healing by primary intention (see Figure 2–2).[24] This is easily illustrated by examining a surgical incision. The incision is cleansed of foreign material and cellular debris, greatly reducing the inflammatory phase. The edges of the incision are physically approximated and held in place with adhesive tapes, biologic tissue adhesives, sutures, or staples, leaving only a small defect to be repaired.[16, 35] Consequently, the body does not need to build a large granulation tissue matrix.[16] This decreases the distance that new blood vessels and keratinocytes must migrate and minimizes bacterial contamination.[21] Wound contraction, as discussed previously, is fastest across linear wounds, such as surgical incisions, further enhancing wound closure. Proliferation, therefore, consists mainly of reepithelialization across the surgical incision and begins as soon as 24 hours after approximation. Wounds heal best by primary closure if the tension across the wound is low and there is good vasculature.[30] In addition to surgical incisions, paper cuts and small cutaneous wounds also heal by primary closure.

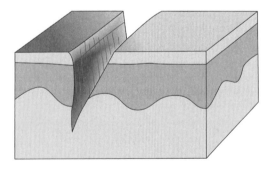

FIGURE 2–2 Healing occurs by primary closure when the edges of the wound can be physically approximated.

Source: Human Diseases: A Systematic Approach 6/e by Mulvihill/Zelman/Holdaway/Tompary/Raymond.

Secondary Closure

When the wound edges cannot be approximated, closure occurs by **secondary closure,** also called healing by secondary intention (see Figure 2–3).[36] A granulation tissue matrix must be built to fill the wound defect.[16, 22] Wound contraction to decrease the size of the defect plays a more important role in healing by secondary closure.[24] In addition, epithelialization must be greater to bridge the wound margins. Whereas primary closure involves principally regeneration and resurfacing of the wound, wounds healing by secondary closure heal by wound repair. Wound repair is a combination of granulation tissue formation (which eventually is converted to scar tissue), wound contraction, and epithelialization from the wound periphery.[5, 37, 38] Secondary closure requires more time and energy and creates more scar tissue than healing by primary closure.[36] The time to wound closure is determined by the rate of wound contraction and the depth of tissue loss.[30] For example, imagine a postal worker is bitten on the leg by a dog, removing a small chunk of epidermis and dermis. It will take time for the postal worker's body to replace this missing tissue and repair the defect left by the bite. The larger or deeper the wound is, the more time it will take to heal. The majority of wounds requiring physical therapy heal by secondary closure.

A severely contaminated wound may also be allowed to close by secondary closure. Suppose a young boy falls off his skateboard, sustaining a deep gash below his knee with bits of asphalt in it. If it is sutured closed, the contaminants would be sealed within a dark, warm, moist environment, providing a perfect opportunity for bacteria to grow and proliferate.[39]

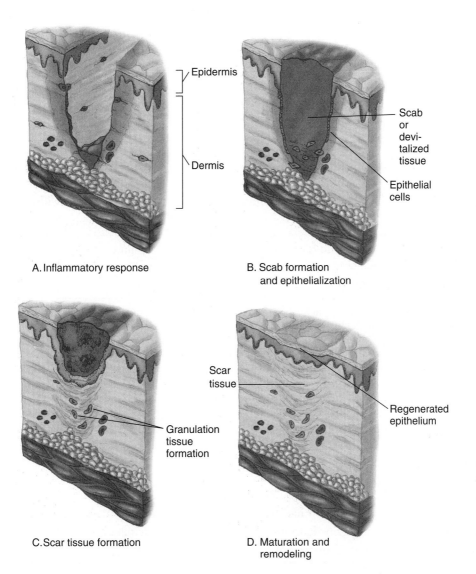

A. Inflammatory response

B. Scab formation and epithelialization

Epidermis

Dermis

Scab or devitalized tissue

Epithelial cells

C. Scar tissue formation

D. Maturation and remodeling

Granulation tissue formation

Scar tissue

Regenerated epithelium

FIGURE 2–3   When healing occurs by secondary closure, granulation tissue must be produced to fill the wound defect before epithelialization and wound closure can occur.

Source: Paramedic Care: Principles & Practice-Trauma Emergencies by Bledsoe/Porter/Cherry.

Healing by secondary closure allows the contaminants to be removed from the area, through cleansing and/or debridement, prior to wound closure to decrease the risk of infection.

Delayed Primary Closure

Occasionally wounds are closed by **delayed primary closure.** This is a combination of healing by primary and secondary closure, also called healing by tertiary intention.[30, 35] If a wound is contaminated,

this technique may be used to decrease the chance of infection.[35] The wound is initially cleansed and observed for several days. Once the wound appears clean, it is surgically closed. Imagine a little boy falls off his bike on a gravel road, creating a laceration in his palm. The emergency room physician cleanses the wound as much as possible but is concerned there may still be some foreign debris within the wound bed. The doctor bandages the wound to allow continued cleaning and inspection of the wound bed. The child is asked to return a few days

TABLE 2–4   Types of Wound Closures

Type of Wound Closure	Description	Normal Progression*
Primary	• Wound is cleaned of foreign material and edges are physically approximated • Also called healing by primary intention	Wound should be closed in 1–14 days
Secondary	• Wound repair follows the three phases of normal wound healing • Also called healing by secondary intention	Signs of progression through the phases of wound healing are noted: • Acute wounds: within 2 weeks • Chronic wounds: within 30 days
Delayed primary	• Wound is cleaned and observed for signs of infection, then closed primarily with sutures • Also called healing by tertiary intention	Wound should be closed within 1–2 weeks of suturing

*Time frames are provided as a general guideline and varies widely based on wound characteristics, local factors, systemic factors, and proper wound management (see Chapter 3 for a detailed discussion).

later. If there are no signs of infection and the wound is free of debris, the physician sutures the wound closed. Because delayed primary closure requires a doctor's expertise, the physician decides if healing by delayed primary closure is appropriate for a given wound. In general, delayed primary closure is performed on surgical wounds or lacerations once they are believed to be free of contamination.[35] Table 2–4 compares the three types of wound closure.

 Checkpoint Question #2

You are working with a patient who had a total knee replacement. Five days after surgery the knee becomes infected and is surgically debrided. One week after debridement the surgeon decides to surgically close the wound. This is an example of what type of healing?

ABNORMAL WOUND HEALING

Failure to move through the inflammatory process, or to do so in an untimely fashion, results in chronic wounds or abnormal wound healing.[37] Abnormal wound healing is assessed clinically if progression is slower than expected or by observing wound and periwound characteristics for an abundance or a reduction of the typical characteristics of each phase of wound healing. The pathophysiology of chronic wounds is not fully understood. Chronic wounds have senescent cells, cells that are mitotically active but are minimally or nonresponsive.[40,41] Chronic wounds have higher levels of MMPs[42] and lower levels of **tissue inhibitors of matrix metalloproteases** (or **TIMPs**) leading to the degradation of the extracellular matrix.[20,23,34,41,43,44] In contrast to acute wounds, chronic wounds contain greater numbers of inflammatory cytokines, and the chronic wound cells within do not respond to growth factors.[20,40] In addition, the current of injury may be arrested in chronic wounds.[45] Wounds presenting with signs of abnormal healing should be examined for underlying causes including local and systemic factors, iatrogenic factors, and certain wound characteristics that may delay wound healing (see Chapter 3). Once identified, interventions that address these causes should promote wound healing. Refer to Section II of this text for more complete details on examination and interventions.

Absence of Inflammation

Inflammation is a necessary and desirable part of wound healing. The goal of the inflammatory phase is to cleanse the wound of debris and set the stage for further healing by calling cells necessary for repair to the injured area. If an individual is unsuccessful in building this inflammatory response, healing cannot progress or will be delayed. Reduced or absent inflammation may be seen in patients who are taking high doses of steroids, patients who are malnourished, patients who are elderly, and patients with immune system disorders, such as HIV or AIDS. Clinically, these wounds present with decreased or absent signs of inflammation: local rubor, calor, tumor, dolor, and functio laesa. It may be necessary to promote an inflammatory response in these wounds using debridement (see Chapter 5) and using electrotherapeutic modalities and physical agents (see Chapter 8).

Chronic Inflammation

In contrast to an absence of inflammation, chronic inflammation is the excessive or prolonged expression of the cardinal signs of inflammation[46] and may be accompanied by fibrosis.[5,8] Whereas acute wound healing, described previously, resolves within 2 weeks, chronic inflammation may continue for months or even years. Cellularly, chronic inflammation is characterized by an influx of lymphocytes, macrophages, and plasma cells,[47] as well as fibroblast proliferation.[48] Chronic inflammation can be self-perpetuating. Lymphocytes and macrophages signal more inflammatory cells into the area, more inflammatory mediators and lysosomal enzymes are produced, and so on. The body cannot build functional, healthy, new tissue in a chronically inflamed environment. By preventing the wound from progressing into the proliferative phase, chronic inflammation causes more harm than good.

There are three common causes of chronic inflammation. First, the presence of a foreign body in the wound bed may result in chronic inflammation.[30,42] The body's attempt to cleanse the wound of items such as a wisp of cotton or debris from a traumatic wound prolongs the inflammatory response as long as these items are present.[47] Second, repetitive mechanical trauma, such as applying a wet-to-dry gauze dressing to a healthy, granulating wound bed, constantly reinitiates the inflammatory process.[30,42] By allowing the dressing to dry out, the gauze becomes adhered to the fragile granular tissue. When the dressing is removed, the granulation tissue is torn away from the wound bed as well, reinitiating the inflammatory process. Third, the use of **cytotoxic agents,** substances that are poisonous to human cells involved in the wound healing process,[49] may perpetuate the inflammatory response.[9,15,28] When solutions created for use on intact skin, such as hydrogen peroxide and povidone-iodine (Betadine), are applied to open wounds, inflammation is prolonged.[28,50,51] Chapter 5 provides additional information on the use of cytotoxic agents.

Hypogranulation or Nonadvancing Wound Edge

Wound repair may be halted by the absence of a successful proliferative phase. A wound that is **hypogranular** fails to build enough granulation tissue to fill the wound defect, resulting in a pothole-type wound. Without the support of a granular matrix, epithelial cells cannot bridge the gap to achieve wound closure, and repair is suspended. Sometimes, epithelial cells continue to multiply and attempt to "turn the corner" and migrate down the sides of the pothole. When the epithelial cells contact the floor of the pothole or each other by making a lip over the edge of the pothole **(epibole),** the keratinocytes believe their migration has been successful, and epithelialization is arrested. A nonadvancing wound edge can also be caused by scar tissue formation around the wound perimeter,[52,53] senescent cells seen in chronic wounds, heavy wound bioburden, repeated trauma from wound dressings, wound dehydration, and local hypoxia.[23,54] Color image 6 provides an example of a hypogranular wound. Hypogranulation seems to occur more frequently in patients with diabetes or malnutrition.

Interventions for hypogranular wounds should be directed toward protecting and enhancing granulation tissue formation. Epithelial cells can be prevented from migrating down the sides of the wound while the granulation tissue matrix is forming by gently wiping the wound edges with gauze with each dressing change. Additionally, lightly filling a pothole-type wound is believed to decrease the risk of premature epithelialization. Serial debridement (refer to Chapter 5) is used to facilitate healing in wounds with a nonadvancing wound edge and to decrease wound bioburden.[55] Serial debridement may also facilitate granulation tissue formation by restarting the inflammatory response in senescent cells within the wound bed.[52] In the extreme, hypogranular wounds may require surgical excision of a small amount of tissue from the wound bed and periwound.

Hypergranulation

In contrast to hypogranulation, **hypergranulation** is when granulation tissue formation continues after the wound defect has been filled. A hypergranular wound appears as a mound of granulation tissue, sometimes termed *proud flesh*, that extends above the surface of the surrounding epithelium.[47] The presence of hypergranulation is a deterrent to epithelialization, as epithelial cells have difficulty climbing up the mound of granular tissue, which can result in a rolled epithelial border.[56] It is debatable which process, hypergranulation or lack of epithelialization, occurs first. The interventions, however, are not debatable.

Hypergranulation can be prevented by protecting fragile epithelial cells from trauma. Types of trauma include inappropriate whirlpool use, maceration, too frequent dressing changes, or adhesives. Certain types of dressings, namely hydrocolloids (see Chapter 7), have been linked to an increased risk of hypergranulation.[56] Therefore, these products should be discontinued if hypergranulation is suspected.

Once present, hypergranulation can be resolved in three ways. First, pressure over the hypergranular tissue causes local ischemia, slowing or reversing the growth of oxygen-dependent granulation tissue. Second, silver nitrate applied to the hypergranular areas essentially cauterizes the pathological tissue, leveling the wound bed to that of the surrounding epithelium.[21, 56] To use silver nitrate, irrigate and debride the wound; then, roll a silver nitrate stick over the hypergranular tissue. The tissue will turn ashen gray in color. Irrigate with saline to stop the chemical reaction prior to bandaging the wound. Third, hypergranular tissue may be surgically excised.[21, 56]

Hypertrophic Scarring

Maturation and remodeling is a careful balance between collagen synthesis and lysis (see Figure 2–4). **Hypertrophic scarring** is due to the overproduction of immature collagen during the proliferative and maturation/remodeling phases of healing. Hypertrophic scars appear as red, raised, fibrous lesions that stay within the confines of the original wound.[25, 57] Hypertrophic scarring is more likely to occur in wounds that cross lines of tension in the skin,[18, 58] or in wounds with a prolonged inflammatory phase, such as large or infected wounds. Burns are also more likely to result in hypertrophic scarring because of their lengthy proliferative phase.[58] Hypertrophic lesions are often associated with contractures because of the

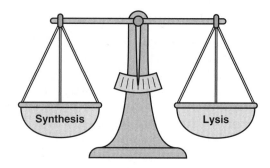

FIGURE 2–4   There is a delicate balance between collagen synthesis and collagen lysis. If the rate of synthesis remains greater than collagen lysis during the maturation and remodeling phase, the patient is likely to develop either hypertrophic scarring or keloids.

random overproduction of collagen.[25] Darker-skinned individuals have a higher predisposition to hypertrophic scarring than those with lighter skin tones.

Usually, these lesions regress, at least partially, without specific interventions.[25, 57] However, there are several intervention options to manage hypertrophic scarring (see Chapters 8 and 14 for further details). First, compression garments worn 23 hours per day can help modify the scar by inducing local ischemia.[25, 48] Second, silicone gel sheets or pads over the scarred areas can be used to modify the scar,[59] possibly by increasing local tissue temperature, causing an increase in the rate of collagen lysis.[57, 58] Third, physical therapists and physical therapist assistants may perform scar mobilization with or without ultrasound application to alter the scar tissue. Fourth, physicians may use repeated steroid injections to modify the scar.[18, 58] Fifth, there is limited evidence that newly developed topical agents, such as those containing allium cepa (Mederma), *may* assist with collagen reorganization.[59] Last, surgery may be used to decrease the tissue tension, thereby reducing the drive for increased rate of collagen synthesis.[18]

Keloids

Like hypertrophic scarring, **keloids** result from excessive immature collagen synthesis and are more common in individuals with more highly pigmented skin and areas of increased tissue tension. However, unlike hypertrophic scarring, keloids extend beyond the confines of the original wound and rarely regress independently.[60]

Keloids are characterized by a growth phase followed by a period of stabilization with possible intermittent periods of growth later on. Keloids are commonly associated with tissue trauma, such as a laceration, surgery, tattoo, ear piercing, or burn. There is a familial predisposition for keloid scarring. Keloids appear as nodular masses of collagen randomly arranged in swirls or clusters of collagen fibers.[57]

Steroid injections with or without surgical excision have been used to treat keloid scarring.[60] Adjuvants to surgical excision include radiation, compression garments, and Z-shaped incisions (Z-plasties) to decrease tissue tension in the affected area.[57, 60] Refer to Chapters 8 and 14 for further information on the treatment of keloids.

Contractures

A **contracture** is the pathological shortening of scar tissue resulting in deformity.[25] Contractures are more likely to occur in patients with wounds, especially burns, crossing a joint. Figure 14–1 provides an example of contracture formation after a burn wound injury. The patient assumes a "position of comfort" during wound healing in an attempt to decrease the stress to the healing integument and the surrounding soft tissue. This promotes adhesions and adaptive shortening of muscles, tendons, and joint capsules, ultimately limiting the patient's movement and potentially inhibiting function of the scarred area.

Contractures are best treated through prevention in at-risk individuals, including patients with burns, wounds crossing one or more joints, and/or limited mobility in the affected area. Interventions for prevention and treatment of acquired contractures may include range of motion exercises and functional activities designed to maintain or restore full movement and function of the area. Educating patients about proper positioning, including avoiding a "position of comfort," is imperative. Splinting may be a useful adjunct for attaining and maintaining ideal positioning.[39] For example, a patient with a burn covering the cubital fossa would likely choose to keep the elbow flexed to decrease stress on the injured areas. If maintained, this would lead to an elbow flexion contracture: limited elbow extension due to adhesion formation. Early prevention activities might include active or active assisted range of motion exercises for elbow extension, requesting the patient to maintain the elbow in an extended position, and possibly a night splint to maintain maximal attainable elbow extension while the patient is sleeping. Additionally, the patient might be asked to use the injured arm functionally for eating, reaching, or dressing. If the patient had difficulty with these activities or if motion was severely limited, a static or dynamic splint might be fabricated to prevent the patient from flexing the elbow beyond a certain point, thereby maintaining the patient's elbow in a more extended position.

Dehiscence

In contrast to hypertrophic scarring, keloids, and contracture formation, wound dehiscence is caused by insufficient scar formation. **Dehiscence** is the separation of wound margins due to insufficient collagen production or tensile strength.[4] A common misconception is that wound infections cause dehiscence. However, it is more likely that the wound edges dissociate before an infection can be established.[61] Perhaps because of decreases in collagen tensile strength or synthesis, longtime steroid users and patients with diabetes mellitus or malnutrition have increased rates of dehiscence.[58, 61–63] Once dehisced, wounds are treated with particular care to decrease or eliminate infection and to protect the wound from unnecessary stress or tension that may disrupt the maturation process.[4] Refer to Chapter 16 for additional information on interventions for surgical wound dehiscence.

☑ *Checkpoint Question #3*

You have been working with a patient with a pressure ulcer daily for the last 3 weeks. Initially, the wound appeared as a crater and was 1.0 cm deep. Today when you remove the bandage, you notice the granulation tissue has risen above the skin surrounding the wound.

a. How would you describe this tissue?
b. What can you do to improve the wound bed?

CHAPTER SUMMARY

 Normal wound healing involves three overlapping phases: inflammation, proliferation, and maturation and remodeling. The inflammatory phase controls bleeding, combats infectious agents that may be present, and attracts cells vital for repair to the zone of injury. The macrophage is vital to this phase of healing. Inflammation is characterized by localized redness, heat, swelling, pain, and decreased function. The proliferative phase involves angiogenesis, granulation tissue formation, wound contraction, and epithelialization. The maturation and remodeling phase reorganizes and increases the strength of the scar tissue up to 2 years after wound closure. Wound closure may be (1) primary, where the wound edges are approximated; (2) secondary, where the wound defect must first be filled with granulation tissue, or (3) delayed primary closure, a combination of the two. Abnormal wound healing is slower than expected or characterized by changes in the typical characteristics of each phase of wound healing. Clinicians must be able to identify both normal and abnormal wound healing characteristics to effectively manage patients with open wounds.

REVIEW QUESTIONS

1. Define the terms *transudate* and *exudate*.
2. Describe the processes by which polymorphonuclear neutrophils (PMNs) arrive at the zone of injury during inflammation.
3. Describe the process of angiogenesis.
4. What is granulation tissue?
5. How does wound contraction occur?
6. Compare and contrast hypertrophic and keloid scarring.
7. Provide two reasons why a wound may be chronically inflamed.
8. Suppose you are working with a patient who sustained burns to the neck and face when trying to relight a pilot light. You notice that he chooses to keep his neck flexed when sitting and lying down.
   a. How may this hinder his recovery?
   b. Describe two interventions you might try to prevent this from happening.
9. Your patient is referred to physical therapy for wound management with a full-thickness pressure ulcer. Describe the normal wound healing process you can expect this patient's wound to undergo during treatment.

PEARSON
myhealthprofessionskit™

Use this address to access the Companion Website created for this textbook. Simply select "Physical Therapy" from the choice of disciplines. Find this book and log in using your username and password to access images, video clips, and additional learning tools.

REFERENCES

Go to myhealthprofessionskit.com to view this chapter's references.

3

Factors Affecting Wound Healing

Chapter Objectives

After reading this chapter, learners will be able to:

1. State the difference between an acute and a chronic wound.
2. Describe wound characteristics associated with delayed wound healing.
3. Compare and contrast colonization and infection.
4. Describe local factors associated with delayed wound healing.
5. Describe systemic factors associated with delayed wound healing.
6. Describe methods to enhance delayed wound healing.

Key Terms

Acute wound	Colonization	Macerated
Chronic wound	Infection	Necrotic

INTRODUCTION

An **acute wound,** for the purposes of this text, is induced by surgery or trauma in otherwise healthy individuals. This type of wound progresses in a predictable time and manner, according to the phases of wound healing outlined in Chapter 2. Because of this, individuals with acute wounds are not normally seen in physical therapy settings *primarily* for wound care. Individuals with infected wounds, surgical wounds, and burns are three notable exceptions. Physical therapy services are more likely to be requested for individuals with chronic wounds.

There are varying definitions for a chronic wound. The Wound Healing Society defines a chronic wound as a wound that does not close in a timely manner or does not maintain this healed state.[1] Other authors refer to a chronic wound as one that has not healed or has not made significant progress in 2–6 weeks.[2] For the purposes of this text, a **chronic wound** is defined as a wound, induced by varying causes, whose progression through the phases of healing is prolonged or arrested because of underlying conditions.[3,4] Although it is not possible to accelerate the normal rate of wound healing,[5] it is possible to improve delayed healing by eliminating deterrents to wound healing and addressing factors complicating wound repair.[6] Several factors have been associated with delayed wound healing. Some of these factors are modifiable; others are not, but may be used to help predict the wound healing prognosis. This chapter reviews wound characteristics as well as local and systemic factors known to adversely affect wound healing. The chapter concludes with a discussion of how inappropriate wound care can delay wound healing.

Many factors are known to adversely affect wound healing. Deterrents to expedient wound healing can be divided into four major categories: (1) characteristics related to the wound itself, (2) local factors within the wounded area, (3) systemic factors related to the individual with the open wound, and (4) inappropriate wound management (see Figure 3–1).

WOUND CHARACTERISTICS

Certain wound characteristics are known to affect the rate of wound healing, including mechanism of onset, time since onset, wound location, wound dimensions, temperature, wound hydration, necrotic tissue or foreign bodies, and infection. Lastly, chronic wounds

exhibit several characteristics that inhibit normal wound healing.

Mechanism of Onset

Surgical wounds generally heal faster than traumatic wounds because there is less cell and tissue damage in surgically induced wounds.[5] Wounds with an insidious onset are usually due to an underlying pathology such as arterial or venous insufficiency. The prognosis is generally not as favorable as with an acute wound. Unfortunately, a nonhealing wound may be the first sign of a serious disease process such as diabetes mellitus or cancer. For patients with comorbidities such as diabetes and vascular disease, a trauma as minor as bumping against a wheelchair leg rest may be just enough stress to upset the delicate balance between deterioration and repair. The added energy required to heal this minor injury may push their body reserves over the threshold, causing a chronic ulceration.

Time Since Onset

Because acute wounds follow a predictable course of healing, time since onset can be helpful in predicting time to wound healing.[7] Unfortunately, the same is not true of chronic wounds. Chronic wounds are not self-limiting.[8] Once a wound fails to progress through the normal phases of wound healing, time since onset cannot be used as a predictor for time to wound healing.[7,9] However, if the clinician can assist a patient's wound into moving forward through the phases of wound healing, the prognosis is improved and predictions can be made. For example, chronic venous insufficiency and neuropathic ulcers of shorter duration—that is, those present for 2 months or less—are more likely to heal than those with a more distant onset.[10–12] Likewise, venous insufficiency ulcers present for less than 1 year had a 64% chance of healing, those present for 1–3 years had a 48% chance of healing, while those present for more than 3 years prior to the start of treatment had just a 24% chance of healing.[13] The clinician must always consider wound characteristics and both local and systemic factors in predicting time to wound healing.

Wound Location

Wounds heal more slowly in some locations than in others. Areas with decreased vascularity, such as the lateral malleolus, heal more slowly than areas with

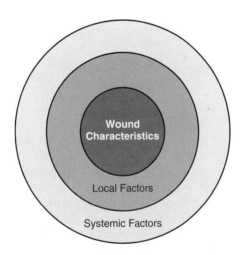

Failure to account for all these factors will result in inappropriate wound management.

FIGURE 3–1   Factors affecting wound healing.

more dense vasculature, such as the head and neck. Wounds over bony prominences, like the greater trochanter, heal more slowly presumably secondary to the increased tissue tension caused by the prominence.[14] Because wound healing can occur through regeneration from epidermal appendages, wounds in areas with fewer epidermal appendages resurface more slowly than other areas.[15] Finally, wounds occurring in areas where the skin is thicker will heal more slowly because of the need to rebuild more tissue.[16]

Wound Dimensions

As discussed in Chapter 2, wound shape, size, and depth affect the rate of healing (see Figure 3–2). Circular wounds close more slowly than square or rectangular wounds, which close more slowly than linear wounds.[17] Because the body needs to repair and rebuild more tissue with larger and full-thickness wounds, these wounds heal more slowly than smaller or more superficial wounds.[9,10,13,18–25]

Clinicians should not make predictions on time to wound closure based solely on wound dimensions because wound size does not account for the many other factors that can contribute to delayed wound healing.[18] However, changes in wound surface area over time can assist with predicting wound healing. For example, an increase in wound size after initiating

interventions for venous insufficiency ulcers was found to be predictive of nonhealing.[26,27] In contrast, a 54% decrease in wound size within 4 weeks of initiating treatment for patients with neuropathic ulcers was 91% sensitive and 58% specific in predicting full wound closure.[28] A 20–40% decrease in wound surface area within 2–4 weeks of initiating treatment is a good indicator that the wound is responding to wound management interventions.[18,21,23] If this reduction is not seen, clinicians should reassess the patient and modify the plan of care or make appropriate referrals.

Temperature

Wound and environmental temperature affect wound healing. Wound healing at 30°C has been reported to be faster than at 20°C.[29] As temperature is further decreased to 12°C, wound tensile strength also decreases. Conversely, maintaining a normothermic wound environment (37–38°C) has been shown to improve wound healing.[30] At these temperatures, the vasculature dilates, tissues are less vulnerable to infection, and tissue oxygen levels are increased.[31]

Wound Hydration

A dry wound progresses through the phases of inflammation more slowly than a moist wound.[29,32–35] If a wound is allowed to air dry, it dehydrates within 2 or 3 hours, leaving a crust consisting of dead cells, proteins such as fibrin, and debris, 0.2–0.3 mm thick on top of the wound bed.[29] Per Jaffe (1984, Clin Dermatol), wound bed desiccation impedes the current of injury, retarding wound healing. Desiccation slows epithelial cell migration by increasing the distance epithelial cells must travel and requiring greater enzyme production to break down the crust, ultimately delaying healing.[36,37] Exposed wounds are also more inflamed and more painful than covered wounds.[38] Covering wounds maintains a moist environment by trapping wound fluids. These fluids stimulate collagen synthesis,[39] induce angiogenesis, and enhance wound contraction.[40] Wound fluids have also been shown to contain growth factors and enzymes important to the healing process (see Figure 3–3).[36,39]

There is a delicate balance between a moist wound and a wet wound.[35,41,42] Too much moisture will also delay wound healing. If a wound is too moist, the periwound will become **macerated**.[37] Consider what happens if you wear a Band-Aid™ while swimming. When you get out of the pool after an hour or so and take the Band-Aid off, you notice the skin surrounding

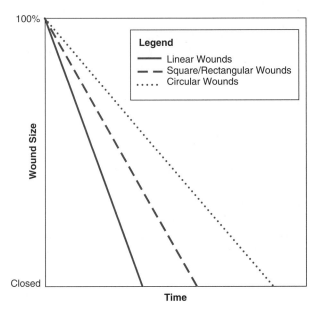

FIGURE 3–2 Wound dimensions affect rate of healing.

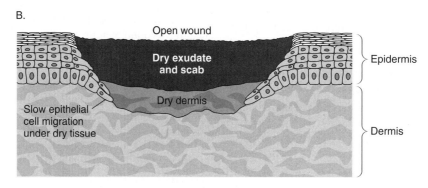

FIGURE 3–3   Wound desiccation retards healing by creating a physical barrier to epithelialization. In contrast, a moist wound environment traps growth factors and enzymes, optimizing wound healing.

the cut is white and wrinkled, almost prunelike. In this case, the Band-Aid trapped moisture too well and your skin became macerated. Macerated skin is more fragile and friable than healthy skin (see white area above open calcaneal wound in color image 11). If not controlled, maceration can lead to an increase in wound size.[37] See Chapter 7 for more information on the use of wound dressings to maximize healing.

Necrotic Tissue or the Presence of Foreign Bodies

Because epithelial cells can only migrate over viable tissue, **necrotic** tissue (dead, devitalized tissue adhered to the wound bed)[43] is an impediment to wound healing[33,42,44] and promotes infection (see color images 15 and 22).[45–47] Dead tissue within a wound bed can change a colonized wound into an infected wound (refer to next paragraph and Chapter 6) by providing food for the microbes present. Foreign bodies or debris

within a wound bed may also contribute to infection and perpetuate the inflammatory response.[8,29] To facilitate healing and decrease the risk of infection, both necrotic tissue and debris should be meticulously debrided from the wound bed.[44,46] See Chapter 5 for more details on wound debridement.

Infection

Wound **infection** is the invasion and multiplication of microorganisms in body tissues.[48] The mere presence of microbes, also known as **colonization,** does not imply that a wound is infected. Certain bacteria and fungi, called microflora, are normally present on intact skin and in the digestive system. Normal skin microflora include *Staphylococcus, Microboccus, Peptococcus, Streptococcus, Acinetobacter,* and yeast. In fact, normal, intact skin may have a bacterial count of up to 10^3 microbes per gram of tissue.[1] These microflora are protective in nature and actually limit invasion by pathogenic, or disease-causing, microorganisms.[48] Chronic wounds have a greater number and variety of microflora than acute wounds.[3,49] However, when the amount of microbes present reaches a critical level, healing will be impaired.[8,44] High concentrations of microorganisms adversely affect wound healing by competing with body cells for oxygen and energy and by secreting cytotoxic substances.[3,16,48] A wound is considered infected if a wound culture contains greater than 10^5 microbes per gram of tissue.[50]

Infection prolongs inflammation, promotes wound dehiscence, increases scarring, and slows wound healing.[2,33] Wound infection causes the body to mount an immune response against the invading organism(s). This response is similar to the cardinal signs of inflammation except on a larger scale (see color image 11).[1] An infection should be suspected if the cardinal signs of inflammation are disproportionate to the size and extent of a wound. After identifying the offending organism(s), the physician will prescribe antimicrobial or antibiotic therapy to combat the infection. Refer to Chapter 6 for more details on the management of infection.

Changes in Chronic Wounds

Chronic wounds exhibit several key differences from acute wound healing. First, cells within chronic wounds are senescent.[4,51,52] While still metabolically active, these cells proliferate at a reduced rate, synthesize fewer proteins, respond less to chemical mediators, and migrate much slower than cells within acute wounds.[51] Chronic wounds also have a dramatic increase in the number of inflammatory mediators,[6] such as tumor necrosis factor α, and matrix metalloproteases (MMPs), as well as a decrease in the number of tissue inhibitors of matrix metalloproteases (TIMPs).[4,53] This imbalance leads to an increased breakdown of the extracellular matrix and inhibits granulation tissue formation.[54] In addition, epithelialization is reduced or arrested, which is recognized clinically as a nonadvancing wound edge.[6] Chronic wounds also have a greater bioburden than acute wounds.[6,51]

All of these changes make healing chronic wounds quite challenging. For example, since growth factors are known to facilitate wound healing, one might think that chronic wound healing would be stimulated by applying a growth factor. However, the senescent cells in chronic wounds do not respond to growth factors.[4] In addition to removing as many barriers to wound healing as possible, serial debridement has shown to facilitate healing in chronic wounds.[4] Perhaps inappropriately termed maintenance debridement, serial debridement decreases wound bioburden and appears to stimulate wound healing in chronic wounds.[4]

 ## *Checkpoint Question #1*

Identify two problems with the following statement:

   If left open to the air, chronic wounds will eventually heal.

LOCAL FACTORS

Circulation, sensation, and mechanical stress are local factors known to affect wound healing.

Circulation

Inadequate blood flow increases the risk of infection.[55,56] Clinicians must be aware that the presence of palpable pulses is not necessarily an indicator of sufficient circulation. It is not enough that blood is delivered to the injured region. The blood must reach close to the wound bed. It is possible to have normal macrocirculation, that is, normal blood flow in the major arteries, but inadequate microcirculation, blood flow to the smaller arterioles and capillaries. It is at this smaller, local level that tissues are actually perfused. Therefore, diseases that impair the microcirculation, such as peripheral vascular disease and diabetes mellitus, are detrimental to wound healing (see Chapters 10, 11, and 13 for more details on arterial, venous, and diabetic ulcers).

Although structural dysfunctions within the vascular system can impair circulation, blood flow may also be affected by conditions that promote a sympathetic response. Circulation is controlled by the sympathetic nervous system,[56] the "fight or flight" branch of the autonomic nervous system. Cold, fear,[33] and pain can all trigger the sympathetic nervous system, thereby causing peripheral vasoconstriction and potentially slowing the wound healing process.[50,56] The astute clinician puts this knowledge into action by attending to patient comfort. Ensuring that the patient is sufficiently warm at rest, during transport, and during treatment is not only good patient care, it is essential practice. Blankets and heat lamps can be helpful adjuncts, especially in whirlpool areas. Because wound care can be frightening to a patient, particularly children, clinicians should attempt to allay these fears by explaining interventions in terms each individual patient can understand. Oftentimes, simple distraction, such as talking with the patient or incorporating a game into an intervention to get a scared child to participate in his care, is enough to calm a patient. Providing a quiet environment for treatment is also beneficial.

Clinicians should monitor patients for expressions of discomfort or pain. Do not assume that if patients do not complain of pain, they are not in pain. Some patients will not be alert enough or able to verbalize their pain. Therefore, clinicians should recognize nonverbal pain complaints such as groaning, fidgeting, physically withdrawing, noncompliance, or even refusing care. Physiological signs of pain or distress, such as increased heart rate or blood pressure, should be monitored, particularly in nonverbal, sedated, or altered patients. Once identified, clinicians must address the issue of pain control and, if unresolved with nonpharmacological approaches, discuss the situation with the attending physician. If pain medication is prescribed, treatment time should correspond with the medication's peak action period to maximize its effectiveness. Whether performing debridement or range of motion, an intervention does not have to be completed in one session. For example, it may be not only improbable, but also impossible for a patient to fully regain elbow extension in one session after a serious burn injury to the volar aspect of the upper extremity. Clinicians should not push patients beyond their pain tolerance. In most cases, it is wiser to progress steadily, gaining patient trust and developing patient rapport, than to insist upon obtaining the last 5 or 10 degrees of elbow extension in one particular session. Refer to Table 3–1 for a summary of methods to improve circulation.

TABLE 3–1   Methods to Improve Circulation

Cause of Impaired Circulation	Interventions
Impaired macro- or microcirculation	• Vascular consult • Medical management
Cold	• Blankets • Heat lamps
Fear	• Explain interventions • Provide rationale, if patient can comprehend • Distraction • Provide a nonthreatening environment • Antianxiety medications
Pain	• Explain interventions • Provide rationale, if patient can comprehend • Distraction • Pain medication • Accept steady improvements when patient tolerance precludes complete resolution during a particular session

Sensation

Sensory deficits cause a failure to recognize and relieve pressure, irritation, or overt trauma.[57] Without adequate sensation, individuals have no signal to warn of tissue damage. This can lead to delayed identification of tissue trauma. Once recognized, the severity of tissue destruction may be underestimated because the individual feels minimal or no pain. As a result, necessary medical assessment and intervention may be neglected or postponed until the damage is irreparable.

Sensory changes not only affect the ability to recognize and obtain proper treatment for tissue damage, but also indirectly retard wound healing. Inadequate sensory input can lead to continued trauma to an injured area. For example, an individual with a complete T10 spinal cord injury has no sensation below the umbilicus. If he is diligent in performing daily skin checks of these insensate areas, he may be able to identify an area of redness under his ischium as soon as it occurs. This redness is called a pressure ulcer and, as the name implies, is due to prolonged, unrelieved pressure (see Chapter 12 for more details on pressure ulcers). In this case, the ulcer is likely due to wheelchair sitting without adequate pressure relief strategies. Because the individual cannot feel the tissue damage to this area, he may continue to traumatize the tissues by prolonged sitting, thereby perpetuating or at least prolonging the problem. Individuals with peripheral neuropathy, diabetes, spinal cord injury, and paresis due to stroke or head injury are particularly at risk for injury and delayed wound healing because of the sensory changes accompanying these diagnoses.

Mechanical Stress

Pressure, shear, and friction are extrinsic factors that have been linked to initiating and perpetuating both neuropathic and pressure ulcers.[58–62] Periwound edema can impede healing by restricting blood flow, as is the case with venous insufficiency ulcers.[63] Tension on wound edges, which may be due to improper suturing or edema, can also delay wound healing.[29] Minimizing adverse mechanical stresses on wounds will enhance healing.[33] Refer to Section III for further details on the effects of mechanical stress on various wound types and specific intervention strategies.

 Checkpoint Question #2

Does wound pain correlate with wound severity?

SYSTEMIC FACTORS

Age, inadequate nutrition, comorbidities, medication, and behavioral risk taking are systemic factors that affect wound healing.[33,64] Some of these factors are modifiable, whereas others are not.

Age

The normal course of aging causes anatomical and functional changes. Decreased macrophage function leads to a slowed immune response.[65] Impaired fibroblast function decreases collagen synthesis and strength.[66] Cellular turnover is also decreased, making repair and regeneration slow with age.[67] Epidermal and dermal atrophy, possibly due to decreased dermal vasculature, makes the skin thinner[67] while decreases in the interdigitations between these two tissue layers make the skin more prone to skin tears and blisters.[65,67,68] Decreases in sweat and oil gland number and activity render the skin dry and impair its barrier function.[67] Pain perception is decreased so that minor trauma may go unrecognized by older patients.[65,67] There is a decrease in the inflammatory response with aging, which slows down the healing process. Vascular responsiveness, the ability to vasodilate and vasoconstrict appropriately, is decreased, affecting the ability of inflammatory cells to reach the injured area.[67]

Older patients are more likely to have coexisting medical problems than younger individuals. These comorbidities may adversely affect wound healing directly, such as peripheral vascular disease, or they may increase the risk of injury. For example, presbyopia, the age-related deterioration of eyesight, may increase the risk of falling or bumping into objects in an older person's path.

The extent and timing of age-related skin changes among individuals are highly variable.[65, 68] However, in general, these changes make aging skin more fragile, more prone to injury, and slower to repair and regenerate after injury. Age-related changes also make older patients more susceptible to infection and make the signs of infection less clinically apparent. Older patients are more likely to be taking more medications than their younger counterparts. Any comorbidities older patients may have should be assessed and addressed to limit the effect these conditions might have on these patients' already impaired wound healing potential. In patients with venous insufficiency ulcers, older age was an independent predictor of poor outcomes and delayed healing.[19] The use of adjuncts to wound healing, such as electrical stimulation and growth factors, should also be considered if healing is delayed.[66, 69] Chapter 17 contains additional information on age-related skin changes.

Inadequate Nutrition

Malnourished patients have an increased incidence of wound complications, including infection and delayed healing.[33, 70–72] Active cells require energy to function, with carbohydrates being the preferred fuel source. If not present, the body will turn to burning amino acids from protein. Because protein is required for cellular repair and regeneration, protein depletion will impair inflammation, immune response, proliferation, and maturation and remodeling.[43] In addition to carbohydrates and protein, vitamins and minerals are also required for wound healing. Fortunately, a patient's recent food intake seems to be more important than food consumed over the course of weeks or even months.[56] Alcohol abuse, drug abuse, and obesity place patients at increased risk for malnutrition. Therefore, health care professionals can positively affect the damage caused by malnutrition by providing appropriate nutritional support and lifestyle education. For this reason, a screening of the gastrointestinal system and a nutritional assessment should be included in the systems review of all patients with, or at risk for,

open wounds. Refer to Chapter 9 for more details on nutrition in wound healing.

Comorbidities

As discussed earlier in this chapter, inadequate tissue perfusion increases the risk of infection.[55, 56] However, for perfusion to be effective, the blood reaching the zone of injury must have enough oxygen content, dissolved in the plasma and combined with hemoglobin, to be released into the tissues.[50] The presence of oxygen is critical to all three phases of wound healing. Oxygen is required for phagocytosis,[56, 73] collagen synthesis, fibroblast replication,[50] growth factor production,[50] angiogenesis,[55] and epithelialization.[56] Therefore, disease processes affecting tissue perfusion, such as peripheral vascular disease,[33] or oxygenation, such as anemia and chronic obstructive pulmonary disease (COPD), are intrinsic factors that can impair wound healing.

Patients who are immunocompromised will have altered wound healing and limited reserves to repair injured tissues.[29] Immunocompromise increases the risk of infection because patients' immune systems are ineffective. Immune system deficiencies may be part of a disease process—as with HIV/AIDS, diabetes, or hypothyroidism—or the normal result of the aging process. Immunocompromise may also be due to steroid use, malnutrition, and chemotherapy or radiation treatment for cancer.[73]

Activity limitation, such as the change of positions while lying, the inability to shift weight while sitting, or extremely limited walking/standing tolerance, is associated with an increased risk of skin breakdown and delayed repair.[74] This would include patients with strength deficits who are unable to turn over in bed or transfer without assistance. Patients' movements may also be restricted by a cast, traction, medical devices (e.g., intravenous or oxygen tubing), or restraining devices. Patients with a decreased desire to move due to pain, depression, or altered cognition will self-restrict their activities, placing them at increased risk for skin breakdown and delayed healing.[75]

By directing interventions toward resolving potential side effects of comorbidities, clinicians can enhance wound healing. Physical therapists should also ensure that concomitant medical diagnoses are attended to, so the adverse effects these conditions have on wound healing can be limited. For example, imagine a patient, Mr. C, with lung cancer and diabetes. Mr. C is severely deconditioned and has developed a sore on his heel from lying in his hospital bed for so long. Given Mr. C's medical diagnoses, the physical therapist believes the wound will require a long time to heal. To enhance wound healing, the therapist's care plan includes direct wound management, but also addresses some of the impairments resulting from Mr. C's lung cancer. The therapist works with Mr. C on positioning, bed mobility, and transfers to alleviate the mechanical stress that seems to have caused the wound: the unrelieved pressure on Mr. C's heel due to limited mobility. To encourage time out of bed, the therapist instructs the nursing staff in the easiest method of assisting Mr. C into a chair. The therapist instructs Mr. C in deep breathing exercises in an attempt to increase tissue oxygenation, thereby enhancing wound healing. Additionally, the therapist discusses the patient's blood sugar control and food intake with the attending physician and the hospital dietitian.

Medication

Certain medications are known to impair wound healing.[5,16,50,72,76] Steroids at doses >30–40 mg/day impair all phases of wound healing.[30,77] They suppress inflammation and the immune system, decrease angiogenesis and epithelialization, and slow cell proliferation. Steroids also decrease collagen synthesis, wound contraction, and wound tensile strength.[78,79] Clinicians should note patients who may be on high doses of steroids, including patients with transplants and rheumatoid arthritis. Chemotherapy is designed to disrupt the cell cycle and, as such, it also delays wound healing.

There is some disagreement as to whether nonsteroidal anti-inflammatory agents (NSAIDs) adversely affect wound healing.[72] By definition, NSAIDs are prescribed to decrease inflammation. Logically, one would assume that this would also decrease the inflammatory phase of wound healing similar to the way steroids impair healing. However, it appears that in therapeutic dosages, there is only minimal evidence

to support this argument.[80] Specifically NSAID use may be associated with a decrease in wound tensile strength.[72,81–83] and recent studies demonstrate that regular NSAID use, particularly nonselective (non-COX-2 inhibitors), results in delayed and abnormal bone healing.[79]

Behavioral Risk Taking

Lifestyle choices, such as alcohol abuse and smoking, adversely affect wound healing (see Table 3–2). Alcohol abuse can lead to malnutrition, thus impeding wound healing. In excess, alcohol can alter judgment and impair coordination, placing alcohol abusers at greater risk for injury. In one study of patients with spinal cord injuries, alcohol abusers were more likely to develop pressure ulcers than nonabusers.[84] Alcohol abusers may also be less likely to obtain medical assistance,[85] allowing wounds to remain untreated until they become serious health problems.

Smoking impairs wound healing in several ways.[5,50,86] First, nicotine reduces tissue perfusion. Second, smoking reduces tissue oxygenation. Third, smoking adversely affects the cellular response to inflammation and wound repair. Smokers have a threefold increase in risk of graft or flap necrosis and a three- to five-fold increased risk of infection compared with nonsmokers.[87] In one study, tissue oxygen levels decreased 30% for one hour after healthy volunteers smoked just one cigarette.[56] In another study, smokers had lower maximal calf blood flow and lower oxygen saturation rates both at rest and after exercise.[86] After 46 hours of smoking cessation, tissue oxygen levels were 10% higher on room air than before stopping smoking.[88]

Clinicians working with patients with open wounds who smoke or abuse alcohol must discuss the adverse effects these behaviors are known to have on wound healing. Patients having difficulty modifying their behavior should be referred to appropriate programs or health care workers. Smoking cessation programs, support groups, and counseling may be beneficial. Ninety-eight percent of companies that provided smoking cessation programs as part of their corporate wellness programs reported a decrease in healthcare costs.[87]

TABLE 3–2   Lifestyle Choices Adversely Affecting Wound Healing

Lifestyle Choice	Effect	Interventions
Alcohol abuse	• Malnutrition • Increases risk of injury • Less likely to seek medical care	• Support groups • Counseling • Inpatient treatment programs
Smoking	Decreases tissue perfusion • Vasoconstrictor • Increases risk for peripheral vascular disease • Increases risk of intermittent claudication Reduces tissue oxygenation • Carbon monoxide has more than 200 time higher affinity for oxygen than hemoglobin, displacing oxygen on RBCs • Hydrogen cyanide interferes with cellular oxygen metabolism • Increases risk of COPD Delays normal cellular response to wounding • Increased platelet aggregation and clot strength • Decreases fibroblast proliferation and their production of extracellular matrix and growth factors • Decreases erythrocyte proliferation • Decreases lymphocyte chemotaxis and function • Increases levels of catabolic enzymes and MMPs • Decreases myofibroblast contraction • Slows epidermal regeneration	• Smoking cessation programs • Support groups • Counseling

 Checkpoint Question #3

Should a patient with an open wound who is undergoing chemotherapy receive physical therapy for wound care? Why or why not?

INAPPROPRIATE WOUND MANAGEMENT

Sometimes, patients' wounds heal regardless of what is done for them. Unfortunately, most of the time, patients are not so lucky. Inappropriate wound management on the part of a health care professional or the patient may adversely affect wound healing. In an attempt to achieve wound healing, patients may try home remedies that are ineffective or even dangerous,

such as one patient who, on the advice of a family member, wrapped her ulcerated limb in kerosene-soaked newspapers for several days. It is the health care professional's duty to determine what the patient is, or is not, doing to care for an open wound and to modify these behaviors appropriately. Alternatively, some patients may not follow recommended treatment regimens. Clinicians must identify and remove barriers to patient adherence. Many times patients may appear to be nonadherent when, in fact, they were given inadequate or incomplete instructions. In some cases, patients may choose not to adhere because they do not understand the rationale for a given intervention and, therefore, fail to see its importance. At times, patients may be unable to adhere with suggested interventions because of limited financial resources or insufficient caregiver support. See Chapter 9 for further details on understanding and enhancing patient adherence.

Failure of a clinician to recognize conditions requiring referral to another health care provider or to follow established guidelines, such as those of the National Pressure Ulcer Advisory Panel, may result in slowed, terminated, or even reversed wound healing. It is the professional responsibility of clinicians to stay abreast of current research and to modify their practice accordingly. Whether due to custom or lack of knowledge, the prevalence of three specific inappropriate wound care practices today warrants further comment.

First, it was once thought that wounds would heal faster if allowed to dry out. This was done either by leaving the wounds open to the air or using a wet-to-dry dressing. Leaving wounds exposed is now known to retard wound healing by allowing a crust to form over the wound bed. Additionally, exposing wounds to the environment allows contaminants and microbes to enter the wound with ease, thereby increasing the risk of infection. A wet-to-dry dressing, when a wound is covered with moistened gauze that is allowed to dry before it is removed, impairs healing by allowing wound desiccation. Additionally, if wet-to-dry dressings are used on granular wounds, removing the dry gauze will traumatize granular tissue that has become adhered to it. As discussed in Chapter 2, this is a common cause of chronic inflammation. Regardless of etiology or severity, wounds heal faster when a warm, moist environment is maintained.[89, 90] See Chapter 7 for further details on dressing selection.

Second, for years antiseptics have been inappropriately used to combat infection in open wounds.[8, 91] Antiseptics, including solutions such as povidone-iodine (Betadine), hydrogen peroxide, and sodium hypochlorite (Dakin's), are antimicrobials designed to reduce bacterial contamination on intact skin.[92] As such, these solutions are quite effectively used as surgical scrubs.[92, 93] However, there is no evidence that antiseptics enhance wound healing.[2, 94] In contrast, there is a plethora of data documenting the detrimental effects these solutions have on open wounds.[33, 91, 95] Antiseptics have been found to be cytotoxic, that is,

they are harmful to living cells, at both the local and systemic levels.[96–99] In an attempt to combat this cytotoxicity, some have professed diluting antiseptic solutions. However, even when significantly diluted, antiseptics continue to be cytotoxic, and they are no longer bactericidal under these conditions.[96] While previously the Agency for Health Care Policy and Research stated that antiseptics should not be used on (pressure) ulcers,[71] the current recommendation takes into account that there are very specific times when an antiseptic may be used. A properly diluted topical antiseptic may be appropriate for a limited period of time as an adjunct in reducing wound bioburden.[100] Clinicians should choose wound care products based on their intended purposes and available literature on their safety and efficacy. See Chapters 5 and 7 for further details on the use of topical agents in wound care.

Third, the overuse of whirlpool for wound care deserves attention. Historically, whirlpool has been almost a standing order for wound care: all wounds received whirlpool regardless of wound characteristics or patient condition. Whirlpool treatment is appropriate for wounds with thick exudate, slough, or necrotic tissue.[71, 100, 101] However, because it increases edema,[102, 103] traumatizes granulating tissue,[101, 104] and retards epithelialization,[101, 105] whirlpool is contraindicated on clean wounds. See Chapter 8 for further details on the appropriate use of whirlpool in wound care.

Education is the key remedy for inappropriate wound management. While clinicians are comfortable educating patients in proper wound management procedures, they may be hesitant to educate other clinicians, especially those who are older, have more experience, hold higher degrees, or have prescriptive powers. New research is performed. Old theories may be disproven. Prior common practices may now be confirmed to be detrimental. It is paramount that clinicians use the same principles of education with all health care providers, regardless of their differences. To best serve a patient's needs, a face-to-face or phone conversation carefully explaining the pros and cons of a certain procedure, along with the presentation of supporting evidence, may be beneficial to alter inappropriate wound management practices to today's standards. This not only serves the immediate patient's needs, it stops a cycle of inappropriate care that might delay healing or cause harm to future patients treated by the same clinician. In addition, this gentle but direct approach promotes a spirit of cooperation, holistic care, and mutual respect among and between disciplines.

CHAPTER SUMMARY

 An acute wound is induced by surgery or trauma in an otherwise healthy individual. A chronic wound is a wound, induced by varying causes, whose progression through the phases of healing is prolonged or arrested because of underlying conditions. Patients with chronic wounds pose a special challenge to medical professionals. Several factors have been associated with delayed wound healing. Wound characteristics, local and systemic factors, and inappropriate wound care can each affect wound healing. Some of these factors, such as infection and the presence of necrotic tissue, are modifiable whereas others, such as age and wound dimensions, are not. What may be considered helpful but not critical interventions for uncomplicated wounds may be essential to the healing process for patients with chronic wounds. Clinicians must recognize and address the factors known to affect wound healing in order to improve delayed wound healing. By staying abreast of current research, clinicians can increase the likelihood of successful outcomes.

REVIEW QUESTIONS

1. How does colonization differ from infection? What medical intervention may be required for each?

2. Do all 80-year-old individuals heal at the same rate? Why or why not?

3. You are working with two patients with open wounds. Patient X is a 20-year-old college student who sustained a laceration to the forehead after falling off her mountain bike yesterday. The wound measures 7.0×0.8 cm and has some debris in the wound bed. Patient Y is a 68-year-old patient with diabetes who noticed a wound on the bottom of his foot 6 months ago. The wound measures 2.5×2.0 cm and is free of necrotic tissue. Which patient's wound do you think will heal faster and why?

4. You are working with a 66-year-old patient with diabetes who has an ulcer on the bottom of his foot. The wound has slowly but steadily decreased in size over the last 3 months using "good" local wound care and non-weight-bearing with crutches. Last week the wound was 0.5 cm in length, 0.4 cm in width, and 0.1 cm in depth, about a quarter of its original size. When you assess the wound today, there are no open areas, only a pink scar where the wound was previously located. The patient wishes to stop using his crutches and begin training for the upcoming Senior Olympic basketball trials. What is your response and why?

PEARSON
myhealthprofessionskit™

Use this address to access the Companion Website created for this textbook. Simply select "Physical Therapy" from the choice of disciplines. Find this book and log in using your username and password to access images, video clips, and additional learning tools.

REFERENCES

Go to myhealthprofessionskit.com to view this chapter's references.

SECTION II

Wound Examination and Interventions

Examination of Patients with Open Wounds

Chapter Objectives

After reading this chapter, learners will be able to:

1. Describe the four aspects of obtaining the history of patients with open wounds.
2. State the key components of the systems review for patients with open wounds.
3. Identify and document wound characteristics.
4. Identify and document periwound and associated skin characteristics.
5. Assess and document circulation.
6. Assess and document sensory integrity.
7. Classify open wounds based on the Integumentary Preferred Practice Patterns.
8. Document goals for patients with open wounds.

Key Terms

Capillary refill	Pitting edema	Slough
Eschar	Semmes–Weinstein monofilaments	Tunneling
Induration	Sinus tract	Undermining

INTRODUCTION

This chapter provides a basic framework for the examination of patients with open wounds. The examination consists of obtaining a history, performing a systems review, and administering tests and measures. During the history, the clinician must obtain the patient's general demographic information, lifestyle and functional status, general medical information, and past and current wound history.[1] Next, the clinician performs a brief review of body systems before focusing on the open wound. The clinician then selects and performs appropriate tests and measures—including wound characteristics, periwound and associated skin characteristics, circulation, and sensation—to establish a diagnosis, to determine a prognosis, and to select appropriate interventions.[1] The chapter concludes with a section on clinical decision making to assist clinicians in these crucial areas of the management of patients with open wounds. Section III builds upon the general patient and wound management information outlined in this chapter and applies it to specific wound types, including wounds due to arterial insufficiency, venous insufficiency, pressure, neuropathy, and burns.

EXAMINATION

The physical therapy examination consists of obtaining a patient history, performing a systems review, and administering tests and measures.[2] The goals of the examination are to determine the physical therapy diagnosis, to identify factors that may contribute to ulceration or abnormal wound healing, and to assist with making a wound healing prognosis.[3] In addition, the examination helps to identify factors that may benefit from referral or consultation with another health care provider. Although presented sequentially in this text for ease of understanding, the three portions of the physical therapy examination are commonly performed concurrently or in an overlapping manner.

History

The physical therapy examination begins by obtaining a focused history of both past and current factors related to the reason the patient is seeing the physical therapist. Relevant information that may be collected is included in Figure 4–1.

Depending on the practice setting, this information may be acquired directly from the patient or from the patient's medical chart, family, caregivers, or nursing staff. In an outpatient setting, clinicians commonly choose to provide patients or caregivers with a medical history questionnaire to screen for key medical conditions and to provide information regarding the patient's chief complaint. When combined with directed questions based on the information provided, this format may provide more accurate information by allowing the patient or caregiver time to contemplate and respond to the questions as well as improve clinician efficiency. For ease of categorization, details of the patient history have been divided into four broad categories: (1) general demographic information, (2) lifestyle and functional status, (3) past and current general medical history, and (4) past and current wound history.

General Demographics

Because the prevalence of many disease processes varies by age,[4] gender, or ethnic background, it is important to obtain general demographic information.[5] Physical therapists should also know the patient's or caregiver's education level. By knowing this information, the therapist can present information and instructions at an appropriate level to maximize learning. In addition, the physical therapist should establish the preferred language for communication with the patient and caregivers. If the therapist is not fluent in this language, a translator should be provided. A short-term alternative solution may include the use of pictures, gestures, or demonstration to improve communication.

Lifestyle and Functional Status

The therapist must gather information regarding the patient's lifestyle and functional status to determine the resources available for wound management and the patient's abilities, respectively.[3] Does the patient live alone? Does the patient live in an apartment or home? Does the patient live in a shelter or is the patient homeless? Is the patient independent with activities of daily living? Does the patient have sufficient vision to inspect for skin and wound changes? Is the patient ambulatory? Does the patient have adequate mobility or dexterity to perform wound care? If not, is someone available to assist with wound care, skin checks, meals, bathing, and so on? Is the patient currently working, and what does this job entail? Does the patient have any behavioral health risks, such as smoking or alcohol abuse, that are known to impair wound healing? Does the patient have any cultural or religious beliefs that may affect therapy?

Answers to these questions may directly impact the plan of care and interventions. For example, a patient living at home who is unable to care for his wound may need to be seen more frequently, have a bandage that allows less frequent dressing changes, have a caregiver instructed in appropriate wound care techniques, or be referred for home health care. An ambulatory patient with a wound on the plantar aspect of the foot may benefit from gait training with an assistive device to unload the affected area and expedite healing. A patient working as a lifeguard would benefit from a wound dressing that is water impermeable. A patient who smokes may benefit from a referral to a smoking cessation program. A female patient who is Muslim and has a pressure ulcer over her sacrum may prefer a female physical therapist. Although insurance should never dictate sound medical practice, this information must also be obtained as it may impact some patient care decisions such as frequency of visits and discharge planning.

Past and Current General Medical History

Physical therapists must obtain information regarding the patient's past and current general medical history to identify conditions that may adversely affect wound

General Demographics
- Age
- Sex
- Race/ethnicity
- Primary language
- Education

Social History
- Cultural beliefs and behaviors
- Family and caregiver resources
- Social interactions, social activities, and support systems

Employment/Work (Job/School/Play)
- Current and prior work (job/school/play), community, and leisure actions, tasks, or activities

Growth and Development
- Developmental history
- Hand dominance

Living Environment
- Devices and equipment (e.g., assistive, adaptive, orthotic, protective, supportive, prosthetic)
- Living environment and community characteristics
- Projected discharge destinations

General Health Status (Self-Report, Family Report, Caregiver Report)
- General health perception
- Physical function (e.g., mobility, sleep patterns, restricted bed days)
- Psychological function (e.g., memory, reasoning ability, depression, anxiety)
- Role function (e.g., community, leisure, social, work)
- Social function (e.g., social activity, social interaction, social support)

Social/Health Habits (Past and Current)
- Behavioral health risks (e.g., smoking, drug abuse)
- Level of physical fitness

Family History
- Familial health risks

Medical/Surgical History
- Cardiovascular
- Endocrine/metabolic
- Gastrointestinal
- Genitourinary
- Gynecological
- Integumentary
- Musculoskeletal
- Neuromuscular
- Obstetrical
- Prior hospitalizations, surgeries, and preexisting medical and other health-related conditions
- Psychological
- Pulmonary

Current Condition(s)/Chief Complaint(s)
- Concerns that led the patient/client to seek the services of a physical therapist
- Concerns or needs of patient/client who requires the services of a physical therapist
- Current therapeutic interventions
- Mechanisms of injury or disease, including date of onset and course of events
- Onset and pattern of symptoms
- Patient/client, family, significant other, and caregiver expectations and goals for the therapeutic intervention
- Patient/client, family, significant other, and caregiver perceptions of patient's/client's emotional response to the current clinical situation
- Previous occurrence of chief complaint(s)
- Prior therapeutic interventions

Functional Status and Activity Level
- Current and prior functional status in self-care and home management, including activities of daily living (ADL) and instrumental activities of daily living (IADL)
- Current and prior functional status in work (job/school/play), community, and leisure actions, tasks, or activities

Medications
- Medications for current condition
- Medications previously taken for current condition
- Medications for other conditions

Other Clinical Tests
- Laboratory and diagnostic tests
- Review of available records (e.g., medical, education, surgical)
- Review of other clinical findings (e.g., nutrition and hydration)

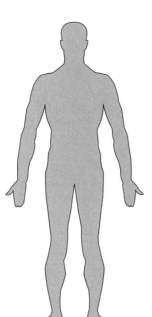

FIGURE 4–1 Types of data that may be generated from a patient/client history. *Source:* Reprinted from American Physical Therapy Association. *Guide to Physical Therapist Practice.* 2nd ed. *Phys. Ther.* 2001;81(1):S36.

healing.[3,6–8] In particular, therapists must ask about the presence of cardiopulmonary diseases, such as hypertension, coronary artery disease, peripheral vascular disease, congestive heart failure, and chronic obstructive pulmonary disease.[9] Likewise, other conditions such as diabetes, cancer, AIDS or HIV, and unexplained weight changes must also be identified. Physical therapists should review the patient's current medications.[10,11] Some medications, such as steroids[12,13] and chemotherapy,[14,15] adversely affect wound healing, whereas others, such as cilostazol or pentoxifylline (Trental), may assist with wound healing.[16–19] Additionally, patients may be taking medication for a medical condition not previously disclosed. The patient may not realize the potential impact this condition, or treatment for this condition, may have on the examination. For example, a patient may be taking pain medication for a preexisting back injury unrelated to his open wound. However, the pain medication may be masking pain associated with the open wound and, therefore, is relevant to the physical therapy examination. Alternatively, the patient may not want the clinician to know of a preexisting condition, such as depression. Obtaining information about a patient's psychological disorders is "as important as screening other body systems"[20] and, therefore, should be included within the past medical history.[1]

The patient must also be questioned about the presence of any allergies,[21–23] particularly to latex, sulfa, and adhesives.[1,24–29] The latex content in many wound care supplies, including gloves and bandages, as well as the increasing prevalence of latex sensitivity require the therapist to specifically question the patient about allergies to latex.[30] Because many topical antimicrobials and antibiotics, such as silver sulfadiazine (Silvadene), are sulfa based, therapists must also specifically inquire about allergies to sulfa or sulfa products.[11,31] Many patients are hypersensitive to the adhesives present in some bandages and tapes used to secure wound dressings. Before applying any adhesive directly to a patient's skin, the patient should be questioned about sensitivities to adhesives. Some wound products, including certain growth factors, contain bovine or porcine material.[11,32] Before using these products the clinician should ask the patient of any known reactions to this type of animal product. Box 4–1 provides a list of sample questions that may guide the physical therapist in taking a patient's medical history. The therapist should ask appropriate follow-up questions as needed to clarify patient responses.

Past and Current Wound History

Physical therapists should question the patient or caregiver about past and current wound history[1,10] as this information can provide valuable insights into wound etiology, interventions, and healing potential. Wounds of acute onset may be due to trauma and generally heal quickly and in accordance with the phases of wound healing described in Chapter 2,

---

> **BOX 4–1   Sample General Medical History Screening Questions**
>
> **Do you have a history of the following medical conditions?**
>
> - High blood pressure
> - Diabetes or high blood sugar
> - Heart disease or heart condition
> - Cancer
> - Peripheral vascular disease
> - HIV/AIDS
> - Stroke or TIA
> - Unexplained weight loss
> - Breathing difficulties
> - Neuropathy or nerve damage
>
> **Are you allergic to any of the following substances?**
>
> - Latex
> - Sulfa
> - Adhesives
> - Animal products
>
> **Please list any other allergies you have.**
>
> **Do you smoke?**
>
> - Number of packs per day:
> - Number of years smoking:
>
> **Do you drink alcohol?**
>
> - Number of drinks per day:
>
> **Do you take drugs not prescribed by a physician?**
>
> - Name of drug(s):
> - Frequency and amount of drug use:
>
> **Please list all medications not previously mentioned that you are currently taking.**

---

whereas chronic wounds or wounds with an insidious onset generally heal more slowly.[33] These wounds may also signal underlying medical conditions, such as venous insufficiency or diabetes. These concomitant medical conditions may impact wound healing,[34] suggest the selection of particular tests and measures, direct referrals to other health care providers, and/or guide interventions. Physical therapists should ask if any tests or diagnostic studies, such as bloodwork, wound cultures, arteriograms, or radiological studies, have been performed and, if so, obtain the results of such investigations. Table 4–1 provides a list of pertinent laboratory tests and reference values.[9,35,36] The patient and caregiver should be asked if the wound has changed.[10] Interventions for wounds that are healing at an appropriate rate will likely remain the same. However, wounds that fail to improve or that are getting worse may require further assessment or alternative intervention strategies.

TABLE 4–1   Reference Values for Laboratory Tests

Test	Normal Value	Possible Significance of Abnormal Values*
• Total red blood cell count	Women: 4.0–5.5 million/mm^3 Men: 4.5–6.2 million/mm^3	If low, may be anemic or may have lost blood volume. If high, may be dehydrated or at risk for blood clots.
• Hematocrit	Women: 38–46% Men: 42–54%	If low, may have anemia, blood loss, or malnutrition. If high, may be dehydrated or at risk for blood clots.
• Hemoglobin	Women: 12–16 g/dL Men: 14–18 g/dL	If low, possible blood loss or nutritional deficiency. If high, possible dehydration or risk for blood clot.
• Total white blood cell count	4,500–11,000/mm^3	If low, at risk for infection. If high, possible infection, inflammatory response, or anemia.
• Platelet (thrombocyte) count	150,000–400,000/mm^3	If low, delayed clotting. If high, potential for blood clots.
• Total lymphocyte count (TLC)	>1,800 cells/mm^3	If low, decreased immune function, may have protein deficiency, can delay wound healing.
• Serum albumin	3.5–5.5 g/dL	If low, may be malnourished, may cause tissue edema, may be sign of metabolic stress or inflammation. Low levels are correlated with pressure ulcer severity. If high, may be dehydrated.
• Serum prealbumin	16–40 mg/dL	If low, may be malnourished, may be sign of metabolic stress or inflammation. Mortality rate increases as prealbumin decreases.
• Serum transferrin	>170 mg/dL	If low, may have protein deficiency or be malnourished. If high, may have iron deficiency.
• Blood glucose	70–110 mg/dL	If high, may have poorly controlled diabetes.
• Urine glucose	Negative	If present, may have poorly controlled diabetes or kidney disease.
• BUN (blood urea nitrogen)	8.0–20 mg/dL	If high, may have kidney disease or be dehydrated. High levels associated with delayed wound healing.
• Creatinine	0.8–1.2 mg/dL	If high, may have kidney disease. Decreases with malnutrition.

*Note this is only a very preliminary list of possible causes of abnormal values. Any abnormal values may adversely affect wound healing. Please refer to other sources for more complete information.

Pain or lack of pain associated with an open wound can provide information regarding wound etiology.[37] There are several options for reliably documenting pain: numerical rating scale (0–10 scale),[38,39] visual analog scale (documenting on a 10-cm line labeled no pain on far left and worst possible pain on far right),[39] verbal pain rating scale (no pain, minimal, moderate, severe, or unbearable pain),[39] or the Wong–Baker FACES rating scale.[40–42] The verbal pain rating scale may be more appropriate with patients who are illiterate,[39] while the FACES scale may be more appropriate for children and patients who are illiterate, whose primary language is not English, or who have communication impairments.[42] Partial-thickness wounds are likely to be painful due to exposed nerve endings. Wounds that extend below the dermis will have little surface pain due to destruction of all cutaneous nerve endings. However, since wounds are seldom all one depth, less severely damaged tissue surrounding a full-thickness wound will still be painful. Patients with wounds caused by arterial insufficiency often have pain due to tissue ischemia.[43,44] This pain often is exacerbated during activities that increase tissue metabolism, such as ambulation.[37] Positions that further compromise tissue perfusion, such as leg elevation, may also increase their pain complaint.

In contrast, patients with wounds caused by venous insufficiency may have pain due to venous hypertension and the resulting peripheral edema.[43] This pain is usually increased with dependency and relieved by elevation or compression.[37,45,46] Patients with wounds that are not painful may have diabetic neuropathy or other nerve damage, such as a spinal cord injury or cerebrovascular accident. Patients without adequate pain control may benefit from a physician's assessment for pharmacological interventions. Patients or caregivers should be asked about currently or previously prescribed oral, intravenous, and topical medications for the wound. Use of an antibiotic may indicate wound infection. Long-term use of an antibiotic without change in wound status may indicate antibiotic resistance or inappropriate antibiotic choice.[7] Box 4–2 provides a list of sample questions that may guide the physical therapist in taking a patient's wound history.[42,47,48] The therapist should ask appropriate follow-up questions as needed to clarify patient responses.

Systems Review

After obtaining the history, the physical therapist performs a brief systems review. The systems review is a limited examination of the anatomical and physiological

---

BOX 4–2   Sample Past and Current Wound History Screening Questions

When did the wound begin?

How did the wound occur?

Have any tests been performed?

- wound culture
- blood tests
- x-ray
- bone scan
- arteriogram
- venous Doppler

Were you previously or are you currently taking any medications, such as antibiotics, for this wound?

Is your wound painful?

- How would you rate the pain on a 0–10 pain scale?
- What medication do you take for pain management?
- How much pain medication do you take and how often?
- Does the medication control your pain?

Does the pain change with:

- elevation?
- dependency?
- activity?

What is currently being done for your wound?

- What, if anything, are you putting on or around your wound?
- How are you wrapping the wound?
- How often do you change the bandage?
- Can you do this by yourself or is someone helping you?
- Are you seeing another health care worker to help manage your wound?

What interventions have been performed in the past? What impact did these interventions have?

Is your wound improving, staying the same, or getting worse?

Have you had any wounds in the past?

- Where was the previous wound(s)?
- How did the previous wound(s) occur?
- Did the wound(s) heal in a timely fashion?
- Did you need to see a medical professional for wound management?
- What interventions were performed?

status of body systems as well as the patient's communication, affect, cognition, language, and learning style.[1,2] Although patients with open wounds will require a comprehensive examination of the integumentary system, wounds cannot be treated in isolation of the patient as a whole.[9,34]

The systems review has four main purposes. First, in combination with the patient history, this brief screening can help the physical therapist identify risk factors or impairments that may require referral to, or consultation with, other disciplines. For example, a patient reporting a nonhealing ulcer on the plantar aspect of the foot who reports the need to urinate four times per night may benefit from a physician's referral to assess for diabetes. Second, the systems review allows the physical therapist to identify risk factors or impairments in areas aside from the integument that may benefit from physical therapy interventions to enhance wound healing. For example, a patient with a sacral ulcer who is unable to independently reposition him- or herself in bed may benefit from therapeutic exercise and mobility training. Third, the systems review may identify signs and symptoms consistent with certain disease processes that may alter physical therapy interventions for wound management. Consider a patient referred to physical therapy with a leg ulcer. The patient has a medical diagnosis of congestive heart failure and presents with pitting edema in bilateral lower extremities. This patient should not be treated with whirlpool as this will exacerbate his or her edema, nor should the patient be treated with compression without prior consultation with his physician because of the potential for systemic fluid overload.[49] Once the patient's heart failure is medically stable, compression therapy may be initiated safely.[49] Fourth, by assessing the patient's communication, affect, cognition, and learning style, the physical therapist can determine patient and caregiver education needs, identify barriers to learning and methods to resolve same, and develop effective ways to disseminate information on wound etiology, prognosis, interventions, outcomes, and prevention of recurrence. The physical therapist should screen the following body systems: cardiovascular/pulmonary, musculoskeletal, neuromuscular, gastrointestinal, urogenital, and integumentary. A more detailed examination is warranted if a particular system is believed to be a contributing factor to ulceration or delayed wound healing.[2,3]

Cardiovascular/Pulmonary System Review

The review of the cardiovascular/pulmonary system should consist of measuring heart rate, blood pressure, and respiratory rate, and assessing for edema.[2,3] Because wounds will not heal without adequate circulation, physical therapists should assess peripheral pulses in patients with extremity wounds. Likewise, since wounds will not heal without adequate oxygenation, physical therapists should perform pulse oximetry measurements in patients at risk for impaired oxygenation.

Musculoskeletal System Review

Impairments in the musculoskeletal system may limit the patient's ability to change positions or create areas of increased pressure. For example, a patient with a T4 spinal cord injury and fixed thoracic kyphosis may develop a wound over the thoracic spinous processes due to unrelieved pressure from prolonged sitting or lying supine. The review of the musculoskeletal system should consist of a gross screening of patient structure/posture, range of motion, and strength.[2,3,50]

Neuromuscular System Review

Activity limitation is associated with an increased risk of skin breakdown and delayed wound healing. Therefore, the review of the neuromuscular system should include a gross assessment of gait and mobility, which may include bed mobility, transfers, and balance.[2,3] It is particularly important to screen the neuromuscular system in patients with pressure ulcers or ulcers on the plantar aspect of the foot.

Gastrointestinal System Review

Although not specifically outlined in the *Guide to Physical Therapist Practice*, the National Pressure Ulcer Advisory Panel strongly recommends a nutritional assessment for all patients with, or at risk for, pressure ulcers.[41] Regardless of wound etiology, inadequate nutrition increases the risk of wound infection and delays wound healing.[51] Likewise, optimal nutrition intake or supplementation is vital to prevent skin breakdown and enhance wound healing for all patients.[52,53] Therefore, it is important for physical therapists to obtain information regarding the patient's gastrointestinal system, including fecal continence. This may be as simple as asking the patient about daily food and water intake or record a 24-hour food and beverage intake history. Nutritional assessment screening tools, such as the Rapid Eating Activity of Patients (REAP) or the Weight, Activity, Variety, and Excess (WAVE), are quick, valid, and easy to administer.[40] Nutritional information may be obtained from medical records, laboratory reports, family, caregivers, or nursing staff. Alternatively, a rough estimate of a patient's nutritional status can be obtained by calculating the patient's body mass index, or BMI. BMI is calculated by dividing the patient's weight in kilograms by his or her height in meters squared. A BMI of 18.5–24.9 is considered normal weight. Lower numbers indicate the patient is underweight, while higher values indicate the patient is overweight or obese. Chapter 9 provides detailed information about the impact of nutrition on wound healing and assessing a patient's nutritional status.

Urogenital System Review

Because of the relationship between incontinence and pressure ulcers, the National Pressure Ulcer Advisory Panel also strongly recommends assessment of the urogenital system for all patients with, or at risk for, pressure ulcers.[41, 54] Another reason for physical therapists to include urogenital system screening in their examination is to identify a key clinical sign of undiagnosed or poorly controlled diabetes or urinary tract infections. Both of these conditions may adversely affect wound healing and warrant further assessment by a physician. Screening of the urogenital system should include asking the patient or caregiver about urinary frequency, difficulty or pain when urinating, and continence.[2]

Integumentary System Review

The integumentary system review consists of a gross examination of exposed skin including skin integrity, skin color, presence of scar formation, as well as hair and nail growth.[2, 3] This system will become the primary focus of the remaining examination.[1] Refer to Chapter 16 for detailed information regarding integumentary screening for lesions other than open wounds.

Tests and Measures

The physical therapist uses the information gathered from the history and systems review to generate a "diagnostic hypothesis."[2] The physical therapist then selects specific tests and measures to rule in or out causes of impairment and functional limitations, to establish a diagnosis, to determine a prognosis, and to select appropriate interventions. Tests and measures performed should also be guided by the known risk factors for ulceration and delayed wound healing. There are 24 categories of tests and measures within the *Guide to Physical Therapist Practice*. It is generally not necessary to perform tests and measures in each category. Physical therapists should select what tests and measures should be performed based on the ability of the information to confirm or reject their diagnostic hypothesis and to support the therapists' judgments about selected interventions and expected outcomes. Likewise, it may be tempting for physical therapists to select only tests and measures that assess integumentary integrity. However, they should remember that only rarely will treating a wound in isolation result in significant improvements or goal attainment.

A thorough discussion of all 24 categories of tests and measures within the *Guide to Physical Therapist Practice* is clearly beyond the scope of this text. This section presents information regarding routine tests and measures performed on patients with open wounds, including integumentary integrity, circulation, and sensory integrity. Anthropometric data is presented in Chapter 9. Additional information regarding diagnosis-specific physical therapy tests and measures, such as the ankle-brachial index or venous filling time, is presented within the corresponding chapters in Section III. Certainly, many other physical therapy tests and measures must be used as part of the physical therapy examination and reassessment, such as range of motion, motor function, and muscle performance. However, because these procedures are performed by physical therapists on a more routine basis, no further explanations are required. Other sources should be consulted for information regarding clinical indications, preferred methods, and interpretation of additional tests and measures that may be required for the examination of patients with open wounds.

Integumentary Integrity: Wound Characteristics

If necessary, the wound is debrided and/or irrigated prior to measurement. Regardless of the method chosen to assess wound characteristics, the clinician must strive for consistency.[41] Because wound size can change with patient positioning, especially tunneling wounds or wounds located on the trunk or pelvis, the patient should be positioned in the same manner each time.[33] Ideally, the same clinician should remeasure the patient each time to improve measurement reliability. A good light source that is able to be manipulated to reduce shadows and glare is beneficial.

During the physical therapy examination, the clinician must identify and document wound characteristics objectively and reliably. The therapist should document wound location, wound size, tunneling or undermining, wound bed, wound edges, wound drainage, and wound odor.[1,8]

Wound Location

The physical therapist must document wound location using anatomically correct terminology. Wound location can provide insights into wound etiology.[6] For example, pressure ulcers commonly occur over bony prominences, such as the ischial tuberosity, whereas arterial ulcers typically develop distally at the tips of the toes.[6,9,55] Location can also have an impact on physical therapy interventions such as positioning and dressing selection.[41] The therapist should document the side (left, right) and body surface of the lesion (anterior, medial, etc.). If multiple wounds exist, it may be helpful to document wounds in relation to anatomical landmarks: "Wound A is located 10 cm superior to the medial malleolus; wound B is located 2 cm superior to the medial malleolus."

Wound Size

Because size is considered to be a major indicator of improvement or decline in wound status,[33,56,57] physical therapists must assess the wound size. Wound size should *not* be estimated, nor should clinicians document wound size in relationship to common objects: "The wound is the size of a quarter." However, the most appropriate method of measuring wound size is an area of intense debate. Wound size can be determined by direct measurement, tracings, photography, volumetric measurement, or percent of total body surface area.

1. **Direct Measurement.** Direct measurement of wound size is performed by measuring the longest length of the wound and the widest width perpendicular to this length (see Figure 4–2).[1,58,59,60,61] Wound surface area is computed by multiplying length by width. Wound depth is measured by placing a probe in the deepest part of the wound bed and noting the point at which the probe is

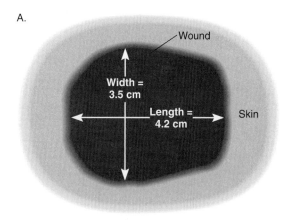

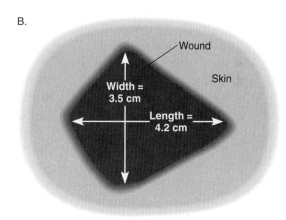

FIGURE 4–2   Measurement of wound size by direct wound measurement. Note there is no change in wound measurements despite a visually appreciable change in wound area.

level with the surrounding intact skin (see Figure 4–3).[61–63] Alternatively, several depth measurements can be performed at standard wound locations using the clock method.[1] When using the clock method, the 12-o'clock position is assigned to the part of the wound located closest to the patient's head. (The clinician may assign the 12-o'clock position to another location, but must document this new reference point.) In addition to the deepest portion of the wound, wound depth is also assessed at varying points around the clock. For example, the clinician may choose to assess wound depth at the 3-o'clock, 6-o'clock, 9-o'clock, and 12-o'clock positions. The clinician documents the measured depth and the corresponding reference position.

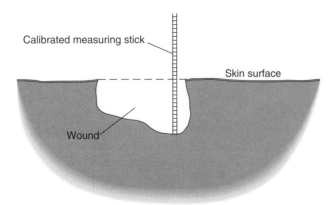

FIGURE 4–3   Direct measurement of wound depth. Documented as: "Wound depth = 1.4 cm."

Direct wound measurement is simple, fast, easy to learn, reliable, and inexpensive.[63–65] The most serious problem with direct wound measurement is that the measurement may not adequately reflect wound size, or changes in wound size, in irregularly shaped or circular wounds. In addition, it is not possible to accurately determine the depth of a wound covered with nonviable tissue. In such cases, clinicians must document this fact, because once nonviable tissue has been removed from the wound bed, wound depth will likely appear to increase (see Figure 4–4).

2. **Wound Tracings.**   Wound tracings can also be used to measure wound size.[1, 62, 66] To perform a wound tracing, a clean, conformable transparency and a permanent, fine-tipped pen are required. There are several commercially available wound tracing sheets, such as E-Z Graph. Most consist of two layers: a wound contact layer and an adhesive permanent layer that can be placed in the patient's permanent record without violating infection control procedures. First, the wound contact layer is cleaned and rinsed to prevent contaminating the wound. The transparency is placed against the wound while the clinician traces the wound. The wound contact layer is then discarded, and the outer permanent layer is affixed within the patient's medical record. Wound surface area is estimated from the tracing as previously described: longest length and widest width perpendicular to this length.[67] Wound depth is assessed using the direct measurement technique.[61, 68] If a commercial transparency is not

available, the clinician may make a wound tracing sheet out of plastic wrap or two sheets of clear transparencies. After cleaning and rinsing the wound contact layer, the wound is then traced and the contact portion of the plastic wrap is discarded. The clinician then photocopies or retraces the uncontaminated, outer layer of plastic wrap onto standard or grid paper to keep as part of the patient's permanent record. Wound tracings should be carefully labeled with the patient's name, date, precise wound location, measured size, and specific wound characteristics (see Figure 4–5).

There are three alternative methods of determining wound surface area from a wound tracing. First, some transparencies have premeasured grid marks, usually in 1-cm^2 increments. The wound surface area may then be determined by counting

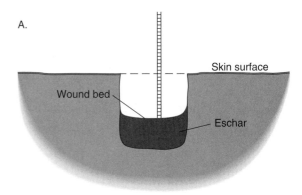

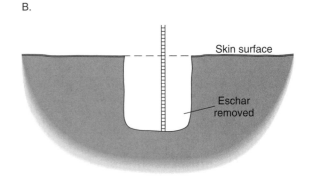

FIGURE 4–4   *A.* Direct measurement of wound depth in a wound covered with eschar. Documented as: "Wound depth measures 1.3 cm. Unable to determine actual wound depth secondary to eschar." *B.* Same wound, but with eschar removed. Documented as: "Wound depth = 2.2 cm."

A.

B.

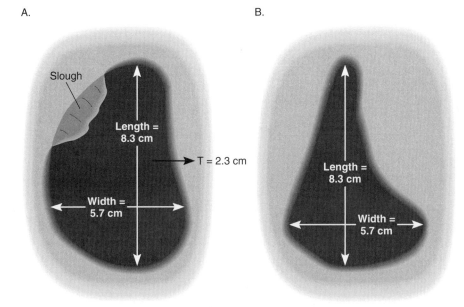

FIGURE 4–5   *A.* Wound tracing to measure wound size. *B.* The same wound is traced 2 weeks later. Note the measurements of wound size remain unchanged despite a decrease in wound area and resolution of tunneling (T).

the number of boxes within the tracing (see Figure 4–6). Boxes that are at least half within the tracing are counted as one full box, while boxes that are less than half within the tracing are disregarded.[69] Although slightly more reliable than calculating wound surface area from tracings using the length by width method, this method is generally considered to be too time consuming and tedious to be used in a clinic setting. Alternatively, wound surface area may be determined by planimetry or digitizing.[64] Planimetry and digitizing are reliable methods of calculating wound surface area.[65,70] Portable digital planimetry, such as Visitrak, MAVIS, and ATOS II, as well as software programs, such as WoundImager™ 2.0, are now available.[71,72] This equipment combines wound tracing with the accuracy of digital planimetry. In addition to calculating wound surface area for the clinician, the software also provides percent changes in surface area and granulation tissue from previous measures. However, because they require expensive equipment, these methods are generally reserved for research purposes.[73] In addition, time saved using this newer technology was noted to range only from a few seconds to 3 minutes.[72]

Like direct wound measurement, wound tracings are simple, fast, easy to learn, reliable, and inexpensive.[61,66,70,73,74] Wound tracings have several advantages over direct wound measurements. The image produced provides a more accurate representation of wound size, especially for irregularly shaped or circular wounds. Wound area determined by wound tracing is more reliable than direct wound measurement.[61] The retained image is also helpful for future comparison, especially if more than one clinician is working with the patient. While calculating the area of a given tracing appears to be reliable, the two key sources of error with wound tracings appear to be visualizing the wound perimeter through the transparency[75] and the ability to accurately trace the wound perimeter.[66,69,76]

3. **Photographic Measurement.** Wound surface area can be determined by tracing the photographic wound image.[67,71] Photographic assessment has two key advantages over direct wound measurements and tracings. First, photographic assessment avoids contact with the patient's wound. Second, the photograph provides additional information including periwound and wound bed characteristics. Wound photographs should include a cue card containing pertinent information including patient name, date, and precise wound location (see color image 4). The clinician would be wise to include a

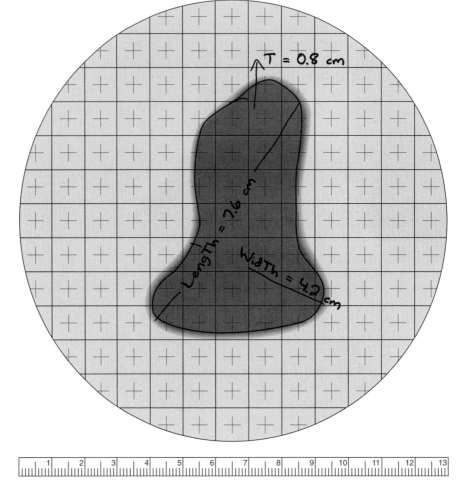

FIGURE 4–6 Wound tracing using graph paper to determine wound area. By the direct measurement of this tracing, wound area is 7.6 cm × 4.2 cm = 31.9 cm² However, by counting the boxes within the tracing, the area is only 25 cm².

measurement guide, such as a ruler, to provide a scaling reference and/or the results of direct wound measurements (see color image 23).[67]

The digital photographic equipment available today allows clinicians with minimal photographic skill and knowledge to obtain fairly consistent, high-quality wound images.[67] However, using photographic tracings to determine wound surface area is prone to errors in scale.[75] Both camera distance from the wound and camera angle can influence the resulting image size.[69] The distance from wound to camera can be held constant by affixing a string to the camera. Alternatively, some cameras used for wound photography have a standard focal distance that is made consistent by adjusting the camera position until two light sources converge into one over the wound. Unfortunately, similar methods to control for camera angle do not exist. Inconsistent lighting conditions may also make photographic wound assessment problematic, and photographic assessment of wound surface area is costly and time consuming.[75] Because of these factors, clinicians should use photography, when available, to provide supplemental information about wound and periwound characteristics,[73,77] but not to determine wound size. Finally, new software technology makes manipulation of digital images easy, and, therefore, unacceptable as a stand-alone record of wound status.

4. **Volumetric Measurement.** Wound size can also be determined by obtaining volumetric measurements, by measuring either the amount of dental or silicone molding[69,78] or saline required to fill the wound void. There are several problems with volumetric wound measurements, however. Molding is time consuming and can be painful to the patient.[78] In addition, it is unclear if the molding material or extrication may have detrimental effects on wound healing.[78] Calculating wound volume by measuring the amount of saline to fill the wound void is also time consuming, inaccurate,[69] and problematic. First, the clinician must ensure adequate removal of any wound exudate or saline prior to filling the wound void. Second, to avoid saline runoff (and therefore miscalculation) the wound must be either positioned with its opening facing directly perpendicular to the line of gravity or covered with a transparent film prior to filling with saline. Third, this method cannot be used with wounds that extend into body cavities or fascial planes because the saline will not be contained within the wound itself. Although volumetric assessment may potentially provide a more complete illustration of wound size by portraying the wound in three dimensions in contrast to the two-dimensional representations of the previously described methods, it is unclear whether this additional information is useful or necessary in determining changes in wound characteristics or making a wound healing prognosis.[78] Therefore, clinicians should not use volumetric measurements for assessing wound size.

5. **Total Body Surface Area.** For wounds covering large surface areas, such as the anterior chest, measurement of wound size, either directly or through tracings, is impractical. In such cases, clinicians would be wise to describe wound size as a percent of total body surface area (TBSA).[79] Total body surface area is a quick, inexpensive, and reliable method of estimating wound size.[80] TBSA is commonly used in patients with burn injuries because of the extensive integumentary damage that can occur with this type of wound. A thorough discussion of estimating wound size as a percent of TBSA is presented in Chapter 14.

Tunneling/Undermining

The entire wound bed should be probed for the presence of tunneling or undermining.[1,33,41,63,68] **Tunneling,** as the name implies, is a narrow passageway created by the separation of, or destruction to, fascial planes. Tunneling is measured by inserting a probe into the passageway until resistance is felt (see Figure 4–7). Tunnel depth is the distance from the probe tip to the point at which the probe is level with the wound edge. Clinicians should use clock terms to identify the tunnel's position within the wound bed[81] to ensure identification and remeasurement at a later time. Tunneling is common in neuropathic ulcerations[68] and surgical wounds (see Figure 4–8). Note some clinicians will use the term tunneling interchangeably with the phrase sinus tract. However, the more accepted use of the phrase **sinus tract** is to describe an elongated cavity that forms allowing purulent material from an abscess to drain to the body surface.[82]

Undermining occurs when the tissue under the wound edges becomes eroded, resulting in a large wound with a small opening. Undermining is measured by inserting a probe under the wound edge directed almost parallel to the wound surface until resistance is felt (see Figure 4–9). The amount of undermining is the distance from the probe tip to the point at which the probe is level with the wound edge.

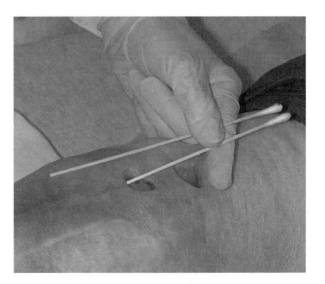

FIGURE 4–7   Tunneling wound.

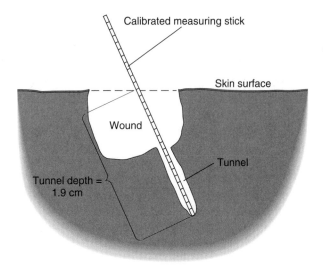

FIGURE 4–8   Cross-sectional schematic of a wound with tunneling. Documentation must include the tunnel's depth and position within the wound bed, most commonly using clock terms: "Wound tunnels 1.9 cm at 3-o'clock position."

Clock terms are also used to identify the area of undermining. Whereas tunneling is thought to include a small portion of the wound base directed in one direction, undermining generally encompasses a wider area.[83] Undermining is more commonly found in patients with pressure or neuropathic ulcers.[62]

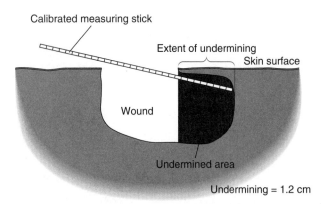

FIGURE 4–9   Cross-sectional schematic of a wound with undermining. Documentation must include the extent of undermining as well as the position within the wound bed, most commonly using clock terms: "Undermining 1.2 cm from 9-o'clock to 1-o'clock positions."

Because tunneling and undermining may not be readily visible, all wounds must be thoroughly probed to identify the full extent of tissue destruction.[68] Wounds presenting with tunnels or undermining heal more slowly than wounds without these characteristics.[84]

Wound Bed

The physical therapist must identify and describe wound bed characteristics.[1,8,34,41,85] The wound bed may contain varying types and amounts of granulation tissue, necrotic tissue, and other structures. As introduced in Chapter 2, granulation tissue is a temporary scaffolding of vascularized connective tissue that fills the wound void. Healthy granulation tissue has a beefy red appearance due to the presence of oxygen-rich capillaries. Granulation tissue that is pale or dusky in color or friable has poor blood supply or may be infected.[59,83,86,87] Therefore, wounds with this type of granulation tissue will likely heal more slowly than wounds with healthy granulation tissue. The physical therapist should document the characteristics of granulation tissue as well as the percent of the wound bed that this tissue occupies.[33]

Necrotic tissue within a wound bed should be described by color, consistency, and percent of the wound bed that the tissue occupies. **Slough** is yellow or tan in color and has a stringy or mucinous consistency.[62] Slough consists of white blood cells, bacteria, and degraded extracellular matrix.[88] **Eschar** is black necrotic tissue[10] that may be either soft or hard.[62] Wounds covered by a thick, black eschar are likely to be full-thickness.[62] Necrotic tissue should also be described as either adherent or nonadherent to the wound bed. Adherence refers to the ease with which the necrotic tissue can be separated from the wound.[83] The greater the depth of tissue destruction, the more adherent necrotic tissue tends to be.[62,83] The physical therapist should document both the characteristics of necrotic tissue and the percent of the wound bed that this tissue occupies.

Other structures found within the wound bed must also be described.[81] For example, a wound may have exposed structures such as fascia, muscle, tendon, joint capsule, or bone. Because of the high risk for osteomyelitis,[50] the care of patients with wounds that probe to bone should be closely coordinated with a physician. The physical therapist must document the type of structure and its characteristics, as well as the percent of the wound bed that these structures occupy. The presence of other items, such as sutures, staples, foreign material, or implants, should also be noted and described. Color image 16 provides an example of how to properly document wound bed characteristics.

Wound Edges

The tissue at the perimeter of the wound is the wound edge.[8,41] The physical therapist should note the following characteristics of the wound edges: distinctness, thickness, color, and attachment to the base of the wound.[62,89] Some superficial wounds present with indistinct wound edges where the wound gradually transitions into intact skin. Generally, deeper wounds have more distinct and well-defined wound margins. Wounds with attached edges are flush with the surrounding tissue, whereas wounds with unattached edges are deep and wound side walls are evident. Wounds with attached edges tend to heal more quickly than wounds with unattached edges.[84,90] The clinician should also note if the wound edges show evidence of epithelialization, scarring, or pigment changes.[34] Chronic wounds may present with thickened or rolled wound edges.

Hyperkeratosis, or callus-like tissue, is commonly seen at the edges of wounds due to diabetes and peripheral neuropathy.[6,8]

Wound Drainage

The physical therapist should assess and document the type, color, consistency, and amount of wound drainage, or exudate (see Table 4–2).[1,41,81,91,92] The type of wound drainage is generally described as one or a combination of the following: serous, sanguinous, or purulent.[81] Serous exudate is a protein-rich fluid with a few white blood cells that is generally seen in the inflammatory phase of wound healing.[86] It ranges in color from clear to pale yellow and has a watery consistency. Sanguinous drainage is red in color when fresh, or dark brown if allowed to dehydrate, and has the consistency of blood or slightly thickened water. Sanguinous drainage results from bleeding at the wound site. Purulent drainage ranges in color from white to pale yellow and has a viscous or creamy consistency. Purulent drainage is generally an indicator of wound

TABLE 4–2   Documentation and Interpretation of Wound Drainage

Drainage	Description	Interpretation
Type	Serous	Normal, transudate
	Sanguinous	Normal acutely or in response to trauma
	Serosanguinous	Normal
	Purulent	Possible infection
	Seropurulent	Possible infection
Color	Clear	Normal
	Pale yellow	Normal
	Red	Fresh blood
	Dark brown	Dried blood
	Blue-green	Probable *Pseudomonas* infection
Consistency	Thin, watery	Normal
	Thick	Possible infection
Amount	None	Desiccated wound bed
	Minimal or moderate	Normal; however, wounds with drainage that is disproportionate to the amount of necrotic tissue may be infected
	Copious	Possible infection, especially if out of proportion to wound size

infection.[86, 93] Certain infections have a characteristic drainage color. For example, *Pseudomonas* infections are usually accompanied by a blue-green drainage (see Chapter 6).[7, 81]

The amount of wound drainage can be categorized as being none, minimal, moderate, or copious. The amount of wound drainage is a subjective measure that may be influenced by several factors. If the type of dressing used is unable to accommodate the amount of wound drainage or if the dressing has not been changed in a long time, the wound may appear to be more heavily draining than it actually is. Conversely, a wound covered with a dressing that absorbs high amounts of fluid or that was recently changed may appear to be draining less than it actually is. Therefore, clinicians should consider both the absorptive capabilities of the wound dressing and the length of time the dressing has remained in place when describing the amount of wound drainage present. The amount of wound drainage can be affected by systemic and local factors: congestive heart failure or dependent positioning may increase wound drainage while dehydration and ischemia may decrease wound drainage.

Wound Odor

After the wound has been debrided and rinsed, the physical therapist should assess for wound odor. Wound odor is a highly subjective measure and, therefore, should only be described as either present or absent.[59] Some clinicians advocate documentation of wound odor in terms of the number of feet away from the wound that the odor can be detected. This is unwise because the odor may not be solely from the wound itself, but also from old bandages, body odor, or incontinence.[94] Conversely, wound odor may be disguised or exacerbated by certain dressings, deodorizers, or topical agents.[94] Wounds with necrotic tissue are likely to have at least a mild odor.[92] Despite its subjective nature, wound odor should be recorded because it is one of the indicators of wound infection.[95] For example, *Proteus* infections have an ammonia-like smell, whereas *Pseudomonas* infections smell "sicky sweet."[86] Wound odor should never be used as the sole indicator of wound status,[8] however. See Box 4–3 and Figure 4–10 for a summary of wound characteristics that should be included in the examination of a patient with an open wound.

BOX 4–3   Wound Characteristics to Include within the Examination of a Patient with an Open Wound

- Wound location
- Wound size
- Wound characteristics
  - Granulation tissue
  - Necrotic tissue
  - Other structures
- Wound edges
  - Attached/unattached
  - Indistinct/well defined
  - Thickened or rolled
  - Hyperkeratosis
- Wound drainage
- Wound odor

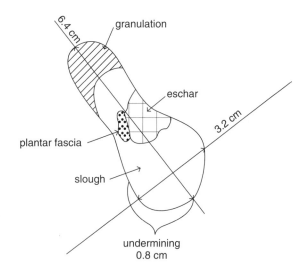

FIGURE 4–10 Wound tracing with completed documentation. **Patient name:** John Doe. **Date:** January 10, 2010. **Clinician:** Jane Smith, PT. **Wound location:** L plantar forefoot over 2nd metatarsophalangeal joint. **Wound size:** 6.4 × 3.2 cm, depth 1.2 cm. **Wound bed:** 25% granulation tissue, 50% yellow adherent slough, 20% black eschar, 5% plantar fascia. **Undermining:** 0.8 cm from 5-o'clock to 8-o'clock positions. **Wound edges:** unattached, circumferentially hyperkeratotic rim. **Wound drainage:** minimal, seropurulent. **Wound odor:** none. **Periwound:** anhydrous.

Checkpoint Question #1

As you remove your patient's bandages, you notice a strong, foul odor.

a. How should you document this information?
b. Is the wound infected?

Integumentary Integrity: Periwound and Associated Skin Characteristics

During the examination, the physical therapist should note the characteristics of the periwound and associated skin,[1,8] including structure and quality, color, epithelial appendages, edema, and temperature.[55] The clinician should compare the periwound and associated skin with skin outside this region and the contralateral side, when possible.

Structure and Quality

The physical therapist should assess the quality of the periwound and associated skin. Normal skin should be continuous, soft, shiny, smooth, pliable, and exhibit elastic recoil. Scaling, rough, or cracked skin is too dry. A slightly waxy appearance, dilated pores, or acne are signs of excessive lipids. For example, normal age-related skin changes may make the skin appear thin, fragile, or transparent.[96] Periwound hydration should be noted. Tissue that is anhydrous will appear dry, scaly, or cracked, whereas tissue that is too moist will appear macerated. Skin turgor can be assessed by lifting up the tissue to be tested between the thumb and index finger. The clinician should note if there is a delay before the skin returns to its normal position. It should be noted that it is normal for older adults to have a momentary delay in the return to normal skin countours due to age-related decreases in skin elasticity.[40] The presence and location of any calluses should be documented. The clinician should inspect for scar formation indicating healing of the current or previous wounds. The quality of scar tissue, including thickness, mobility, and color, should also be assessed. The therapist should note the presence of any deformities and describe any deviations. For example, varicosities suggest venous insufficiency,[97] and skin rashes may indicate hypersensitivity[98] or a fungal infection.[99]

Color

The physical therapist should describe the color of the periwound and associated skin in relation to both neighboring skin and comparable skin on the contralateral side.[89] Normal skin should have an even skin tone throughout, which may range from pale white to dark brown or black, depending on ethnicity and the amount of melanin present. Erythema should be described as either blanchable (turns white when the clinician applies digital pressure) or nonblanchable. Erythema is an indicator of inflammation (see color image 3), but, if out of proportion to the size and extent of the wound, may indicate infection (see color image 11). The amount of erythema should be quantified if possible by measuring how far the redness extends from the wound edge. Nonblanchable erythema indicates ischemic damage due to unrelieved pressure (see Chapter 12). Skin that appears lighter or paler than surrounding tissue may indicate decreased blood supply or newly formed scar tissue that has not yet regained normal pigmentation. Skin that is blue in color generally represents areas of severe and/or prolonged ischemia[100–102] (see Chapter 10). Long-standing venous insufficiency may cause hyperpigmentation of intact skin (see Chapter 11).[103]

Epithelial Appendages

The physical therapist should assess for the presence and quality of epithelial appendages, including hair and nail growth.[60] Areas of long-standing ischemia may be unable to support hair growth.[104] This is particularly evident in the lower extremity. Prolonged ischemia also increases the risk of nail fungal infections, making them appear thick and yellow.[101] However, because trophic changes alone are insufficient to diagnose arterial insufficiency,[44] these findings should be confirmed with further testing.

Edema

Because of their effect on function and association with wound infection, the therapist should assess for edema and **induration,**[89] edema that is hard or firm. Edema is a localized or generalized accumulation of interstitial fluid and may be described as either pitting or nonpitting. To assess for **pitting edema** the clinician should firmly press a thumb or index finger into the affected area and hold for 5 seconds.[105,106] If a depression remains within the tissue upon removal of pressure, pitting edema is present. Pitting occurs as the interstitial fluid moves away from the applied pressure, and slowly returns upon release of this pressure.[100] Pitting edema may be quantified on a 1 to 3+ scale or 1 to 4+ scale,[40,105,106] ranging in degree from minimal to severe (see Table 4–3). Long-standing edema will progress from pitting to nonpitting as a result of tissue fibrosis.[100,107] Quantification of edema by circumferential measurements is fast, simple, and reliable.[108] Both affected and unaffected sides should be measured and referenced to a bony landmark for consistency and ease of reassessment (see Table 4–4).[108] Volumetric displacement may be used to quantify edema;[109] however, the increased time, instrumentation,[109] potential for wound contamination,[109] and potential for error make this method less preferable.

Temperature

The physical therapist should assess periwound temperature. An increase in temperature is an indicator of inflammation[110] or infection,[111] whereas a decrease in temperature may reflect impaired circulation.[112,113] Prior to testing, the patient should rest supine with the area to be examined uncovered for approximately 5 minutes to allow the local skin temperature to stabilize with the ambient environment. Since the dorsum of the hand is more sensitive to temperature changes than the fingertips, skin surface temperature can easily be assessed by lightly palpating with the back of the hand. The temperature of the area of interest should be compared with more proximal body segments and the contralateral side, if possible. Palpation of temperature differences is a qualitative assessment of peripheral circulation and should be recorded as increased, normal, or decreased. Clinicians may attempt to quantify temperature differences. Fever strips are readily available, but they do not register skin temperatures below 95°F and there are no studies documenting the reliability or validity of such measurements. An infrared thermometer may provide a more quantitative, reliable, and valid measure of temperature changes in the feet and digits,[113,114] but this device is not readily available in most clinics. Because infrared thermometers measure temperature to the nearest 0.1°F, temperature should be measured after 15 minutes to allow normalization of skin temperature.[113] A left to right difference of more than 4°F (2.2°C) in the same location is considered clinically significant.[110] Because, in most instances, precise quantification of temperature changes is not required to develop a plan of care or assess interventions, palpation of skin temperature differences is satisfactory. See Box 4–4 for a list of periwound and associated skin characteristics to include in the examination of a patient with an open wound.

Circulation

Peripheral pulses should be assessed for all extremity wounds. Diminished or absent pulses likely represent more proximal arterial occlusion[101] and indicate poorer wound healing outcomes.[115] Pulses should be assessed with the patient resting supine and are graded on a 0 to 3+ scale ranging from absent to accentuated (see Table 4–5).[116] Although a 0–4+ scale for describing pulses has been mentioned in the literature,[43,104] there is poor intertester agreement.[117] By decreasing category choices, reliability may be improved. Palpating pulses, particularly pedal pulses, requires skill and practice. It is estimated that 0.10% of the population congenitally lacks a posterior tibial artery and up to 2% lacks a dorsalis pedis artery.[117] While pulses are

TABLE 4–3   Classification of Pitting Edema

Grade	Verbal Descriptor	Amount of Indentation
1+	Barely perceptible depression	<2 mm
2+	Easily identifiable depression, rebounds in <15 seconds	2–4 mm
3+	Depression rebounds in 15–30 seconds	5–7 mm
4+	Depression lasts for >30 seconds	>7 mm

TABLE 4–4   Sample Chart for Circumferential Measurements

Date:

Left	LE Location	Right	Left	UE Location	Right
	Dorsal MTP (metatarsophalangeal joint)			Proximal palmar crease	
	A = Lateral malleolus			A = Ulnar styloid process	
	B = +10 cm			B = +8 cm	
	C = +20 cm			C = +16 cm	
	D = +30 cm			D = +24 cm	
	E = +40 cm			E = +32 cm	
	F = +50 cm			F = +40 cm	
	G = +60 cm			G = +48 cm	
	H = +70 cm			H = +56 cm	

Clinician Signature/Credentials:

Note all girth measurements are documented in cm. Measurements B–H represent the distance in cm from the midpoint of the lateral malleolus and ulnar styloid process.

generally palpable if the pulse pressure is greater than 80 mm Hg, they may be difficult to palpate even with normal circulation because overlying tissues and pulses may be missed up to 8% of the time.[117] Therefore, the absence of palpable pulses should be followed up with more sensitive testing devices, such as a Doppler ultrasound, to more accurately assess perfusion.[50, 118]

Clinicians may assess **capillary refill** as an indicator of surface arterial blood flow in patients with extremity wounds. To assess capillary refill, first observe the color of the patient's digits. Then push against the distal tip of the digit to be examined with enough pressure to blanch the skin and hold for 3 seconds, thereby emptying surface vessels of

BOX 4–4   **Periwound and Associated Skin Characteristics to Include within the Examination of a Patient with an Open Wound**

- Structure and quality
- Color
- Epithelial appendages
- Edema
- Temperature

TABLE 4–5   Pulse Examination

Pulse Grade	Characteristics
0	Absent pulse
1+	Diminished pulse
2+	Normal pulse (easy to palpate)
3+	Bounding or accentuated pulse

blood.[116,119] Capillary refill time is recorded as the amount of time required for digit surface color to return to normal after the removal of pressure. Normal capillary refill time is less than 3 seconds.[40,119,120] Capillary refill measurements have been shown to be valid and reliable.[121,122] However, some studies have shown capillary refill is not predictive of peripheral arterial disease or impaired healing.[123] Refer to Chapters 10 and 11 for further details regarding the assessment of circulation in patients with arterial and venous insufficiency.

Sensory Integrity

The ability to perceive light touch acts as an early warning system to alert individuals to minor irritation or overt trauma. Impaired light touch sensation is a risk factor for ulceration and reulceration.[8,68] In addition, the inability to perceive integumentary trauma or the pain of an open wound decreases the likelihood of patient compliance with recommended prevention and wound management regimens. For example, a patient with a complete spinal cord injury will be unable to recognize the development of an ulcer over the ischial tuberosity due to unrelieved pressure from prolonged wheelchair sitting until tissue damage becomes visible when performing a skin check. Likewise, a patient with a full-thickness hand burn may be unable to feel a developing pressure ulcer under a splint. Impaired sensory integrity is the most significant risk factor for the development of ulcers in patients with diabetes. Alarmingly, many of these patients are not even aware they lack the ability to perceive light touch because of the slow, progressive onset of neuropathy. Physical therapists should assess sensory integrity in all patients with diabetes, peripheral neuropathy, or burns. Because a nonhealing or slow-healing ulcer may be the first sign of diabetes, physical therapists should also assess the sensory integrity of all patients with foot ulcers or chronic lower extremity wounds.[50]

The gold standard for assessing light touch sensation is **Semmes–Weinstein monofilaments** (see Figure 4–11). Monofilaments are reliable,[124] valid,[125] inexpensive, and clinically useful.[65,126–128] Monofilaments are pieces of nylon, similar to different gauges of fishing wire, that extend perpendicularly from a plastic rod. Each monofilament is carefully calibrated to create a precise amount of pressure before bending. To assess sensory integrity, the clinician should hold the end of the rod to dampen the effect of his or her hand vibration.[129] With the patient's vision

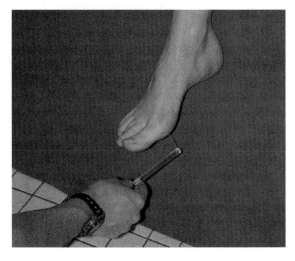

FIGURE 4–11 When assessing sensory integrity, apply the monofilament perpendicular to the skin with enough pressure to cause the filament to bend.

occluded, the filament should be applied gradually over 1–2 seconds with enough force to cause the filament to bend, then removed over 1–2 seconds so that a repeatable and consistent force is produced.[129,130] It may be wise to assess each test location three times. It has been proposed that a patient must be unable to perceive half of the test locations before categorizing sensory deficits.[131] However, it would seem prudent to classify the patient by the highest monofilament that any portion of the test area is unable to perceive.[126,132] Normal light touch sensation varies with anatomical location. For example, individuals can perceive lighter touch on the tips of the fingers than on the thorax.[130] Because of the preponderance of patients with diabetes and diabetic foot ulcers seen by physical therapists, Table 4–6[133] provides the normative values and interpretations for light touch sensation on the foot. Patients who are unable to perceive 10 grams of pressure on their foot should be considered at risk for ulceration or reinjury due to insensitivity.[134] Because sensory assessment over thick callus may be inaccurate,[130,132] the clinician should attempt to assess noncallused skin when possible. If a thickly callused area is assessed, the clinician should document the presence and location of the callus(es) along with the test results.

Vibration testing has also been used to assess sensation. However, clinicians are unable to consistently

TABLE 4–6   Interpretation of Sensory Testing

Normal light touch

• **Foot:** able to perceive 4.17 monofilament, which is equal to 1 gram of pressure.

• **Hand:** able to perceive 2.83 monofilament, which is equal to 72 mg of pressure.

Monofilament	Pressure Produced (grams)	Interpretation of Inability to Perceive Monofilament
4.17	1	Decreased sensation
5.07	10	Loss of protective sensation
6.10	75	Absent sensation

apply the tuning fork with a controlled amount of force,[129] potentially invalidating test results. In addition, monofilaments have been found to be superior to vibration testing for identifying sensory neuropathy.[125, 135] Most importantly, it may be difficult to use vibration testing as a learning tool to educate patients on the need for skin checks and the ramifications of sensory loss, as patients may not be able to make the interpretative or functional leap that loss of vibration sensation equates to a loss of protective sensation.

The website for this textbook contains a documentation template for the examination of a patient with open wounds.

Checkpoint Question #2

Your patient presents with a wound superior to her medial malleolus that began insidiously 6 months ago. Her pedal pulses are 1+. She is able to perceive the 5.07 but not the 4.17 monofilament. The wound has a moderate amount of thick, purulent drainage that has a blue tint to it. What is your interpretation of these findings?

CLINICAL DECISION MAKING

The physical therapist must synthesize the information in the history, systems review, and tests and measures to make clinical judgments. This should tell the therapist whether physical therapy is indicated and whether the patient would benefit from a referral or consultation with another health care provider (see Figure 4–12). If the physical therapist believes that physical therapy interventions are appropriate for a given patient, the therapist must then establish a diagnosis and determine the prognosis, outcomes, and plan of care.

Diagnosis

The diagnostic process (examination, evaluation, and diagnosis) consists of organizing signs and symptoms into categories to help determine the prognosis, plan

of care, and necessary interventions. The Integumentary Preferred Practice Patterns are diagnostic classifications that describe the elements of patient management and provide a system for classifying integumentary disorders. Physical therapists can readily place patients with open wounds into the appropriate practice pattern based on the extent of

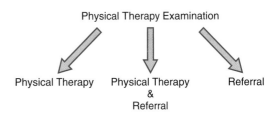

FIGURE 4–12   Clinical decision making.

tissue damage determined in the examination. The level of integumentary involvement within the Integumentary Preferred Practice Patterns ranges from prevention and risk factor reduction, to superficial skin involvement, to impaired integument involving destruction into fascia, muscle, or bone.[2, 3] Consistent with the other practice patterns within the *Guide to Physical Therapist Practice*, the Integumentary Preferred Practice Patterns provide information to assist with classification, including inclusion and exclusion criteria, and a list of ICD-9-CM codes related to each classification. In addition, the patterns suggest information that should be gathered during the physical therapy examination, including applicable tests and measures, and possible intervention strategies.

The Integumentary Preferred Practice Patterns provide a uniform language and method for physical therapists to assess and manage patients with, or at risk for, open wounds (see Box 4–5). Recall from Chapter 2 that superficial wound healing occurs through regeneration of epidermal tissues and as such, no scar formation occurs.[136, 137] Partial-thickness wounds heal by way of both regeneration from remaining epidermal appendages and repair leading to minimal scar tissue formation.[136, 137] Full-thickness wounds heal by way of repair with scar tissue formation.[136, 137] While the Integumentary Preferred Practice Patterns are well known to physical therapists, other disciplines may use alternative systems for certain types of wounds. Three

common wound-specific classification systems exist. The staging system,[41] described in Chapter 12, is used by physicians, nurses, and reimbursement analysts to classify pressure ulcers. The Wagner classification system,[138] described in Chapter 13, is used by surgeons and podiatrists for classifying diabetic foot ulcerations. The depth of burn injuries, described in Chapter 14, may be classified by physicians and surgeons in terms of degree[81] (e.g., third-degree or full-thickness burn). Each method of classification describes the level of tissue destruction and attempts to guide intervention strategies. To better coordinate patient care among different disciplines, physical therapists would be wise to use these alternative systems in tandem with the preferred practice patterns when working with patients with pressure ulcers, diabetic foot ulcers, or burns.

Successful management of patients with open wounds requires more than a thorough examination and proper classification[10] within the Integumentary Preferred Practice Patterns. For example, consider two patients, Mr. J and Mr. K, who present for physical therapy examinations under state direct access laws. Both patients complain of having a nonhealing lower extremity open wound. Based on the examination findings of the depth of tissue involvement, the physical therapist makes the same diagnosis of "Impaired Integumentary Integrity Associated with Partial-Thickness Skin Involvement and Scar Formation" (practice pattern 7C) for both patients. However, whereas Mr. J's wound is due to venous insufficiency, Mr. K's wound is due to arterial insufficiency. Interventions that may be appropriate for Mr. J, such as applying compression to control edema, are contraindicated for Mr. K.[116, 139] Applying compression to an arterial insufficient limb will only further compromise Mr. K's circulation and hasten tissue destruction. Therefore, the therapist must not only make a physical therapy diagnosis, but also accurately determine wound etiology[6, 139] and address risk factors contributing to ulceration and delayed wound healing,[6, 139] either through physical therapy interventions or referral to the most appropriate health care practitioner.

Wound etiology may be previously identified by a physician. For example, the patient may be referred to physical therapy for wound management with the diagnosis of "venous insufficiency ulcer." In such instances, the physical therapist should perform

---

BOX 4–5   Integumentary Preferred Practice Patterns

Pattern A: Primary Prevention/Risk Factor Reduction for Integumentary Disorders

Pattern B: Impaired Integumentary Integrity Associated with Superficial Skin Involvement

Pattern C: Impaired Integumentary Integrity Associated with Partial-Thickness Skin Involvement and Scar Formation

Pattern D: Impaired Integumentary Integrity Associated with Full-Thickness Skin Involvement and Scar Formation

Pattern E: Impaired Integumentary Integrity Associated with Skin Involvement Extending into Fascia, Muscle, or Bone and Scar Formation

examination procedures to verify wound etiology. Any inconsistencies in examination findings should be reported to the physician. For patients with burn injuries, surgical wounds, or traumatic integumentary damage, determining wound etiology is generally quite simple. In contrast, chronic wounds or wounds of insidious onset pose a greater challenge. To facilitate identification of wound etiology, typical characteristics of various types of ulcers presented in Section III are described using the 5PT method: pain, position, presentation, periwound, pulses, and temperature.

Prognosis

To make a prognosis, the physical therapist must predict the optimal level of improvement and determine the frequency and duration of physical therapy, the types of interventions required, and the time required to reach this optimal level. Unfortunately, there is a paucity of research available to guide clinicians in making scientifically grounded judgments regarding wound healing prognosis. In general, wounds that are deeper or involve a greater amount of tissue loss will take longer to heal than wounds that are more superficial or smaller in size[33,79,140–148] because the body must repair and rebuild more tissue. An analysis of wound healing curves suggests that the rate of wound closure (decrease in wound size) is slow initially. The rate increases dramatically during wound contraction, before slowing again during epithelialization (see Figure 4–13).[57] Research to date suggests that a 20–40% decrease in wound surface area within 2–4 weeks of initiating treatment is a good indicator that a wound is responding to wound management interventions and full closure will follow.[33,145,146] Wounds that do not decrease in size or show evidence of healing within 2 weeks should be reassessed for alternative or adjunctive interventions.[33,41,146]

It is critical for the physical therapist to consider more than just the practice pattern diagnosis and wound size to accurately predict the potential for wound healing. Acute wounds, such as surgical incisions and lacerations, follow the normal phases of wound healing and a predictable and expedient course to full wound closure. However, as discussed in Chapter 3, chronic wounds no longer follow this normal wound healing progression and time since onset cannot guide predictions for time to wound closure.[141,149] The physical therapist must also take into consideration the wound characteristics, local factors, and systemic factors affecting wound healing presented in chapter 3 when determining a wound healing prognosis. For example, one study found the average healing time for wounds due to diabetes (neuropathic ulcers) was 12 weeks while the average healing time for ischemic wounds (arterial insufficiency ulcers) was 16 weeks.[145] Additionally, consider Miss T

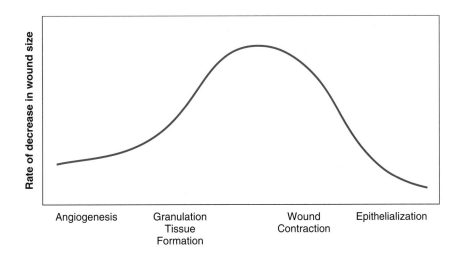

FIGURE 4–13   Wound healing curve.

and Miss V, two patients with right-hand burns. After examining each patient, the physical therapist makes the same diagnosis of "Impaired Integumentary Integrity Associated with Full-Thickness Skin Involvement and Scar Formation" (practice pattern 7D) for both. The therapist believes the best dressing choice for both is to use topical antimicrobial "X" and to cover the wound with a gauze dressing. The therapist tells both patients to change their dressings twice daily (as the antimicrobial effectiveness is 12 hours per the manufacturer's directions for product use) and to make follow-up appointments in the clinic in 3 days. This plan of care may be appropriate for Miss V. However, Miss T is right-handed, lives alone, and cannot identify anyone to assist her with her dressing change. Therefore, if the therapist does not modify this plan of care for Miss T, wound healing will likely be delayed.

Interventions

Interventions are defined as "purposeful and skilled interaction"[2] of the physical therapist or physical therapist assistant with the patient/client and related caregivers as needed to attain the stated prognosis. Physical therapy interventions involve a tripartite approach of coordination, communication, and documentation; patient/client-related instruction; and procedural interventions. In addition, the physical therapist must perform periodic reexaminations based on changes in patient or wound status.

The remainder of Section II provides information regarding interventions for local wound care, including debridement, infection control, dressing and bandage selection, and the use of modalities as adjuncts to wound healing. Section II also provides insights into patient education, enhancing patient adherence, and interdisciplinary collaboration for the successful management of patients with open wounds. Section III presents detailed information on physical therapy interventions based on specific wound etiologies, including wounds due to vascular insufficiency, pressure, diabetes, burns, lymphedema, and selected miscellaneous wounds. Although clearly beyond the scope of physical therapy, common medical and surgical interventions based on wound etiology are also presented to provide the clinician with a better understanding of the valuable roles these disciplines play.

Goals and Outcomes

Physical therapy interventions are directed toward achieving certain objectives. In cooperation with the patient and/or caregiver, the physical therapist must state anticipated goals and expected outcomes that are specific, measurable, and time dependent. Each Integumentary Preferred Practice Pattern provides many examples of anticipated goals and functional outcomes for the management of patients with, or at risk for, open wounds. In general, the goal is for complete wound healing; however, this may be neither necessary nor possible.[41] In some cases, the goal of wound management may be to prepare the wound for surgical closure or to attain a stable wound that the patient or caregiver can manage independently. Consider a 19-year-old patient referred to physical therapy after sustaining a partial-thickness wound on his forearm in a road bike accident. The physical therapist may consider the patient's young age, good social support, and unremarkable medical history in determining that physical therapy should be discontinued prior to complete wound healing. In conjunction with the patient, the physical therapist may set the following three goals to be attained in two visits: (1) the wound bed will be free of foreign debris, (2) the patient's college roommate will be independent with performing dressing changes as instructed, and (3) the patient will be able to state the signs and symptoms of a decline in wound status or infection, which would require further medical assessment. In this case, a normally healing wound no longer requires skilled physical therapy.

In contrast, consider a 45-year-old hospice patient referred to physical therapy with a full-thickness wound on his heel due to prolonged pressure. The physical therapist must consider that this patient is terminally ill and will likely be unable to heal the wound. In this case, the therapist, along with the patient's caregiver, may set the following goals to be attained in four visits: (1) an appropriate dressing will be determined to minimize the risk of infection, control wound drainage, and minimize patient discomfort with dressing changes; (2) the patient's wife will be independent with dressing changes; and (3) the patient's wife will be independent in repositioning the patient to minimize the risk of further skin breakdown.

Boxes 4–6 and 4–7 provide examples of goals that might be helpful when working with patients with wounds.

BOX 4–6   Sample Goals

The following chart includes some examples of objective and measurable goals that might be helpful when working with patients with wounds. *Note:* Time frames have intentionally not been included.

- Wound bed will contain at least _____ % granulation tissue.
- Wound bed will have less than _____ % necrotic tissue.
- Maceration will be resolved.
- Wound will decrease in size to:_____.
- Wound surface area will decrease _____ %.
- Wound will be clinically free of the signs and symptoms of infection to allow wound healing progression.
- Wound will be ready for surgical closure.
- Wound will progress to the proliferative phase of wound healing as evidenced by epithelialization and granular budding.
- Clean and stable open wound to decrease/eliminate (choose) the need for skilled physical therapy interventions.
- Immature scar will be evident.
- Wound will be completely closed with resurfaced epithelium.
- Wound will be completely closed with fully restored skin/barrier function.
- Patient will be able to tolerate _____ minutes of sitting/standing/lying (choose) without a decline in skin integrity.
- Patient will ambulate with appropriate footwear without erythema or change in skin structure.

BOX 4–7   Sample Behavioral Goals for Patients with Open Wounds

The following chart includes some examples of objective and measurable behavioral goals that might be helpful when working with patients with wounds. *Note:* Time frames have intentionally not been included.

- Patient/caregiver will verbalize the signs/symptoms of infection or decline in wound status and identify correct action if needed.
- Patient/caregiver will verbalize/demonstrate (choose) proper:
  - wound care techniques
  - independent monitoring of skin
  - edema/pressure control methods
- Patient/caregiver will be able to manage wound independently.

 Checkpoint Question #3

Revise the following goals to make them appropriate for documentation purposes.

a. The wound will be closed.

b. Increase granulation tissue.

c. Enhance circulation.

d. Decrease infection.

e. Patient will understand proper wound care.

CHAPTER SUMMARY

The three components of the examination are the history, systems review, and tests and measures. Clinicians must be able to objectively and reliably describe open wound characteristics such as location, size, tunneling, undermining, wound bed, wound edges, drainage, and wound odor. The clinician should also note the characteristics of the periwound and associated skin including structure and quality, color, epithelial appendages, edema, and temperature. Last, the clinician must assess the patient's circulation and sensory integrity. By integrating the information from the examination, the physical therapist must classify the wound and determine whether the patient would bene- fit from physical therapy, referral to another health care provider, or both. If the patient is a candidate for physi- cal therapy, the therapist must determine the prognosis, select appropriate interventions, and set specific, objec- tive, measurable, and time-dependent goals.

REVIEW QUESTIONS

Use color image 6 to answer the following questions.

1. Document the characteristics of the wound, peri-wound, and associated skin as you would in a patient's chart.

2. How would you classify this wound?

3. Write two goals for changes in wound characteristics.

myhealthprofessionskit

Use this address to access the Companion Website created for this textbook. Simply select "Physical Therapy" from the choice of disciplines. Find this book and log in using your username and password to access images, video clips, and additional learning tools.

REFERENCES

Go to myhealthprofessionskit.com to view this chapter's references.

5

Debridement

Chapter Objectives

After reading this chapter, learners will be able to:

1. Describe why necrotic wounds should be debrided.
2. Use the red–yellow–black descriptions of wound bed characteristics to guide general wound interventions.
3. Differentiate between sharp, autolytic, enzymatic, mechanical, and surgical debridement.
4. Explain the indications and contraindications for sharp debridement in a physical therapy setting.
5. Differentiate between serial instrumental and selective sharp debridement.
6. Describe the basic steps involved in sharp debridement.
7. Explain the indications and contraindications for autolytic debridement.
8. Describe the basic steps involved in autolytic debridement.
9. Explain the indications and contraindications for enzymatic debridement.
10. Describe the basic steps involved in enzymatic debridement.
11. Explain the indications and contraindications for mechanical debridement.
12. Describe the basic steps involved in mechanical debridement.
13. Describe biologic debridement.
14. Explain the indications and contraindications for surgical debridement.
15. Determine the most effective method(s) of debridement for individual patients with necrotic wounds.
16. Set appropriate debridement goals for patients with necrotic wounds.
17. Recognize the benefits of a collaborative approach to debridement.

Key Terms

Autolytic debridement	Nonselective debridement	Surfactants
Biologic debridement	Selective debridement	Surgical debridement
Debridement	Selective sharp debridement	Wet-to-dry dressing
Enzymatic debridement	Serial instrumental	Wound cleanser
Incision and drainage	debridement	Wound cleansing
Mechanical debridement	Sharp debridement	Wound scrubbing

INTRODUCTION

In most cases, the desired outcome of wound management is wound healing: the wound bed is completely resurfaced with epithelium, and the tissue is remodeled so that its strength approaches normal. An interim step in this process is to obtain a clean, moist, warm, granular wound bed while protecting the periwound and intact skin. The combination of debridement, bacterial control, and exudate management, sometimes referred to as wound bed preparation, facilitates the achievement of this short-term goal and, as such, is standard procedure in wound management.[1] This chapter provides an in-depth analysis of wound debridement. Bacterial control is discussed in Chapter 6 while exudate management through the use of wound dressings and bandaging is discussed in detail in Chapter 7.

Debridement is the removal of necrotic tissue, foreign material, and debris from the wound bed. In general terms, debridement decreases the risk of infection and enhances wound healing.[2,3] Most chronic wounds require some form of debridement.[4-6] Debridement is generally described as being either selective or nonselective. **Selective debridement** involves the removal of specific areas of devitalized tissue[7] and may include sharp, enzymatic, or autolytic debridement. **Nonselective debridement** is the removal of nonspecific areas of devitalized tissue[7] and may include mechanical and surgical debridement. The risks of not debriding include infection, osteomyelitis, sepsis, amputation, and even death.[8] Although some authors contend that wound debridement is "the single most important factor in wound management,"[9,10] it is important for clinicians to remember that debridement is just one of the many interventions necessary to attain wound healing. In fact, because wound debridement is the standard of care, there are no studies comparing patients receiving some form of debridement with patients without debridment.[11] Debridement does not preclude the need to address other issues that may be deterrents to wound healing.[12] As discussed in Chapter 3, systemic factors such as comorbidities and malnutrition, local factors such as tissue loads and circulation, and wound etiology must still be identified and addressed. The value of collaboration between various health care disciplines, the patient, and caregiver to create and implement the most effective care plan cannot be overstated.

ROLE OF DEBRIDEMENT IN WOUND MANAGEMENT

Debridement plays a vital role in wound management.[1,13-20] This section describes the many purposes of debridement. Next, the contraindications and considerations for performing debridement are discussed in general terms. Finally, this section provides an outline of how to prepare for this procedure.

Purposes for Debridement

There are no less than seven reasons for debridement[21,22] (see Box 5–1). First, devitalized tissue provides an excellent medium for bacterial growth.[5] Its presence is associated with increased bacterial colonization,[10,23] but not necessarily wound infection.[8] At least one study indicates that devitalized muscle, fat, and skin are as conducive in supporting bacterial growth as a nutrient broth.[10] After debridement, this bioburden is decreased,[6,23,24] allowing the patient's own immune system to be more effective and decreasing the risk of infection.[2,18,25-27] Second, topical antimicrobials have difficulty penetrating devitalized tissue and, therefore, are more effective once necrotic tissue has been removed.[28] Third, the bactericidal activity of leukocytes is decreased in samples with devitalized tissues when compared with samples without devitalized tissue.[10] This may be because necrotic tissue creates an anaerobic environment that reduces the ability of the body to phagocytize and opsonize bacteria, foreign material, and debris.[10] So, debridement improves the body's own defenses against infection.[29] Fourth, recall that one of the goals of the inflammatory phase of wound healing is to rid the wound of necrotic tissue, foreign material, and cellular debris. As long as devitalized tissue remains within the

---

BOX 5–1   Purposes for Debridement

- Decrease bacterial concentration within the wound bed and the risk of infection
- Increase the effectiveness of topical antimicrobials
- Improve the bactericidal activity of leukocytes
- Shorten the inflammatory phase of wound healing
- Decrease the energy required by the body for wound healing
- Eliminate the physical barrier to wound healing
- Decrease wound odor

wound bed, the inflammatory response will be perpetuated.[8] Debridement of these substances can minimize the inflammatory phase and allow the wound to progress to the proliferative phase of wound healing.[6,30] Fifth, devitalized tissue within the wound bed increases the energy needed for wound healing. The bacteria within devitalized tissue compete with the body's cells for nutrients and oxygen, decreasing the energy available.[25] If the tissue is exogenously debrided, more of the patient's energy reserves can be directed toward building new tissue and closing the wound defect. Sixth, devitalized tissue acts as a physical barrier to wound healing by inhibiting wound contraction and epithelialization.[6,20,28] Epithelial cells can only migrate over living tissue. Therefore, rather than simply crawling across a granular wound bed, epithelial cells must dive under devitalized tissue, producing enzymes to solubilize and digest this material. This not only requires more energy, but also increases the distance epithelial cells must travel, ultimately prolonging the time needed for wound healing.[31] Finally, one of the additional benefits of debridement is a decrease in wound odor. Although certainly not vital to the healing process, this can have a dramatic effect on patient and caregiver perceptions of wound progress and decrease potential patient embarrassment when interacting with others.

General Indications for Debridement

Although wound classification using the preferred practice patterns, the International NPUAP/EPUAP Pressure Ulcer Classification system (previously known as the staging system), or other methods provides insights into the depth of tissue destruction, it does not adequately direct interventions based on wound bed characteristics. As described previously, a short-term goal of wound management is generally to obtain a clean, moist, warm, granular wound bed while protecting the periwound and intact skin.[1] Therefore, debridement is indicated when there is necrotic tissue, foreign material, or debris within a wound bed.[4] Recall from Chapter 4 that necrotic tissue should be described in terms of its consistency, color, adherence, and percent of the wound bed that it occupies. Because of the various presentations of necrotic tissue, clinicians may choose to use the red–yellow–black system[32] to assist in determining appropriate management strategies for the wound bed (see Table 5–1).

The red–yellow–black system provides a means of describing the wound bed and suggests intervention strategies based on three general wound bed presentations.[33] A black wound bed is covered with eschar[24,34,35] and likely indicates a full-thickness wound.[2,36,37] The necrotic tissue present is generally thick and adheres to the wound bed. Eschar may be moist, but will be dry and leathery if allowed to dehydrate.[8,35,38] The treatment goal for a black wound is debridement of devitalized tissues.[24,34] A yellow wound is a draining wound covered with slough, a collection of fibrin, pus, and proteinaceous material.[24,35] A yellow wound may result from partially removed eschar of a black wound or may represent a more superficial wound in which there was not enough tissue destruction to create a thick eschar.[32] The moisture content of the slough promotes bacterial growth, putting a yellow wound at increased risk for infection. The periwound is at increased risk for maceration due to the quantity of exudate accompanying this type of wound. A yellow wound may also be due to topical agents or dressing residue remaining within the wound bed. In this circumstance, the yellow appearance should resolve after irrigation and removal of these substances. The treatment goals for a yellow wound are to remove the nonviable tissue, absorb the exudate,[39] and protect the surrounding tissue from excess

TABLE 5–1   Using the Red–Yellow–Black System to Describe the Wound Bed

Color	Wound Bed Description	Treatment Goals
Red	Pale pink to beefy red, granulation tissue	• Protect wound • Maintain warm, moist environment • Protect periwound
Yellow	Moist, yellow slough May vary in adherence	• Debride necrotic tissue • Absorb drainage • Protect periwound
Black	Thick, black, adherent eschar	• Debride necrotic tissue

moisture. A red wound is a granular wound.[34] This type of wound is said to be "red and ready to heal" because the pale pink to beefy red wound bed need only proliferate to fill the wound void so that epithelial cells can migrate across the wound defect. The treatment goal for a red wound is to protect the fragile granular tissue and epithelium.

In the original scheme of the red–yellow–black system, these colors were believed to represent a healing progression. Appropriate wound management was believed to transform a black wound into a yellow wound before ultimately progressing into a red wound.[39] In clinical practice, however, it is sometimes possible to remove all of the eschar from a black wound by way of sharp debridement, exposing a red, granular base. In this case, the wound would never be categorized as a yellow wound. Alternatively, it is possible for wounds to digress from a red wound to a yellow or black wound due to a decline in status or inappropriate wound management. Placement of a wound into one of these three categories is not always straightforward. Wounds may present with a combination of these three color types. For example, a wound bed may consist of 75% black eschar and 25% yellow slough. In such cases, it was originally suggested that the most serious color category should be treated first.[32] In this scenario, the wound would be treated as a black wound and debridement would be appropriate. However, the clinician should appropriately address all portions of the wound bed and not just the most severe. Therefore, appropriate wound management in this example should also include absorption of excess exudate, debridement of necrotic tissue, and protection of the periwound.

Blisters and calluses may also require debridement.[2,13] The fluid components within burn blisters alter the bactericidal activity of neutrophils[40] and inhibit fibrinolysis.[41] Whether due to a burn or friction, if a blister breaks open spontaneously, it will likely create a larger wound. Therefore, large fluid-filled blisters, blisters over joints, and burn blisters should be debrided (see color image 20). Refer to Chapter 14 for further details regarding burn care. Calluses should be debrided to eliminate localized areas of increased pressure (see color image 8).[13] This is particularly important on the plantar aspect of the foot where pressure points increase the risk of ulceration in people with diabetes. Cracks and fissures within callused areas provide a path by which bacteria can enter the body.[42] By debriding calluses as they

form and routinely applying moisturizing lotions, the risk of infection can be decreased.[13] Refer to Chapter 13 for further details on the management of neuropathic ulcerations.

General Contraindications for Debridement

The clinician should be aware of the following general contraindications for *all* methods of debridement within the physical therapy setting. Debridement of red, granular wounds is contraindicated.[43] Not only do these wounds not have devitalized tissue to remove, but any attempts to debride will only disrupt the healing process and delay wound closure. The clinical practice guidelines for the treatment of pressure ulcers state that stable, hard, dry eschar in ischemic limbs "should not be debrided."[2] If this type of wound starts to exhibit signs and symptoms of infection or progression (e.g., becomes tender, boggy, fluctuant, malodorous, or exhibits crepitous), the guidelines suggest that immediate referral to a vascular surgeon and debridement is warranted.[2]

Debridement in a physical therapy setting is contraindicated when there is an urgent need for surgical debridement[2,44-46] for two reasons. First, potentially limb and lifesaving procedures would be delayed by continued debridement within a physical therapy setting. Second, if more wide-ranging debridement is imminent, debridement in a physical therapy setting would be redundant. Debridement of muscles, tendons, ligaments, capsules, fascia, bones, nerves, and blood vessels is beyond the scope of physical therapy and requires surgical intervention. Similarly, gangrenous tissue requires surgical debridement. Large category/stage III and IV pressure ulcers (see Chapter 12) with significant undermining, tunneling, or sinus tracts are best managed surgically.[2,8,35,38] Because of the wide-ranging necrosis that occurs with electrical burns, this type of injury generally requires surgical debridement initially, until the extent of tissue destruction is known.

See Table 5–2 for a summary of the general indications and contraindications for debridement.

General Considerations for Debridement

The clinician must take into consideration the characteristics of the wound, the status of the patient, existing practice acts, and his or her own skills when determining whether debridement is appropriate and what

TABLE 5–2 General Debridement Indications and Contraindications

Debride	Do Not Debride
• Necrotic tissue (eschar, slough)	• Granular tissue
	• Viable tissue
• Foreign material	• Stable, hard, dry eschar in ischemic limbs*
• Debris	
• Residual topical agents	• Urgent need for surgical debridement gangrene, osteomyelitis
• Blisters	• Electrical burns
• Callus	• Deeper tissue muscle, tendon, ligament, capsule, fascia, bone, nerves, blood vessels

*See the section "General Contraindications for Debridement" in this chapter.

method(s) to use.[14] Wound characteristics that influence this decision include wound etiology, wound size, presence of infection, amount of necrotic tissue present, and other characteristics of the wound bed, such as the presence of tendons or tunneling into body cavities.[2,3] In order to determine whether the type of debridement chosen is successful, the clinician must set goals for this intervention and assess progress regularly. For example, one goal may be "The wound will be free of black eschar within 2 weeks of initiating debridement." Note that because wound size is likely to increase after initial debridement,[11,47] especially if there is a significant amount of devitalized tissue or undermining, clinicians should be wary of using changes in wound size alone to judge progress at this point in the healing process.

The patient's general health, nutrition, and concomitant medical conditions must also be considered. For example, if the patient's care plan includes palliative measures because death is imminent, debridement is not consistent with this care plan and should not be initiated or continued.[2] More specifically, the presence of immunosuppression, thrombocytopenia, or the use of anticoagulants must also enter into the decision-making process.[2,45,48] In addition, the setting the patient is in, whether it be outpatient, long-term care, or acute care, must be considered.[2] Because debridement may elicit pain or patient apprehension, the clinician should ensure adequate pain control and explain procedures thoroughly prior to initiating this intervention.[2,49,50]

There are two clinician characteristics that must be taken into account when determining what method of debridement is most appropriate.[2,3,14] First and foremost, current local laws and practice acts influence what type of health care provider may perform what type of debridement. Clinicians are encouraged to contact their state professional organization for the most current information. Second, clinician knowledge and skill level, both in wound management and with the various forms of debridement, must be considered. Wound management is a specialized area of practice and, regardless of a health care provider's professional training, clinicians who have not mastered the necessary skills should not participate in this facet of patient care.

Preparing to Debride

Box 5–2 provides a step-by-step guide for preparing for debridement. As with all other types of intervention, the clinician must follow accepted standard precautions at all times. Of note is the standard use of clean, rather than sterile, gloves. Clean gloves in combination with sterile equipment (forceps, scissors, and scalpel) are sufficient[2] because there is a very low probability that the clinician's hands will come into direct contact with the wound bed (refer to Chapter 6 for further

---

BOX 5–2 Steps to Prepare the Patient for Debridement

1. Assemble equipment and supplies that may be needed.
2. Position the patient comfortably, allowing for visualization of the wound bed. An aide may be needed to assist with attaining and maintaining this position.
3. Use proper posture and body mechanics to allow safe technique and minimize fatigue.
4. Ensure sufficient lighting of the involved area.
5. Wash hands and don clean gloves.
6. Remove the old bandage and discard according to facility policies.
7. Discard soiled gloves and apply clean gloves.
8. Inspect the wound to determine if debridement is necessary and, if so, what method is most appropriate. The wound may need to be irrigated with normal saline to provide more accurate inspection.
9. Remove soiled gloves.
10. Explain the procedure to the patient.
11. Don clean gloves and initiate debridement technique.

information regarding clean and sterile technique). Once the method of debridement is chosen, the clinician must explain the procedure to the patient. This is particularly important when sharp instruments, such as scissors and scalpels, may be used, as uninformed patients may erroneously fear intolerable pain, disfigurement, or even amputation. By calmly explaining the rationale for this procedure, patient anxiety and fear can be lessened. Specific procedures for each debridement method are provided in the following section.

☑ *Checkpoint Question #1*

You have a wound management referral for a 72-year-old nursing home resident with an ulcer over his sacrum. The ulcer measures 3.0 × 2.6 cm and is 50% eschar and 50% slough. Based on the red–yellow–black system, what are your general treatment goals?

METHODS OF DEBRIDEMENT

 There are four primary methods nonphysician health care providers can use to debride wounds: sharp, autolytic, enzymatic, and mechanical. Although seldom used in the United States at this time, biologic debridement with the use of maggots is gaining in popularity. This section provides detailed information regarding each of these techniques including indications, contraindications, and specific procedures for each method. Protocols for these techniques are also included. In addition, the role of surgical debridement in wound management is elucidated (see Table 5–3).

Sharp Debridement

Sharp debridement involves using forceps, scissors, or a scalpel to selectively remove devitalized tissue, foreign material, and debris from a wound bed.[51,52] Sharp debridement is the fastest and most aggressive form of debridement[18,31,38] outside of surgery.[18,31] Because of this, vigorous and repeated sharp debridement of necrotic tissue and debris is the standard of care for many patients with open wounds.[53] It may also be the most controversial method. Sharp debridement may be performed by physicians and podiatrists. Physical therapists,[3,14,17,46,54,55] physical therapist assistants, enterostomal nurses, nurse practitioners, registered nurses (and in a few states LPNs), and physician assistants may also perform sharp debridement *where allowed by law.* Clinicians should review the laws and practice acts governing sharp debridement in their state.[14] While no physical therapy practice act specifically prohibits sharp debridement, most fail to specifically mention sharp debridement, either as an intervention available to physical therapists or as one that is prohibited. Several states currently require evidence of continuing education, certification, or mentored performance of sharp debridement prior to independent performance of this procedure.[14,56] Some state

TABLE 5–3   Methods of Debridement

Method		Definition
Selective	**Sharp**	The use of forceps, scissors, or a scalpel to selectively remove devitalized tissue, foreign material, and debris
	Autolytic	Maintaining a warm, moist wound environment to allow endogenous enzymes to digest necrotic material
	Enzymatic	The use of exogenous enzymes to remove devitalized tissue
Nonselective	**Mechanical**	The use of force to remove devitalized tissue, foreign material, and debris
	Surgical	The use of scalpels, scissors, or lasers in a sterile environment by a physician or podiatrist to remove necrotic tissue, foreign material, and debris

practice acts defer to facility policy and procedures and that these must reflect a certain competence level prior to skill performance. Given the controversy involved with sharp debridement and the potential need for physician consultation and/or interventions when treating patients with open wounds, it would be prudent for all physical therapists, regardless of direct access legislation, to obtain a specific physician order for sharp debridement prior to commencement. The Centers for Medicare and Medicaid Services have determined that sharp debridement is a key component of active wound management and, as such, is reimbursable under Medicare guidelines.[57] The disadvantages of sharp debridement are the skill required for this technique and the potential for procedure-related pain.

Indications

Sharp debridement is indicated when there is a large amount of necrosis, callus, advancing cellulitis or sepsis, or thick, adherent eschar.[2,13,14] In addition, sharp debridement may be used on wounds with any amount of necrotic tissue.[1,4,5,12] Chronic wounds are likely to require repeated bouts of debridement because necrotic tissue and wound bioburden tend to re-accumulate within the wound bed.[2,4,13] Color images 8 and 9 provide an excellent example of plantar foot wounds pre- and postdebridement.

Contraindications

Sharp debridement is contraindicated when the area of debridement cannot be adequately visualized because of extensive tunneling or undermining, when the material being debrided cannot be identified, when the clinician is out of his or her comfort zone, or when clinician competency has not been demonstrated. Sharp debridement should not be performed on uninfected ischemic ulcers with low ankle-brachial indexes (refer to Chapters 4 and 10 for further details) prior to successful revascularization.[2,13] This recommendation stems from the fact that, without sufficient blood supply, ischemic ulcers are unlikely to heal; sharp debridement would probably increase the wound size rather than promote wound closure. Sharp debridement should be used with caution on patients who are immunosupressed, thrombocytopenic, or on anticoagulants.[2,48] Sharp debridement may not be indicated for patients with life-threatening diseases or conditions in which wound closure is not consistent with the plan of care.[2,58] Physical therapists should not perform sharp debridement on hypergranular tissue. Although this tissue is not conducive to wound healing, sharp debridement of hypergranular tissue may be considered surgery and is beyond the scope of physical therapy. As discussed in Chapter 2, physical therapists may try to eliminate hypergranular tissue using silver nitrate sticks or compression, or they may request surgical debridement.

Termination

Sharp debridement should be terminated if the clinician becomes fatigued, the patient reports pain that is not adequately controlled, there is a decline in patient status or tolerance to the technique, there is extensive bleeding, a new fascial plane is identified, or there is nothing remaining that should be debrided.[2,6,28,59] Given the clinician's usual time constraints, extensive debridement should only be undertaken when time permits.

Procedure

The American Physical Therapy Association (APTA) has defined two types of sharp debridement: serial instrumental debridement and selective sharp debridement (see Table 5–4). **Serial instrumental debridement** uses instruments such as forceps and scissors to remove loosely adherent necrotic tissue. This technique usually occurs over a number of visits and creates minimal bleeding or pain.[2,4,60] Serial instrumental debridement is sometimes inaccurately referred to as "maintenance debridement."[48] Serial instrumental debridement does not just maintain the wound's status quo, but rather is a vital component of controlling chronic wound bioburden and promoting wound healing. In addition, the erroneous use of the term "maintenance" may be perceived by third-party payers as a nonskilled and nonrequired procedure, thereby limiting reimbursement for this medically necessary component of wound management. Because water or saline softens necrotic tissue and makes it more amenable to debridement, serial instrumental debridement commonly requires prior tissue preparation by way of nonspecific debridement, such as whirlpool, irrigation, or pulsatile lavage.[60] In contrast, **selective sharp debridement** uses scissors or a scalpel to cut along the border of viable and nonviable tissue and does not require prior tissue preparation.[7,60] This boundary can only be determined on a macroscopic level, which may cause bleeding because of the small amount of circulation at the edges of nonviable tissue. Therefore, the use of hemostatic agents, such

TABLE 5–4   Contrasting Types of Sharp Debridement

Sharp Debridement	Guidelines
Serial instrumental debridement	• Uses instruments such as forceps and scissors to remove loosely adherent necrotic tissue • Generally occurs over a series of visits • Minimal bleeding or pain • May need prior tissue preparation • **Qualified providers*** 　Physician 　Podiatrist 　Physical therapist 　Physical therapist assistant
Selective sharp debridement	• Uses scissors or a scalpel to cut along the line of demarcation between viable and nonviable tissue • Does not require prior tissue preparation • Hemostatic agents may be required to control bleeding • Generally requires pain management • Followed by dry dressing for the first 8–24 hours if significant bleeding occurs with procedure • **Qualified providers*** 　Physician 　Podiatrist 　Physical therapist

*Enterostomal nurses, nurse practitioners, registered nurses, and physician assistants may also perform sharp debridement where allowed by law after competency has been demonstrated.

as Gelfoam or silver nitrate, may be required to control bleeding.[3] If selective sharp debridement causes significant bleeding, a dry dressing should be used for the first 8–24 hours after the procedure to control bleeding and minimize hematoma formation. If minimal to moderate bleeding occurs, the clinician may apply pressure with a gauze pad until the bleeding is controlled or use an alginate dressing.[3,35] Selective sharp debridement generally requires one or only a few sessions to complete.[21] Because this technique requires greater knowledge, skills, and abilities, it is the position of the APTA's House of Delegates that selective sharp debridement can be performed only by a physical therapist, and *not* by a physical therapist assistant.[14,61] The procedure for serial instrumental debridement is similar; however, hemostatic agents and topical pain medication are not required. A sample debridement protocol is provided in Box 5–3.

The patient is prepared for debridement as previously described. Once the clinician determines that sharp debridement is indicated, the procedure should be explained at a level appropriate for each individual patient. This is particularly important when the clinician is using sharp instruments, such as scissors or scalpels. The necessary instruments and supplies should be opened. For selective sharp debridement, the clinician generally requires forceps, scalpel, iris scissors, gauze squares, additional gloves, and a wound dressing. Clinicians must refrain from the use of inappropriate instruments, such as suture sets, for debridement. Silver nitrate sticks and an absorbable gelatin sponge, such as Gelfoam or other hemostatic agent, should also be available. Topical pain management may be achieved with a physician's prescription for 2% lidocaine or EMLA® cream (eutectic mixture of local anesthetics consisting of lidocaine 2.5% and

BOX 5–3   Sample Sharp Debridement Protocol
1. Prepare the patient for debridement.
2. Explain the specific procedure to the patient.
3. Open necessary equipment and supplies. This may include:
forceps   gauze squares
scalpel   a wound dressing
iris scissors   additional gloves
4. For selective sharp debridement, silver nitrate sticks and/or an absorbable gelatin sponge should be available.
5. Ensure adequate pain control; use physician-prescribed topical or systemic pain medications if necessary.
6. Don clean gloves.
7. Identify devitalized tissue, foreign material, and debris to be debrided.
8. Remove as much of these tissues/materials as possible, applying tension and using a layered approach.
9. Rinse the wound with saline.
10. Assess changes in wound status and perform any necessary wound measurements.
11. Dispose of sharp instruments and infectious waste.
12. Remove and dispose of soiled gloves. Don clean gloves.
13. Apply wound dressing.
14. Remove and dispose of soiled gloves.
15. Initial and date wound dressing.
16. Wash hands.
17. Provide any necessary posttreatment instructions.
18. Complete documentation.

prilocaine 2.5%),[49, 62–64] if necessary.[65] Topical lidocaine provides quick onset of relief and lasts approximately 20 minutes. Because it has a slower onset of action, EMLA cream should be applied to the wound area and covered with an occlusive dressing or plastic wrap for 30–45 minutes prior to debridement.[64] Delayed hypersensitivity reactions and allergic contact dermatitis have been reported with the use of topical lidocaine in both prescription dosages and over-the-counter dosages.[66] Sensitization may increase with repeated exposure.[66] Therefore, clinicians must ask patients if they have a history of adverse reactions to lidocaine and monitor for these adverse effects. These products should be discontinued and the physician of record notified if any adverse effects are noted. Patients receiving intravenous or intramuscular pain medications should be scheduled for debridement during peak medication action time. Once preparations are completed, the clinician should begin by identifying the tissue to be debrided. It may be helpful to visualize which tissues are normally found in the involved location.

When performing debridement, the clinician should hold the scalpel and scissors parallel to the wound surface and debride in layers to keep from incising healthy underlying tissues. Using the forceps to apply gentle traction to the devitalized tissue may assist in its removal. When removing a callus, the clinician should apply tension to the skin with the nondominant hand, being careful to remain clear of the sharp instruments. Upon completion, the clinician should rinse the wound with saline and assess the effect of this procedure. All sharp instruments and infectious waste must be disposed of according to facility policy. The clinician should provide the patient or caregiver with any posttreatment instructions, and the wound should be observed for signs of infection or bleeding.

Because of the significant damage that can be inflicted using this technique, such as inadvertently severing a tendon or blood vessel, clinicians are encouraged to have supervised practice with sharp debridement.[67] There are several methods to provide practice in a safe, nonthreatening environment. The most basic technique would be to review available anatomy texts or dissection videos, in combination with the basic science section of this text, to recall structure location, depth, and presentation of all involved tissues. In addition, experience with cadaver dissection should be mandatory prior to performing selective sharp debridement in the clinic.[68] Cadaver dissection provides learners with a unique opportunity to observe human anatomy in three dimensions and familiarize themselves with the instruments of debridement. Structured laboratory activities can assist novice clinicians in proper setup and technique. Three commonly used scenarios to practice debridement include removing the white, pithy part of a peeled orange without rupturing the inner membrane (see Figure 5–1),[69] melting wax from a candle onto a candle of a different color and then using a scalpel to remove only this outer layer of wax,[28] or using the various instruments to remove selected portions of tissue from a sample of pigs' feet obtained from the butcher or supermarket (see Figure 5–2). A mentor may prove beneficial for novice clinicians. Advanced continuing education courses or certifications in wound management may also provide novice clinicians with the opportunity for supervised practice. Regardless of the

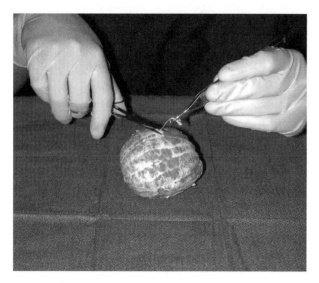

FIGURE 5–1 Use the forceps to lift devitalized tissue. Hold the scissors flush with the patient to avoid piercing the patient with the sharp end of the scissors.

method of practice chosen, all clinicians who may perform sharp debridement should be required to pass a sharp debridement competency.[21] Clinicians deemed competent—either through certification as a wound specialist or by a physician or podiatrist with expertise in wound management—should then evaluate the

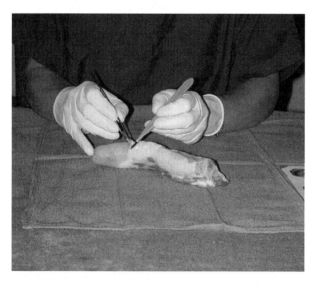

FIGURE 5–2 When debriding with a scalpel, hold the blade level with the tissue to be debrided to avoid cutting into deeper, healthy tissues.

competency of other clinicians within their facility. See Table 5–5 for a sample debridement competency.

Autolytic Debridement

Wound fluid contains endogenous enzymes, neutrophils, growth factors, and macrophages.[8] **Autolytic debridement** uses the body's own (endogenous) enzymes, including collagenase, to digest necrotic tissue by applying a moisture-retentive dressing, such as a sheet hydrogel, semipermeable foam, or hydrocolloid (see Chapter 7), and leaving it in place for several days.[2,6,12,20,26,30,70] Moisture-retentive dressings have been found to be more effective in autolytic debridement than simple gauze dressings.[18] The wound fluid trapped beneath the dressing softens and liquefies necrotic tissue.[9,24,71] In addition, the growth factors and inflammatory cells within the wound fluid may hasten the inflammatory and proliferative phases of wound healing. It is important that clinicians (and patients/caregivers) do not mistake wound fluid for an infectious process. It is normal and desirable to have a localized collection of wound fluid beneath the dressing. When the dressing is removed, there may be an odor due to the softened necrotic tissue or product residue. The wound should be rinsed with normal saline prior to assessing the wound bed.

Autolytic debridement is consistent with the moist wound healing model described in Chapter 3 and is considered the most conservative method of debridement. It is also the least invasive and least painful method. Autolytic debridement is easy to teach to patients and caregivers and requires minimal clinician and patient/caregiver time. Autolytic debridement also does not introduce any potentially cytotoxic substances to the wound bed and may reduce costs over the long term.[11] The disadvantages of autolytic debridement are that it requires time for the body to debride itself[35] and does not allow frequent visualization of the wound bed. Although some clinicians may be concerned that covering a wound in a warm, moist environment may promote bacterial growth, the rate of infection using moisture-retentive dressings (2.6%) has been found to be lower than when traditional gauze dressings are used (7.1%).[72]

Indications

Autolytic debridement can be used on all wounds regardless of etiology as long as the wound contains necrotic tissue. It is particularly useful for patients

TABLE 5–5   Sample Debridement Competency

Criteria	Competent
Clinician Knowledge	
1. Ensures written or verbal orders for sharp debridement from attending physician unless practicing under direct access legislation.	_____
2. Verbalizes tissues that are not to be debrided, including tendons, capsule, muscle, ligament, bone, viable tissue, ischemic tissue, and eschar due to electrical injuries without specific physician approval.	_____
3. Verbalizes when procedure should be terminated.	_____
4. Verbalizes need for dry wound dressings for first 8–24 hours after selective sharp debridement causing bleeding.	_____
Patient Education	
1. Informs patient of procedure to be performed and rationale.	_____
2. Informs patient/caregiver to notify clinician of any changes in wound status after procedure.	_____
Clinician Technique	
1. Positions patient appropriately.	_____
2. Dons appropriate personal protective equipment.	_____
3. Selects appropriate equipment.	_____
4. Identifies tissues to be debrided.	_____
5. Demonstrates the following techniques:	_____
a. Lifting away nonviable tissues with forceps	_____
b. Crosshatching eschar	_____
c. Removing callus	_____
d. Separating viable and nonviable tissues with scissors or scalpel (physical therapists only)	_____
6. Disposes of devitalized tissues and soiled bandages according to facility policy.	_____
7. Disposes of sharp instruments in approved sharps container.	_____
Clinician Documentation	
1. Documents patient education and understanding of same.	_____
2. Documents wound status. Objective measurements included at least weekly or more frequently if changes occur.	_____
3. Documents performance of debridement, changes as a result of debridement as well as patient response.	_____

Comments:

_____

_____

Clinician: _____

Preceptor: _____

Date: _____

who cannot tolerate other forms of debridement.[70] Autolytic debridement is frequently used in home care or long-term care settings. Patients with open wounds who are receiving palliative treatment may benefit from this form of debridement because of its ease and painlessness.[58]

Contraindications

Autolytic debridement is contraindicated in infected or deep cavity wounds.[6, 48, 73] Autolytic debridement is not appropriate when sharp or surgical debridement is mandated (e.g., gangrene or necrotic tendon) unless the latter interventions are not consistent with the patient's overall plan of care.[2]

Termination

Although technically no longer called autolytic debridement, the use of moisture-retentive dressings can continue after the wound bed is rid of necrotic tissue, foreign material, and debris.[74] Autolytic debridement should be discontinued in favor of alternative methods if the amount of necrotic tissue fails to decrease in the expected amount of time.

Procedure

Box 5–4 provides a sample protocol for autolytic debridement. The clinician may choose to use only autolytic debridement for an uninfected, necrotic wound. Alternatively, the clinician may choose to perform sharp debridement and/or mechanical debridement during dressing changes followed by autolytic debridement between sessions. If so, eschar should be crosshatched to increase the wound's surface area and allow greater penetration of the body's own enzymes (see Figure 5–3).[26, 28] In general terms, the moisture-retentive wound dressing should be at least 2 cm larger than the wound and should absorb enough wound fluid to allow the dressing to remain in place for approximately 72–96 hours. Because of the pooling of wound fluid under the dressing, the periwound must be protected with a skin sealant to prevent maceration or fungal infection.

Enzymatic Debridement

Enzymatic, or chemical,[75] **debridement** is the use of a topical exogenous enzyme to remove devitalized tissue.[1] Enzymatic debridement is a form of selective

---

> **BOX 5–4   Sample Autolytic Debridement Protocol**
>
> 1. Prepare the patient for debridement.
> 2. Explain the specific procedure to the patient.
> 3. Open necessary equipment and supplies. This may include:
>   forceps   skin sealant
>   scalpel   moisture-retentive dressing
>   additional gloves
> 4. Ensure adequate pain control.
> 5. Don clean gloves.
> 6. Identify devitalized tissue, foreign material, and debris to be debrided.
> 7. If present, crosshatch eschar with scalpel.*
> 8. If using sharp or mechanical debridement in combination with autolytic debridement, remove as much of these tissues as possible following the respective protocol. Rinse the wound with saline.
> 9. Apply a skin sealant to the periwound.
> 10. Assess changes in wound status and perform any necessary wound measurements.
> 11. Dispose of sharp instruments and infectious waste.
> 12. Remove and dispose of soiled gloves. Don clean gloves.
> 13. Apply moisture-retentive wound dressing and ensure adequate seal.
> 14. Remove and dispose of soiled gloves.
> 15. Initial and date wound dressing.
> 16. Wash hands.
> 17. Provide any necessary posttreatment instructions.
> 18. Complete documentation.
>
> *In accordance with state law and clinician practice act.

---

debridement that requires a physician's prescription.[57] In the past, several different enzymes were approved for use in patients with open wounds, including fibinolysin, papain-urea, streptokinase, and collagenases. However, currently only collagenase (trade name Santyl) is available and FDA approved for use as an enzymatic debriding agent.[22, 76] Collagenase is an endogenous matrix metalloprotease (MMP).[76] Exogenous collagenase is derived from a bacterial strain of *Clostridium histolyticum.* Collagenase is sometimes considered a selective debridement because this agent only digests type I, or denatured, collagen.[77] It is believed that collagen filaments may anchor necrotic

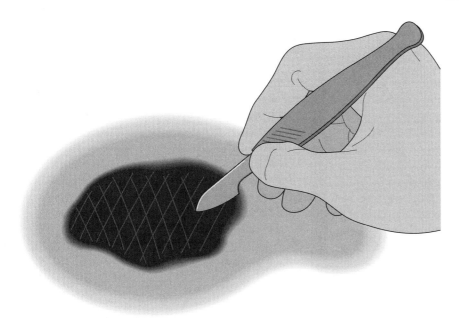

FIGURE 5–3 Crosshatching an eschar-covered wound. To crosshatch, a scalpel is used to score eschar or necrotic tissue in lines at an angle to one another in order to increase wound surface area.

tissue and debris to the wound bed.[77] In addition to promoting wound debridement, collagenase and its degraded products appear to promote cell migration, which may further enhance wound healing.[76]

There is sufficient evidence to recommend the use of collagenase for wound debridement.[2,22] Several studies demonstrate collagenase effectively debrides wounds and increases the amount of granular tissue.[78,79] A computer model comparing the effects of autolytic debridement with enzymatic debridement reported the likelihood of achieving a clean wound within 2 weeks of using autolytic debridement was only 50% compared to 70% using collagenase.[80] Collagenase also debrided wounds faster than a sham ointment.[22] In contrast, a study comparing chronic venous insufficiency ulcers treated with compression and either autolytic debridement or collagenase demonstrated no significant differences in outcomes.[81]

Enzymatic debridement requires less skill than sharp or surgical debridement but takes more time to achieve the same results. However, enzymatic debridement is less painful than other methods of debridement (except autolytic)[70] and is easy to instruct patients and caregivers in how to perform. Enzymatic preparations can be expensive. This cost factor may prohibit the use of enzymes for wounds with minimal necrotic tissue or wounds that may be expediently debrided by other methods, especially since there appears to be no clear improvement in wound healing time when comparing enzymatic and sharp debridement.[53]

Indications

Enzymatic debridement is indicated for infected and uninfected wounds with necrotic tissue.[2,6] This method may be appropriate for patients who cannot tolerate sharp debridement as an adjunct to sharp or mechanical debridement between treatment sessions and in home care or long-term care settings.[22,70] Patients who fail to respond to autolytic debridement may benefit from the "boost" provided by exogenously supplied enzymes. In most cases, enzymatic debridement may be used on infected wounds in combination with appropriate systemic or topical antimicrobial therapy.[22] For example, polymyxin B may be used in combination with collagenase to decrease infection and the amount of devitalized tissue present in a wound bed.[79] Enzymatic debridement, in combination with serial instrumental debridement, may be used intermittently in the care of chronic wounds.[77] Collagenase may be particularly effective in this role, as it has been shown to decrease wound bioburden, enhance epithelial cell migration, promote angiogenesis, and stimulate granulation tissue formation.[20,48]

Contraindications

Enzymatic debridement is contraindicated in wounds with exposed deep tissues,[6] including ligament, tendon, capsule, blood vessels, nerves, or bone. Because of the time required for enzymatic debridement, this method is not appropriate when sharp or surgical debridement is required.[2,22] Enzymes are not recommended for use on facial burns.[82] Enzymes cannot debride calluses.[43] Enzymatic debridement is not indicated in wounds that are free of necrotic tissue. Liquefaction of necrotic material within the wound bed without regular irrigation may provide an ideal environment for bacterial proliferation. Therefore, exogenous enzymes should not be applied to wounds being autolytically debrided.[2] Because collagenase is inactivated by heavy metal ions and acidic solutions, it should not be used in combination with dressings, topical agents, or solutions containing silver, iodine, acetic acid, or hydrogen peroxide.[6,20,22,76,77]

Termination

Although the manufacturer may state that collagenase can continue to be used once necrotic tissue has been removed, it is more cost effective to terminate enzyme use once satisfactory debridement has occurred. If the amount of devitalized tissue within the wound bed is not effectively reduced within 2 weeks of product use, enzymatic debridement should be discontinued in favor of alternative treatment methods.[2,48]

Procedure

It is important to follow the manufacturer's guidelines for product indications, contraindications, dosage, and method of application. Box 5–5 provides a sample protocol for enzymatic debridement. There are several key points that should be made. The clinician must verify the physician's prescription and apply the enzyme only to the areas to be debrided. Eschar should be crosshatched prior to application of the enzyme to enable greater penetration.[6,9,26,28,30,82] Collagenase works best in a moist environment, so the wound should be kept covered. If necessary, a saline-moistened gauze or hydrogel can be applied along with the enzyme.[22]

Many clinicians fear there may be an increased risk of infection with enzymatic debridement because of the softening of devitalized tissue.[28] It appears, however, that collagenase actually reduces wound bioburden, even in the absence of clinical infection.[23] As with all patients with open wounds, clinicians need to observe for the signs and symptoms of infection. A topical antimicrobial may be used in combination with collagenase in the case of infection.[22] It also may be prudent to use prophylactic topical antimicrobial therapy when using enzymatic debridement on patients who have small burns or who are immunosuppressed, such as those who are malnourished or HIV positive.[30,83]

BOX 5–5   Sample Enzymatic Debridement Protocol

1. Verify physician's order.
2. Prepare the patient for debridement.
3. Explain the specific procedure to the patient.
4. Open necessary equipment and supplies. This may include:

scalpel	gauze squares	skin sealant
enzyme	wound dressing	
tongue blade	additional gloves	

5. Ensure adequate pain control.
6. Don clean gloves.
7. Identify devitalized tissue, foreign material, and debris to be debrided.
8. If using sharp or mechanical debridement in combination with enzymatic debridement, remove as much of these tissues as possible following the respective protocol. Rinse the wound with saline.
9. If present, crosshatch eschar with scalpel.*
10. Assess changes in wound status and perform any necessary measurements.
11. Remove and dispose of soiled gloves. Don clean gloves.
12. Apply enzyme to remaining devitalized tissue, foreign material, and debris areas with a tongue blade. A topical antimicrobial may be used in conjunction with the enzyme.
13. Apply wound dressing.
14. Dispose of sharp instruments and infectious waste.
15. Remove and dispose of soiled gloves.
16. Initial and date wound dressing.
17. Wash hands.
18. Provide any necessary posttreatment instructions.
19. Complete documentation.

*In accordance with practice act.

Mechanical Debridement

Mechanical debridement involves the use of force to remove devitalized tissue, foreign material, and debris from a wound bed. Mechanical debridement is a type of nonselective debridement that includes wet-to-dry dressings, scrubbing, wound cleansing, wound irrigation, pulsatile lavage, and whirlpool.[6, 20, 25] The use of hydrogen peroxide on superficial wounds may also be considered a form of mechanical debridement because of the force created by the product's effervescence (see Chapter 6 for more details on the use of hydrogen peroxide, and Chapter 8 for information concerning wound irrigation, pulsatile lavage, and whirlpool).

Wet-to-Dry Dressings

Wet-to-dry dressings entail applying a single layer of fluffed saline-moistened gauze to a necrotic wound, covering with more gauze, and then allowing the dressing to dry for 8–24 hours.[74] As the dressing dehydrates, the gauze adheres to the wound bed, trapping wound exudate, foreign material, and debris within the interstices. When the dressing is dry, it is torn away at a right angle from the wound surface, thus lifting any material adhering to the gauze off of the wound bed. There is a danger of periwound maceration[6] and fungal infection if the saline-moistened gauze is placed on intact skin that is not first protected with a moisture barrier or skin sealant. Even when used appropriately, wet-to-dry dressings are nonselective and less effective than enzymatic and autolytic debridement.[80]

Wet-to-dry dressings are only indicated for wounds with 100% devitalized wound beds. There are two reasons why this type of debridement is contraindicated for wounds with granular tissue or exposed deeper tissues.[74] First, any viable tissue in the wound bed will also adhere to the gauze. Granulation tissue may even begin to grow into the gauze before the wound bed dehydrates. Thus, when the dry dressing is torn from the wound bed, it will remove adhered viable tissue along with the necrotic tissue, ultimately delaying rather than enhancing wound healing. New epithelial cells and granular tissue are particularly fragile and highly vulnerable to this type of trauma. The tearing-away of healthy tissue can be quite painful[6, 20] and cause bleeding as well. Second, because it encourages wound bed desiccation, the wet-to-dry procedure does not follow the basic wound management principle of moist wound healing previously described. As such, this procedure delays wound healing when used on granulating wounds. Tissues with high collagen contents, such as tendons, fascia, and joint capsule, are especially vulnerable to dehydration and can be irreparably harmed if a moist environment is not maintained.

Wet-to-dry dressings were the standard in wound care over 30 years ago. Unfortunately, this archaic and generally contraindicated intervention continues to be used. A recent study[74] found wet-to-dry dressings to be the most frequently ordered dressing, accounting for 42% of all dressing orders. To make matters worse, the majority of these wounds contained more than 75% granulation tissue. It is extremely important that clinicians know the current treatment standards and guidelines for treating patients with open wounds and use this information to educate patients, physicians, and other clinicians who may be unaware of practice changes and the negative impact improper care can have.

Scrubbing

Wound scrubbing is the use of a sponge, brush, or gauze along with a fluid to break the adherence of devitalized tissue and debris from the wound bed. As with wet-to-dry dressings, scrubbing is nonselective and can remove or traumatize any tissue within the wound bed, making it contraindicated for granulating wounds. If scrubbing is the debridement method of choice, it is suggested that the clinician use a high-porosity sponge (90 pores per square inch) and as little force as possible to minimize trauma.[39, 84] Water or saline is an appropriate solution for scrubbing. When scrubbing a wound, the clinician should begin at the wound center and gradually work out to the wound margin to avoid contaminating the cleansed areas.[85] Clinicians may choose to use scrubbing for superficial wounds that are highly contaminated with foreign material or bacteria, such as if a young runner were to fall on a cinder track, obtaining a "road rash" abrasion. The clinician must weigh the benefits of the rapid removal of this potentially infectious bacteria and debris against the likelihood of trauma caused by this technique. In this scenario of a young, healthy patient, the benefits likely outweigh the risks, and the clinician may choose to scrub the wound on the initial visit. Although it may be appropriate to begin using nonselective debridement, the clinician should change to a more selective form of debridement as soon as possible.

Wound Cleansing

Wound cleansing is an area of both confusion and intense controversy. For the purposes of this text, **wound cleansing** is defined as the delivery of a wound cleanser to the wound surface using mechanical force to remove lightly adhered necrotic tissue, debris, and bacteria.[85] A **wound cleanser** is a commercially available solution that commonly contains **surfactants,** substances that lower the surface tension of loose particulate matter on the wound bed. Some wound cleansers also contain an antiseptic and therefore have antimicrobial properties. Although meant to accelerate wound healing by debridement and removal of bacteria from the wound bed, the risks of wound cleansers clearly outweigh any potential benefits in almost all circumstances. First, wound cleansers are not regulated by the Food and Drug Administration, and manufacturers are not required to prove either safety or efficacy. All wound cleansers have been found to contain cytotoxic agents that delay wound healing by killing or incapacitating human cells.[85, 86] Second, because wound cleansing is nonselective, it has the same limitations as other forms of mechanical debridement. Third, surfactants can only remove loosely adherent material from the wound bed, and therefore are not efficient debriding agents for partial-thickness or full-thickness necrotic wounds. Wound cleansers were designed for use on acute, minor integumentary injuries or for cleaning intact skin, not for long-term use on chronic wounds.[2, 87] The National Pressure Ulcer Advisory Panel suggests clinicians only *consider* the use of wound cleansers (as defined above) to clean pressure ulcers with debris, confirmed infection, or high bacterial colonization.[2] While a timeline was not provided, clinicians would be wise to discontinue the use of wound cleansers as soon as possible: when the signs and symptoms of infection have improved or, at most, within 2 weeks.

Refer to Table 5–6 for a summary of the three types of mechanical debridement discussed in this chapter.

TABLE 5–6   Contrasting Types of Mechanical Debridement*

Method	Important Points
Wet-to-dry dressings	• Fluffed saline-moistened gauze is applied to a necrotic wound and allowed to dry for 8–24 hours before being torn away from the wound bed
	• Nonselective form of debridement
	• Should be used only on wounds containing 100% devitalized tissue
Scrubbing	• Use of a sponge, brush, or gauze with a fluid to remove devitalized tissue and debris from the wound bed
	• Nonselective form of debridement
	• Use of a high-porosity sponge, water, or saline, and as little force as necessary to minimize trauma
	• May be used on superficial wounds that are highly contaminated
	• May be used on wounds with 100% devitalized tissue
Wound cleansing	• Use of a wound cleanser and mechanical force to remove lightly adhered necrotic tissue, debris, and bacteria
	• Cytotoxic
	• Delays wound healing
	• Rarely appropriate

*Also includes wound irrigation, pulsatile lavage, and whirlpool (see Chapter 8).

Checkpoint Question #2

Your 85-year-old patient with Alzheimer's disease has an ulcer over her greater trochanter. The ulcer measures 3.6 × 3.2 cm and is 100% eschar covered. The patient is confused, restless, and easily agitated during your examination. Is sharp debridement appropriate? Why or why not?

Biologic Debridement

Biologic debridement, sometimes referred to as maggot therapy, was approved by the FDA in 2004 as a live medical device for the debridement of necrotic tissue in nonhealing necrotic wounds.[88,89] While it is still seldom used in the United States, an increasing number of physicians and facilities are trying this method of debridement. Approximately 300 centers in the United States currently utilize maggot therapy[90] for biologic debridement. A physician's prescription is required and a single vial, containing 250–300 larvae, costs approximately $98.00 U.S.[91] It is estimated that approximately 10 larvae will be needed to debride 1 cm^2 of wound surface area.[92] First, the wound perimeter is protected with a dressing such as a hydrocolloid. Then the sterile maggots are placed within the wound and retained within the wound bed with a netting and covered with an absorbant dressing.[93] Alternatively, the maggots are placed within the wound and not contained with a dressing.[94] At least one report suggests that this "free-range" approach yields superior results.[95] One to two applications of maggots are performed over 3–7 days.[88] The dressing is then removed and the maggots rinsed away, discarded in a biohazard container.[88]

Maggots assist with wound debridement in two ways. First, the larvae produce and release enzymes that degrade and liquefy necrotic tissue and biofilms without harming viable tissue.[48,88,89,93,96] Second, the larvae ingest necrotic tissue and bacteria, thus physically removing these deterrents to wound healing from the wound bed.[89] Enzymes within the larvae's gastrointestinal system kill ingested bacteria,[89,93] including methicillin-resistant *Staphyloccocus aureus*, group A and B *streptococcus*, and *Pseudomons*.[97] Increased local wound partial pressures of oxygen have been noted in wounds treated with maggots.[89] Additionally, biologic debridement may decrease wound odor, control wound exudate, increase the amount of granulation tissue, and stimulate epithelialization.[88,98,99] Biologic debridement may be faster than autolytic and enzymatic ddebridment.[70] Maggots are unaffected by oral and intravenous antibiotics.[88]

Problems associated with using maggot therapy for biologic debridement include the potential for psychological stress from having live creatures crawling on an individual and reports of increased pain in nondiabetic patients.[100] According to surveys of patients with open wounds, 23–25% of patients would never consider biologic debridement.[94,101] Of those that stated they would try maggot therapy, they would only do so if it was known that wound healing would be significantly faster than more traditional methods.[94] Biologic debridement is the least preferred method of debridement of an infected ulcer.[102] While there is a growing body of literature to support the use of biologic debridement in pressure ulcers,[2,103] neuropathic ulcers,[99,104] traumatic wounds,[105] and a variety of chronic leg ulcers,[106] claims cannot currently be made that biologic debridement will consistently hasten wound healing or control infections.

Surgical Debridement

Surgical debridement is the use of scalpels, scissors, or lasers[9,20] in a sterile environment by a physician or podiatrist to remove necrotic tissue, foreign material, and debris from the wound bed. By taking a patient into the carefully controlled operating room environment, the risk of infection is less than if the same procedure were to be performed in a clinic or at the bedside. The advanced knowledge, skill, and training of physicians and podiatrists allow more extensive exploration of the wound bed and debridement of deeper structures, such as infected bone or nonviable tendons, in addition to more superficial tissue layers. Early surgical debridement can prevent amputation and even loss of life due to sepsis.[96] For example, early surgical debridement of burn eschar is associated with increased survival rates.[82] The disadvantages of surgical debridement include the physical and emotional stress of surgery and the high cost.[70] In addition, surgical debridement is somewhat imprecise,[9,30] in that it frequently sacrifices healthy tissue along with nonviable tissue.[64] Because surgical debridement is outside of the scope of physical therapy, only a cursory review of this method of debridement has been provided. However, information regarding surgical debridement should be included in physical therapy curricula so these clinicians can have a better understanding of the basic indications and interventions that may be required for holistic and appropriate patient management.[67]

Indications

Along with sharp debridement, surgical debridement is the fastest and most aggressive method of debridement.[70] It is indicated in the presence of ascending cellulitis, osteomyelitis, extensive necrotic wounds, wounds with extensive undermining, or wounds in which the degree of undermining cannot be determined.[2, 13, 44, 107, 108] Surgical debridement is also required when necrotic tissue is near vital organs and structures or when the patient is septic.[8]

Contraindications

Despite its many benefits, surgical debridement is not indicated for every patient with necrotic wounds. Patients who are unlikely to survive such a stressful procedure or patients with palliative care plans are generally not surgical candidates.[2, 58] Surgical debridement is contraindicated when another form of debridement will suffice.[70]

Procedure

Surgical debridement techniques vary widely depending on the type of wound and the type of nonviable tissue to be removed. Many times the physician or podiatrist will excise the nonviable tissues along with a wide margin of healthy tissues to ensure the removal of as many microorganisms as possible. In addition, this wide excision removes senescent cells, such as keratinocytes, which may be responsible for a nonadvancing wound edge on a hypogranular wound.[29] Surgical debridement of some wounds, such as burns, generally involves tangential excision of burn eschar by sequentially shaving with a dermatome, a cutting instrument used to remove a thin layer of skin, until healthy, vascular tissue is reached.[82] If a deep space infection is suspected, an **incision and drainage** may be performed. This procedure involves surgical exploration, drainage, and debridement.[109] Tissues such as tendon, fascia, and dura act as free grafts for living cells to grow across regardless of their viability. Therefore, if these structures are clean, the physician or podiatrist may choose to leave them in place within the wound bed rather than surgically remove them.[10] The wound is generally thoroughly irrigated during surgery to assist with the removal of any remaining microbes. The physician or podiatrist may choose to close the wound at the time of surgery (primary closure) if confident that all of the devitalized tissue and microbes have been removed and the wound edges can be approximated. Alternatively, the physician or podiatrist may choose to place a graft, a flap, or allow the wound to heal by secondary or delayed primary closure. During the surgical procedure, the physician or podiatrist will usually perform a tissue biopsy to better establish the presence and type of infection. This is followed by appropriate antimicrobial therapy. Ideally, surgical debridement is performed only once. However, patients with extensive wounds, such as full-thickness burns to the entire trunk and upper extremities, may require multiple surgical procedures.

Refer to Table 5–7 for a summary of the advantages and disadvantages of different methods of debridement. Figure 5–4 provides an alogrithm to assist with clinical decision making for wound debridement.

TABLE 5–7 Advantages and Disadvantages of Different Methods of Debridement

Sharp	**Advantages**
	Expedient, can be used on wounds with any amount of necrotic tissue
	Disadvantages
	Requires skilled personnel, may be painful
Autolytic	**Advantages**
	Allows for debridement outside of skilled care, easy to instruct patient/caregiver, can be used on wounds with any amount of necrotic tissue, virtually pain free, may be lower in cost than other methods
	Disadvantages
	Requires more time than other methods, should not be used on infected wounds

TABLE 5–7   Continued

Enzymatic	**Advantages**
	Faster than autolytic debridement, allows for debridement outside of skilled care, easy to instruct patient/caregiver, virtually pain free, can be used on both infected and uninfected wounds
	Disadvantages
	Requires more time than sharp or surgical debridement, may be costly
Mechanical	**Advantages**
	Removes loosely adhered devitalized tissue, foreign material, and debris
	Disadvantages
	Nonselective, traumatizes wound bed, may be cytotoxic
Surgical	**Advantages**
	Sterile environment, fast, can fully explore wound and address all tissue layers
	Disadvantages
	Physical and emotional stress, high cost, sacrifices some healthy tissue, requires skilled personnel

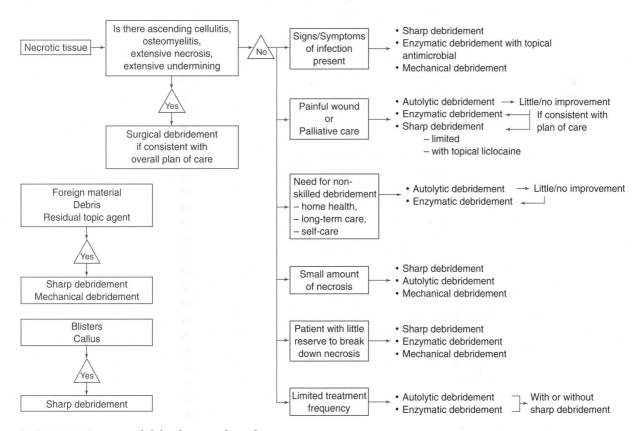

FIGURE 5–4   Wound debridement algorithm.

DEBRIDEMENT AS A COLLABORATIVE EFFORT

Debridement, like other aspects of patient care, should be a collaborative effort. Collaboration enhances treatment effectiveness and efficiency and contributes to increased patient/caregiver satisfaction. Two examples will help illustrate the importance of this point. Consider Mr. D, a 32-year-old patient with a T10 spinal cord injury and a nonhealing ulcer over his right ischium. Mr. D is admitted to the hospital because he has a fever that is believed to be due to a wound infection. You receive a referral for physical therapy for wound care. During your initial examination, you find a 100% necrotic ulcer that is 4.0 × 5.0 cm with a depth of 1.5 cm. After your sharp debridement the wound's size is unchanged, but the wound bed now contains 50% granulation tissue and 50% adherent yellow slough. After obtaining the physician's order, you culture the wound, apply an enzyme to the remaining necrotic tissue, and then apply a wound dressing. Because you believe it will take at least 2 days for the enzyme and antibiotics to take effect, you discuss Mr. D's care with his nurse. You provide written instructions as to how and when to change Mr. D's dressings, inform the nurse of any precautions or warning signs to be aware of, and set up your next visit in 3 days. You instruct both the patient and the nurse in proper positioning and the use of pressure-relieving devices to avoid pressure and shear to the affected area. You request a dietary consult because of the presence of a nonhealing (pressure) ulcer (refer to Chapter 12 for more information regarding pressure ulcers). By collaborating with different disciplines, addressing causative factors, and combining different methods of debridement, the plan of care becomes more efficient and effective. Appropriate delegation of non–physical therapy tasks (dressing changes) to qualified nursing personnel lowers overall patient cost and allows you to see other patients in need of physical therapy services.

Similarly, consider Mrs. W, a 51-year-old referred to physical therapy by her primary care physician. She has ulcers on the tips of her left second and third toes. During your interview, you find that Mrs. W is a two-pack-a-day smoker and has a history of coronary artery disease. Your examination findings include no palpable pedal pulses bilaterally, capillary refill of 5 seconds, an ankle-brachial index of 0.4 on the left and 0.7 on the right, and wounds that are 90% necrotic. You determine that Mrs. W has significant left lower extremity ischemia and that debridement by a physical therapist is contraindicated. You discuss your findings with Mrs. W's primary care physician and arrange for a vascular consult. The vascular surgeon performs a lower extremity bypass and assists Mrs. W in finding a smoking cessation program before referring her back to you for wound care. When you see the patient 2 days after surgery, the wounds are still 90% necrotic, but her circulatory status is vastly improved. You determine that the patient would benefit from mechanical debridement (irrigation with saline) to soften the necrotic tissue prior to sharp (serial instrumental) debridement. In this situation, Mrs. W was best served by an interdisciplinary approach as well as a combination of debridement methods.

CHAPTER SUMMARY

Debridement is the removal of necrotic tissue, foreign material, and debris from the wound bed. Debridement enhances wound healing by reducing the wound bioburden, improving the ability to fight infection, shortening the inflammatory phase of wound healing, decreasing the energy required for wound healing, and removing physical barriers to wound healing. Clinicians may choose from one or a combination of debridement methods, including sharp, autolytic, enzymatic, and mechanical debridement. In some instances, the clinician may request a consult for surgical debridement. When determining the most effective means of debridement, the clinician must consider the characteristics of the wound, the status of the patient, current state laws, existing practice acts, and his or her own skills.

REVIEW QUESTIONS

1. Your 85-year-old patient with Alzheimer's disease has an ulcer over her greater trochanter. The ulcer measures 3.6 × 3.2 cm and is 100% eschar covered. The patient is confused, restless, and easily agitated during your examination. Explain why you would or would not choose to use autolytic, enzymatic, and mechanical debridement for this patient.

   Use the following scenario to answer questions 2–6.

   Two weeks ago your 48-year-old patient cut her forearm on a piece of gardening equipment.

The wound increased in size and became infected. She was given a prescription for antibiotics and referred to physical therapy for wound management including enzymatic debridement with collagenase and polymyxin B that same day. The wound measures 4.5 × 2.3 cm, and the deepest point is 0.3 cm. The wound bed is 90% yellow slough and 10% granular tissue. There is a moderate amount of thick, yellow drainage. There is bright red erythema extending 0.4 cm from the wound, and the forearm is swollen and feels warm to the touch. The patient reports she has a fever and had a tetanus booster just last year. The patient's past medical history is unremarkable.

2. Do you agree with the specifics of this referral? Why or why not?

3. Are there any other methods of debridement you would use in combination with enzymatic debridement? If so, what methods would you use and why?

4. Write a debridement goal for this wound to be accomplished in 1 week.

5. After two visits (over 5 days), the patient reports she no longer has a fever. The wound size is unchanged. The wound bed is 30% slough, 50% granular tissue, and 20% exposed extensor tendons. There is minimal serosanguinous drainage, the wound has no odor, and the periwound erythema and edema have resolved. Should your interventions change? Support your rationale.

6. Describe the benefits or limitations to changing to sharp, autolytic, or mechanical debridement. Which of these three interventions would you suggest to the referring physician?

myhealthprofessionskit

Use this address to access the Companion Website created for this textbook. Simply select "Physical Therapy" from the choice of disciplines. Find this book and log in using your username and password to access images, video clips, and additional learning tools.

REFERENCES

Go to myhealthprofessionskit.com to view this chapter's references.

6

Management of Infection

Chapter Objectives

After reading this chapter, learners will be able to:

1. Identify factors that increase the risk of wound infection.
2. Compare and contrast the clinical signs of inflammation and infection.
3. Describe three methods used to diagnose wound infections.
4. Define biofilms and describe how they affect wound healing.
5. Describe the procedures for performing aerobic and anaerobic swab cultures.
6. Define microbial sensitivity and resistance, and describe their relevance in the management of wound infection.
7. Describe the advantages, disadvantages, and application of topical and systemic antimicrobial therapies.
8. Describe the adverse reactions associated with the use of antiseptic solutions on open wounds.
9. Identify acceptable uses for antiseptic solutions.
10. Describe four methods to prevent infections in open wounds.
11. Explain the indications and procedures for clean and sterile technique.
12. Perform wound management procedures to minimize the risk of wound contamination and infection.

Key Terms

Abscess
Aerobes
Anaerobes
Antibacterial
Antibiotics
Antifungal
Antimicrobial
Antiseptic
Bactericidal
Bacteriostatic
Biofilms

Clean technique
Colonization
Complement system
Contamination
Critical colonization
Disinfect
Fluid aspiration
Gram-negative
Gram-positive
Infection
MRSA

Nosocomial infection
Resistance
Resistant
Sensitive
Standard precautions
Sterile technique
Sterilization
Swab cultures
Tissue biopsy
Universal precautions
VRE

6

INTRODUCTION

Infection control is an important part of all therapeutic interactions, especially wound management procedures. Clinicians must understand and practice safe techniques to reduce the risk of infecting a patient with an open wound, eliminate wound infection when present, and prevent cross-contamination. By controlling wound infection, wound healing is enhanced and scarring is minimized.[1–4] This chapter begins by defining infection and detailing the typical signs and symptoms of wound infection. Next, methods of diagnosing wound infection are reviewed followed by detailed information regarding the use of antimicrobials and debridement to manage infection. The chapter concludes with a thorough presentation of methods to prevent infections, including hand washing, standard precautions, sterile and clean techniques, and proper wound care techniques.

DEFINING INFECTION

To properly manage wound infections, there must first be a consensus as to what constitutes an infected wound. The body has two main lines of defense against infection. The first line of defense consists of surface barriers. Body surfaces, such as the skin and digestive tract, normally contain a small number of resident bacteria and fungi called microflora.[5] This presence of nonreplicating microbes is called **contamination.**[3,6] Normal skin microflora include *Staphylococcus, Micrococcus, Peptococcus, Streptococcus, Acinetobacter,* and yeast.[3,7] Intact skin may be contaminated with a bacterial count of up to 10^3 microbes per gram of tissue without any adverse tissue reaction within an individual.[8,9] In fact, resident microflora protect the body from pathogenic, or disease-causing, organisms.[3,10,11] In addition to the normal microflora, the skin and body's immune system help protect against infection. The skin's normal pH of 5.5 creates a slightly acidic environment, discouraging microbial growth, and the layers of epithelial cells and lipids present in the skin form a protective barrier against microbial invasion (see Chapter 1).[6]

The second line of defense consists of cellular and chemical defenses, discussed in Chapter 2. Immune cells—such as polymorphonuclear neutrophils, Langerhans' cells, macrophages, and NK cells—also help defend the body against infection by destroying pathogenic microorganisms.[12] The inflammatory response helps direct many of these cells and chemical mediators to dispose of pathogens. Fever, caused by the systemic response to pyrogens, also helps inhibit microbe multiplication.[12] Last, antimicrobial proteins help boost these defenses by destroying microbes directly or inhibiting their ability to reproduce.[12] Interferons are proteins made by virally infected host cells and some lymphocytes. These proteins are then secreted and used by nearby cells to manufacture protective proteins, which then help block viral reproduction and mobilize the immune system. The **complement system** is a group of over 30 normally inactive circulating plasma proteins.[5] The complement system is activated by recognizing antibodies on the surface of a pathogen or one of the proteins; for example, C3 can be triggered spontaneously. Once activated, a cascade of events occurs in which proteins are produced that "complement," or enhance, the body's immune response. This results in direct pathogen destruction via opsonization and a boost in the body's inflammatory response.

Wound **colonization** occurs if the microflora adhere to the body's surface and replicate, forming colonies, but do not adversely affect the individual or cause a host response.[3,6] **Critical colonization** is the theoretical turning point at which the increasing number of bacteria becomes a bioburden and adversely affects the individual.[6,13,14] Wound **infection** occurs when microorganisms multiply and invade viable body tissues.[14–16] While contamination and colonization are normal occurrences, critical colonization and infection are not.[6,13] Previously, it was believed that microbial concentrations needed to exceed 10^5 microorganisms per gram of tissue for infection.[7,16–18] When such a high concentration of pathogens is present, the body will mount an inflammatory response, but this is generally insufficient.[9,19] Therefore, the body requires outside assistance to successfully combat the offending organisms.

However, recent research reveals that there is no magical critical cutoff point for infection. Rather, infection is best represented as part of a continuum (see Figure 6–1).[3,6] While wound infection generally does correlate with 10^5 microbes per gram of tissue,[2,6,20] bacterial quantity is only one of three key pieces required. In addition, certain types of bacteria are more detrimental than others and their mere presence in any quantity is deemed worthy of intervention for infection.[6] For example, beta-hemolytic *Streptococcus*[7,16,21] is a particularly virulent strain of bacteria that produces exotoxins (see below) and spreading factors that allow this strain of bacteria to

		Description	Interpretation	Effect
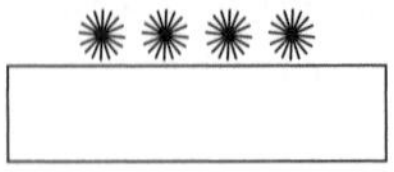	**Contamination**	Presence of microbes on wound surface	Normal	None
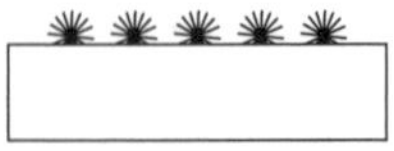	**Colonization**	Presence of replicating microbes on wound surface	Normal	None
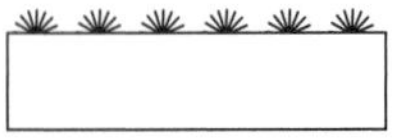	**Critical Colonization**	Increasing wound bioburden reaches critical point and begins to adversely affect host	Abnormal	Plateau in wound healing or decline in wound status
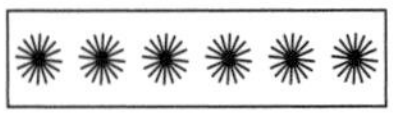	**Infection**	Replicating microbes invade viable body tissues	Abnormal	Decline in wound status, signs and symptoms of infection likely

FIGURE 6–1   Continuum of wound infection.

cause infection at very low concentrations. Third, the host's resistance to the invading organism must also be considered (see Figure 6–2).[1,11] Examples of people with decreased resistance to infection include individuals who are immunocompromised or have diabetes.[3]

High concentrations of microbes adversely affect the host in four ways.[3,10,14] First, the microbes compete with host cells for available oxygen and nutrients.[22] Second, bacterial exotoxins, proteins released from gram-positive and gram-negative bacteria during growth,[14] may be cytotoxic, inactivating or modifying host cell processes and ultimately resulting in host cell dysfunction or death.[21,23] For example, some bacteria produce enzymes that destroy host cell membranes and structural proteins, causing extensive damage. Third, bacterial endotoxins, molecules within the walls of certain types of bacteria (gram-negative bacteria),[14] may activate host inflammatory processes, increasing production of matrix metalloproteases

(MMPs) and inducing changes such as fever, bleeding, and clotting.[14,22,23] Fourth, wound infections delay, and may even prevent, wound healing.[1,2,11]

Factors That Increase the Risk of Infection

Infection-causing microbes may be endogenous (part of the normal microflora) or exogenous (from the environment). An infection that is acquired while an individual is hospitalized is called a **nosocomial infection.**[24] Any break in the skin's integrity provides a pathway for microbes to enter the body. Besides an overt open wound, skin integrity may also be compromised by dry and cracked skin, callus, or maceration. Additionally, the skin may be stripped of its natural lipids or stratum corneum by harsh soaps or strong adhesives.[5,25]

Factors predisposing individuals with open wounds to infection can be divided into two categories: host

$$\text{Wound healing} = \frac{(\text{number of bacteria} \times \text{bacterial virulence}) + \text{interaction between microbes}}{\text{host resistance} + \text{modifying factors}}$$

Modifying factors include host's overall health; presence of underlying pathologies, such as diabetes or peripheral vascular disease; steroid use; presence of nonviable tissue; and proper wound management.

FIGURE 6–2   Equation for wound healing.

characteristics and local factors. Individuals with an increased risk of infection include persons with diabetes, malnutrition, or obesity; steroid users; immunocompromised individuals; and older adults.[1–3,6,20,26–28] Healing and resistance to infection go hand in hand: rapid wound repair lowers the risk of infection.[3] Granulating wounds are more resistant to infection than nongranulating wounds, and tissues with adequate perfusion are more resistant than ischemic tissues.[3,27] Therefore, local factors increasing the risk of wound infection include ischemia, presence of necrotic tissue or foreign debris within the wound bed (including dressing residue such as gauze), and chronic wounds.[14,20–22,29] Exposed wounds are more likely to be infected than wounds covered with occlusive or gauze dressings (see Chapter 7 for details regarding wound dressings).

Signs and Symptoms of Infection

Histologically, infection is characterized by the presence of bacteria within healthy, viable tissue and the presence of host polymorphonuclear neutrophils.[20] Clinically, the signs and symptoms of infection are a result of the struggle between the body's immune system and the invading organisms. This response is similar to the cardinal signs of inflammation reviewed in Section I: rubor, calor, tumor, dolor, and functio laesa (see Table 6–1).[3] Unfortunately, it is not possible to objectively quantify these clinical signs to definitively diagnose a wound infection. However, if the wound is infected, these signs are typically excessive or disproportionate to the size and extent of integumentary damage due to the increasing wound bioburden.[7,8,16,30] Because of the similarities in presentation, normal inflammation is sometimes mistaken for wound infection. A decline in wound status despite appropriate care is an additional clue that infection may be present.[2,3,14,21] Because bacteria do not invade host tissues in critically colonized wounds, these wounds will not demonstrate the typical signs and symptoms of infection and a decline in wound status may be the only indicator of heavy bioburden.[14] This section compares and contrasts the signs and symptoms of inflammation and infection.[18,31] Color images 3 and 10 provide examples of inflamed wounds. Color image 11 provides a drastic example of an infected wound.

Rubor

An inflamed wound has a well-defined erythemal border, and the amount of erythema is proportional to the size and extent of the wound. In contrast, an infected wound has a poorly defined erythemal border, and the amount of erythema is disproportionate to the size and extent of the wound.[2,20,32] An infected wound may also have proximally directed erythemal streaking.

Calor

An inflamed wound will have a localized increase in temperature.[2,20] In patients with infected wounds, this response will be magnified and warmth will extend farther away from the site of injury.[32] They may also present with a systemic increase in temperature (i.e., a fever).[20,32]

Tumor

Inflamed wounds have a small amount of edema that is proportional to the size and extent of the wound. In infected wounds, the amount of swelling is disproportionate to the size and extent of the wound.[32] In addition, tissue around the wound may be indurated.[2] The clinician should be aware that edema may also be a sign of other pathologies, including venous insufficiency, lymphatic dysfunction, and congestive heart failure. To attempt to differentiate swelling due to infection from other pathologies, clinicians should perform a complete history, including screening for preexisting conditions, and identify if any patterns of edema are present. Infection-related edema is confined to the wounded area, has a rapid onset, and occurs in conjunction with other signs of infection. In contrast, edema related to congestive heart failure is bilateral and appears first, and is more severe in the lower extremities. The edema of venous insufficiency or mild lymphatic dysfunction is less severe upon first rising in the morning and generally increases with dependency.[33] Edema due to lymphatic dysfunction is generally of slower onset and may be bilateral, or may present after surgical trauma (e.g., surgical removal of lymph nodes during a mastectomy or radiation to the axilla).[33]

Dolor

Inflamed wounds may be painful. However, an increase in pain level is consistent with wound infection.[2,21,32,34,35] In patients who are immunocompromised, the only sign of wound infection may be pain[16] (or an increase in previous pain level).

Functio Laesa

An inflamed wound may cause a temporary decrease in function of the affected area. In contrast, patients with infected wounds generally do not feel well systemically.

TABLE 6–1   Comparing and Contrasting Wound Inflammation versus Infection

Characteristic	Inflammation	Infection
Rubor	• Well-defined erythemal border • Proportionate to the size and extent of the wound	• Poorly defined erythemal border • Disproportionate to the size and extent of the wound • May have red streaks leading from the wound
Calor	• Local increase in temperature	• Greater amount of localized tissue temperature increase spreading over a wider surface area • Patient may be febrile
Tumor	• May be slightly swollen • Proportionate to the size and extent of the wound	• Swelling is disproportionate to the size and extent of the wound • May be indurated
Dolor	• May have pain that is proportional to extent of tissue involvement	• New onset or increase in pain
Functio laesa	• May have a temporary decrease in function of the affected area	• Malaise • Patient may feel sick
Drainage	• Amount is proportionate to the size and extent of the wound • Thin consistency • Serous or serosanguinous	• Amount is disproportionate to the size and extent of the wound; may be copious • Thick, purulent, or creamy consistency • May be white, yellow, green, or blue in color • May have a distinctive odor
Decline in wound status	• Follows normal phases of wound healing if treated appropriately	• Plateau in wound healing • Changes in granulation tissue: decrease in amount; friable, cobblestone-like appearance; or color change

They may have lower than normal energy levels or a feeling of malaise.[5] In addition to tachycardia, there may be hypotension, altered mental status, or altered function of the affected area.[20]

Drainage

Drainage from inflamed wounds generally differs from infected wounds in amount, consistency, color, and odor.[36]

Amount

Inflamed wounds have drainage that is proportional to the size and extent of the wound. Infected wounds, however, have drainage that is disproportionate to the size and extent of the wound and, at times, may be copious.[14,21,35] Quantification of the amount of wound drainage is hindered by the type of wound dressing used and the time since the bandage was last changed. Newly infected wounds may require more frequent dressing changes or more absorptive dressings to handle the increased wound drainage.

Consistency

Drainage from inflamed wounds is usually thin or the consistency of blood, whereas infected wounds have thick, viscous, purulent, or creamy drainage.[34,37] Purulent drainage is commonly seen in *Staphylococcus aureus* infections.[21]

Color

Drainage from inflamed wounds is generally serous (clear or slightly yellow in tint) or sanguineous (red, as from fresh blood, or brown, if allowed to dry out). Infected wounds may have drainage that is white, yellow, green, or blue.[13]

Odor

Dead tissue and old bandages will have a foul odor, regardless of whether the wound is inflamed or infected; therefore, clinicians should *not* use odor as a predictor of infection.[21,38] After being rinsed with saline, inflamed wounds should not have an odor unless there is necrotic tissue present. In contrast, infected wounds frequently are malodorous even when free of necrotic tissue.[2,13,30] Certain infections have a characteristic aroma. *Proteus* infections have an ammonia-like smell, whereas *Pseudomonas* infections smell "sickly sweet" and are usually accompanied by a bright blue or green drainage.

Decline in Wound Status

Inflamed wounds *should pass* through the normal phases of wound healing in a predictable fashion if treated appropriately. In contrast, an infected or critically colonized wound will exhibit a plateau or even a decline in wound status.[2,6,14,21,35,39,40] For example, a newly infected wound that was previously healing may increase in size. New onset of undermining or tunneling may be noted in infected wounds because of bacterial toxins digesting healthy host tissue.[21,30] Chronic wounds may exhibit more subtle signs of infection. For example, granulation tissue may become friable, easily traumatized, or take on a cobblestone-like appearance.[6,14,16,21,40,41] The amount of granulation tissue may decrease or the color may change from beefy red to pale or bright red.[14,21,35] Color image 19 provides an example of an infected wound with poor-quality granulation tissue. An infected wound may also have no evidence of epithelialization at the wound margins.[7]

Silent Infections

The clinician should be aware that an infection may be clinically "silent," that is, unapparent.[18,34] Individuals who are immunocompromised or who have inadequate perfusion to the involved area are not only at greater risk for infection but also less likely to exhibit the classic signs of infection because of their tempered immune responses. Two examples will help illustrate the concept of silent infections. First, an **abscess** is a localized collection of pus composed of devitalized tissue, microbes, and white blood cells within body tissues. The body is able to contain the microbes and prevent them from spreading but is unable to destroy the microbes. Unless the abscess forms a sinus tract and drains to a body surface, the infection might go unnoticed because it is walled off from the rest of the body. A second example is a patient with severe arterial insufficiency and a gangrenous toe. This patient may be unable to mount a sufficient response to an infection because of the inadequate blood flow to the region. Hence, the classic signs of infection might not be evident in this patient. However, because infection delays or prevents wound healing, wounds that fail to heal despite appropriate interventions or show a decline in wound status should be assessed for infection. When a silent infection is suspected, the clinician may need to assess for some of the systemic effects infections can have on the body, such as elevated white blood cell counts, fever, increased heart rate, increased respirations, fatigue, and confusion.[31] Additionally, patients with intact sensation may report an increase in pain when infection arises.

Biofilms

Information to this point has been presented with the basic understanding that microbes are free living organisms. New research suggests that interactions between different strains of microorganisms can adversely affect wound healing. **Biofilms** are communities of microorganisms that attach to the wound surface, encasing themselves in an extracellular polysaccharide matrix or glycocalyx.[3,29,42,43] The glycocalyx allows microbes to survive in wound environments that would otherwise be unfavorable and may protect the microbes from the effects of antiseptics and topical antimicrobials.[3,9,42] Leukocytes may also become trapped within the biofilm, making them ineffective.[44] Intercellular communication between organisms within a biofilm activates certain genes that increase bacterial virulence and **resistance,**[21,44–46] making them respond less predictably[44] to pharmacological interventions. Biofilms are thought to be 50–100 times more resistant to a drug than free-living bacteria.[44] If individual bacterial organisms break away from the biofilm, they may maintain this resistance to antimicrobials,[42,44,45] leading to delayed wound healing and infection. Biofilms are also able to modulate cell growth.[46] By slowing the rate of microbe replication, antimicrobials become less effective in eradicating these communities.[7,45]

Because biofilms are multimicrobial,[29] the different types of bacteria may actually work synergistically. Rather than competing for resources, bacteria that consume different nutrients are more likely to survive and the presence of oxygen-consuming aerobic organisms may promote the growth of anaerobic organisms.[13,21] Biofilms are generally found on devitalized tissue[7] and implanted devices,[7] such as catheters, as well as within the gastric mucosa, such as *Helicobacter pylori* (*H. pylori*) infections.[44] Up to 60% of chronic wounds may have biofilms.[29] In contrast, biofilms have been found in only about 6% of acute wounds.[29] While biofilms may not constitute an infection based solely on quantity of microbes, they clearly adversely affect wound healing[7] and contribute to the development of microbial resistance.

In summary, an infection should be suspected if the cardinal signs of inflammation are disproportionate to the size and extent of the wound; if drainage is purulent, copious, malodorous, or has an uncharacteristic color; if there is a sudden increase in pain; or if the wound fails to heal in a timely manner. Because infection can be limb- and life-threatening if not recognized in a timely fashion, patients with open wounds who present with these signs and symptoms should be assessed for wound infection.[2]

Checkpoint Question #1

Your patient's wound presents with copious amounts of thick, blue-green drainage. Is this wound likely to be inflamed or infected? Defend your answer.

DIAGNOSING WOUND INFECTION

Because the signs and symptoms of infection are similar to the cardinal signs of inflammation, and there is always the possibility of silent infection, observation alone is insufficient to accurately diagnose a suspected infection. Wound cultures are needed to confirm the presence or absence of infection. Wound cultures are various ways of sampling fluid and/or tissue from the affected area. From this wound sampling, laboratory tests are used to identify the type and quantity of any microbes present.

Wound Cultures

If an infection is suspected, the wound should be cultured to identify the offending organism(s) so that appropriate intervention strategies can be implemented. A culture involves placing a microorganism in an environment conducive for cell growth, commonly on an agar plate or in a broth. Several methods of wound culturing exist; however, the gold standard is a **tissue biopsy**.[2,16,18,34] Tissue biopsies are performed by a physician or podiatrist and involve removing a sample of living tissue from the wound for examination.[22] A bone biopsy is the gold standard to diagnose and appropriately treat osteomyelitis.[16] **Swab cultures** are a reliable method that can be used by clinicians to quantify the number and type of bacteria present on a wound.[16] The benefits of a swab culture over a tissue biopsy include simplicity, lack of trauma to the wound bed, and avoidance of a surgical procedure.[18] In addition, swab cultures may be performed by physical therapists, physical therapist assistants, occupational therapists, and nurses without a physician's order. Because swab cultures sample the wound surface (along with fluid expressed from the wound surface or areas of tunneling or undermining), the key disadvantage of this technique is that test results may only reflect surface contamination or colonization rather than the infecting microorganism. There are two types of swab cultures: one for aerobic microorganisms and one for anaerobic microorganisms (see Figure 6–3). Aerobic wound cultures are the standard culture procedure because oxygen-metabolizing

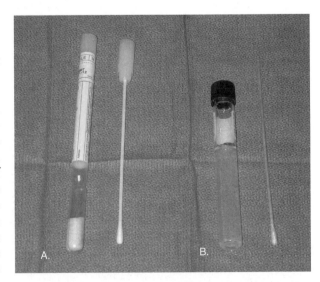

FIGURE 6–3   Aerobic and anaerobic swab cultures. *A.* Aerobic culture. *B.* Anaerobic culture.

microbes are more likely to be present in most wounds. However, deep, tunneling wounds, wounds with undermining or sinus tracts, or wounds that are occluded by thick layers of topical agents provide an oxygen-depleted environment that may allow proliferation of anaerobic microbes. Wounds with these characteristics should be cultured for both aerobic and anaerobic microorganisms.

To perform a swab culture, first debride and rinse the wound as able.[21] For an aerobic culture, rotate the end of an alginate-tipped applicator over a 1-cm^2 viable wound surface area for 5 seconds while applying enough pressure to express tissue fluid (see Figure 6–4A).[2, 47] Because necrotic tissue harbors surface bacteria and, by definition, an infection can only occur in viable tissue, only viable tissue should be swabbed, not exudate, eschar, pus, or slough.[2, 16, 48] There is some debate as to whether cotton- or rayon-tipped applicators may inhibit the growth of some types of bacteria. Therefore, current recommendations are that alginate-tipped applicators be used.[21] If the wound surface is dry, the swab should be moistened with saline prior to swabbing.[22] For wounds with a larger viable surface area, swab the wound in a 10-point pattern while slowly rotating the tip and applying pressure to express tissue fluid (see Figure 6–4B).[22] Both the 10-point and 1-cm^2 methods have been found to correlate with tissue biopsy results.[21, 47, 49] For an anaerobic culture, the applicator should be used to thoroughly probe tunnels and any areas of undermining. The swab culture or tissue biopsy is then taken to a laboratory within 2 hours of sampling for further processing to identify the organism(s).[16] Boxes 6–1 and 6–2 provide step-by-step procedures for performing aerobic and anaerobic swab cultures.

Fluid aspiration is an alternative method to diagnose a wound infection[16] and represents a sort of middle ground between a tissue biopsy and wound culture. To perform this procedure, the physician uses a needle to draw up 1.0 mL of fluid within the wound area for analysis in the laboratory. The advantage of fluid aspiration is that this procedure assesses bacteria present within the tissues rather than surface colonization, which may be sampled by a swab culture. However, fluid aspiration is only successful if there is sufficient fluid to sample. Additionally, there are several potential dangers to performing this procedure including the spread of infection

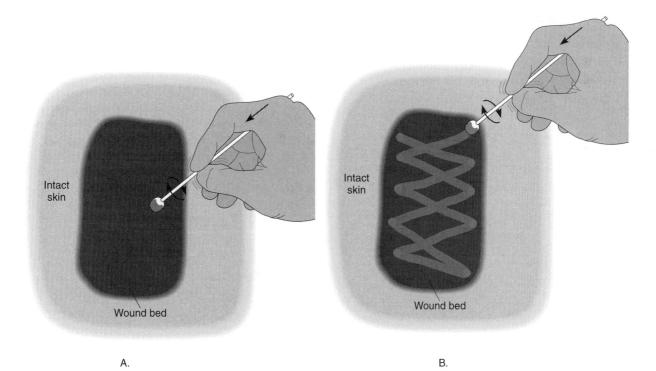

A.   B.

FIGURE 6–4   Aerobic swab culture technique. *A.* The culturette is rotated over a 1-cm^2 of viable wound surface area for 5 seconds while applying enough pressure to express tissue fluid. *B.* Alternatively, the culturette is rotated while moving in a 10-point pattern across viable tissue within the wound bed while applying enough pressure to express tissue fluid.

BOX 6–1   Steps to Perform a Swab Culture for Aerobic Microorganisms

Indications

1. Patient exhibits signs and symptoms of infection.
2. Patient presents with a nonhealing wound despite appropriate wound management.

Procedure

1. Obtain physician's order for wound culture.
2. Debride necrotic tissue per protocol and rinse with saline.
3. Remove and discard soiled gloves.
4. Obtain a culturette and label it with the date, patient's name, identification number, and site cultured.
5. Don clean gloves.
6. Using the applicator, apply gentle pressure to express tissue fluid.
   - Swab a 1-cm^2 area of viable wound surface for 5 seconds.*
   - Rotate the applicator while traveling over the wound bed.
   - Swab into wound tunnels if present.
7. Securely replace the applicator into the culturette.
8. Squeeze the ampoule of fluid at the bottom of the culturette to bathe the applicator.
9. Place the culturette in a biohazard bag labeled with the patient's name, identification number, and site cultured.
10. Remove and discard soiled gloves.

   - Perform separate cultures on each wound.
   - Complete any necessary documentation.
   - Send the culture to the laboratory for processing.

*Alternatively, follow a 10-point pattern to sample viable areas of the wound bed. This method may be preferable for larger wounds or wounds with little nonviable tissue.

BOX 6–2   Steps to Perform a Swab Culture for Anaerobic Microorganisms

Indications

1. Patient presents with a deep, tunneling wound that exhibits signs and symptoms of infection.
2. Patient's wound presents with undermining or sinus tract and signs and symptoms of infection.
3. Patient does not present with signs and symptoms of infection but has a nonhealing, deep, tunneling wound despite appropriate wound management.

Procedure

1. Obtain physician's order for wound culture.
2. Debride necrotic tissue per protocol and rinse with saline.
3. Remove and discard soiled gloves.
4. Obtain an anaerobic culture test tube and label it with the date, patient's name, identification number, and site cultured.
5. Don clean gloves.
6. Using a calcium-alginate-tipped applicator, apply gentle pressure to express wound fluid.
   - Swab a 1-cm^2 area of viable wound surface for 5 seconds.*
   - Rotate the applicator while traveling over the wound bed.
   - Swab into wound tunnels, undermined areas, and sinus tracts if present.
7. Securely replace the applicator into the agar at the base of the culture test tube. If necessary, break off any portions of the applicator that do not fit within the length of the culture test tube. Securely close the cap of the culture test tube.
8. Place the culture in a biohazard bag labeled with the patient's name, identification number, and site cultured.
9. Remove and discard soiled gloves.

   - Perform separate cultures on each wound.
   - Complete any necessary documentation.
   - Send the culture to the laboratory for processing.

*Alternatively, follow a 10-point pattern to sample viable areas of the wound bed. This method may be preferable for larger wounds or wounds with little nonviable tissue.

along the needle tract, fistula formation, and damage to underlying structures from the needle. For these reasons, fluid aspirations are performed less often and are primarily reserved for diagnosing wound infections in abscesses.

It is also possible to use blood tests to determine the organism causing an infection. Serology involves identifying microbes by the presence of serum antibodies within the infected individual. However, because this method is less accurate and more time consuming than wound cultures, it is seldom used in the management of open wounds.

Since it is neither possible nor feasible to culture all wounds, the clinician should examine each wound for the clinical signs and symptoms of infection during every visit and, if present, discuss with the attending physician if a wound culture should be performed. Clinicians should also instruct patients and caregivers in the signs and symptoms of wound infection and tell them to contact their health care provider as soon as possible if these occur.[50] Because of the possibility of a silent infection, wounds that have not made significant progress in 2–6 weeks of appropriate wound management should also be cultured.[2,51]

Microbe Identification

In the laboratory, several methods are used to identify the microbe(s) from the wound culture: shape, means of reproduction, response to staining, and the environment in which they grow best. Offending microbes are most commonly bacteria, but may also be viruses or fungi. Bacteria are unicellular organisms ranging in size from 0.2 to 10.0 mm in diameter. Bacteria have a rigid cell wall, lack a nuclear membrane, and require nutrients from an external medium, such as the human body, to survive.[5] Bacteria are named by their genus (e.g., *Pseudomonas*) and species (e.g., *aeruginosa*). The genus name may describe the shape of the bacteria: spherical bacteria are called *cocci*, helical bacteria are called *spirilla*, and rod-shaped bacteria are called *bacilli*. All bacteria reproduce by cellular division. Bacteria that divide in chains are identified by the prefix *strept-*, and bacteria that divide in clusters are identified by the prefix *staphyl-*. Some bacteria, such as *Bacillus anthracis* (anthrax), form spores when faced with harsh environmental conditions. Spores represent a stasis-like condition that enables bacteria to exist indefinitely. When favorable conditions arise, the spores germinate and then metabolize and reproduce as before. Organisms that are stained by crystal violet are called **gram-positive** bacteria. Bacteria that are not stained by crystal violet, but are stained by safranin, are called **gram-negative.**[10] Recall that both gram-positive and gram-negative bacteria are capable of secreting exotoxins that can cause extensive damage to host tissues,[14] while only gram-negative bacteria produce the less destructive endotoxins.[5,23] Gram-negative bacteria also tend to adhere better to the wound surface.[13] Last, bacteria are identified by the environment most conducive for their growth: oxygen-rich or oxygen-free. Bacteria that require an oxygen-rich environment to survive are called **aerobes;** those that cannot survive in an oxygenated environment are called **anaerobes.** Some bacteria have the ability to adapt their metabolism to either oxygen-rich or oxygen-free environments. For example, *Staphylococcus aureus* is a spherical-shaped, gram-positive bacteria that divides in clusters. *Staphylococci* are aerobic bacteria, that is, they prefer an oxygenated environment. However, they are facultative anaerobes, meaning they are also able to survive in an oxygen-depleted environment, if necessary. Among all possible bacteria, wounds with *Staphylococcus aureus*, *Pseudomonas aeruginosa*, or beta-hemolytic *Streptococcus* are most likely to become infected.[34]

In addition to bacteria, intact skin and open wounds may be infected by fungi. The most common skin and nail fungal infections are tinea and the yeast-like *Candida*.[52] Like bacteria, many fungi are part of the normal microflora present on the skin's surface. Normally, fungi are kept in check by a healthy immune system and by competing for food with colonizing bacteria. However, patients taking **antibiotics** to fight bacterial infections are vulnerable to fungal infections.[10] For example, women who are taking an antibiotic for strep throat may develop a vaginal yeast infection because the antibiotic lowers the local bacterial counts, leaving the colonizing fungi without competition for food. In wound care, patients using antibiotics long term, such as patients with large surface area burns, may develop a fungal overgrowth on or around the open areas. Other factors that increase the risk of fungal infections include moist, occluded areas of skin, and diseases that attack the immune system, such as AIDS.[10] Although the etiology is unclear, individuals with diabetes also have an increased incidence of nail fungal infections.[23,52,53] Tinea infections appear as red, scaling patches with fissuring and itching. *Candida* infections present as red, papular skin rashes accompanied by burning or itching. Refer to Chapter 16 for additional information on the examination and treatment of superficial fungal infections.

MANAGING WOUND INFECTIONS

There is a significant relationship between a decrease in bacterial load and a decrease in wound size.[6, 54] After identifying the offending organism, the physician must determine the most appropriate intervention(s) to reduce the wound's bioburden: antimicrobial therapy, debridement, or a combination of the two.

Antimicrobial Therapy

An **antimicrobial** agent is a substance that is able to destroy unicellular microorganisms.[3] Antimicrobials may be delivered to the infected individual either topically or systemically. In some cases, antimicrobials are delivered directly to the wound by means of antimicrobial-impregnated beads.[55] **Antibacterial** agents are types of antimicrobials that are effective against bacteria. Antibacterials act by inhibiting the bacterial synthesis of proteins, cell walls, proteoglycans, or nucleic acid or by interfering with cellular metabolism.[10] Antibacterial agents may be **bactericidal,** causing irreparable damage to bacteria resulting in bacterial death, or **bacteriostatic,** inhibiting bacterial cell growth while present.[23] **Antifungal** agents are types of antimicrobials that target the cytoplasmic membranes of yeasts and molds.[23] There are several possible reasons to initiate antimicrobial therapy. Although most commonly used to treat infections and reduce wound bioburden, antimicrobials may also be used prophylactically to prepare for graft placement or to improve quality of life by decreasing wound odor, inflammation, and pain.[56]

There are numerous classes of antimicrobials—including penicillins, cephalosporins, erythromycins, aminoglycosides, tetracyclines, quinolones, and sulfonamides—that work in various ways to kill bacteria.[10, 57] The physician must choose the right antibiotic for the type of microorganism present in a particular wound infection to effectively reduce bacterial counts. He or she must consider how effective an antimicrobial is (e.g., how well it kills the offending microbe, decreases the rate of infection, or decreases microbial load). The physician must also consider how safe the antimicrobial is, that is, whether it retards healing or causes adverse reactions to the patient.[58]

Sensitivity and Resistance

A particular antimicrobial is only effective against certain types and strains of microbes. Therefore, prescribing the wrong type of antimicrobial for a given infection would not be therapeutic and would substantially increase the cost of wound care. Antimicrobials have a spectrum of effectiveness. Some are only effective against gram-positive bacteria, and some are only effective against gram-negative bacteria. However, broad-spectrum antimicrobials, sometimes called "super drugs," are able to destroy many varieties of bacteria, including gram-positive, gram-negative, and other bacteria.[57] In addition to an antimicrobial's normal spectrum of action, the physician must know if the bacterial strain is sensitive to a given drug. Determining microbial sensitivity is the second part of the wound culturing process. After culturing and identifying the offending microorganism, smears of microbe cells are placed in an environment conducive to bacterial growth, such as agar plates, where they are subjected to various antimicrobials. Bacterial smear samples that are unable to grow in the presence of a certain antimicrobial are considered **sensitive** to the drug, whereas bacteria that continue to multiply are considered **resistant.**[10]

Bacterial resistance occurs when bacteria produce enzymes that inactivate the antimicrobial, alter cell metabolism, or alter cell permeability to prevent antimicrobial entry into the bacterial cell.[10, 59] Bacterial resistance may be natural or acquired. Natural resistance is an inherent lack of sensitivity of a certain bacterial strain to a particular antimicrobial beyond the antimicrobial's normal spectrum of activity. Acquired resistance occurs when bacteria that were previously sensitive to a certain drug become resistant to the antimicrobial. As previously discussed, this may be seen with biofilms. In some instances, acquired resistance can be overcome by increasing the dosage of the antimicrobial. This is called relative acquired resistance.[60] Premature antimicrobial cessation may lead to recurrence of infection and promotes bacterial resistance.[26] Patients who feel their infection has been resolved may discontinue antimicrobial use. To enhance compliance and improve outcomes, clinicians should counsel patients on the rationale for antimicrobial use and specifically instruct patients to continue to follow prescribed information until advised otherwise.[59]

The two most prevalent strains of resistant bacteria are **MRSA** (methicillin-resistant *Staphylococcus aureus*) and **VRE** (vancomycin-resistant *Enterococci*) MRSA is a gram-positive bacterial strain that emerged in the United States in the 1970s.[61] Whereas *Staphylococcus aureus* once was sensitive to penicillins, such as methicillin, MRSA is a strain of bacteria that has developed a resistance to this class of drugs and many others.[10,61,62] MRSA is more common in the United States than in Canada (26% vs. 3%), with the highest percentage of cases being nosocomial and occurring in intensive care units. Risk factors for MRSA infections include increasing age, diabetes, immunosuppression, malnutrition, recent surgery, immobility, large surface area burns, prior exposure to broad-spectrum antimicrobials, or significant debility.[26,62,63] However, community-acquired infections are becoming increasingly prevalent in certain populations, including prisons, contact sports such as football and wrestling, military personnel, and individuals with AIDS.[26,61,64] Community-acquired MRSA is typically sensitive to a wider variety of antimicrobials than nosocomial MRSA.[65] MRSA can live on environmental surfaces for hours to days.[26] In hospitals, spread of MRSA is typically through environmental contact (contact with contaminated surfaces or contaminated staff members).[26] In contrast, community-acquired MRSA appears to be spread through person-to-person sharing of personal items (towels, close contact).[26] MRSA infections may cause cellulitis, osteomyelitis, and abscesses.[65] Similarly, VRE emerged in the United States in 1989.[66] This strain of bacteria was once sensitive to vancomycin, but it is no longer. VRE infections are more commonly seen in surgical wounds and urinary tract infections.

Patients at greatest risk for MRSA or VRE infections include those who are critically ill, are severely immunosuppressed, have prolonged hospitalizations, or have received multiple antimicrobial therapies.[26] Although resistant strains of bacteria have become more prevalent, they have not become more resistant.[10,60] That is, there are more cases of resistant bacterial infections, but these resistant bacteria have not developed additional resistances to alternative therapies. For example, mupirocin (Bactroban) continues to be an effective bactericidal for MRSA, and ampicillin–amoxicillin continues to be effective against VRE.[10]

Since infections can be clinically silent and are readily eradicated with antimicrobial treatment, why isn't the use of broad-spectrum antimicrobials to cover a wide variety of potential offending organisms a standard intervention for all patients with open wounds? First, there is no evidence to support that uninfected wounds heal any faster with antimicrobial therapy.[67,68] Second, the solution is not to use broad-spectrum antimicrobials wantonly. If used inappropriately, any antimicrobial can actually encourage exposed microbes to build a resistance to traditional therapies.[26,69] In the United States

over 150 million antibiotic prescriptions, the equivalent of about 50 million lb, are written annually.[69] There is evidence to suggest that the misuse of antibiotics, such as prescribing an antibacterial to attempt to combat a common cold virus rather than a bacterial infection, is not only ineffective, but may lead to the development and perpetuation of resistant strains of bacteria.[13,24,59] Antibiotics are the second most frequently prescribed medication, and it is believed that up to 50% of these prescriptions are unnecessary.[7] To add to the problem, in the United States an additional 24.6 million lb of subtherapeutic dosages of antibiotics are given to livestock yearly to build muscle bulk faster to increase the amount of meat that can be sold for human consumption.[70] This widespread use of antibiotics in animals can promote the emergence and virulence of antibiotic-resistant bacterial strains.[69,70] The European Union and other countries have since banned the use of many antibiotics for animal growth promotion, resulting in a significant decline in antibiotic resistance. However, a 2003 study in the United States predicted a ban on the use of growth-promoting hormones in pigs would cost the pork industry $4.50 per pig ($700 million over 10 years), essentially allowing economic interests to continue this unsafe practice. Most important, antimicrobials, especially when given systemically, can have a variety of adverse reactions, ranging in severity from a minor rash to death.

Adverse Reactions

Antimicrobial use, either topical or systemic, is not without risks and should not be initiated without clear goals in mind and guidelines on when to terminate or modify therapy. Generally, adverse reactions are infrequent and the adverse reactions resulting from systemic antimicrobials tend to be more severe than with topical antimicrobials. Mild skin reactions, such as rashes and localized areas of irritation and inflammation, may be seen with topical antimicrobial use.[22] These skin reactions commonly result from an allergic response to one of the components of an antimicrobial preparation, such as sulfa. Therefore, during the initial examination, it is important for clinicians to question the patient about any known allergies. Although some patients may be aware of this allergy from prior experience with prescribed antibiotics, such as penicillin, many more patients may have undiagnosed sensitivities to sulfa drugs. Clinicians should suspect a sulfa allergy if a patient presents with ascending redness and increasing inflammation from the site of topically applied sulfa-containing antimicrobials such as silver sulfadiazine. If severe, allergic reactions may cause hives, difficulty breathing, and even anaphylactic shock.[10] Because some topical agents—such as neomycin (for up to 50% of patients), gentamicin, bacitracin, and lanolin-containing ointments[22]—are known to cause delayed sensitivity, prolonged use of these agents is not recommended.

Systemic antimicrobials may create a more generalized skin reaction. A sulfa allergy should be suspected if a patient receiving sulfonamide medications develops a generalized skin rash, pruritus, or ascending erythema.[10] Systemic antimicrobial use may also produce a wide range of adverse reactions. Gastrointestinal irritation, stomach cramps, nausea, vomiting, and diarrhea[71] are frequent. Photosensitivity is a common side effect, especially with tetracyclines, sulfonamides, and fluoroquinolones.[10] Some patients may experience fever.[71] Antimicrobial adverse reactions may be toxic, causing permanent hearing loss, hepatitis, and kidney damage.[71]

Patients experiencing minor adverse reactions may choose to discontinue their antimicrobials without consulting a clinician and because of the potential severity of these reactions. Therefore, in addition to asking patients if they are taking their antibiotics as prescribed, clinicians should routinely question patients about any potential adverse reactions and report these findings to the attending physician. If an adverse reaction is suspected, the clinician should discontinue the antimicrobial and contact the attending physician. Physicians may minimize these adverse reactions by changing to a different antimicrobial that is still effective.

Topical Antimicrobial Therapy

Topical antimicrobials are applied to the wound surface and reapplied regularly. The goal of topical antimicrobial therapy is to provide an agent to destroy the offending organism(s) with relatively few adverse reactions. Topical antimicrobial therapy, such as the use of bacitracin or triple antibiotic ointment, is familiar to clinicians and most laypeople. Topical antimicrobial medications have been shown to penetrate the wound bed to the site of infection, inhibiting bacterial growth.[8] Clinicians should be aware that not all topical agents have antimicrobial properties. For example, the typical "first aid cream" does not contain an antimicrobial and, therefore, would not effectively combat an infection. Although typically ointments or creams, antimicrobial solutions may also be used. Ointments are oil-in-water preparations available in tubes or single-use packets.

Creams are oil-in-water emulsions (i.e., they contain more water than oil) available in tubs and tubes. Antimicrobial creams typically feel soothing when applied to the wound surface. The antimicrobial properties of ointments are generally effective for 8–24 hours, while creams are generally effective for 8–12 hours.

Several types of antimicrobial-impregnated wound dressings are currently available. Antimicrobial dressings are any category of wound dressing that contains an active ingredient to decrease wound bioburden, such as iodine or silver (refer to Chapter 7). Historically, iodine-containing dressings were cytotoxic. However, newer formulations of cadexomer iodine allow the iodine to be released in lower levels over time. These newer products appear to be effective antimicrobials, including eradication of MRSA, VRE, and *Staphylococcus aureus*, without significantly delaying wound healing.[2,6,21,72,73] While topical agents containing silver have been used for decades, silver has recently been incorporated into virtually all classes of dressings flooding the wound care market. Silver has even been incorporated into some compression garments and stockings marketed toward patients with diabetes or venous insufficiency. Silver is known to be a broad-spectrum antimicrobial that is effective against aerobic, anaerobic, gram-positive, and gram-negative bacteria, as well as yeast, fungi, and viruses.[6,21] However, not all silver preparations are antimicrobial. For example, a recent study showed that colloidal silver solutions, including those currently available in the wound care market, had no antimicrobial effects.[74] Sensitivity to silver is rare.[21] However, in addition to a local allergic reaction, systemic toxicity has been reported with the use of silver dressings on large surface area burns.[75] Silver kills microbes in many ways including inhibition of cellular respiration, denaturing bacterial nucleic acids, and altering cell membrane permeability.[21,22,76] Perhaps because of silver's multiple binding sites[76] and multimodal attack on microbes, resistance is rare.[76] However, resistant strains of *Escherichia coli* and *Pseudomonas aeruginosa* have been found.[22]

There is minimal nonmanufacturer-sponsored research available to support or refute the safety and efficacy of topical antimicrobial-incorporated wound dressings.[77] Additionally, there are multiple potential problems with the delivery of antimicrobials via a wound dressing. First, antimicrobial dressings cost more than the equivalent standard dressing, increasing the cost per dressing change. For example, iodine or silver wound dressings vary from $10.00–27.80 per dressing. Second, the gratuitous use of broad-spectrum antimicrobials may contribute to the development of resistant strains of bacteria.[76] Third, if the dressing is not in direct contact with the wound bed (e.g., if another dressing is used as the wound contact layer and secured with an antimicrobial-impregnated roll gauze), antimicrobial effectiveness would presumably be reduced. Fourth, a recent study comparing the effects of an antimicrobial gauze to standard gauze in colonized cavity wounds found a reduction in wound bioburden without any improvements in wound healing.[78] Because other means of combating and preventing infections have been proven effective, clinicians should carefully weigh the potential benefits of antimicrobial-impregnated dressings with the known risks of wanton antimicrobial use.

Despite these problems, short-term use of topical silver or cadexomer iodine may be warranted in some situations in conjunction with addressing underlying wound pathology and contributing factors, regular debridement, and moist wound healing strategies.[2, 6, 36, 73, 79] New research now shows that topical honey or honey-impregnated dressings may assist with controlling wound bioburden. Patients who might benefit from short-term use of these products include patients with high wound bioburden and those at high risk of infection, such as a patient with a full-thickness burn or an individual who is immunocompromised.[7, 22] Please refer to Chapter 7 for more information on wound dressings containing silver, cadexomer iodine, and honey.

Advantages and Disadvantages

The benefits of topical antimicrobial therapy include lower cost than systemic therapy and ease of application. The obvious advantage of topical antimicrobials over nonantimicrobial topical agents, such as an amorphous hydrogel (see Chapter 7), is that topical antimicrobials will reduce bacterial load when used appropriately. Because topical antimicrobials are applied directly to the wound bed and do not rely on local circulation, they may be more appropriate than systemic antibiotics to treat infections in wounds with compromised circulation. Tables 6–2 and 6–3 provide an overview of the most widely used topical antimicrobial agents and their recommended uses.[6, 36, 57, 80] The disadvantages of topical antimicrobial therapy include increased cost when compared to nonantimicrobial topical agents, the need for frequent applications (one to three times per day), sensitivity or allergic reaction, and the potential for microbes to become resistant to the drug, particularly with prolonged use.[6] To reduce the risk of developing resistance, it is recommended

that topical antimicrobial use be limited to infected wounds. Treatment should be discontinued when the signs and symptoms of infection are no longer present.[2, 6] There are a couple of exceptions to this rule. First, prophylactic antimicrobial therapy may be appropriate for patients with open wounds who are at risk for infection and wounds grossly contaminated with foreign debris. Second, the National Pressure Ulcer Advisory Panel suggests a 2-week trial of antimicrobial therapy for nonhealing wounds to guard against the possibility of silent infections.[2] Third, some antifungal agents, such as oxiconazole nitrate, are to be applied to intact skin and nails and *not* to open wounds. Therefore, clinicians must have a thorough knowledge of the product to ensure successful outcomes.

Application

Antimicrobials lose their effectiveness over time. While ointments and creams are typically effective for several years, antimicrobial solutions may become ineffective in as little as 2 weeks after production. Because of this very limited shelf-life, clinicians should check the expiration date prior to application. Box 6–3 provides step-by-step directions for the application of antimicrobial ointments and creams. Antimicrobial containers are sterile prior to opening, and the clinician should make every effort to prevent contamination of the remaining supply. When using an antimicrobial ointment, a small amount of ointment should be applied to a sterile impermeable surface, sterile applicator, or sterile glove, and the tube should be recapped. Similarly, when using a cream, a sterile tongue applicator or sterile glove should be used to extract the amount necessary. Although typically only a thin layer (one-sixteenth to one-eighth of an inch, or 16–30 mm) of antimicrobial is required, clinicians should refer to individual product directions. The clinician is warned against using larger amounts as this would needlessly increase treatment cost and could make complete removal of the antimicrobial difficult during the next dressing change. Excessively thick applications, especially of antimicrobial creams, create a more occlusive environment that may increase the risk of fungal infections. Contaminated applicators should not be redipped; rather, a new applicator or sterile glove should be used if more antimicrobial is needed. The ointment or cream is then applied directly to the wound. Alternatively, the clinician may choose to apply the antimicrobial to the contact layer of the wound dressing. This method is particularly useful when the

TABLE 6–2   Topical Antibacterial Agents Commonly Used in Wound Care

Topical Antibacterial	Properties

Bacitracin	• Availability: ointment
	• Effectiveness: gram-negative and gram-positive *cocci* and *bacilli*
	• Resistance: rare
	• Application: 1–5 times per day
	• Adverse reactions: patients may develop a delayed hypersensitivity
	• Common uses:
	  ◦ Superficial and partial-thickness wounds
	  ◦ Facial burns (may leave open to air or cover)
	  ◦ Use as a sulfa-free alternative for burn patients who are allergic to sulfa (as an alternative to silver sulfadiazine)

Gentamicin sulfate 0.1% (Garamycin)	• Availability: ointment or cream
	• Effectiveness: gram-negative bacteria, *Streptococci* and *Staphylococci*
	• Resistance: common
	• Application: 1–4 times per day
	• Adverse reactions:
	  ◦ Should not be used on patients who are allergic to sulfa
	  ◦ Patients can develop a sensitivity
	  ◦ Ototoxicity and nephrotoxicity, especially with prolonged use or large surface area wounds
	  ◦ Erythema
	  ◦ Pruritus
	• Common uses:
	  ◦ Superficial and partial-thickness wounds
	  ◦ Because of side effects, should not be used prophylactically, and use should be discontinued as soon as signs of infection have resolved

Mafenide acetate 0.5% cream (Sulfamylon) or solution	• Availability: cream or solution
	• Effectiveness:
	  ◦ Broad-spectrum antimicrobial effective against gram-positive and gram-negative bacteria including *Pseudomonas aeruginosa*
	  ◦ Penetrates wound eschar
	• Application: 1–2 times per day
	• Adverse reactions:
	  ◦ Should not be used on patients who are allergic to sulfa or are pregnant
	  ◦ May develop fungal overgrowth
	  ◦ May inhibit keratinocytes and fibroblasts
	  ◦ Higher rate of sensitivity
	  ◦ May be more painful than silver sulfadiazine
	  ◦ Rash, itching, hives
	  ◦ May cause systemic reactions such as acidosis or hyperventilation with prolonged use or over large surface areas

TABLE 6–2   Continued

Topical Antibacterial	Properties
Mafenide acetate 0.5% cream (Sulfamylon) or solution	• Common uses: 　○ Burn wounds 　○ Readily penetrates wound eschar (good on nose and ear burns) 　○ May leave open to air (face, ears) or cover
Mupirocin (Bactroban)	• Availability: ointment or cream • Effectiveness: gram-negative and gram-positive organisms including MRSA • Application: 3 times per day • Adverse reactions: burning, stinging • Common uses: generally reserved for patients with MRSA to reduce potential for resistant bacterial strain development
Neomycin sulfate	• Availability: ointment or cream • Effectiveness: broad-spectrum antimicrobial particularly effective against gram-negative and some gram-positive bacteria • Resistance: common • Application: 1–3 times per day • Adverse reactions: 　○ Should not be used on patients who are allergic to sulfa 　○ May cause skin rashes 　○ If applied to large areas may cause ototoxicity, neurotoxicity, and nephrotoxicity • Common uses: superficial and partial-thickness wounds
Polymyxin B sulfate	• Availability: ointment • Effectiveness: gram-negative organisms • Should not be used on patients who are allergic to sulfa • Apply 1–3 times per day • Common uses: 　○ Superficial and partial-thickness wounds 　○ Burns
Polysporin powder	• Availability: powder combination of bacitracin and polymyxin B sulfate • Effectiveness: broad-spectrum antimicrobial • Adverse reactions: 　○ See main ingredients 　○ Should not be used on patients who are allergic to sulfa • Apply 1–3 times per day • Common uses: mixed with collagenase for use on infected, necrotic wounds
Silver sulfadiazine 1% cream (Silvadene, SSD Cream, Thermazene)	• Availability: cream • Effectiveness: broad-spectrum antimicrobial especially effective against gram-negative bacteria (*E. coli*, *Enterobacter*, *Klebsiella*), gram-positive bacteria (*S. aureus*), and *Candida albicans* • Resistance: rare

(Continued)

TABLE 6–2   Continued

Topical Antibacterial	Properties

Silver sulfadiazine (continued)	• Application:
	  ◦ 1–2 times per day
	  ◦ Feels soothing/cooling
	  ◦ Forms a loose film over the wound bed that must be removed with each dressing change
	• Adverse reactions:
	  ◦ Should not use on patients who are allergic to sulfa or are pregnant
	  ◦ May develop cutaneous sensitivity (rash)
	  ◦ May be toxic to keratinocytes and fibroblasts
	  ◦ May get fungal overgrowth
	• Common uses:
	  ◦ Most widely used topical agent for burns
	  ◦ Wounds of all depths/sizes

Triple antibiotic (Neosporin)	• Availability: ointment containing a blend of neomycin, bacitracin, and polymyxin B sulfate
	• Effectiveness:
	  ◦ May provide broader-spectrum coverage than each drug individually
	  ◦ May enhance epithelialization
	• Adverse reactions: should not be used on patients who are allergic to sulfa
	• Common uses:
	  ◦ Superficial and partial-thickness wounds
	  ◦ Facial burns (may leave open to air or cover)

wound bed is very moist, making it difficult to apply the antimicrobial directly to the wound surface, or when the wound is painful to the touch. When using this alternative indirect application, the clinician should be careful to limit antimicrobial contact to the wound surface, as prolonged contact with intact skin may cause maceration and increase the cost of dressing changes. The wound is then covered with a wound dressing, typically gauze. Clinicians should follow package inserts for manufacturer-recommended antimicrobial application and dressing change frequencies.

An alternative means of using topical antimicrobials to combat wound infection is to surgically implant polymethylmethacrylate antimicrobial-impregnated beads within the wound bed after surgical debridement (color image 11).[55] Such beads provide a slow, sustained release of antimicrobial medication directly to the site of infection; as such, antimicrobial bead implants may be superior to topically applied ointments and creams. Antimicrobial

bead implants are most commonly used in deep partial-thickness or full-thickness diabetic foot infections. Although the bead implants may be removed (or fall out of the wound bed), they may remain indefinitely. The bead implants serve as a biological spacer, reducing the need for the body to build granulation tissue to fill the wound void,[55] potentially decreasing wound healing time.

Antiseptic Agents

An **antiseptic** agent is an antimicrobial solution that prevents infection by killing microorganisms.[3,81] See Table 6–4 for a list of antiseptic agents. Historically, antiseptic agents were a standard of wound care. Chlorine-based agents were added to whirlpools, and povidone–iodine soaks were applied to wound beds. Although the Food and Drug Administration (FDA) has approved povidone-iodine products for short-term use in superficial, acute wounds, the FDA has

TABLE 6–3   Commonly Used Topical Antifungal Agents

Topical Antifungal	Properties
Nystatin (Mycostatin)	• Availability: cream or ointment • Effectiveness: *Candida* • Resistance: possible • Application: 1–3 times per day

Oxiconazole nitrate (Oxistat)	• Availability: cream or lotion
	• Effectiveness: tinea
	• Application:
	  ○ 1–2 times per day
	  ○ Usually continued for 2–4 weeks
	• Adverse reactions:
	  ○ Pruritus
	  ○ Burning
	  ○ Dermatitis
	  ○ Maceration
	• Common uses: to combat fungal infections on *intact* skin and nails

Miconazole (Lotrimin)	• Availability: cream, ointment, or spray
	  ○ Topical
	  ○ May be given intravenously for severe infections
	• Effectiveness: tinea
	• Adverse reactions: pruritus

BOX 6–3   Application of Topical Antimicrobials

1. Confirm the presence of infection (or appropriate rationale for use) and physician's order for specific antimicrobial medication.
2. Assemble and open necessary supplies.
3. Confirm the antimicrobial belongs to the patient and check the expiration date to ensure it is not expired.
4. Prepare the patient.
   a. Explain the procedure to the patient.
   b. Position patient comfortably while allowing access to the wound.
5. Prepare the wound.
   a. Wash hands and don clean gloves.
   b. Remove the old bandage and discard according to facility policies.
   c. Change gloves.
   d. Inspect the wound.
   e. Perform any necessary irrigation or debridement and note changes in patient/wound status postintervention.
   f. Perform any necessary wound measurements.
   g. Change gloves.

6. Apply topical antimicrobial.
   a. If ointment: squeeze the necessary amount onto a sterile impermeable surface, sterile applicator, or sterile glove.
   b. If cream: use sterile applicator or sterile glove to obtain the necessary amount.
   c. Recap the ointment or cream.
   d. Protect the surrounding intact skin with a skin sealant.*
   e. Apply specified amount to wound surface or to contact layer of wound dressing.
   f. Change gloves.
7. Apply outer layer of wound dressing.
8. Remove and discard soiled gloves.
9. Initial and date wound dressing.
10. Wash hands.
11. Provide any necessary posttreatment instructions.
12. Complete documentation.

*Refer to Chapter 7.

TABLE 6–4   Antiseptic Agents

Antiseptic	Properties

Acetic acid (0.25–0.5%)	• Effectiveness:
	  ◦ Gram-positive and gram-negative bacteria
	  ◦ Particularly effective against *Pseudomonas aeruginosa*[*]
	  ◦ Solution effective for only 2 weeks
	• Adverse reactions:
	  ◦ Cytotoxic to human cells[*]
	  ◦ When diluted to a level that is noncytotoxic, solution is no longer bacteriostatic[†]
	  ◦ Irritates intact skin[*]
	  ◦ May cause acidosis when used on large surface area wounds
	• Acceptable uses:
	  ◦ *Pseudomonas* infections
	  ◦ If infection persists after 2 weeks, use should be reassessed

Chloramine-T	• Effectiveness:
	  ◦ *Pseudomonas aeruginosa*
	  ◦ *Staphylococcus aureus*
	  ◦ *E. coli*
	  ◦ *MRSA*
	• Adverse reactions:
	  ◦ Prolongs inflammatory phase of healing[‡]
	  ◦ Delays collagen synthesis[‡]
	  ◦ Damages fibroblasts[‡‡]
	• Acceptable use: short-term pulsed lavage in heavily colonized or infected wounds in a 100–200 ppm solution[‡‡]
	• Historical use: whirlpool additive

Chlorhexidine gluconate (Hibiclens)	• Effectiveness: broad-spectrum antimicrobial
	• Adverse reactions:
	  ◦ Causes irritation and sensitization
	  ◦ Increases inflammatory response[‡]
	  ◦ Delays epithelialization[‡]
	• Acceptable uses:
	  ◦ Cleanser for intact skin (avoid eyes)
	  ◦ Surgical scrub
	  ◦ Hand-washing solution for health care workers
	  ◦ Perisurgical skin prep

Dakin's solution (sodium hypochlorite, bleach)	• Effectiveness:
	  ◦ Bactericidal
	  ◦ Virucidal
	  ◦ Fungicidal[*]
	• Adverse reactions:
	  ◦ Cytotoxic to human cells[*,§]

TABLE 6–4   Continued

Antiseptic	Properties
Dakin's solution (sodium hypochlorite, bleach)	∘ When diluted to level that is not cytotoxic to human cells (0.005%), is only bacteriostatic[†] ∘ Reduces neutrophil migration[§] ∘ Delays angiogenesis and epithelialization[*] ∘ May cause acidosis when used on large surface area wounds[*] • Acceptable use: cleaning surfaces of inanimate objects
Hydrogen peroxide (3.0%)	• Effectiveness: minimally bactericidal[*,‖,¶] • Solution must be protected from direct light • Adverse reactions: ∘ Cytoxic to human cells even when diluted 1:50 or 1:100,[‖,¶] at which point solution is no longer bactericidal[†,††] ∘ May cause oxygen embolus[#] ∘ Impairs microcirculation[*] • Acceptable uses: ∘ Removing dried blood and exudate over superficial wounds such as pin sites and sutures ∘ Rinse with normal saline after use
Povidone–iodine (Betadine)	• Effectiveness: gram-positive and gram-negative bacteria[*] • Adverse reactions: ∘ Causes sensitization[*] ∘ At 0.001%, solution is still cytotoxic and only bacteriostatic[†,††] ∘ Can cause systemic toxicity after prolonged use on large surface area wounds[**] ∘ Delays epithelialization[**] ∘ Reduces wound tensile strength by 79%[†] ∘ Some studies show wounds treated with povidone–iodine were more likely to be infected than wounds treated with saline[**] • Acceptable uses: ∘ Surgical scrub on intact skin[**] ∘ 1.0% solution may be appropriate for short-term use on acute wounds[**]

[*]Ward RS, Saffle JR. Topical agents in burn and wound care. *Phys Ther.* 1995;75(6):526–538.

[†]Lineaweaver W, Howard R, Soucy D, et al. Topical antimicrobial toxicity. *Arch Surg.* 1985;120:267–270.

[‡]Brennan SS, Foster ME, Leaper DJ. Antiseptic toxicity in wound healing by secondary infection. *J Hosp Infect.* 1986;8:263–267.

[§]Kozol RA, Gillies C, Elgebay SA. Effects of sodium hypochlorite (Dakin's solution) on cells of the wound module. *Arch Surg.* 1988;123:420–423.

[‖]Brown CD, Zitelli JA. A review of topical agents for wounds and methods of wounding: Guideline for wound management. *J Dermatol Surg Oncol.* 1993;19:732–737.

[¶]Mertz PM, Ovington LG. Wound healing microbiology. *Dermatol Clin.* 1993;11(4):739–747.

[#]Sleigh JW, Linkter SPK. Hazards of hydrogen peroxide. *Br Med J.* 1985;291:1706.

[**]Burks RI. Povidone–iodine solution in wound treatment. *Phys Ther.* 1998;78(2):212–218.

[††]Rabenberg VS, Ingersoll CD, Sandrey MA, Johnson MT. The bactericidal and cytotoxic effects of antimicrobial wound cleansers. *J Athletic Train.* 2002;37(1):51–54.

[‡‡]Kloth LC, Berman JE, Laatsch LJ, Kirschner PA. Bactericidal and cytotoxic effects of chlroamine-T on wound pathogens and human fibroblasts in vitro. *Adv Skin Wound Care.* 2009;20(6):331–345.

been unable to document that such use is associated with any improvements in wound healing criteria.[58] In the past, it was generally believed that antiseptic agents would reduce the rate of infection and speed wound repair. However, research over the past decade has clearly illustrated the dangers of these traditions. Although antiseptic agents are broad-spectrum antimicrobials, they are also cytotoxic to fibroblasts, keratinocytes, and neutrophils.[4, 6, 16, 82–88] Antiseptics increase the duration and intensity of the inflammatory response, delay epithelialization, and retard wound contraction.[4, 87] As such, they delay wound healing and avoidance of these substances is a component of prudent wound management.[22, 89] Recall from Chapter 5 that the National Pressure Ulcer Advisory Panel states that antiseptic agents and surfactants should not be used in the standard treatment of open wounds (pressure ulcers).[2] Therefore, if clinicians decide not to follow these guidelines, they must clearly document their rationale.

The primary use of antiseptic agents is to decrease bacterial growth on inanimate objects.[73] The secondary use of antiseptic agents is to reduce bacterial concentrations on intact skin.[73] In this capacity, antiseptic agents may be used as a surgical scrub for clinicians to prevent contaminating a surgical field, for health care worker hand washing such as in the workplace, and for cleansing the patient's intact skin prior to invasive techniques and blood tests. Despite the plethora of research available about the hazards of applying antiseptics to open wounds, many health care providers are either ignorant of these dangers or reluctant to change previous practices. Clinicians who receive orders for the inappropriate use of antiseptics should educate the referral source on alternative, more efficacious intervention options. Table 6–4 provides an overview of the most widely used antiseptic agents, including their effectiveness, adverse reactions, and acceptable uses.

In rare cases, antiseptic agents *may* be appropriate for short-term use on open wounds.[2, 6, 21, 90] Two examples may help to identify these cases. First, patients with wounds infected with *Pseudomonas* may benefit from short-term use of acetic acid soaks. However, if the infection lasts longer than 2 weeks, the clinician should reculture the wound and reconsider the effectiveness of this regimen,[91] as the risks of continued antiseptic treatment likely outweigh the potential benefits. Second, patients with acute open wounds due to an animal bite or farming accident

may benefit from short-term (2–7 days) use of an antiseptic solution, such as povidone–iodine. The rationale behind this recommendation is that these wounds are typically multimicrobial. As such, it may be beneficial to destroy everything within the wound bed initially to prevent infection. The antiseptic should be discontinued shortly (within 2–7 days) to prevent delays in wound healing that are associated with the use of antiseptics on open wounds.[6]

When applying an antiseptic solution to an open wound, the wound is first irrigated with saline and debrided if necessary. Next, the wound is typically rinsed with the solution and then the wound cavity is lightly filled with solution-moistened gauze and covered by a secondary gauze dressing. Again, it is important to note that research to date on the use of antiseptic agents on open wounds demonstrates that these solutions are cytotoxic to human cells, delay wound healing, and have limited efficacy.[3, 83] The clinician should remember that, in almost every circumstance, more effective interventions exist. For example, the clinician may prefer to use a broad-spectrum antimicrobial to assist with reducing bacterial load without compromising the repair process.

Systemic Antimicrobial Therapy

In addition to topical therapy, systemic antimicrobials, commonly referred to as **antibiotics,** may be prescribed just as oral penicillin may be prescribed for strep throat. Physicians typically prescribe antibiotics for patients with sepsis or signs of advancing infection[16, 68] despite the use of topical antimicrobials.[2, 6, 21, 88] Deep space infections also require antibiotic therapy.[2, 38] Antibiotics may be prescribed in isolation or in combination with topical antimicrobial therapy. Some authors contend that oral antibiotics do not reach adequate tissue levels and, therefore, have no effect on bacterial growth at the site of wound infection.[8] This is particularly important in patients with decreased tissue perfusion and local ischemia.[6, 10, 21, 55] In these patients, revascularization is key to wound and limb healing.[55, 92] An alternative treatment option for severe infection is for the physician to prescribe a stronger dose of systemic antibiotics and administer it intravenously.[10, 93] The use of intravenous antibiotics is more expensive and disruptive to the patient's lifestyle than oral antibiotics. However, the recent ability to perform intravenous therapy on an outpatient basis and the increase in the prevalence of resistant infections have led to a substantial increase in the use of this intervention. When determining the appropriate antibiotic for a given patient's infected wound, the physician must consider the type(s) of microorganism(s) causing the infection, the sensitivity of the microorganism(s) to different antimicrobial agents, cost, and the adverse reactions antimicrobial therapy may have.

Advantages and Disadvantages

Similar to topical antimicrobials, the advantages of systemic antibiotics include reduction in bacterial load and ease of application for oral medications. In fact, because antibiotics do not require a dressing change to apply and laypeople are familiar with antibiotic regimens (take all of the medication prescribed, rather than taking the drugs as needed), adherence with oral antibiotics may be higher than with topically applied medications. The disadvantages of systemic antibiotics include more frequent and more severe adverse reactions, the development of resistant bacterial strains, problems with missed doses, higher cost, and, for intravenous medications, disruption in patient lifestyle.[10] Clinicians can help mitigate these factors by querying patients about their medication use and educating them on the importance of following prescribed instructions.

Debridement

Because necrotic tissue and foreign material increase the risk of wound infection, debridement plays a vital role in the management of wound infections. Debridement can help prevent wound infection and assist in resolving an existing infection (see Chapter 5).[2, 16] Regular debridement of necrotic tissue and removal of exudate from the wound surface helps reduce bacterial bioburden[94] and can transform a chronic, recalcitrant, infected wound into an actively healing wound.[16, 30] Regular debridement may increase the effectiveness of topical antimicrobials and antibiotics.[7] Prior to the development of antimicrobial therapy, debridement, particularly amputation, was the only intervention for wound infections. Sharp debridement should only be performed by appropriately trained and certified health care personnel. Surgical debridement, the removal of necrotic and infected tissues most commonly with a portion of healthy tissue along the wound margins,[94] is limited to physicians and podiatrists. Surgical debridement continues to be an important intervention when the offending microbe is resistant to other interventions, when infection is rapidly progressing, or when the antimicrobial cannot reach the site of infection (as with an abscess or decreased tissue perfusion).[2, 55] Surgical debridement is required in the presence of osteomyelitis or sepsis.[55] The preferred treatment strategy for osteomyelitis includes surgical excision of the infected portions of bone along with a short course of intravenous antibiotics.[1, 2, 55] This is followed by oral antibiotics for a total of 4–6 weeks of antimicrobial therapy.[68] Multiple surgeries may be required to eradicate osteomyelitis.[55] Successful treatment of an abscess requires incision and drainage. Surgical debridement is required for deep space abscesses. Refer to Chapter 5 for further details regarding the advantages, disadvantages, and methods of debridement.

 Checkpoint Question #2

Miss Smith presents with the following prescription for physical therapy: "PT evaluate and treat, acute second-degree burn dorsal right foot, apply silver sulfadiazine bid." The amount of inflammation is proportional to the size and extent of the wound, there is minimal serous drainage, and the wound is 50% eschar covered. When you follow up with the patient 3 days later, you notice an increase in inflammation and ascending erythema from the wound site but no other objective or subjective changes.

a. What is the most likely cause of these new findings?
b. What changes in treatment do you recommend?

Clinical Application

Although there are hundreds of different types of microorganisms, only a few are responsible for the majority of wound infections. By knowing the wound etiology, one can reasonably narrow down the type of microorganism. If an infection is suspected, a wound culture or tissue biopsy is taken, and the physician will immediately prescribe a broad-spectrum antimicrobial based on the wound's etiology. For example, infections in pressure ulcers are commonly due to *Streptococci*, *Staphylococci*, and/or *Escherichia coli*. In addition to these three microbes, chronic or full-thickness infected pressure ulcers may also be caused by gram-negative bacilli and anaerobes.[95] Cellulitis infections are most commonly the result of a *Staphylococcus aureus* infection, but may also be due to *Streptococcus aureus*.[69] In the immunocompromised patient, cellulitis may also be due to gram-negative bacilli, such as *Pseudomonas aeruginosa*. Diabetic (neuropathic) ulcer infections average four to five different types of microorganisms and typically result from uncontrolled growth of the natural microflora.[1,6,69] These infections are commonly caused by *Staphylococcus aureus*,[38] followed by *Streptococci* strains,[22,96] gram-negative bacilli, and anaerobes.[95] Ninety-six percent of all cases of acute osteomyelitis and 45% of chronic osteomyelitis are caused by *Staphylococcus aureus*.[69]

After a few days, when the culture and sensitivity results are known, the physician will fine-tune the antimicrobial based on the sensitivity of the cultured organism(s) to the various types of antimicrobial agents.[26,97] Combination therapy may result in fewer cases of resistance than monotherapy[98] and should be used when the offending microbes cannot be effectively covered with one drug. For example, the combination of rifampin and vancomycin has been found to be more effective in the treatment of chronic osteomyelitis than either drug used in isolation.[98] In this way, it is possible to combat the infection immediately, thus avoiding potential spread of the infective process while minimizing the risk of antimicrobial resistance by limiting the exposure to ineffective or inappropriate antimicrobials.

PREVENTING INFECTIONS

In order to prevent wound infections, clinicians should first target ways to decrease the risk of wound formation.[68] For patients with existing open wounds, clinicians should vigilantly follow proper infection control guidelines to minimize the chance of infection.

Preventing Open Wounds

The best way to prevent wound infections is to actively prevent wound occurrence. By being aware of the risk factors for ulcer development, and constantly assessing for changes in risk factors (and addressing these factors), the incidence of open wounds can be markedly reduced. Keys to wound prevention include aggressive management of medical conditions known to increase the risk of wound formation, such as diabetes mellitus,[68] malnutrition, obesity, and incontinence.[99] Proper positioning of patients with impaired mobility and proper foot care for patients with diabetes[52,68] also reduce the risk of skin breakdown. Clinicians should work to protect the barrier function of the integument by treating dry skin, avoiding harsh soaps and detergents, and limiting the use of adhesives directly on the skin. The incidence of fungal infections may be reduced by the judicious use of antibiotics as well as proper skin and wound care. Refer to Section III for specific risk factors for wounds of various etiologies.

Preventing Infections in Open Wounds

Once a wound exists, the single most important means of preventing wound infections is to meticulously follow proper infection control procedures.[4,63] This includes hand washing, standard precautions, the appropriate use of either sterile or clean technique, and proper wound care procedures.[2,5,100]

Hand Washing

Hand washing with water, 3–5 mL of soap, and friction for at least 10–15 seconds will remove debris and transient microbes from the skin and is acceptable for most casual patient interactions.[5] Health care workers should use a consistent technique to ensure that all surfaces of the wrists, hands, fingers, and nails have been cleaned (see hand washing video clip). Antiseptics such as antimicrobial soaps or alcohol-based hand rubs remove and destroy microbes from deeper layers of the skin and can help prevent infections. Health care workers should wash their hands with an antimicrobial soap or alcohol-based hand rub before and after invasive procedures such as wound care (see using a hand sanitizer video clip).[5] Alarmingly, health care practitioners may perform proper hand hygiene as little as 50% of the time.[100] Because the main mode of transmission of MRSA is via hand contact, especially with health care workers who have become contaminated by contact with colonized or infected patients or contaminated items,[26] proper hand-washing procedures are essential.[23,63,100]

Standard Precautions

 Universal precautions, or blood and body fluid precautions, are an approach to infection control in which all blood and body fluids are managed as if they are contaminated. Contamination is defined as the presence or anticipated presence of blood or other potentially infectious waste.[16] **Standard precautions** incorporate the concept of universal precautions along with hand washing and personal protective equipment to reduce the risk of transmission of microbes.[81] Gloves serve as a barrier to prevent gross contamination and should be worn during all wound care procedures because of the reasonable expectation of contact with blood or wound fluid.[5] Gloves should be changed between procedures on the same patient and promptly after touching contaminated materials. Clinicians should recognize that wearing gloves is not a substitute for proper hand-washing procedures. Clinicians must wash their hands both before and after glove use. If there is danger of a splash injury, clinicians should wear either a face shield or mask covering the nose and mouth along with protective eyewear covering the anterior and lateral portions of the eyes.[5] Specially treated gowns that are impermeable to fluids may be used to protect clothing and skin if these are at risk for contamination with blood and wound fluids. The reader is encouraged to watch the videos for the proper methods of donning and doffing of personal protective equipment.

Contact isolation procedures should be followed for patients who have MRSA or VRE wound infections.[100] If possible, wound care equipment, such as modalities, should be dedicated to the individual patient or group of patients with MRSA.[5] If this is not possible, equipment must be disinfected prior to use by another patient. Outpatients or patients who must be transported who have MRSA- or VRE-infected wounds must have wounds covered during transport.

Sterile and Clean Techniques

Wound care procedures are performed using one of two techniques: clean or sterile. Unfortunately, there is a lack of consensus within the literature as to the definitions of, and indications for, these two procedures. The inconsistent use of these terms and the introduction of new terminology, such as the "no-touch" technique, can be a source of tremendous confusion for wound care clinicians. **Sterilization** is a procedure that destroys all microbes from the area of interest. Instruments, gloves, linens, gowns, and the like can be sterilized in specialized settings using steam, dry heat, or liquid chemicals. Although a truly sterile environment is impossible outside of the surgical suite, for the purposes of this text, **sterile technique** is defined as the use of sterile equipment,[50] including gloves, wound dressings, and instruments, in an attempt to significantly reduce exposure to microorganisms.[101] When using sterile technique, sterile–sterile guidelines should be followed, that is, only sterile items may contact the patient's wound. Sterile technique requires hand washing and the meticulous setup and maintenance of a sterile field, including topical agents, wound dressings, and linens.[81] Any contact between nonsterile surfaces, other than the patient's wound, should be avoided. The many intricacies of sterile technique preclude the use of this technique by patients and lay caregivers within the home care setting. Box 6–4 reviews basic guidelines for following sterile technique. The reader is encouraged to watch the videos on how to properly perform sterile techniques.

BOX 6–4   Guidelines for Sterile Technique

- Use sterile gloves, instruments, topical agents, and wound dressings.
- Maintain gloved hands above waist level and in line of sight.
- Touch the wound bed only with sterile items (sterile–sterile technique).
- Open wound dressings immediately prior to use and observe to prevent inadvertent contamination.
- May apply noncontact wound bandages (e.g., stockinette) using clean technique, as these layers will not directly contact the wound.
- Discard sterile supplies appropriately if they become contaminated, and obtain new sterile supplies.

Clean technique is defined as procedures designed to reduce the overall number of microorganisms or prevent the risk of transmitting microorganisms from one locale to another.[101] Like sterile technique, clean technique requires hand washing, sterile instruments, and preventing contamination of supplies.[101] In contrast, clean technique involves the use of clean (boxed, rather than sterile) gloves and the maintenance of a clean, rather than sterile, field. Clean gloves are not free of bacteria; rather, they are free of gross contamination and have a low bioburden. When using clean technique, clinicians should handle wound dressings as little as possible and try to contact only the outer surface or edge of the dressing to minimize the risk of contamination. Because whirlpools, ultrasound heads, and carbon-rubber electrodes are **disinfected** rather than sterilized, these are considered clean procedures.[26] Clean technique requires less knowledge and skill than sterile technique. Additionally, clean technique creates less waste and lowers treatment costs.[67, 102] See Box 6–5 for definitions of important terms and Box 6–6 for examples of sterile, clean, and contaminated supplies.

There is limited research available to guide clinicians in choosing the most appropriate technique. Traditionally, sterile technique was believed to be of prime importance in preventing wound infection, and all wound care was performed using this technique. However, when these two techniques were compared in postoperative wounds, no differences in the rate of infection or wound healing were found.[102, 103] It is now believed that sterile technique is not warranted for most wound care. In fact, the Clinical Practice Guidelines for the Treatment of Pressure Ulcers recommends the use of clean technique for the care of pressure ulcers.[2] For these reasons, clean technique is now the standard technique for wound management. Sterile technique is generally reserved for wounds that require packing, large surface area wounds, severe burns, and wounds in patients who are immunosuppressed. Clinicians are encouraged to examine their facilities' guidelines regarding the use of sterile technique if they are not in line with current recommendations.

Proper Wound Care Procedures

 Clinicians must follow procedures that reduce the risk of contaminating the patient, the equipment, other patients, and personnel. When working with a patient with multiple wounds, proper wound care procedures must also be followed to prevent spreading infection from an infected to an uninfected wound. Most wound supplies, except moisturizers and noncontact layers of wound dressings such as compression bandages, come standard in sterile containers. Clinicians should open wound supplies just

BOX 6–5	**Defining Terms**
Contamination	Presence or anticipated presence of blood, wound fluid, or other potentially infectious waste
Clean	Free of gross contamination
Disinfect	To clean a surface with an antimicrobial
Sterile	Environment free of microbes

BOX 6–6	**Examples of Sterile, Clean, and Contaminated Supplies**
Sterile	• Sterile gloves • Sterile towels/sheets • Debridement kits • Suture sets • Newly opened bandages and the inner surfaces of their wrappers • Newly opened topical agents

Clean	• Clean (boxed) gloves
	• Bandage scissors
	• Wound measuring sheets
	• Modalities
	• Clean bandages
	  ○ Stockinette
	  ○ Tubular bandages
	  ○ Elastic netting
	  ○ Most compression wraps
	• Linens
	• Moisturizers

Contaminated	• Any item that contacts the patient's wound or wound drainage • Old bandages • Used bandage scissors • Any moist item placed on a water-permeable surface

prior to use to minimize contamination from the environment. If using clean technique, any remaining supplies that can be used during future visits should remain within their clean, dry original containers and then be sealed in a plastic container labeled with the patient's name or identification number and reserved for use on the same patient. Labeled medication must then be stored according to Joint Commission for the Accreditation of Healthcare Organizations (JCAHO) standards. These items should not be housed on multiple patient treatment carts. To decrease the risk of cross-contamination, topical agents should also be reserved for single patient use and labeled appropriately.

To minimize the risk of infection and reduce bacterial bioburden, wounds should be kept covered except during wound examination and management procedures.[16] Moisture-retentive dressings, discussed in Chapter 7, are associated with lower infection rates than gauze dressings. Wound dressings should be changed if they become contaminated or ineffective. There are four common ways in which this occurs. First, wound contamination can occur if a dressing slips such that it no longer covers the wound bed, or if a channel develops, providing a passage for microbes and foreign debris from the environment into the wound bed. Second, water-permeable dressings, such as gauze, may be contaminated if they get wet. Third, urine or stool frequently contaminate sacral or perineal wounds covered with permeable dressings. Last, dressings should be changed if strike-through is evident, or impending, because of the potential for contaminants to enter the wound by osmotic forces.

Clinicians should sequence wound management procedures to minimize the risk of wound contamination or cross-contamination.[81] The clinician or delegated personnel should gather anticipated supplies before the treatment session. The necessary quantity of any topical agents, such as antimicrobial ointments, creams, or gels, should be placed on an impermeable sterile surface, such as the inside of a plastic debridement kit or a coated bandage wrapper. If these items are placed on a noncoated wrapper or surface, such as a gauze square, strike-through of any microbes beneath this surface can occur in as little as 30 seconds,[104] contaminating the topical agent and potentially infecting the patient. If additional supplies are required during wound management procedures, the clinician must either ask an assistant to obtain and open them or remove his or her gloves, obtain and open the supplies, and then reglove with new gloves. If a patient has multiple wounds, the most infected wound should be treated last, and gloves should be changed in between wounds.[104] Two different sets of supplies should be used if the clinician suspects only one wound is infected or if the areas are infected by different organisms. The use of gloves is discouraged when handling noncontaminated supplies, such as unopened bandages, pens, and photographic equipment, to prevent the clinician from mistakenly believing these gloves are still clean and may be used subsequently for wound management. Gloves must be removed and hands washed upon completion of wound management procedures, before leaving the treatment area, and before performing any necessary documentation.[81] The treatment area must be thoroughly disinfected between patients.[81]

To prevent potential injuries and contamination, clinicians must properly dispose of all infectious waste and sharps prior to leaving the treatment area. Infectious waste—bandages and supplies that are heavily soiled with blood or wound fluids—should be disposed of according to facility policy in appropriately labeled biohazard containers, such as red bag trash. Contaminated sharp instruments, such as disposable forceps and scalpels, scalpel blades, and wooden applicators, must be disposed of in closeable, puncture-resistant, leakproof, biohazard-labeled containers, such as a sharps container.

 Checkpoint Question #3

What personal protective equipment should be used in the following clinical situations?

a. When removing a patient's wound dressings
b. When debriding over a whirlpool
c. When debriding a patient with second-degree burns over his trunk and upper extremities
d. When measuring or culturing a wound
e. When cleaning up wound supplies after a wound treatment session

CHAPTER SUMMARY

Wound infections occur when microorganisms invade and multiply within body tissues. Infections delay or prevent wound healing. Although similar to the cardinal signs of inflammation, the classic signs and symptoms of wound infection are disproportionate to the size and extent of the wound and may be clinically silent. Tissue biopsies, swab cultures, and fluid aspirations are used to diagnose wound infections and identify the offending microbe(s). Based on the sensitivity and resistance of the microorganisms, the physician prescribes topical and/or systemic antimicrobial therapy to eradicate the infection. Excessive and inappropriate use of antimicrobials contributes to resistant bacterial strains. However, nonhealing ulcers may benefit from a 2-week trial of a topical broad-spectrum antimicrobial to guard against the possibility of a silent infection. Wounds with devitalized tissue or foreign debris should be debrided to help prevent and control infection. Once a standard in the prevention and management of infection, the use of antiseptic solutions is now known to retard wound healing. Therefore, antiseptics should be reserved for use on intact skin. The four keys to preventing infections in open wounds are hand washing, personal protective equipment, the appropriate use of clean or sterile technique, and proper wound care procedures.

REVIEW QUESTIONS

1. Your patient, Mr. V, is a 58-year-old accountant with a history of a coronary artery bypass graft using a left saphenous vein graft, and a nonhealing ulcer on his right lower leg. Previous wound treatment included wet-to-dry dressings for 6 months and twice-daily povidone–iodine soaks for the last 3 months. On examination you find an ulcer measuring 2.3 × 4.5 cm with a 0.2-cm depth. The wound bed contains 100% pale granulation tissue with a 0.4-cm perimeter of erythema.

The wound is mildly tender to probing and there is a mild increase in skin temperature within a 1-cm radius of the wound. There is no evidence of edema. Mr. V's ankle-brachial index is 0.9. The old bandages have a yellow-brown tinge as well as a small amount of dried blood.

   a. What portions of this patient's examination and history might lead you to suspect a wound infection?

   b. What portions of this patient's examination and history might lead you to suspect inflammation?

   c. Based on the information provided, does the wound appear to be infected or inflamed?

   d. What changes in treatment do you recommend?

   e. Would you use clean or sterile technique when treating Mr. V's wound?

2. Your patient is a 52-year-old with a history of rheumatoid arthritis. She presents with a lateral forearm ulcer sustained while gardening one week ago. The ulcer measures 1.0 × 0.5 cm with a 2.0-cm erythemal border. The wound is 50% granular and 50% yellow slough. While probing, you find a 3.0-cm tunnel at the 12-o'clock position and are able to milk a moderate amount of thick, white material from the tunnel. The periwound is indurated and painful to palpation. She has been washing the wound daily with soap and water before applying first aid cream and a Band-Aid. The patient reports her forearm has been getting progressively sorer over the past 2 days.

   a. Based on the information provided, does the wound appear to be inflamed or infected? Defend your answer.

   b. What wound management procedures are appropriate for this patient at this time?

   c. Would you use clean or sterile technique when treating this patient's wound?

Use this address to access the Companion Website created for this textbook. Simply select "Physical Therapy" from the choice of disciplines. Find this book and log in using your username and password to access images, video clips, and additional learning tools.

REFERENCES

Go to myhealthprofessionskit.com to view this chapter's references.

7

Dressing Selection and Bandaging

Chapter Objectives

After reading this chapter, learners will be able to:

1. Describe the benefits of maintaining a moist wound environment.
2. Describe the main properties of moisture-retentive wound dressings.
3. Describe the properties of the nine main categories of wound dressings: gauzes, impregnated gauzes, semipermeable films, hydrogels, semipermeable foams, hydrocolloids, alginates, composite, and antimicrobial dressings.
4. Discuss the indications, precautions, and contraindications for each of the nine main categories of wound dressings.
5. Discuss considerations when choosing charcoal, honey-impregnated, and collagen wound dressings.
6. Describe methods to protect periwound tissues.
7. Describe the indications for the use of skin sealants and moisture barriers.
8. State the indications and precautions for the use of moisturizers.
9. Describe the indications and contraindications for the use of tissue adhesives.
10. Describe the potential role of growth factors, biological dressings, and skin substitutes in wound healing.
11. Examine factors that should be considered prior to choosing a wound dressing.
12. Choose appropriate wound dressings and bandaging techniques based on wound, patient, and setting characteristics.
13. Describe the objectives of comprehensive wound management and their clinical implications.
14. Describe the role of wound dressings in comprehensive wound management.
15. Describe proper bandaging procedures for all types of wound dressings.

Key Terms

Alginate	Hydrogels	Primary dressing
Biologic dressings	Impregnated gauzes	Secondary dressing
Biosynthetic dressings	Moisture barriers	Semipermeable film
Composite dressings	Moisture-retentive dressings	Semipermeable foam
Gauze	Moisture vapor transmission rate	Skin sealants
Granuloma	Moisturizers	Skin substitutes
Hydrocolloids	Occlusion	Tissue adhesives

INTRODUCTION

Ideally, the desired outcome of wound management is wound healing: the wound bed is completely resurfaced with epithelium, and the tissue is remodeled so that its strength approaches normal. An interim step in this process is to obtain a clean, moist, warm, granular wound bed while protecting the periwound and intact skin. Wound dressings and debridement can facilitate the achievement of this short-term goal and, as such, are standard procedures in wound care. This chapter expands on the concept of moist wound healing introduced in Chapter 3 by providing an in-depth analysis of wound dressings and bandaging. Wound debridement is discussed in detail in Chapter 5.

This chapter begins with an overview of the rationale behind moist wound healing and the functions of wound dressings. This is followed by detailed information regarding the nine major categories of wound dressings. Due to their unique features, charcoal, honey-impregnated, and collagen dressings are presented separately. Next, skin care and periwound management principles are presented. Newer advances in wound management, such as growth factors and biologic dressings, are introduced. Building on this information is a section on clinical decision making to enhance the clinician's ability to integrate wound management concepts. The chapter concludes with a section providing location-specific tips for bandaging open wounds.

MOIST WOUND HEALING

A moist wound heals three to five times faster than a dry wound.[1] Creating a moist wound environment facilitates all three phases of wound healing.[2] Moist wound healing decreases the intensity[3] and length of the inflammatory phase.[4] By preventing scab or crust formation over the wound bed, a moist wound environment eliminates the energy and time that would have been required for the body to solubilize these materials.[5] A moist environment also traps endogenously produced enzymes within the wound bed,[6] facilitating autolytic debridement.[7,8] Moist wound healing hastens the proliferative phase of wound healing.[9] By eliminating the barriers presented by scabs, necrotic tissue, and debris, keratinocyte travel time and distance across the wound surface are greatly reduced.[6] A moist wound environment preserves endogenously produced growth factors[6] within the wound fluid.[2] These growth factors, including cytokines, interleukins, and colony-stimulating factors, promote cell growth, proliferation, or activity.[10] Moist wound healing increases fibroblast proliferation and collagen synthesis,[2] as well as the proliferation and migration of keratinocytes.[3,4] Angiogenesis and full-thickness wound contraction occur earlier and require less time when a moist environment is maintained.[4] Moist wound healing may also reduce patient pain complaint.[1,3,8,11,12] Finally, if a moist environment is maintained throughout wound healing, the maturation and remodeling phase may result in a more cosmetically appealing scar.[2,3]

The exact amount of moisture required to maximize wound healing is unknown. A wound that is too dry will result in crust formation and lack the endogenously produced enzymes and growth factors that facilitate wound healing. However, a wound that is too wet can also delay healing.[5] For example, if a wound is too wet, the wound fluid will not only pool over the wound surface, but also flow onto the intact periwound, causing maceration.[5,9] Macerated skin is easily recognized as white or silvery and may have a wrinkled appearance (recall from Chapter 3 what happens after wearing a Band-Aid™ when swimming). When skin is too moist, it becomes more permeable to irritating substances and more readily colonized by microorganisms. For example, consider a patient with a pressure ulcer over his sacrum. If the skin surrounding the ulcer is macerated, uncontrolled perspiration or incontinence may cause a skin rash, create additional ulceration, or increase the risk of infection, resulting in a new or larger wound. In addition, macerated skin is more friable and more easily torn by friction. In the previous example, friction on macerated tissues may occur from improperly performed transfers or sliding down in the bed when the head of the bed is raised. However, improperly applied wound dressings may also cause friction between the dressing and the patient's skin.

A simple food analogy can assist with determining whether or not a moist wound environment is being maintained. A dry wound, which presents with a crust or eschar and has no wound fluid, is like raw pasta. In contrast, a wet wound, which presents with maceration of the surrounding tissue, is like pasta that has been cooked too long, taking on a soft and mushy consistency. During a discussion with Heather Hettrick, then of New York University's Physical Therapy Department, a perfectly moist wound is like perfectly cooked al dente pasta: pasta that is neither crunchy nor mushy. Moist wound healing is accomplished through the use of wound dressings.

Functions of Dressings

Exposed wounds are more inflamed, more painful, and more fibrotic than wounds covered with a dressing. Exposed wounds also develop a thicker crust and have lower collagen content than covered wounds.[7] Wound dressings should provide an optimal environment for wound healing. In many respects, dressings should mimic the functions of the skin described in Chapter 1. The ideal dressing should create a moist wound environment.[8,13–19] If a wound is too wet, the dressing will absorb excess exudate. If a wound is too dry, the dressing will donate moisture to the wound bed. Wound dressings should also provide thermal insulation,[19] for wounds heal faster if the environment is maintained between 37°C (normal body temperature) and 38°C.[3,17,20] Maintaining a warm environment enhances tissue perfusion by causing the microvasculature to vasodilate.[21,22] In addition, this temperature range increases oxygen saturation and decreases hemoglobin's affinity for oxygen.[21] Greater tissue oxygen levels enhance many key wound healing processes, including phagocytosis, resistance to infection, granulation tissue formation, wound contraction, epithelialization, and scar tissue formation.[20,23,24] Because wound temperature decreases with each dressing change and may remain decreased for up to 90 minutes after a dressing change,[25] wound dressings should be chosen that minimize the frequency of dressing changes whenever possible.[13,26] Wound dressings should provide a barrier to microorganisms to protect against infection.[14,17,19] Wound dressings should also protect exposed nerve endings, decreasing the pain associated with an open wound.[7]

Some additional functions that wound dressings can provide include hemostasis, edema control, and the elimination of dead space within a wound bed.[13] Dead space is best described as the void left by a wound cavity, tunneling, or undermining (see Figure 7–1). Dead space within a wound must be eliminated to prevent premature wound closure and abscess formation. The ideal wound dressing should assist the body with the removal of necrotic tissue, foreign material, and debris.[14] Finally, wound dressings should also provide adequate gas exchange between the wound and the environment.[14,19]

Wound dressings are generally divided into two basic types: primary and secondary. A **primary dressing** comes into direct contact with the wound and, therefore, is sometimes called the contact layer. A **secondary dressing** is placed over a primary dressing to provide increased protection, cushioning, absorption, or occlusion. In many instances, a primary dressing may be used without an added secondary dressing. A Band-Aid™ is an example of a primary dressing that does not require a secondary dressing. In contrast, consider the dressing typically applied immediately after donating blood. The primary dressing, a small gauze square or adhesive bandage, is placed over the donation site. The secondary dressing, a self-adhesive elastic bandage, is placed over the primary dressing to assist with hemostasis and edema control.

Moisture-Retentive Dressings

Although moist wound healing can be attained with traditional gauze dressings, moisture-retentive dressings are better suited to provide and maintain

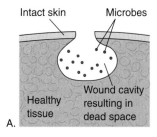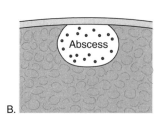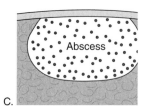

FIGURE 7–1   Abscess formation due to dead space. *A.* Wound presenting with a large wound cavity and small opening. Note the wound is colonized by a small number of microbes as expected. *B.* If the wound is not lightly filled, it is likely that it will prematurely close prior to granulation tissue formation, leaving a potential space and sealing in the colonizing organisms. *C.* In the presence of a warm, moist, dark environment, the normal colonizing bacteria will multiply, causing an abscess and potentially increasing the size of the "wound."

an ideal wound healing environment. **Moisture-retentive dressings** are specialized synthetic or organic dressings that are typically more occlusive than gauze.[27] **Occlusion** describes the ability of a dressing to transmit moisture vapor and gases from the wound bed to the atmosphere.[28] A truly occlusive substance, such as latex, is impermeable to water, vapor, and bacteria. In contrast, a truly nonocclusive substance, such as air, is completely permeable to water, vapor, and bacteria. Wound dressings fall somewhere along this continuum. There are different classes of moisture-retentive dressings, which vary in absorptive capabilities, cost, durability, composition, and the ability to allow gas exchange. However, all moisture-retentive dressings help contribute to obtaining and maintaining a moist wound environment and, therefore, facilitate wound healing.

Moisture-retentive dressings have a lower **moisture vapor transmission rate** than gauze.[4, 14] That is, they are better able to trap wound fluid rich in enzymes, neutrophils, growth factors, and macrophages within the wound bed. As such, lower moisture vapor transmission rates are associated with faster wound healing and lower pain complaints.[4, 29–31] Additionally, moisture-retentive dressings facilitate autolytic debridement,[3] usually within 72 to 96 hours.[7] The occlusive nature of many moisture-retentive dressings allows the patient to bathe, do the dishes, or swim without contaminating the wound or changing the dressing. Moisture-retentive dressings also stimulate granulation tissue formation, collagen synthesis, and epithelialization.[28] Moisture-retentive dressings maintain wound temperature better than gauze dressings[22] and are better able to protect the wound from trauma and bacterial contamination.[30]

Most moisture-retentive dressings are adhesive, precluding the need for tape or a secondary dressing, such as roll gauze. They are also more elastic and may conform better to body contours than gauze. Whereas gauze dressings tend to slide down or roll up over time, moisture-retentive dressings stay in place. Moisture-retentive dressings are more expensive per application than gauze dressings. However, because they are designed to stay in place for several days, moisture-retentive dressings require fewer dressing changes and less clinician time,[31] consistently resulting in lower overall wound care costs (see Box 7–1).[14, 29, 32, 33]

BOX 7–1   Properties of Moisture-Retentive Dressings

- Maintain moist wound environment
- More occlusive than traditional gauze dressings
- Facilitate autolytic debridement
- Associated with lower infection rates than traditional gauze dressings
- Conform well to skin surface contours
- Result in nontraumatic removal from wound surface
- Designed to stay in place for 3–7 days
- Require less clinician/caregiver time
- Associated with higher one-time cost but lower overall wound costs than traditional gauze dressings
- Can be used on granular (red) or necrotic (yellow or black) wounds
- Can be used on superficial, partial-thickness, and full-thickness wounds
- Have varied absorptive capabilities
- Lower patient pain complaint
- Come in a variety of shapes and sizes

Common Fears Associated with the Use of Moisture-Retentive Dressings

Infection

When moisture-retentive dressings were first introduced to wound care, clinicians were afraid their use would increase the rate of wound infection. Clinicians believed that maintaining a moist, warm, dark wound environment for several days would provide an ideal environment for microbes to multiply unchecked. In fact, wounds treated with occlusive dressings have been found to have lower infection rates (2.6%) than those treated with nonocclusive, gauze dressings (7.1%).[2, 4, 34] There are four possible explanations for this. First, occlusive dressings serve as a bacterial barrier. Some types of moisture-retentive dressings (specifically hydrocolloids) have even been found to be effective barriers against methicillin-resistant *Staphylococcus aureus* (MRSA),[6, 34] hepatitis B, HIV-1, and *Pseudomonas aeruginosa*.[6, 8] Many moisture-retentive dressings are impermeable to urine and stool; therefore, these dressings reduce the risk of wound contamination and the need for dressing changes when patients with perineal ulcers have episodes of incontinence. Second, because moisture-retentive dressings require less frequent dressing changes, the risk of cross-contamination during dressing changes is reduced.[6] Third, by retaining macrophages and neutrophils, moisture-retentive dressings facilitate the neutralization of microorganisms. Fourth, the preservation of endogenous enzymes within the wound fluid facilitates the removal of the necrotic tissue and debris microbes feed upon.

The risk of infection when using moisture-retentive dressings can be further reduced by following a few simple guidelines. Moisture-retentive dressings should be changed if their barrier properties become compromised. That is, if the edge seal is no longer intact or a channel develops between the body surface and the dressing, a new dressing should be applied. These channels provide a pathway for bacteria to enter the wound bed and flourish in the warm, moist environment (see Figure 7–2). If strike-through occurs or wound fluid reaches close to the edge of the dressing, the dressing should also be replaced. Because of the potential for subclinical or silent infections in patients who are immunosuppressed, moisture-retentive dressings should be used with caution on these individuals.[3,7] It may be wise to initially perform more frequent dressing changes (e.g., the clinician may choose to change the dressing after 3 days, rather than 5–7 days) when using moisture-retentive dressings on this population to allow for wound inspection. Moisture-retentive dressings should be discontinued if the signs and symptoms of infection are detected. To avoid a more serious infection, moisture-retentive dressings are contraindicated in wounds known to be infected. There are three exceptions to this rule: Semipermeable foams and alginates (discussed later in this chapter) may be used on infected wounds with caution; antimicrobial dressings (discussed later in this chapter), by definition, are appropriate for use on infected wounds. Because wounds with copious drainage may be infected, the use of moisture-retentive dressings should be carefully monitored in these types of wounds.[3] Moisture-retentive dressings should be removed after a specified period of time (typically within 5 to 7 days) or as often as is demanded by the accumulation of fluid within the dressing. All wounds, whether treated with traditional or moisture-retentive dressings, should be monitored for the signs and symptoms of infection.

Wound Bed and Surrounding Skin

Clinicians initially feared that the adhesive backing of many moisture-retentive dressings would traumatize the fragile wound bed. However, while the adhesive allows the dressing to adhere to intact skin, the interaction of the dressing with wound fluid prevents the dressing from adhering to the wound bed. The adhesive used in moisture-retentive dressings is less tacky than traditional silk tape. Therefore, dressing removal does not pose as significant a threat when applied to healthy skin. However, skin breakdown has been noted if adhesive moisture-retentive dressings are changed too frequently.[35] To further reduce the risk of skin trauma when removing moisture-retentive dressings, the edge of the dressing should be lifted up near the corner and then stretched longitudinally to decrease the dressing's adhesion to the skin's surface.

Many clinicians were concerned that trapping wound fluid within a dressing for several days would lead to maceration of the surrounding intact skin. However, this risk is decreased in two ways. First, when used appropriately, moisture-retentive dressings are able to achieve a

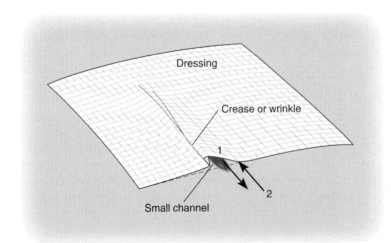

FIGURE 7–2   Wrinkles or creases in a wound dressing provide a pathway for (1) wound fluid to escape from under the dressing and (2) for microbes from the environment to enter the wound bed, increasing the risk of wound infection. A similar pathway is formed if strike-through occurs or if wound drainage accumulates near the edge of a dressing.

moist, rather than wet, wound environment. Moisture-retentive dressings with higher rates of moisture vapor transmission decrease the pooling of fluid within the dressing.[2, 14] Many of these dressings have the ability to wick moisture away from the wound and periwound, similar to the way fabrics like Cool-Max are able to wick perspiration away from the skin. Second, topical skin protectants, in the form of barriers or sealants, should be applied to all intact skin covered by moisture-retentive dressings. These products provide a protective coating over intact skin, preventing maceration if wound fluid stays in contact with the skin. At least one author states that although maceration may be a side effect of the use of moisture-retentive dressings, maceration is not consistently associated with an increase in adverse occurrences nor with delayed wound healing.[4] Additional information on the use of skin protectants is presented later in this chapter.

Checkpoint Question #1

Describe why the following two statements are false.

a. Although it may be desirable to cover wounds during the day, they should be left open to air at night.

b. A draining wound is infected and should not be bandaged with a moisture-retentive dressing.

THE CONTINUUM OF WOUND DRESSINGS

There are several thousand wound management products available on the market today that are purported to facilitate wound healing. It is easy for clinicians and students to become overwhelmed by the multitude of wound care manufacturers and products on the market today. The secret to demystifying wound care products is to understand the basic properties of the nine main categories of wound dressings. Wound dressing categories can be represented as a continuum of occlusion, with traditional gauze dressings being the least occlusive wound dressing and hydrocolloids being the most occlusive (see Figure 7–3). Wound dressing categories can also be represented as a continuum of absorptive capabilities (see Figure 7–4). Although dressings within each category are not identical (e.g., they may vary slightly in structure and absorptive capabilities), they possess many of the same properties. Clinicians can successfully manage patients with open wounds by understanding wound etiology, basic wound healing principles, and the basic properties of the major categories of wound dressings.[14, 15, 27]

This section provides detailed information on the properties of the nine main categories of wound dressings on the market today: gauze dressings, impregnated gauze dressings, semipermeable films, hydrogels, semipermeable foams, hydrocolloids, alginates, composites, and antimicrobial dressings. Wound dressings containing charcoal, honey, and collagen may take many of these forms but are considered separately because of

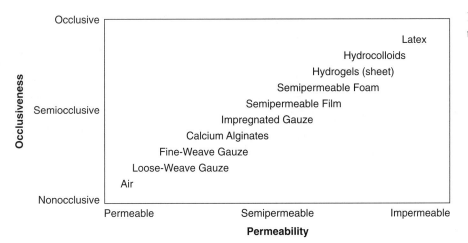

FIGURE 7–3 Occlusion continuum of wound dressings.

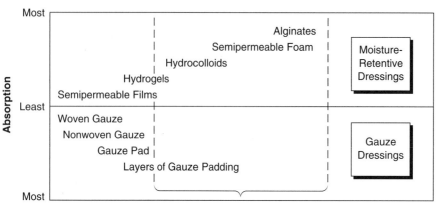

FIGURE 7–4 Absorption continuum of moisture-retentive wound dressings.

their unique qualities. Enzymatic debriding agents are presented in Chapter 5, while topical antimicrobials, antifungals, and cleansers are presented with the management of infection in Chapter 6. Because compression is required to address the etiology of venous insufficiency ulcers, compression dressings are discussed in Chapter 11. Boxes provide information on approximate dressing cost. It should be noted that dressing cost varies based on dressing size and any additional dressing features, for example, a dressing may cost more if it contains an adhesive border. Dressing reimbursement is a much more complex topic and is based on HCPCS dressing codes and local coverage decisions that change annually. Clinicians should contact individual insurers and examine local coverage decisions to determine if a specific dressing class is reimbursable and at what rate. Several online resources are available.[36]

Gauze Dressings

Traditionally, wound dressings were made from woven or nonwoven gauze. **Gauze** dressings continue to be the most readily available wound dressings in use today. Woven gauze is made from cotton yarn or thread that is woven like fabric. In contrast, nonwoven gauze is made from synthetic fibers pressed together. Nonwoven gauzes typically have greater absorbency than woven gauzes. Gauze dressings with a loose weave have large pores. Loose-weave gauze aids in the mechanical debridement of wet-to-dry dressings by trapping foreign material, debris, and slough within the large pores.[37] However, if a loose-weave gauze is applied to a granular wound, granulation tissue and keratinocytes may also become enmeshed within the dressing.[21]

When the dressing is removed, these fragile new tissues will be dislodged, delaying wound healing. By using a finer weave with smaller pores, the risk of traumatizing the wound bed during dressing changes is reduced.

Gauze is highly permeable and relatively nonocclusive. Therefore, gauze dressings may promote desiccation in wounds with minimal exudate unless used in combination with another dressing or topical agent. Gauze may be used as a primary or secondary wound dressing. Gauze dressings are inexpensive for one-time or short-term use.

Gauze dressings come in many forms: squares, sheets, rolls, and packing strips (see Figure 7–5). Gauze squares are generally included in debridement

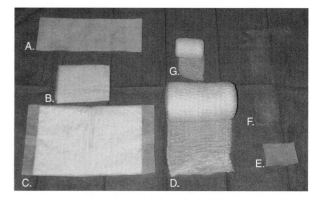

FIGURE 7–5 Gauze products labeled counterclockwise, from top left: *A.* nonadherent gauze, *B.* 3 × 4-inch gauze square, *C.* absorbent gauze pad, *D.* six-ply gauze roll, *E.* bismuth-impregnated gauze, *F.* petrolatum-impregnated gauze, and *G.* two-ply roll gauze.

kits. Gauze rolls are typically two- or six-ply. The more layers, the greater the absorbency, padding, and dressing bulk. Gauze packing strips may be 1/4 to 2 inches in width to accommodate for a variety of wound and tunnel sizes. So-called burn gauzes are available in large sheets or vests and can be up to 50-ply to absorb the massive amounts of drainage from full-thickness burns. Multilayer gauze dressings typically consist of an outer nonocclusive layer, which allows gas exchange; a middle antishear layer that moves with the patient; and a nonadherent contact layer, which allows absorption of wound exudate and wicks moisture away to reduce the risk of maceration.[38] Many manufacturers market gauze squares and roll gauzes that are impregnated with antimicrobials. Based on current research regarding the use of topical antimicrobials, it would seem prudent for clinicians to avoid (or at least limit) the use of such products to reduce the potential for the development of resistant microorganisms (refer to Chapter 6).

Common Uses

Gauze dressings can be used on both infected and uninfected wounds of any size, shape, depth, or etiology. Although gauze may not be the best choice of dressing, gauze dressings can be modified to be safe with any wound type. For example, if used on a nondraining or minimally draining wound, a topical agent can be applied to the wound bed to help maintain a moist wound environment or the gauze may be premoistened with normal saline. Alternatively, if used on a highly draining wound, additional layers can be used to aid in absorption. Gauze dressings can be used alone or in combination[14] with topical antimicrobials, enzymes, growth factors, amorphous hydrogels, alginates, semipermeable foams, or semipermeable films.

There are several scenarios in which gauze is the dressing of choice. If a wound requires daily or more frequent dressing changes, gauze is the most economical choice. Therefore, gauze is commonly used on infected wounds or wounds being treated with enzymatic debriding agents. Because roll gauze dressings avoid adhesives, they may be the most appropriate secondary dressing for patients with fragile integument. Patients with large wounds or wounds in irregularly shaped areas may be best treated with gauze dressings because gauze is inexpensive and can easily be secured in place. Gauze packing strips are commonly used to prevent premature closure and wick away exudate in tunneling or undermining wounds.[16,21,39]

Precautions/Contraindications

Woven gauze may require more force to remove than nonwoven gauze, potentially traumatizing the wound bed. Additionally, woven gauze may leave a residue or lint within the wound bed. The body may respond to this foreign material by forming a **granuloma**.[3,21,38] Therefore, clinicians would be wise to use nonwoven gauze with a fine weave on wounds that are not 100% necrotic. If gauze dressings are allowed to dehydrate, they will adhere to the wound bed, causing trauma upon removal.[16,22,40] If a gauze dressing appears to be adhered to the wound bed, the clinician should first moisten the dressing with saline prior to removal. The clinician should also consider using a topical agent, a saline-moistened gauze, an impregnated gauze wound contact layer, a moisture-retentive dressing, or a combination of these methods to maintain a moist wound environment and prevent this from occurring again.[14,40]

When using roll gauzes, clinicians should be cautious to prevent the bandage from causing a tourniquet-like effect. Roll gauze should be applied snugly but without tension and arranged on a slight angle rather than straight across. The dressing should be changed if the gauze rolls up, causing constriction, or slides down, exposing the wound. If used as a secondary dressing, gauze dressings should be changed when strike-through occurs to reduce the risk of wound contamination.

Telfa dressings are nonadherent gauze dressings with little absorptive capabilities. These dressings should be reserved for use on superficial, nondraining wounds closed by primary or secondary intention, such as those in which a typical Band-Aid™ would suffice. When used on more significant wounds, this type of dressing promotes maceration by maintaining wound exudate close to the wound and periwound surface, potentially resulting in an increase in wound size or severity. See Box 7–2 for a summary of gauze dressings.

Impregnated Gauze Dressings

Impregnated gauzes are mesh gauze dressings into which materials such as petrolatum, hydrogel (see hydrogel section later in this chapter), saline, bismuth, or zinc have been incorporated (see Figure 7–5 E and F). This type of dressing is used as the wound contact layer and requires a secondary dressing, typically regular gauze. Impregnated gauzes are nonadherent, allowing pain-free and trauma-free removal. They may also mildly increase the occlusiveness of a standard gauze dressing,[7] potentially improving the dressing's ability

BOX 7–2	Gauze Dressings
Benefits	• Universally available • Have a low one-time cost • Can be used on infected and uninfected wounds • Can be used alone or in combination with other classes of dressings and topical agents • Can add more layers to increase absorption capabilities • Provide cushioning • Keep adhesives off patients' skin (roll gauze)
Limitations	• Costly over time • May adhere to wound bed • May leave particulate matter in wound bed • Highly permeable • Require more frequent dressing changes • Have a higher infection rate than occlusive dressings
Common Uses	• Infected wounds • Wounds requiring packing • Wounds requiring frequent dressing changes • Highly exudating wounds
Common Examples* **(Roll gauze)**	• Bulkee • Conform • Elastomull • EXU-DRY • Kerlix • Kling • Nu-Gauze
Approximate Cost†	• Gauze squares: $0.10 • Gauze pads: $0.20–3.99 • Roll gauze: $0.75–5.40

*This is a noninclusive, alphabetical list of products and should not be considered an endorsement of any brand/manufacturer.

†Actual cost may differ based on product size/characteristics, manufacturer, and distribution contracts. Dressing reimbursement is based on local coverage decisions and is not considered here.

to maintain a moist wound environment. Some authors suggest that impregnated gauzes should not be used because studies have shown that spreading a thick layer of the impregnated substances, such as petrolatum, directly over a wound bed creates a physical barrier to epithelialization. However, when these materials are incorporated into mesh gauze sheets, there are no studies supporting the theory that wound healing is impaired. Clinically, petrolatum-impregnated gauzes may facilitate wound healing by preventing wound bed trauma during dressing changes. Zinc-impregnated gauzes, such as paste bandages (Unna's boot), are used primarily in the treatment of venous insufficiency ulcers and are described in Chapter 11.

Common Uses

Petrolatum-impregnated gauzes may be used as a wound contact layer on granulating wound beds in combination with a secondary gauze dressing. They can be used with or without a topical agent, such as an amorphous hydrogel or antimicrobial. Impregnated gauzes may also help prevent exposed tendons or tendon sheaths from dehydrating[41] or adhering to the primary dressing. Because petrolatum-impregnated gauzes allow pain-free removal, these dressings are commonly used on burn wounds.[42] Before being placed on the burn, a topical antimicrobial, such as silver sulfadiazine, is typically applied to these dressings either prophylactically or to treat an existing infection.

Precautions/Contraindications

There are times when impregnated gauze dressings may be inappropriate. Xeroform gauze is impregnated with a combination of bismuth and petrolatum. Bismuth has mild antimicrobial properties and has been used prophylactically to prevent wound infection. However, bismuth is also cytotoxic to inflammatory cells[43] and may be a sensitizing agent, that is, it may cause irritation, dermatitis, or an increased inflammatory response. Patients with venous insufficiency ulcers are particularly prone to such responses. Clinicians must weigh these potentially adverse responses against the potential benefits of bismuth's antimicrobial properties. Similarly, iodine-impregnated gauze packing strips are cytotoxic to human cells and only mildly antimicrobial. Clinicians must carefully weigh the potential advantages against this product's inherent dangers. See Box 7–3 for a summary of impregnated gauze dressings.

BOX 7–3	**Impregnated Gauze Dressings**
Benefits	• Decrease trauma to wound bed during dressing changes • Decrease pain of dressing changes • May increase occlusiveness of gauze dressing
Limitations	• More costly than plain gauze • Require secondary (gauze) dressing • Present a barrier to keratinocyte migration if highly impregnated • Have minimal absorptive capabilities
Common Uses	• Burn wounds • Granulating wounds • Epithelializing wounds • Wounds with exposed deep tissues • Wounds that bleed easily • Painful wounds
Common Examples*	• Adaptic (petrolatum) • Aquaphor gauze (petrolatum) • CURAFIL hydrogel (hydrogel) • Invacare oil emulsion (petrolatum) • Vaseline gauze (petrolatum) • Xeroflo (bismuth) • Xeroform (bismuth)
Approximate Cost†	• $1.07–3.45

*This is a noninclusive, alphabetical list of products and should not be considered an endorsement of any brand/manufacturer.
†Actual cost may differ based on product size/characteristics, manufacturer, and distribution contracts.

Semipermeable Films

Semipermeable film wound dressings are thin, flexible sheets of transparent polyurethane with an adhesive backing. Film dressings are permeable to water vapor, oxygen, and carbon dioxide, but impermeable to bacteria and water.[8,14,44-46] Film dressings, which are similar to kitchen plastic wrap, have little absorptive capabilities.[14,21] It is normal for a brownish fluid to accumulate beneath the dressing. Clinicians should not assume this fluid to be a sign of infection. The transparent quality of film dressings allows visualization of the wound bed. However, as fluid pools within the dressing, the wound bed becomes obscured. Film dressings are highly elastic and conformable to body contours and are available in a variety of sizes. Like all adhesive moisture-retentive dressings (see Figure 7–6), the adhesive reacts with wound fluid to prevent adhesion to the wound bed while allowing the dressing to stick to dry, periwound skin. Film dressings do not significantly insulate the wound.[47]

The film dressing should be secured to a 1- to 2-cm border of intact skin. Larger film dressings can be difficult to apply. Semipermeable film dressings should be applied without tension or wrinkles and may normally be left in place up to 5–7 days. If a channel develops, the dressing should be changed to prevent wound contamination. Because of their inability to manage large amounts of fluid, film dressings should not be used on cavity wounds or wounds with moderate to heavy drainage. Semipermeable film dressings vary in adhesiveness and may cause trauma to the periwound upon removal.[8,48] Therefore, these dressings should not be applied to patients with frail skin.

Common Uses

Semipermeable film dressings are commonly used on superficial wounds such as skin tears, lacerations, and abrasions. They may also be used on partial-thickness wounds, sutured wounds, and donor graft sites. Films may be used on red granular wounds and yellow slough-covered wounds with minimal drainage.[21] An amorphous hydrogel covered by a semipermeable film can be used to soften black eschar-covered wounds. Semipermeable film dressings may be used in areas of friction[21] to allow shearing forces to occur between the dressing and the support surface instead of the skin and the surface. Because film dressings are waterproof, they may be used to cover intravenous catheter sites or wounds to allow bathing. Semipermeable films have also been used to cover wounds prior to ultrasound treatment.

Precautions/Contraindications

To prevent maceration, a skin sealant (refer to the following section on moisturizers, skin sealants, and moisture barriers) must be applied to all areas of intact skin that will be covered by the film dressing. To prevent bacteria from entering the wound bed, clinicians must be sure to obtain a good edge seal. Film dressings will not adhere to wet or oily skin. If a channel or wrinkle forms, the edge seal is no longer intact, and the dressing must be changed. If the edge of a film dressing begins to separate from the intact skin, this area may be trimmed leaving the remainder of the dressing intact as long as the wound bed remains safely covered. Semipermeable films should not be used on infected wounds.[1,14] Refer to Box 7–4 for a review of semipermeable film dressings.

Sheet Hydrogels

Hydrogels are 80–99% water- or glycerin-based wound dressings that are available in sheets, amorphous gels, or impregnated gauzes (discussed previously).[1,8,44,49] Hydrogels are able to absorb a minimal amount of fluid by swelling. They are also able to donate moisture to dry wounds.[8,49-51] Hydrogels are permeable to gas and water, making them less effective bacterial barriers than semipermeable films or hydrocolloids.[46,47] They may dehydrate easily,[47] particularly if water based. When applied to the skin or wound, they feel cool and may decrease wound site pain.[1,8,49]

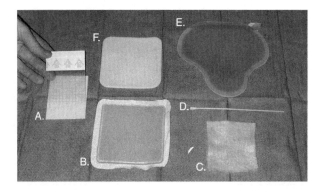

FIGURE 7–6 Moisture-retentive dressings labeled counterclockwise, from top left: *A.* semipermeable film, *B.* sheet hydrogel, *C.* sheet alginate, *D.* alginate-tipped applicator, *E.* hydrocolloid, and *F.* semipermeable foam.

BOX 7–4	Semipermeable Film Dressings
Benefits	• Moisture retentive • Encourage autolytic debridement • Reduce friction • Allow visualization of wound bed • Waterproof • Cost less over time
Limitations	• Adhesive may traumatize periwound upon removal • Cannot be used on highly exudating wounds • Can be difficult to apply, especially larger sizes • Should not be used on infected wounds
Common Uses	• Skin tears • Donor sites • Areas of friction • Abrasions • Over intravenous catheters to allow bathing/whirlpool • Over wounds for ultrasound treatment
Common Examples*	• BIOCLUSIVE • Cutifilm • Opsite • Polyskin • Tegaderm semipermeable film
Approximate Cost†	• $0.50–9.10

*This is a noninclusive, alphabetical list of products and should not be considered an endorsement of any brand/manufacturer.
†Actual cost may differ based on product size/characteristics, manufacturer, and distribution contracts.

Because almost all hydrogels are nonadhesive, they require a secondary dressing.

Common Uses

Sheet hydrogels are indicated for minimally or moderately draining wounds.[50] They are commonly used on superficial and partial-thickness wounds such as abrasions, skin tears, blisters, donor sites, radiation burns, thermal burns, pressure ulcers, diabetic ulcers, mastitis, and surgery sites. Amorphous hydrogels may be used over wounds as a coupling agent for ultrasound.[52] Sheet hydrogels can provide padding and may be used within total contact casts and splints to decrease pressure and shear forces. Amorphous hydrogels, available in tubes or spray bottles, can be used on dry wounds to obtain a moist wound environment.[17,49,51] Hydrogels are particularly effective at softening eschar to facilitate autolytic debridement.[8,53–55]

Precautions/Contraindications

Hydrogels are not able to absorb significant amounts of fluid and, therefore, should not be used on heavily draining wounds.[14] In addition, they absorb fluid fairly slowly,[7] so they are not usually appropriate for bleeding wounds. Sheet hydrogels should not be used on infected wounds. A skin sealant (refer to the following section on moisturizers, skin sealants, and moisture barriers) should be used to protect the periwound skin from maceration. An alternative method to reduce the potential of periwound maceration is to time the sheet hydrogel to the size of the wound. See Box 7–5 for a summary of hydrogel dressings.

BOX 7–5	Hydrogel Dressings	
Benefits	• Moisture retentive • Encourage autolytic debridement • Reduce pressure • Non- or minimally adherent	
Limitations	• May dehydrate • Cannot be used on highly exudating wounds • Generally require secondary dressing • Should not be used on infected wounds	
Common Uses	• Minimally to moderately exudating wounds • Pressure ulcers • Blisters • Abrasions • Skin tears • Burns (thermal and radiation) • Donor sites • Coupling medium for ultrasound • Padding for splints and total contact casts • Amorphous hydrogels can be used to soften eschar and provide a moist environment to dry wounds	
Common Examples*	**Sheet**	**Amorphous**
	• AQUASORB • Carradres • CarraSmart hydrogel • CURAGEL • Elastogel • Polyderm • Spenco 2nd Skin • Vigilon	• Biolex gel • Carrasyn gel • Carrington gel • CURAFIL gel • IntraSite gel • SAF-GEL
Approximate Cost†	• $2.75–10.00	• $9.00–34.00

*This is a noninclusive, alphabetical list of products and should not be considered an endorsement of any brand/manufacturer.
†Actual cost may differ based on product size/characteristics, manufacturer, and distribution contracts.

Semipermeable Foams

Semipermeable foam wound dressings are made of polyurethane foam with a hydrophilic wound side and a hydrophobic outside.[8] They are permeable to gas but not to bacteria.[1,19] Semipermeable foams have relatively high moisture vapor transmission rates. However, some semipermeable foams have a film backing to decrease the rate at which moisture vapor can escape, thereby increasing the amount of moisture that can be retained.[14] Some foam dressings are thin; others are thicker and provide more cushioning and absorption. Semipermeable foams provide thermal insulation[23] and come in both adhesive and nonadhesive forms.[1,8,14] The adhesives used in foam dressings are not as tacky as those used in semipermeable film dressings and hydrocolloids and, therefore, are less likely to cause trauma to frail skin upon removal. Adhesive foam dressings should be secured to a 1- to 2-cm border of intact skin. Nonadhesive foams require a secondary dressing. Foam dressings are easy to apply and remove. Semipermeable foam dressings are good to use on pressure ulcers. One study stated that stage II and stage III pressure ulcers treated with a semipermeable foam (Epilock) healed faster and with lower cost than similar ulcers treated with saline-moistened gauze.[56]

Common Uses

Semipermeable foams can be used on wounds with minimal to heavy exudate.[1,8] They are generally reserved for granulating or slough-covered partial- and full-thickness wounds. Semipermeable foams may be used on donor sites, ostomy sites, minor burns, diabetic ulcers, and venous insufficiency ulcers. If they are used on infected ulcers, foam dressings should be changed daily.

Precautions/Contraindications

Semipermeable foams are not indicated for dry or eschar-covered wounds. Because arterial ulcers tend to be very dry, semipermeable foams are not generally indicated for these wounds. Nonadhesive foams should be used on patients with fragile skin integrity. Foam dressings, particularly thicker foams, tend to roll in areas of high friction. Therefore, they may not be ideal for use in situations such as heel ulcers in a patient who is bed-bound. A skin sealant (refer to the following section on moisturizers, skin sealants, and moisture barriers) should be used to protect the periwound skin from maceration. See Box 7–6 for a review of semipermeable foam dressings.

Hydrocolloids

Hydrocolloids contain hydrophilic colloidal particles such as gelatin, pectin, and carboxymethylcellulose with a very strong film or foam adhesive backing.[8] This class of dressings varies greatly in absorption abilities, with different brands absorbing somewhere between 75% and 647% of their weight in fluid.[57] Hydrocolloids absorb exudate slowly by swelling into a gel-like mass. Upon removal, a residue commonly remains

within the wound bed.[21] Because this residue may have a foul odor, it is often mistaken as a sign of infection.[3] Hydrocolloids should be secured to a 1- to 2-cm border of intact skin. Hydrocolloids come in a variety of sizes and precut shapes. Several hydrocolloids have beveled edges to reduce the tendency for the dressing to roll when placed in high-friction areas. Hydrocolloids provide thermal insulation to the wound and are impermeable to water, oxygen, and bacteria.[50] The most highly studied hydrocolloid, DuoDerm, is an effective barrier against urine, stool, MRSA, hepatitis B, HIV-1, and *Pseudomonas aeruginosa*.[6,34] Wounds dressed with hydrocolloids have lower infection rates than wounds covered with gauze, semipermeable films, sheet hydrogels, or semipermeable foams.[4,46,58]

Common Uses

Hydrocolloids are indicated for partial- and full-thickness wounds.[50,59] They may be safely used on both granular and necrotic wounds. Several hydrocolloids come in a butterfly shape, designed for use over sacral and coccygeal pressure ulcers. Although used most often to treat pressure ulcers, hydrocolloids are also used on minor burns and venous insufficiency ulcers. In addition to the standard sheet hydrocolloids, hydrocolloid pastes and powders are also available to fill the cavities of heavily exudating wounds.[50]

Precautions/Contraindications

Hydrocolloids without beveled edges are likely to roll if placed in high-friction areas.[59] Hydrocolloids absorb fluid slowly, so they are not appropriate for managing bleeding wounds[7] or heavily draining wounds.[50] Because of the occlusive nature of hydrocolloids, these dressings are contraindicated in infected wounds.[1,14] Additionally, the rate of anaerobic infections is higher under occlusive dressings such as hydrocolloids. Occlusion may contribute to silent infections, so hydrocolloids should be used with caution on immunosuppressed patients. The use of hydrocolloids has been associated with hypergranulation. Because hypergranular tissue delays wound healing, these dressings should be discontinued at the first sign of hypergranulation. Hydrocolloids should not be used on dry wounds, such as arterial ulcers, third-degree burns,[50] or wounds with minimal drainage. Hydrocolloids should not be used on wounds with exposed tendon or fascia[50] to avoid dessication of these structures. Because of the strong adhesive backings of most hydrocolloids, these dressings should only be used

BOX 7–6	Semipermeable Foam Dressings
Benefits	• Moisture retentive • Encourage autolytic debridement • Provide thermal insulation • Many provide cushioning • Available in both adherent and nonadherent forms • Absorb moderate amounts of exudate
Limitations	• Adhesive may traumatize periwound upon removal • May roll in areas of friction • Should not be used on infected wounds unless changed daily
Common Uses	• Minor burns • Skin grafts • Donor sites • Ostomy sites • Pressure ulcers • Venous insufficiency ulcers • Neuropathic (diabetic) ulcers
Common Examples*	• ALLEVYN • CURAFOAM • Cutinova foam, thin, cavity • Epi-lock • Flexzan • HYDRASORB • LYOFOAM, with/without carbon • Mitraflex • Optifoam
Approximate Cost†	• $4.29–16.81

*This is a noninclusive, alphabetical list of products and should not be considered an endorsement of any brand/manufacturer.

†Actual cost may differ based on product size/characteristics, manufacturer, and distribution contracts.

on patients with good skin integrity.[59] A skin sealant (refer to the following section on moisturizers, skin sealants, and moisture barriers) should be used to protect the periwound skin from maceration. Refer to Box 7–7 for a review of hydrocolloid dressings.

Alginates

Alginate wound dressings are salts of alginic acid extracted from certain types of brown seaweed[1] and converted into calcium/sodium salts.[44,60] Alginates have a soft, cotton-like appearance and can be either woven or nonwoven. When placed within the wound bed, alginate dressings react with serum and wound exudate to form a hydrophilic gel.[61,62] This gel provides a moist wound environment and may trap bacteria, which can then be washed away during dressing changes.[61] Clinicians should be careful not to confuse this gel-like state for infection. Alginates and sheet dressings made from carboxymethycellulose have similar qualities and forms, therefore, these two dressings are sometimes referred to as hydrofiber dressings.[8,14]

BOX 7–7	**Hydrocolloid Dressings**	
Benefits	• Moisture retentive • Encourage autolytic debridement • Impermeable to urine, stool, bacteria • Provide thermal insulation • Waterproof • Some have beveled edges to prevent dressing from rolling up • Provide moderate absorption	
Limitations	• Will likely traumatize fragile periwound upon removal • Leave residue within wound bed • May cause hypergranulation • May roll in areas of friction • Should not be used on infected wounds	
Common Uses	• Pressure ulcers • Burns • Venous insufficiency ulcers • For use on periwound to attach adhesive tape in the case of large wounds	
Common Examples* (sheets)	• Comfeel • Cutinova • DuoDerm regular, extra thin, CGF • Replicare • Restore regular, extra thin • Tegaderm hydrocolloid regular, thin • Ultec	Also available in paste and powder form
Approximate Cost[†]	• $5.45–18.00	

[*]This is a noninclusive, alphabetical list of products and should not be considered an endorsement of any brand/manufacturer.

[†]Actual cost may differ based on product size/characteristics, manufacturer, and distribution contracts.

Alginates are highly permeable and nonocclusive. Therefore, they require a secondary dressing, most commonly gauze. Alginates are available in three forms. Alginate sheets may be placed on wound beds to absorb drainage. Alginate ropes are used to lightly fill wound tunnels or areas of undermining.[39,50] Alginate-tipped applicators can be used to probe wounds, fill wound cavities and tunnels, perform swab cultures,[63] and measure wound depth. Alginate-tipped applicators are superior to cotton swabs because they do not cause the body to mount an inflammatory response if wisps are left behind in the wound bed.[14] Additionally, alginates may stimulate macrophage activity.

Common Uses

Alginates are purported to absorb up to 20 times their weight in exudate;[64] therefore, these dressings are indicated for moderately or highly draining wounds.[1,8] Alginates are typically used on partial- and full-thickness draining wounds, such as venous insufficiency ulcers, pressure ulcers, neuropathic ("diabetic") ulcers, and burns. A comparison of alginates and gauze packing strips for cavity wounds found lower overall cost, decreased pain with dressing changes, and less frequent dressing changes with alginate dressings.[39] Since infected wounds tend to have significant amounts of drainage, alginates are ideal primary dressings for these types of wounds.[1,14,65] When used on infected wounds, dressings should be changed at least daily. Alginates can be used on both granular and slough-covered wounds. Although some authors suggest premoistening alginate sheets when treating dry, eschar-covered wounds,[60] there is little advantage to this technique, and the cost per dressing change is significantly increased. Therefore, alginates are not indicated for use on dry or minimally draining wounds.[14]

Precautions/Contraindications

Alginate dressings are not recommended for use on full-thickness (also known as third-degree) burns.[50] Because of the risk of desiccating tissues with high collagen contents, alginates should not be used on wounds with exposed tendon, joint capsule, or bone.[50]

Alginates are not recommended for use in neonates born at less than 38 weeks of gestation as the dressing's absorption of sodium and calcium can alter neonate electrolyte balance.[8] A skin sealant (refer to the following section on moisturizers, skin sealants, and moisture barriers) should be used to protect the periwound skin from maceration. See Box 7–8 for a summary of alginate dressings.

Composite Dressings

Composite, or combination, **dressings** are multilayer dressings that can be used as primary or secondary wound dressings.[14] Most composite dressings have three layers. The inner contact layer is nonadherent, preventing trauma to the wound bed during dressing changes. The middle layer absorbs moisture and wicks it away from the wound bed to prevent maceration while

BOX 7–8	**Alginate Dressings**	
Benefits	• Encourage autolytic debridement • Highly absorbent • Can be used on infected and uninfected wounds • Biocompatible • Nonadherent	
Limitations	• Require secondary dressing • Use with extreme caution with exposed tendon, capsule, or bone to prevent desiccation	
Common Uses	• Highly exudating wounds • Venous insufficiency ulcers • Tunneling wounds • Swabs used to probe, fill, and measure wound depth	
Common Examples*	• ALGISITE M • CURASORB • Cutinova alginate • Kaltostat • Maxsorb • Restore CalciCare • Sorbsan	Available in sheets, ropes, and on applicators
Approximate Cost†	• $4.50–15.00	

*This is a noninclusive, alphabetical list of products and should not be considered an endorsement of any brand/manufacturer.
†Actual cost may differ based on product size/characteristics, manufacturer, and distribution contracts.

maintaining a moist wound environment. This middle layer may consist of a hydrogel, semipermeable foam, hydrocolloid, or alginate. The outer layer serves as a bacterial barrier and is commonly composed of a semipermeable film. The number of composite dressings on the market today continues to grow exponentially. However, the clinician should remember that composite dressings are merely a combination of moisture-retentive and/or gauze dressings packaged in a different way. Because composite dressings are prepackaged, they have less flexibility in terms of indications for use, and buying and storing these dressings can be quite costly. Most clinicians in general wound care practice are better able to meet the wound dressing needs of their patients by using one of the major categories of wound care products reviewed previously or combining dressings on-site based on individual patient needs.

Antimicrobial Dressings

Silver and cadexomer iodine are broad-spectrum antiseptic agents (see Chapter 6) that have been incorporated into virtually all classes of dressings (see Figure 7–7). Because the vast majority of dressings and anecdotal evidence addresses the use of silver, this will be the focus of the information provided unless otherwise noted. The rate and percentage of silver released from a dressing depends on many factors, including the form of silver within the dressing, wound characteristics (depth, surface area, amount of wound moisture), and type of dressing.[66–68] It appears that dressings with free silver release greater than 20 mg/l have the best results.[69] The increased availability of silver dressings may be due to technological advancements, new research about delayed wound healing associated with biofilms and critically colonized wounds, and, perhaps most importantly, very aggressive marketing strategies by product manufacturers.

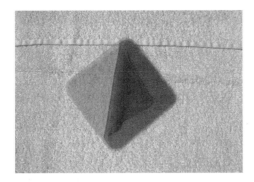

FIGURE 7–7   Moisture-retentive dressings. Example of a sheet hydrogel impregnated with silver.

Clinicians must obtain all relevant information and use sound judgment when choosing wound care products. Despite widespread use, several authors as well as a 2009 *Cochrane Review* report there is no sound research to date to support the use of silver-impregnated dressings.[69–71] While silver undoubtedly is able to kill multiple types of microorganisms in isolation, such as in a lab or experimentally produced wound inoculated with just one strain of bacteria, there is little research to support that silver is effective against multiple organisms within the same wound or against biofilms.[67,72,73] Second, there is no evidence that silver's antimicrobial abilities are effective in the presence of slough or necrotic tissue.[67] Third, silver dressings should be used with caution in epithelializing and granulating wounds because silver is cytotoxic to fibroblasts and single layers of epithelial cells in vitro as well and retards wound epithelialization in vivo.[73] Fourth, while silver dressings (and cadexomer iodine dressings) have been shown to consistently decrease wound bioburden, there is no evidence that prophylactic use of antimicrobial-impregnated dressings (or topical agents) will enhance wound healing in uninfected wounds.[69, 74–76] Fifth, manufacturers' claims and manufacturer-sponsored research, as always, must be carefully examined. For example, one manufacturer may tout its product's ability to kill microbes faster than the competition. While one product may be bactericidal in vivo in just 45 minutes compared to the 2 hours required by a competing manufacturer's product, this distinction between products is not clinically relevant.[73] Alternatively, manufacturers may market their product as the fastest release of silver on the market, but there is no research to support that this accelerates the rate of wound healing.[73] Last, silver dressings cost more than standard moisture-retentive dressings, driving up total wound care costs. This cost may be acceptable if the silver dressing facilitates wound healing. However, two recent studies comparing a silver dressing with a non-silver-containing moisture-retentive dressing in patients with chronic ulcers found no significant difference in wound healing or infection.[77,78]

Common Uses

Silver has been incorporated into virtually all classes of dressings including gauze, semipermeable films, hydrocolloids, semipermeable foams, and alginates, as well as cloth or fabric dressings.[79, 80] Dressings containing silver may be primary or secondary dressings, adhesive or nonadhesive, and vary greatly in absorptive capabilities based on the class of dressing it has been incorporated into. Silver dressings are FDA-approved for use on partial- and full-thickness wounds. The National Pressure Ulcer Advisory Panel's updated guidelines for the treatment of pressure ulcers states that silver-impregnated dressings should be considered for pressure ulcers that are heavily colonized in patients at high risk of infection.[81]

Precautions/Contraindications

Release of silver ions can result in a blue-black wound bed discoloration due to insoluble silver sulfide precipitation.[68,71] This should not be mistaken for eschar. Silver dressings should only be used short term and discontinued once infection is controlled.[81,82] Clinicians must read manufacturer labels carefully when using silver dressings and monitor for signs of hypersensitivity or adverse reactions.[68] Some dressings require premoistening with water prior to use. Saline should not be used, as it deactivates the silver.[82] Cadexomer iodine dressings should not be used in patients that are sensitive to iodine, patients with thyroid disease, or in patients with large cavity wounds.[81] As with any other intervention, antimicrobial dressings should be discontinued and alternate treatments initiated if no improvements in wound status are noted after 1 or 2 weeks of use.[83,84] Refer to Box 7–9 for a review of antimicrobial dressings.

BOX 7–9	Antimicrobial Dressings: Specifically Silver Dressings

Benefits	• Broad-spectrum antimicrobial
	• Proposed methods of action
	  ◦ Binding damages bacterial cell membrane
	  ◦ Interferes with bacterial ATP synthesis
	  ◦ Impairs bacterial DNA replication
	  ◦ Reduces MMP levels

Limitations	• Paucity of research support • High cost • Cannot be used in combination with electrical stimulation • Must be removed prior to MRI • Not recommended for neonates due to potential toxicity
Common Uses	• Partial- and full-thickness chronic wounds • Burns • Donor sites • Neuropathic foot ulcers • Pressure ulcers • Traumatic wounds • Venous insufficiency ulcers
Common Examples*	• Acticoat • Actisorb • Aquacel AG • Arglaes • Contreet • SilvaSorb
Approximate Cost†	• $10.00–27.80

*This is a noninclusive, alphabetical list of products and should not be considered an endorsement of any brand/manufacturer.
†Actual cost may differ based on product size/characteristics, manufacturer, and distribution contracts.

Checkpoint Question #2

Your patient presents with a granular, traumatic wound on the lateral lower leg. You are currently bandaging the wound twice weekly with a hydrocolloid. How might you modify this dressing if:

a. the wound bed appears dry on your next visit?

b. the periwound is macerated and there is strike-through evident on the hydrocolloid?

Charcoal Dressings

Charcoal has been incorporated into several classes of wound dressings. The key function of charcoal dressings is to control wound odor by absorbing odor-producing gases released by bacteria and absorb wound drainage.[14, 81,85–87] While charcoal dressings do not enhance wound healing more than any other type of moisture-retentive dressing, they may improve quality of life in patients by allowing them to feel more comfortable participating in social interactions without the fear of unpleasant wound odor.[14, 87] This is particularly important in patients in whom wound debridement is not consistent with the overall plan of care, such as those with end-stage cancer and an infected pressure ulcer.

Honey-Impregnated Dressings

Topical honey and honey-impregnated dressings have reemerged in the last several years. Again, new information regarding infection, colonization, biofilms, and bacterial resistance may be driving this resurgence. Honey, specifically *Leptospermum* aka Mankua, appears to assist with wound healing in several ways (see Box 7–10).[70, 88–90] The National Pressure Ulcer Advisory Panel's revised guidelines suggest honey be considered to control wound bioburden and wound odor.[81] Honey may decrease wound-related pain, reduce wound healing time, and improve scar tissue formation.[90] Due to its high osmolality, honey may cause a mild stinging sensation when first applied.

Collagen Dressings

Collagen is the most abundant protein in the body.[91] Collagen dressings are a class of dressings that contain collagen from various animal or human sources that may promote wound healing in a variety of ways (see Box 7–11).[1, 19, 92–95] Collagen has been incorporated into sheets, ropes, and pad wound dressings and can be applied topically as a gel, paste, powder, or as particles. Collagen dressings, particularly pastes and powders, may be difficult to apply and require a secondary dressing to ensure a good edge seal.[7] Once

> **BOX 7–10   Purported Ways in Which Honey Improves Wound Healing**
>
> - Antimicrobial
>   - Creates acidic wound environment
>   - May be effective against antibiotic-resistant strains of bacteria
> - Decreases wound-related pain
> - Stimulates angioblasts, fibroblasts, and monocytes
> - Reduces inflammation and edema
> - Osmotic action controls wound drainage
> - May contain or stimulate growth factors

> **BOX 7–11   Purported Ways in Which Collagen Dressings Assist with Wound Healing**
>
> - Stimulate macrophages, angioblasts, keratinocytes, and platelets
> - Protect host growth factors
> - Provide a scaffolding for host cell proliferation and migration
> - Maintain healthy wound moisture levels by donating fluid or absorbing drainage
> - May encourage healthier balance between MMPs and TIMPs within wound
> - Common examples[*]
>   - BIOSTEP
>   - Promogran
>   - Puracol
> - Approximate cost[†]: $17.10–36.61
>
> [*]This is a noninclusive, alphabetical list of products and should not be considered an endorsement of any brand/manufacturer.
> [†]Actual cost may differ based on product size/characteristics, manufacturer, and distribution contracts.

in place, collagen dressings adhere to the wound bed but not to the periwound. Although generally left in place until the wound is resurfaced underneath, collagen dressings may be changed anywhere from daily to weekly. Collagen dressings have been used for acute and chronic wounds that are partial or full-thickness including burns, neuropathic (diabetic) ulcers, pressure ulcers, surgical wounds, and venous ulcers. The National Pressure Ulcer Advisory Panel's revised guidelines suggest collagen dressings be considered for nonhealing category/stage III or IV pressure ulcers.[81] Collagen wound dressings are contraindicated for patients who are sensitive to collagen or any of its components, such as bovine or porcine tissue.[21] Clinicians should read the product insert for specific information. At least one study comparing a collagen dressing to a hydrocolloid demonstrated no benefit to the collagen dressing despite a nearly 40% higher cost of wound management.[95] At this time, more research is needed before collagen can be considered a standard wound dressing.

SKIN AND PERIWOUND CARE

To this point, this chapter has focused on wound dressings. However, it is also critical for clinicians to protect the skin and periwound skin using moisture barriers or skin sealants and to manage dry skin with moisturizers. Tissue adhesives are alternatives for acute primary wound closure. Because clinicians may encounter tissue adhesives when performing skin and scar management, these are included in this section. Silicone dressings used for scar management are addressed in Chapter 14.

Skin Sealants and Moisture Barriers

Skin sealants and **moisture barriers** are two types of skin protectants (see Box 7–12). These substances form a protective layer or coating over the skin, preventing water, topical agents, and wound or body fluids from causing skin breakdown.[12,50,85] Skin sealants are generally alcohol-based wipes used on intact periwound skin.[50] Skin sealants make the skin surface slightly tacky, providing a better edge seal for adhesive dressings while simultaneously protecting the skin from the adhesive.[21] The alcohol within sealants can cause a mild stinging sensation if allowed to contact open skin in patients with intact sensation. Spray skin sealants are commonly used over category/stage I pressure ulcers to protect intact skin.[50] In contrast, moisture barriers are ointments or creams that contain petrolatum, dimethicone, and/or zinc oxide. Although moisture barriers can be used on periwound skin, they are primarily used to prevent rashes and skin breakdown in areas of incontinence.[96,97] Moisture barriers make the skin surface slightly oily, preventing any adhesives

BOX 7–12	Skin Sealants and Moisture Barriers
Benefits	• Protect the skin from maceration • Minimally protect the skin from adhesives
Limitations	• May build up around the wound edge • Cream version cannot be used with adhesive dressings
Common Uses	• Any time moisture-retentive dressings are used • When adding a topical agent to the wound bed • On macerated periwound/perineum
Common Examples*	• Aloe Vesta protective barrier spray/ointment • Bard's protective barrier film wipes • Hollister moisture barrier skin ointment • Sensi-Care protective barrier • Skin Prep
Approximate Cost	• Wipes $0.21–0.28/wipe. • Ointments $2.10–2.80/oz.
*This is a noninclusive, alphabetical list of products and should not be considered an endorsement of any brand/manufacturer.	

from sticking to the skin and precluding their use in combination with adhesive wound dressings. While skin sealants and moisture barriers are designed for use on intact skin, some moisture barriers may be safely applied to rashes and broken skin. Clinicians should carefully read the manufacturers' directions for use before applying moisture barriers to nonintact skin.

The following three examples will help illustrate why the periwound tissue of all wounds should be protected. First, consider a patient with a moderately draining wound. The clinician should use a dressing designed to absorb this amount of drainage, such as a hydrocolloid, with the goal of leaving the dressing in place for about 5 days. Because of the moist wound environment created and maintained by the hydrocolloid, a skin sealant should be applied to protect all of the intact skin that will be covered by the dressing from maceration and from the adhesive within the hydrocolloid. Next, consider a patient with a nondraining wound. The clinician would need to add moisture to the wound bed to create a moist wound healing environment. The clinician may choose to use an amorphous hydrogel, an impregnated gauze, a gauze square, and a roll gauze and change the dressing daily. As the bandage and the patient move, it is unlikely that the hydrogel added to the wound will stay directly over the wound bed; rather, it will also come into contact with the periwound skin. The gauze square will become moist and may cause maceration in areas where it contacts the periwound skin. In this case, a skin sealant applied to the periwound skin will help protect the skin from the moist environment required to maximize wound healing. Last, consider a patient with Alzheimer's disease who is frequently incontinent of bowel and bladder and has developed a perineal rash but no open wounds. This patient's skin breakdown would be best managed with a moisture barrier.[96]

Moisturizers

Sebum normally maintains skin hydration and provides a protective layer that helps to minimize fluid loss through the skin. Excessive bathing, soaps that strip the skin of natural oils, low environmental humidity, poor hydration, smoking, and sun exposure all increase the risk of dry skin.[98] Older adults are more likely to have dry skin due to the slower rate of skin cell turnover and decreased water and fat emulsions produced by their skin.[98,99] Individuals with diabetes also have an increased prevalence of dry skin.[100] Dry skin can lead to inflammation, cracking, scaling,

and even fissuring of the skin. Once the barrier function of the skin is lost, there is an increased risk of infection. Moisturizers, creams, and lotions are used both to prevent dry skin and to help restore the skin's normal level of hydration. In addition to treating the dry skin itself, clinicians should identify and address the reason for a patient's dry skin. For example, the patient may need to change the type of soap used, bathe less frequently, or drink more noncaffeinated beverages.[99,101]

Moisturizers are a key component to basic skin care[102] and are the most effective means of preventing and treating dry skin. Moisturizers help restore the barrier function of the epidermis, provide a soothing protective film over intact skin, and increase the water content of the epidermis.[102] Moisturizers may slow evaporative moisture loss through the skin, thereby maintaining skin hydration and appearance.[102] Clinicians should choose moisturizers without perfumes or alcohols because these substances may cause skin reactions. Petrolatum-containing moisturizers form a protective layer over the skin and penetrate the stratum corneum, making them particularly effective in the management of calluses, dry skin in individuals with diabetes, and burn scars. Moisturizers should be applied to intact skin twice daily. Because of the risk of fungal infections, moisturizers should not be applied between the toes. Ointments are mixtures of water and oil, typically lanolin. Ointments, like moisturizers, form an occlusive protective layer over the skin, enhancing their ability to relieve dry skin. Creams and lotions consist primarily of water, making them less occlusive and less effective in the treatment of dry skin. These substances require more frequent applications and may provide only temporary relief of dry skin.

Tissue Adhesives

Tissue adhesives, also known as skin glues, are rarely used in the physical therapy setting. However, clinicians should be aware of their benefits and limitations, especially since many are now available over the counter to the general public. Tissue adhesives are specially formulated compounds that allow primary wound closure without the use of staples or sutures.[103–105] As such, they decrease treatment time, are associated with less pain, and do not require a follow-up visit for removal.[104,106] When compared to traditional primary wound closure, there is no difference in scar cosmesis[104,106] or infection rates.[103,107,108] Tissue adhesives are associated with a clinically insignificant 4% increase in wound dehiscence rates.[103, 108] They are appropriate for acute linear wounds without tissue loss.[107] To decrease the risk of infection, tissue adhesives should not be used in heavily contaminated wounds, puncture wounds, or wounds more than 12 hours old.[108] To decrease the risk of dehiscence, creams, adhesives (such as an adhesive bandage or steri-strips), and antimicrobial ointments should not be used in combination with tissue adhesives.[107] When compared to wounds closed with sutures, wounds closed with tissue adhesives have 12 times less tensile strength immediately after application.[104] However, after 1 week, there is no difference in wound tensile strength.[104] Therefore, wounds crossing a joint should not be treated with tissue adhesives[108] because of the potential for dehiscence from high tensile forces.[109] Wounds with exposed deep tissues should not be treated with tissue adhesives.[104]

THE FUTURE OF WOUND MANAGEMENT

A new wave of wound management products, surpassing the use of gauze and moisture-retentive dressings, is emerging. Advances in biomedical engineering have led to the ability to harvest growth factors to aid in chronic wound healing. Technological innovations have allowed wound management to move beyond skin grafts, the most widely used means of providing early wound coverage, to biosynthetic dressings and skin substitutes. Although these interventions are not yet standards in wound management, their limited use to date continues to show tremendous promise. This section provides a brief overview of these exciting advances.

Growth Factors

Growth factor is an all-encompassing term including cytokines, interleukins, and colony-stimulating factors.[91, 110] Recall from Chapter 2 that growth factors are growth-promoting substances that increase or enhance cell size, proliferation, or activity. Because endogenous growth factors have been isolated in healing wounds, it is believed that these substances assist with wound healing. In animal models, the addition of growth factors accelerates collagen deposition, increases wound tensile strength, and enhances epithelialization.[10] In humans, wounds treated with topically applied epidermal growth factor (EGF), fibroblast growth factor (FGF), or platelet-derived growth factor (PDGF) improved significantly more than wounds treated with a placebo.[14, 110] Becaplermin gel and small intestinal submucosa are two examples of these products on the market today.

Becaplermin (Regranex) gel contains PDGF and has been approved for use on diabetic foot ulcers that extend into, but not through, the subcutaneous tissue.[111] PDGF is the most extensively researched growth factor used for wound management and has been found to stimulate migration of inflammatory cells and fibroblasts into the wound area, enhance collagen deposition, and increase granulation tissue formation.[50] A measured quantity of Regranex is applied directly to the wound and covered with saline-moistened gauze. After 12 hours, the dressing is rinsed with saline and a new moist dressing without Regranex is applied to the wound. These two dressing changes are repeated daily. When used in combination with debridement, pressure relief, and standard wound care, this product has been shown to enhance wound healing.[111] Because patients exposed to large amounts of becaplermin gel were found to have a five-time increased risk of developing cancer, the Food and Drug Administration has placed a black box warning on this product to limit its use to three tubes or less.[112]

A wound dressing made from freeze-dried porcine small intestinal submucosa, Oasis,[113] contains an acellular matrix of collagen (Types I, III, and IV) and growth factors (TGF-β and FGF-2).[114] This dressing has been used to facilitate wound healing in partial-thickness ulcers due to arterial insufficiency, diabetes, pressure, surgery, trauma, and venous insufficiency.[110, 115] A recent study of patients with mixed arterial and venous insufficiency ulcers demonstrated a statistically significant increase in wound healing rates and percentage of healed wounds when comparing wounds treated with Oasis versus wounds treated with petrolatum-impregnated gauze.[115] The National Pressure Ulcer Advisory Panel recently concluded that while some studies suggest growth factors, such as PDGF, may assist with wound healing, there is insufficient evidence at this time to recommend the use of growth factors for pressure ulcer treatment.[81]

Oasis is shipped in dry form and has a shelf-life of up to 1 year. The thin sheet is trimmed to the size of the wound, leaving a slight overlap with the periwound, then rehydrated and molded over the wound bed (see Figure 7–8). If the wound is infected or there is significant drainage, Oasis should be fenestrated. The wound

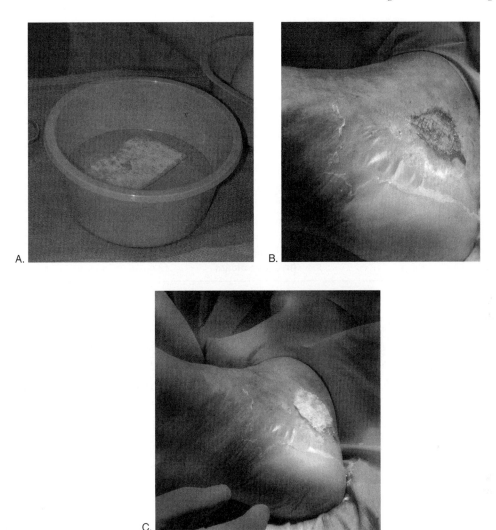

FIGURE 7–8 Surgical placement of Oasis on a patient with a chronic ulcer inferior to his medial malleolus. In many cases, Oasis may be applied in the clinic setting. *A.* Oasis dressing being rehydrated prior to application. *B.* The wound is scored by the surgeon, causing minimal bleeding to provide a better environment for the dressing. *C.* The Oasis is cut to size and placed over the wound bed. A moist dressing will be applied over the Oasis.

is then covered with a moist compression dressing. Oasis placement can take place in the clinic or as part of a surgical procedure, such as surgical debridement. During subsequent dressing changes, any loose edges are trimmed and additional layers of Oasis may be applied. Oasis and becaplermin appear to be equally effective in facilitating neuropathic wound healing.[116]

Numerous growth factors have shown promise in stimulating delayed wound healing. At this time, the use of growth factors to facilitate delayed wound healing is extremely costly and limited to chronic wounds that are recalcitrant to standard interventions. Current research is directed toward determining the therapeutic concentrations of individual growth factors required to enhance wound healing. It appears that different growth factors may work in combination with one another or at different phases of wound healing.[3,110,117] Future studies will likely search for the ideal combination(s) of growth factors necessary to maximize healing potential and to determine the relative value of using growth factors on different wound types (acute, chronic, and caused by various etiologies).[117] Table 7–1 reviews promising growth factors under investigation in clinical trials.[50,110,118–123]

TABLE 7–1 Promising Growth Factors to Enhance Wound Healing

Growth Factor	Preliminary Research
Fibroblast Growth Factor (FGF-1 and FGF-2)	• Appears to stimulate angiogenesis and improve wound perfusion, granulation tissue formation, and wound contraction in pressure ulcers • Component of Oasis
Granulocyte Macrophage–Colony Stimulating Factor (GM-CSF)	• Increases granulation tissue formation • Venous ulcers healed significantly faster with growth factor than placebo • May assist with healing of infected neuropathic ulcers
Interleukin 1β (IL-1β)	• Investigations currently examining effect on healing of infected pressure ulcers
Keratinocyte Growth Factor (KGF)	• May assist with wound epithelialization but not wound contraction • May not significantly improve wound closure rate
Platelet-Derived Growth Factor (PDGF)	• Increases angiogenesis and granulation tissue formation • Stimulates migration of inflammatory cells and fibroblasts • Increases rate of healing in wounds due to pressure, venous insufficiency, and neuropathy • FDA-approved product currently available
Transforming Growth Factor-Beta (TGF-β)	• Appears to increase angiogenesis, granulation tissue formation, and epithelialization in venous insufficiency ulcers • Component of Oasis

Biosynthetic Dressings and Skin Substitutes

Biologic dressing and **biosynthetic dressings** are derived from natural tissues. These dressings are believed to be superior to moisture-retentive dressings because they restore the skin's natural barrier properties, preventing evaporative water loss, heat loss, protein and electrolyte loss, and bacterial contamination.[19] Biological and biosynthetic dressings encourage autolytic debridement and help create a healthy granular wound bed.

Skin grafts have been used to provide skin coverage for wounds with extensive surface areas, large full-thickness burns, and chronic wounds that failed to heal with traditional interventions (see Chapter 14). Although they can successfully lead to wound closure, skin grafts have certain limitations. Allografts (tissue grafts taken from a cadaver) and xenografts (tissue grafts taken from an animal, usually a pig)[19] are very costly and have a short shelf-life. Clinicians must also be aware of differing cultural and religious beliefs regarding the use of animal and neonatal tissues, and informed consent should be obtained prior to the use of these products.[124] Autografts (tissue grafts taken from an unaffected area of the patient and transferred to the affected region) are also problematic in that a new wound is created and the supply of new grafts can be extremely limited in cases of large surface area wounds, such as burns.

Recent advances in tissue engineering have led to the ability to produce **skin substitutes** that do not create an immune response from the patient and can be used for temporary or extended wound coverage. Clinical indications for the use of tissue-engineered skin products include nonhealing, uninfected partial- and full-thickness venous insufficiency ulcers, neuropathic ulcers, burns, and traumatic wounds.[125, 126] The National Pressure Ulcer Advisory Panel's most recent guidelines state that while there appears to be some evidence to support the use of these dressings for neuropathic (diabetic) ulcers, there is currently not enough data at this time to recommend their use for pressure ulcers.[81] The primary goal of skin substitutes is to achieve rapid wound closure and restore normal skin function. These products generally consist of bilayered systems that approximate the structure and function of human epidermis and dermis. Table 7–2 describes several skin substitutes currently on the market.[21, 50, 126–132] Because biosynthetic dressings and skin substitutes are generally reserved for use in highly specialized areas of wound care, such as burn clinics, a complete account of these products is beyond the scope of this text. The reader should refer to other sources for detailed information regarding these promising new products.[125, 130, 133–135]

TABLE 7–2   Skin Substitutes

Skin Substitute	Description
Alloderm	• Acellular dermis • Used for permanent coverage of partial-thickness burns and soft tissue replacement
Apligraf	• Also known as Graftskin, bilayered matrix containing cultured neonatal keratinocytes and fibroblasts on Type I bovine collagen, contains granulocyte/macrophage colony-stimulating factor • Used for permanent coverage of nonhealing neuropathic, pressure, or venous insufficiency ulcers, chronic wounds, and full-thickness burns
Biobrane	• Synthetic dermis, temporary skin substitute comprised of an inner nylon layer and outer silicone layer with added bovine collagen • Most commonly used for temporary coverage of partial- and full-thickness burns
Dermagraft	• Cultured neonatal fibroblasts in a polyglycan mesh • Used as a skin substitute for burns and neuropathic ulcers
Epicel	• Epidermal substitute consisting of cultured autogenous keratinocytes • Used for permanent coverage of large deep partial-thickness or full-thickness wounds
GRAFTJACKET	• Human acellular dermal tissue matrix
Integra	• Collagen glycoaminoglycan dermal matrix covered with an outer silicone layer; requires thin skin graft over it for definitive closure • Used for permanent coverage of full-thickness burns
Transcyte	• Inner nylon layer containing neonatal fibroblasts covered with an outer silicone mesh layer • Used for temporary coverage of partial- and full-thickness burns

Checkpoint Question #3

Your 55-year-old patient sustained a partial-thickness volar forearm wound 3 days ago in a boating accident. She has a history of osteoarthritis. The wound is uninfected and measures 3.4 × 4.0 cm. Which of the following dressings is *not* appropriate at this time for this patient? Why?

a. Amorphous hydrogel with a gauze dressing
b. Semipermeable film
c. Semipermeable foam
d. Growth factor with a gauze dressing

CLINICAL DECISION MAKING

After becoming familiar with the basic properties of the main categories of wound dressings, the clinician must select an appropriate wound dressing based on the information obtained during the wound examination. In most cases, the desired outcome of wound management is wound healing: the wound bed is completely resurfaced with epithelium, and the tissue is remodeled so that its strength approaches normal. An interim step in this process is to obtain a clean, warm, moist granular wound bed while protecting the periwound and intact skin. There are two key questions the clinician must answer to determine the most appropriate local wound care:

1. Is the wound draining or nondraining?
2. Is the wound granular or necrotic?

After these two key questions are answered, the clinician must consider other factors affecting local wound management to finetune the choice of the most appropriate wound dressing.

Draining or Nondraining

Because a moist wound environment enhances wound healing, the dressing selected must assist with obtaining and maintaining this type of environment. The key clinical decision point, therefore, is determining whether the wound is draining or nondraining. A draining wound requires a dressing with the ability to absorb moisture[22] and protect the surrounding tissue from maceration.[9,13,15] A nondraining wound requires a dressing that provides moisture or prevents evaporative fluid loss.[9,13,15,22] Since moisture will be added to the wound bed, as with a hydrogel, a skin sealant is also required to protect the surrounding tissues of nondraining wounds. Prior to removing a wound dressing, the clinician should always check to see when the dressing was applied. This can help determine the amount of wound drainage and the ability of the current dressing to handle this moisture content.

Granular or Necrotic

A granular wound requires a dressing that will protect the wound bed from trauma. In contrast, a necrotic wound requires debridement. The clinician must determine the most appropriate method(s) to accomplish the removal of necrotic tissue (see Chapter 5).

The type of debridement used helps to determine the most appropriate wound dressing. If autolytic debridement is indicated, a moisture-retentive dressing should be selected and remain in place for several days.[81] If enzymatic debridement is desired, a gauze dressing is typically most appropriate because the dressing must be changed one to three times per day. If the clinician wants to use a dressing to mechanically debride the wound, a wet-to-dry gauze is the dressing of choice.[40]

Wound Dressing Decision Grid

By considering the first two key decision points and the characteristics of the main categories of wound dressings, the clinician can develop a wound dressing decision grid (see Table 7–3). Wounds can be grouped into four categories: (1) granular and nondraining, (2) granular and draining, (3) necrotic and nondraining, and (4) necrotic and draining.

Granular and Nondraining

A granular and nondraining wound is healing as expected. The granulation tissue and periwound should be protected. To attain a moist wound environment, moisture may need to be added, as with an amorphous hydrogel, or a more occlusive dressing may be needed to better retain the wound's moisture content.

Granular and Draining

If a wound is granular and draining, the granulation tissue and periwound should be protected. To obtain a moist, but not wet, wound environment, a more absorptive dressing should be applied. Since there is no necrotic tissue to be solubilized, the most common reason for a granular wound to be heavily draining is the presence of an infection. Excessive drainage from a granular wound or friable granulation tissue may be the only sign of a silent infection in patients who are immunocompromised or patients with chronic wounds. If the wound is not infected, the drainage indicates that the dressing may need to be changed more frequently or be slightly more absorptive.

Necrotic and Nondraining

The necrotic, nondraining wound requires debridement and softening of eschar. To attain a moist wound environment, moisture may need to be added,

TABLE 7–3   Wound Dressing Decision Grid

Wound Description	Short-Term Goals	Debridement Options	Dressing Options*
Granular, nondraining	1. Obtain/maintain moist environment 2. Protect surrounding tissue	NA	Gauze[†] Impregnated gauze[†] Transparent film Hydrogel
Granular, draining	1. Observe for infection 2. Absorb exudate 3. Protect surrounding tissue	NA	Gauze Alginate Semipermeable foam Hydrocolloid[†]
Necrotic, nondraining	1. Soften eschar 2. Remove eschar 3. Obtain/maintain moist environment 4. Protect surrounding tissue	1. Surgical 2. Sharp 3. Enzymatic 4. Autolytic[‡]	Gauze[†] Impregnated gauze Transparent film Hydrogel Hydrocolloid
Necrotic, draining	1. Observe for infection 2. Absorb exudate 3. Remove eschar 4. Protect surrounding tissue	1. Surgical 2. Sharp 3. Enzymatic 4. Autolytic[‡]	Gauze Alginate Semipermeable foam Hydrocolloid[‡]

*Skin sealant should be applied to intact periwound as needed.
[†]With topical agent, such as an amorphous hydrogel.
[‡]If not infected.

as with an amorphous hydrogel, or a more occlusive dressing may be needed to better retain the wound's moisture content. Enzymatic debridement of a necrotic, nondraining wound may accomplish two goals: (1) the active enzyme can assist with debridement, and (2) the enzyme preparation may assist with attaining and maintaining a moist wound environment. The surrounding tissue should be protected with a skin sealant.

Necrotic and Draining

A necrotic, draining wound requires debridement, absorption, and protection of the surrounding tissue. The clinician should observe the wound for signs of infection both because a necrotic wound has a higher bioburden than a granular wound and because the wet wound bed provides an ideal environment for these microbes to proliferate.

Other Considerations

After using the two key decision point questions as a guide for determining dressing options, the clinician should consider a few other factors before making a definitive dressing selection.[136,137]

Wound Infection

A clean or colonized wound can be safely bandaged with any type of wound dressing, though moisture-retentive dressings are generally more conducive to wound healing than gauze dressings. Infected wounds should not be occluded and should be rebandaged at least daily. Therefore, infected wounds may be best covered with gauze dressings. Infected wounds that are draining heavily may require additional gauze layers, an alginate, or semipermeable foam for increased absorption.

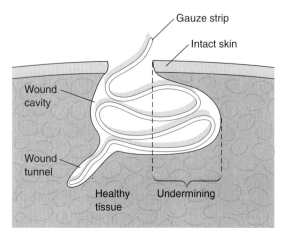

FIGURE 7–9 Cross section of a wound with undermining and tunneling. To prevent abscess formation and promote granulation tissue formation, the wound cavity should be lightly filled with a strip of gauze or alginate rope if there is significant wound drainage.

Wound and Skin Characteristics

Small wounds can be managed successfully with either gauze dressings or moisture-retentive dressings. However, large wounds are more conducive to gauze dressings. Deep wounds require light filling to prevent abscess formation (refer to Figure 7–9). This may be accomplished with gauze packing strips, gauze, alginates, or hydrocolloid particles along with a secondary dressing. Tunneling wounds are generally best managed with gauze dressings and more frequent dressing changes. Adhesives and adherent dressings should be avoided in patients with poor skin integrity.

If a wound is draining more than the current dressing can absorb, periwound maceration may be evident. Therefore, the clinician should choose a more absorbent dressing, perform more frequent dressing changes, and/or use a skin sealant.

Frequency of Dressing Changes

If the patient or caregiver is unable or unwilling to perform dressing changes, a moisture-retentive dressing may be more appropriate than gauze because it is designed to stay in place for several days. Gauze dressings are best for frequent dressing changes. Generally speaking, the optimal dressing for an uninfected wound may be the one that requires the least frequent dressing change.[12,22,25,26] Because periwound skin can be damaged if an adhesive moisture-retentive dressing is changed too frequently,[35] these dressings should be used only if the dressing is intended to stay in place for at least 3 days.

Availability of Dressings

The choice of wound dressings is dictated, in part, by the availability of wound care products. If a certain category of dressings is not available, the clinician must choose the next best alternative. *In general*, there are only minimal differences between various wound dressings within each of the nine main categories presented earlier. Therefore, it is usually acceptable for one type of semipermeable film dressing to be substituted for another semipermeable film dressing.

Cost

Clinicians must consider the economic impact of their choice of wound management. For example, it would not be fiscally responsible or clinically applicable to use a hydrocolloid for a wound that requires daily dressing changes. For one-time dressing changes, gauze dressings are less expensive. However, if an occlusive dressing can be used and left in place for several days, the overall cost of wound management (product cost plus the cost of skilled personnel to perform the dressing change) is reduced.[32]

Wound Location

Wounds in highly mobile areas, such as the palm, may be best managed with adherent moisture-retentive dressings. Similarly, wounds in areas that are not conducive to wrapping, such as sacral wounds, also are more easily bandaged with adherent moisture retentive dressings. Digital wounds may be more easily wrapped with gauze. Refer to the next section for location-specific bandaging tips.

☑ *Checkpoint Question #4*

Your patient presents with a wound on the lateral fifth metatarsal measuring 1.2 × 1.3 cm and 0.5 cm deep. The wound has copious drainage that is milky white. The periwound is warm to the touch and there is erythema noted up to 3 cm away from the wound. Which of the following dressings is *not* appropriate at this time? Why?

a. Amorphous hydrogel with a gauze dressing
b. An alginate with a gauze dressing
c. A hydrocolloid
d. A bulky gauze dressing

Comprehensive Wound Management

Although the focus of this chapter has been the philosophy of moist wound healing, wound dressings comprise only a portion of comprehensive wound management. The importance of examining and treating the patient as a whole cannot be overstated. The clinician must look beyond the wound and periwound characteristics. To achieve lasting wound closure, the health care team must identify and control wound etiology, contributing factors, and infection. The basic tenets of wound management are recapped in Table 7–4.

BANDAGING PROCEDURE

Box 7–13 provides a step-by-step guide for general wound bandaging. As with all other types of interventions, the clinician must follow accepted standard precautions at all times. Wound bandaging occurs after debridement, modality, and irrigation procedures have been completed. Some wound dressings, such as hydrocolloids and gauze, may leave a residue within the wound bed that must be removed with each dressing change. Because alginate residue is biocompatible, it need not be meticulously removed with each dressing change. In most cases, it is sufficient to use clean technique.[21,81,138] However, sterile technique is indicated for patients with extensive burns, immunosuppression, or wounds requiring filling. If gloves become contaminated during wound care procedures such as debridement or measuring, they should be discarded and clean gloves should be donned prior to bandaging to ensure that the outer bandage is free of contaminants.

Adherent Occlusive Dressings

Adherent occlusive dressings (semipermeable films, adherent semipermeable foams, hydrocolloids, and composite dressings) are commonly used on small- or medium-sized uninfected wounds provided that the patient's skin integrity can tolerate the dressing's adhesive properties. Because these dressings are conformable and have some elasticity, they will move along with the patient without traumatizing the wound bed, making adherent occlusive dressings ideal for hands, arms, legs, and trunk wounds. As discussed previously, butterfly-shaped adherent occlusive dressings are ideal for uninfected sacral and coccygeal pressure ulcers. After preparing the wound site, the clinician places the occlusive dressing over the wound bed, ensuring there is about a 1- to 2-cm border of intact skin to provide an adequate edge seal. The clinician should ensure there are no wrinkles or creases in the dressing as these may provide a channel for microbes to enter the wound bed. To enhance dressing adhesion, it is recommended that the clinician apply gentle pressure to the dressing perimeter. The warmth of the clinician's hands molding the dressing to the patient's skin may also increase the dressing's adherence. The clinician should remove and discard his or her gloves and provide the patient/caregiver with any necessary posttreatment instructions.

The clinician should initial and date the wound dressing. Writing on the wound dressing provides an important means of determining how much the wound has drained as well as how well the dressing has stayed in place. This process is particularly important when more than one person is participating in dressing

TABLE 7–4   Comprehensive Wound Management

Objective	Clinical Implication
Granular wound bed	• Debride necrotic tissue • Protect granular tissue
Moist wound bed	• Add moisture to dry wound bed • Absorb moisture from wet wound bed • Keep wound covered
Warm wound environment	• Cover with wound dressing
Manage infection	• Prevent contamination • Keep wounds covered • Use universal precautions • Use sterile technique when indicated • If infected, use topical antimicrobials and systemic antibiotics as directed by physician
Eliminate dead space	• Lightly fill wound cavity, tunnels, and undermining
Healthy periwound and intact skin	• Apply moisturizers to anhydrous or calloused intact skin • Apply skin sealant to protect from maceration

Manage tissue loads	• Prevent trauma (pressure, friction, and shear) to wound bed
	• Unload affected areas
	  ◦ Positioning
	  ◦ Cushions
	  ◦ Supports
	  ◦ Assistive devices

Control contributing factors	• Educate patient and caregivers
	• Involve appropriate health care professionals to address factors known to delay wound healing:
	  ◦ Malnutrition
	  ◦ Impaired circulation
	  ◦ Impaired oxygenation
	  ◦ Immunocompromise
	  ◦ Activity/mobility limitations
	  ◦ Behavioral risk taking

Enhance patient's ability to heal	• Stimulate healing of recalcitrant wounds:
	  ◦ Serial instrumented debridement
	  ◦ Electrotherapeutic modalities
	  ◦ Physical agents
	  ◦ Mechanical modalities
	  ◦ Growth factors
	  ◦ Skin substitutes

changes. For example, suppose a physical therapist applies a semipermeable foam dressing on Monday, expecting the dressing not to be changed until the next visit on Friday. However, on Thursday, the patient's home health nurse changes the dressing because strike-through is apparent. If the dressing is not initialed and dated at that time, the physical therapist might erroneously conclude the following day that the wound is not draining very much at all. As a result, the physical therapist might change to a less absorptive dressing, the exact opposite of what the situation actually requires.

Nonadherent Dressings

After preparing the wound site, the clinician places an appropriately sized nonadherent moisture-retentive dressing or gauze dressing over the wound. The dressing must then be secured in some fashion. Although the simplest means of securing a dressing may be to tape the dressing in place, this should be avoided whenever possible.[12] The adhesives used in tapes are far more aggressive than the adhesives used in adherent occlusive dressings. Application and removal of tape, especially if done repeatedly, will traumatize even the healthiest of skin. If tape *must* be used, foam, cloth, or hypoallergenic paper tape should be chosen.[16] Preferable methods of securing nonadherent dressing include roll gauze, self-adherent elastic wraps (such as Coban or Co-flex), and elastic netting (such as Surgiflex and stretch net). The clinician removes and discards his or her gloves, initials and dates the outer dressing, and provides the patient/caregiver with any necessary posttreatment instructions.

Wounds with dead space, such as deep cavities, tunnels, or undermining, should be filled to prevent premature wound closure and abscess formation (see Figure 7–9).[13,81] After preparing the wound site, the

---

BOX 7–13	**General Bandaging Procedure**

1. Assemble equipment and supplies that may be needed.
2. Position the patient comfortably, allowing for visualization of the wound bed, proper posture and body mechanics, and sufficient lighting of the involved area.
3. Explain general procedure to patient.
4. Wash hands and don clean gloves.
5. Note date on old bandage prior to removal and discard according to facility policies.
   a. To remove adhesive dressings, lift up corner and stretch dressing longitudinally to decrease dressing's adhesion to the skin's surface.
   b. To remove a gauze dressing that is adhered to the wound bed, moisten with saline prior to removal unless performing wet-to-dry dressing on a wound that is 100% necrotic.
6. Remove and discard soiled gloves.
7. Open necessary bandaging supplies.
8. Apply clean gloves.
9. Inspect the wound to determine appropriate interventions (such as debridement, modality, or irrigation). The wound may need to be rinsed with normal saline to provide a more accurate inspection.
10. Explain procedure(s) to the patient and perform appropriate intervention(s).
11. Note changes in wound/patient status postintervention.
12. Apply skin sealant to periwound.
13. Apply topical agents to the wound bed as indicated/prescribed.
14. Remove and discard soiled gloves.
15. Don clean gloves.
16. Apply wound dressing. Ensure primary dressing completely covers wound bed. About 1–2 cm perimeter of adherent moisture-retentive dressings should be in contact with intact skin to provide a good edge seal.
17. Remove and discard soiled gloves.
18. Initial and date wound dressing.
19. Wash hands.
20. Provide any necessary posttreatment instructions.
21. Complete documentation.

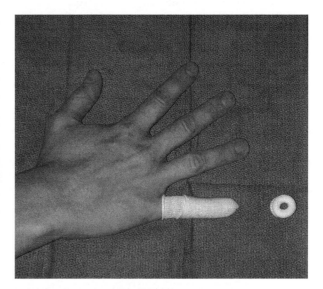

FIGURE 7–10   Finger wrapped with tubular gauze.

clinician must choose the most appropriate material to fill the dead space: alginate rope or gauze packing strips. Alginate ropes should be considered if the wound has moderate to copious drainage. Alginate rope packing is not appropriate for minimally or nondraining wounds; wounds with deep tunnels; or wounds with exposed deep tissues, such as tendon, capsule, nerve, vessels, or bone. Appropriately sized gauze packing strips may be used to fill wounds with any amount of drainage and of any depth, regardless of the type of tissues exposed. Because packing strips are made of small-weave gauze, they are unlikely to disturb the wound bed. However, if the gauze packing strip adheres to the wound bed or removal causes bleeding, the clinician should consider changing to hydrogel-impregnated or saline-moistened gauze packing strips.[81] This can be achieved either by using prepackaged materials or by having the clinician moisten the gauze strip manually. Large wounds with extensive cavities or undermining may require filling with small-weave roll gauze or gauze sponges. To prevent maceration of periwound tissue, care should be taken to ensure that packing material is confined to within the wound bed.[37] Because roll gauzes may be removed in one continuous piece, these are preferable to packing with numerous gauze squares.[81] If gauze squares are used for wound filling, the clinician must ensure that every gauze square is removed with each dressing change by carefully documenting the number of squares used and removed. All packing material must be removed at each dressing change to decrease the risk of infection and minimize the inflammatory response to these substances. (In some cases, it may be acceptable to leave packing material in place while changing the secondary dressing. This may allow patients or caregivers to safely change wound dressings outside of skilled treatment sessions. However, when using this approach, the wound must be carefully monitored for adverse effects.)

To fill a wound, the clinician should use sterile instruments and packing materials. Sterile gloves should be worn if the clinician anticipates contacting the packing material with a gloved hand. For example, some clinicians prefer to hold an applicator in one hand and handle the packing material with forceps in the other, whereas other clinicians prefer to hold the packing material in hand. A sterile alginate applicator or sterile gloved hand should be used to *loosely* fill the wound cavity, tunnel, or undermined area with the material chosen. Local ischemia can be created by packing a wound too tightly, delaying

wound healing.[21] Cotton-tipped applicators should not be used because of the potential for wisps of cotton to remain within the wound bed, causing an inflammatory response or granuloma.[3,21,38] A small amount of packing material, called a tail or wick, should be left outside of the wound cavity or tunnel to allow easy identification of this material during the next dressing change. This tail also provides a means of wicking fluid out of the cavity. After filling the wound cavity, the wound bed should be covered with an appropriate dressing, such as a gauze pad with or without a nonadherent gauze. The dressing should then be secured using roll gauze, self-adherent elastic wraps, elastic netting, or hypoallergenic paper tape.

Tricks of the Trade

This section provides clinicians new to wound management with specific bandaging suggestions for various body locations including the fingers, hands, legs and arms, trunk, abdomen, and ankles and feet.

Fingers

When bandaging finger wounds, each digit should be wrapped individually. After preparing the wound site, the wound bed is covered with an appropriately sized gauze square (cut to size if necessary) secured with roll gauze. When wrapping the digits, the clinician should strive to keep the amount of bandaging to a minimum. This will encourage functional use of the hand, permit range of motion exercises, and allow appropriate splint fit if necessary to prevent contracture formation. Tubular dressings, such as finger bobs or elastic netting, can be used to secure the dressing rather than roll gauze. Tubular dressings are quicker and easier to apply than roll gauze, allow more freedom of movement, and seem to stay in place better than roll gauze (see Figure 7–10). Because tubular dressings are clean dressings, they cannot be used if sterile technique is required.

Hands

Occlusive dressings may be appropriate for small wounds covering only a portion of the hand. Because these dressings are conformable and have some elasticity, they will move along with the patient without traumatizing the wound bed. If the wound is infected or covers a larger area, roll gauze dressings are required. To prevent dressing slippage, the clinician should apply the roll gauze in a figure-eight fashion around

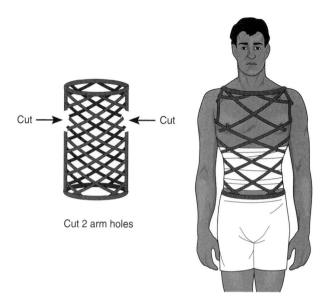

FIGURE 7–11   A vest can be made out of elastic netting to help secure trunk bandages.

the patient's wrist and hand. The clinician should strive to minimize bandage bulk to encourage functional use of the extremity, permit range of motion exercises, and allow appropriate splint fit if necessary.

Legs and Arms

Similar to hand wounds, occlusive dressings may be appropriate for uninfected extremity wounds. Nonadherent dressings should be chosen if the patient's skin integrity is poor or if the patient has a significant amount of body hair in the wound region. Gauze dressings and nonadherent occlusive dressings may be secured with roll gauze, self-adherent elastic wraps, or elastic netting. Roll gauze should be applied snugly, but without tension, and on a slight angle to prevent compromising circulation to the extremity. To decrease the likelihood of gauze slippage, the extremity should be wrapped beyond the point at which limb girth begins to taper. For example, when wrapping the lower leg, if the gauze stops at the widest portion of the calf, rather than above the bulk of the calf, it will likely slide down as the patient ambulates. Elastic netting or a self-adherent elastic wrap may also be used over the roll gauze, if necessary.

Trunk

Trunk wounds requiring a secondary dressing may be secured with roll gauze, a vest fashioned from elastic netting (see Figure 7–11), or both. Short-stretch compression wraps may be used with caution to ensure adequate respiratory capacity. Trunk wounds covering a large area may be best covered with a burn vest. A burn vest is a multi-ply gauze sheet dressing with a nonadherent contact layer, a head hole, and ties located at both midaxillary lines to secure the dressing.

Abdomen

Bandaging abdominal wounds without applying tape directly to the patient's skin can be difficult. The clinician may choose to bandage abdominal wounds like trunk wounds. However, because of the greater amount of subcutaneous fat and skin folds in the abdominal region, the wound edges tend to be pulled apart, slowing wound healing. One method of correcting this is to apply Montgomery straps to either side of the wound bed. These are minimally adhesive strips with ties on one side (see Figure 7–12). After placing a primary dressing, such as a foam or gauze pad, over the wound bed, the straps are tied together, creating an external suture that decreases the amount of tension across the wound bed. Alternatively, a hydrocolloid dressing can be placed on the intact skin on each side of the wound (see color image 7). After placing the primary dressing over the wound bed, tape is applied from the dressing to the hydrocolloid, avoiding the patient's skin. The primary wound dressing can be changed as often as necessary, while the hydrocolloid is left in place for up to 1 week.

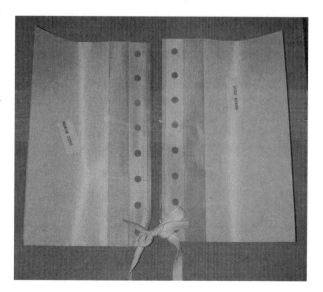

FIGURE 7–12   Montgomery straps.

Ankles and Feet

Ankle wounds can be bandaged like hand wounds. However, because of the dependent position of the lower extremity, many times these wounds drain more significantly, requiring dressings with greater absorptive capabilities. Thick gauze pads (such as ABD pads), sheet hydrogels, and thick foams may be used on plantar wounds to provide additional protection from the pressure of weight bearing and the shearing forces of ambulation. The clinician should ensure there is adequate room in the patient's footwear to accommodate for wound bandages. Temporary footwear, such as an enclosed postoperative shoe or a Darco shoe, may be required. Chapter 13 provides additional information on therapeutic footwear options. An assistive device should be strongly considered for patients with plantar or digital wounds and patients with decreased sensation or proprioception.

CHAPTER SUMMARY

Wound dressings play a key role in wound management. Wound dressings have several functions, including maintaining a moist wound environment, providing thermal insulation, creating a barrier against infection, controlling bleeding and edema, eliminating dead space, assisting with debridement, and reducing pain. There are nine main categories of wound dressings: gauze, impregnated gauze, semipermeable films, hydrogels, semipermeable foams, hydrocolloids, alginates, composite dressings, and antimicrobial dressings. Wound dressings can be considered along a continuum of occlusion and absorptive capabilities. The use of moisture-retentive dressings, specialized synthetic or organic dressings, on uninfected wounds may be more effective and less costly than traditional gauze dressings. Recent advances in bioengineering have led to the emergence of growth factors and biologic/biosynthetic dressings to enhance wound healing. A wound decision grid can assist clinicians with choosing appropriate dressings for individual wounds. After choosing a wound dressing, clinicians must secure the dressing in such a way as to minimize periwound trauma and maximize patient mobility and function. Although wound dressings are a vital component to obtaining a moist wound environment, the clinician must look beyond local wound characteristics and identify and control wound etiology, contributing factors, and infection in order to achieve lasting wound closure.

REVIEW QUESTIONS

1. You are covering a softball tournament when you are asked to treat a 20-year-old player with an abrasion on her lateral thigh sustained when sliding into home plate. Her medical history is unremarkable except for surgery to repair a torn anterior cruciate ligament 3 years ago.
   a. Describe how you might use a gauze dressing to cover this wound. What are the advantages and limitations of this dressing?
   b. Describe how you might use a semipermeable film to cover this wound. What are the advantages and limitations of this dressing?

2. You are working with a patient with a diabetic foot ulcer on her fourth toe that just had antimicrobial beads surgically implanted after surgery for osteomyelitis (see color image 12). How would you bandage this wound?

3. You are working with a patient who has a sacral pressure ulcer with minimal serous drainage. You are dressing the wound with a skin sealant and a hydrocolloid. How often should you change the dressing?

4. Your 71-year-old patient has a wound over her lateral forearm due to an improperly fitting splint that began approximately 1 week ago. The wound is 100% black eschar covered and measures 2.0 × 2.6 cm. The patient has a history of rheumatoid arthritis requiring multiple joint replacements and long-term oral steroid use. The periwound skin appears slightly thinned but otherwise healthy. The patient reports no pain and the wound was previously treated by leaving it open to the air.
   a. Describe what interventions you would use to manage this patient's wound at this time.
   b. One week later the eschar has been removed to reveal a 100% granular wound bed with minimal drainage and measuring 1.8 × 2.5 cm with a depth of 0.4 cm and a tunnel of 1.3 cm extending proximally from the 12-o'clock position. Describe what interventions you would use to manage this patient's wound at this time.

PEARSON
myhealthprofessionskit

Use this address to access the Companion Website created for this textbook. Simply select "Physical Therapy" from the choice of disciplines. Find this book and log in using your username and password to access images, video clips, and additional learning tools.

REFERENCES

Go to myhealthprofessionskit.com to view this chapter's references.

8

Electrotherapeutic Modalities, Physical Agents, and Mechanical Modalities

Chapter Objectives

After reading this chapter, learners will be able to:

1. Explain the purpose and effects of wound irrigation, whirlpool, pulsed lavage, electrical stimulation, ultrasound, negative pressure wound therapy, and hyperbaric oxygen.
2. Explain the indications, contraindications, advantages, and disadvantages of wound irrigation, whirlpool, pulsed lavage, electrical stimulation, ultrasound, negative pressure wound therapy, and hyperbaric oxygen.
3. Describe proper procedure for performing wound irrigation, whirlpool, pulsed lavage, electrical stimulation, ultrasound, and negative pressure wound therapy.
4. Describe the potential of ultraviolet, low-intensity laser, and monochromatic infrared energy to enhance wound healing.
5. Identify when adjunctive interventions should be considered for wound healing.
6. Choose appropriate modalities and physical agents to enhance wound healing based on wound presentation, wound etiology, and patient status.

Key Terms

Current of injury
Galvanotaxis
Hyperbaric oxygen therapy (HBO)

Low-intensity laser therapy
Negative pressure wound therapy (NPWT)
Pulsed lavage

Transcutaneous oxygen monitoring (TCOM)
Vacuum-Assisted Closure (VAC)

INTRODUCTION

Chronic wounds and wounds that fail to progress through the phases of wound healing as expected may require additional interventions to enhance wound healing. There is significant research and consensus on the use of most standard interventions such as saline irrigation, whirlpool, and the previously described concept of moist wound healing. However, there is less research to support the use of adjunctive therapies, specifically modalities and physical agents, used to facilitate healing in chronic wounds or wounds that fail to respond to standard care. There are several general problems in the literature on the use of adjunctive therapies to enhance wound healing (see Box 8–1).

Prior to expanding to adjunctive interventions, the clinician must first ensure that all standard care practices for wound characteristics, local factors, and systemic factors are employed and performed appropriately. As with medical care in general, too often patients and clinicians seek a magic bullet—a single pill (or in wound management, a modality)—that will fix all the problems related to impaired wound healing without addressing the complexities of each individual patient, such as tissue perfusion, infection, wound bed factors, immune status, nutrition, pressure, neuropathy, economic factors, psychosocial issues, medications, and other disease processes. Next, because wounds are dynamic, interventions must be altered based on changes in wound characteristics. This makes research particularly problematic when the endpoint is the time to wound closure rather than the time to reach the treatment goal of a particular modality. Without the use of consistent approaches to confirm or refute a study's findings, it is difficult to extrapolate the effect of the intervention, particularly if study results are contradictory. Because most adjunctive interventions are currently recommended only for chronic or recalcitrant wounds, it is not known whether adjunctive therapies may, in fact, accelerate the normal rate of healing and decrease overall wound care costs and patient morbidity. Manufacturer sponsorship of research is particularly controversial. Suggested methods to address the problems associated with this include prospective mandatory trial registration with an obligation to publish all results as well as requiring authors to declare the lack of competing interests.[1]

Despite these problems, clinicians can use the following information to make sound clinical judgments on the use of modalities and physical agents to enhance wound healing. This chapter represents a compilation of current research and is designed to provide specific, scientifically grounded information on the use of modalities and physical agents to promote wound healing.

BOX 8–1   Problems with Research to Support Adjunctive Interventions

- Patient-related variables
  - Comorbidities (e.g., diabetes, peripheral vascular disease)
  - Nutrition status
  - Immune status
  - Adherence
  - Psychosocial and economic issues
- Wound-related variables
  - Wounds of various etiologies or only one etiology
  - Inadequate wound description (depth of tissue involvement, granular, necrotic, or infected)
  - Wound chronicity (chronic, acute, or unchanging)
  - Prior interventions
  - Wounds are dynamic (interventions need to change as wound changes)
- Treatment-related variables
  - Differing modality parameters (technique, intensity, frequency, or duration)
  - Combining of modality with dressing
  - Inclusion/exclusion and documentation of other interventions (e.g., unloading, controlling blood sugars, nutritional supplementation, moist wound healing, debridement, exercise)
- Research-related problems
  - Inadequate sample size
  - Inadequate control group
  - Paucity of randomized controlled trials
  - Reliance on case studies or case series and the inability to determine causal effects or generalize results
  - Data interpretation (e.g., statistical vs. clinical significance)
- Manufacturer-sponsored research
  - Selective reporting of positive outcomes
  - Inappropriate comparisons
  - Data interpretation
  - Restrictions on publication and information sharing
  - Lack of information regarding intervention costs

MODALITIES AND PHYSICAL AGENTS TO ENHANCE WOUND HEALING

This section provides detailed information on the purposes and effects of various modalities used to enhance wound healing, including wound irrigation, whirlpool, pulsed lavage, electrical stimulation, ultrasound, hyperbaric oxygen therapy, and other promising modalities. Additional information is provided on the procedures, indications, contraindications, advantages, and disadvantages for each procedure.

Wound Irrigation

Wound irrigation is the use of fluid to remove loosely adherent cellular debris, surface bacteria, wound exudate, dressing residue, and residual topical agents.[2–4] Wound irrigation facilitates debridement, assists with achieving and maintaining a moist wound environment, and enhances wound healing. Although not technically a modality, wound irrigation is closely related to other forms of hydrotherapy, such as whirlpool and pulsed lavage. It is presented here for comparison and continuity.

Wound irrigation is sometimes referred to as wound cleansing.[5,6] However, this terminology is particularly confusing as the recommended irrigant solution for wound cleansing is not, in fact, a wound cleanser (see Chapter 6 for cytotoxicity and other information regarding wound cleansers and antiseptics), but rather saline or potable water.[5,6]

Indications

Wound irrigation is a standard component of treatment for all types of wounds.[6–8] In fact, gentle irrigation, bandaging, and protection are the only direct wound interventions indicated for healing granular wounds.

Contraindications/Precautions

Wound irrigation is not indicated in wounds with active, profuse bleeding.

Method

Wounds and the surrounding skin should be irrigated upon initial examination and with each dressing change.[5] The most common irrigant solution is normal saline.[2] However, regular tap water is an acceptable alternative,[9] with no additional risk of wound contamination if a clean water source is available.[5,10,11] In fact, irrigation with regular tap water may result in faster wound healing[12] and lower treatment cost than irrigation with saline. To be effective, wound irrigation must use minimal force.[10] Simply pouring saline from a bottle onto the wound or using a bulb syringe will "water the wound" but will not effectively remove surface pathogens or prevent the development of infection. However, too much force will traumatize the wound bed and may actually drive foreign debris and surface pathogens through the wound surface. It is also theorized that high irrigation pressures will impair the ability to resist infection.[13] Wounds should be irrigated with pressures between 4 and 15 psi.[5,8] This is equivalent to using a 35-mL syringe with a 19-gauge angiocatheter or a Waterpik at the lowest setting (6.0 psi).[14] Pressurized saline canisters that provide acceptable irrigation pressures are also available. Recent recommendations suggest that pressures between 10 and 15 psi are most effective for preventing infection.[4] Irrigation may be performed alone or in combination with other modalities including whirlpool, ultrasound, and electrical stimulation. Irrigating a wound after whirlpool treatment has been shown to remove four times as much bacteria as whirlpool alone.[15,16]

Prior to wound irrigation, the clinician should explain the procedure to the patient. Next, the patient should be positioned comfortably to provide the clinician with easy access to the affected area. Any dressings present should be removed. The patient should be draped for modesty, and toweling or water-impermeable padding should be placed to absorb the irrigant. To protect from a splash injury, the clinician must use appropriate barrier devices, including gloves, protective eyewear or face shield, moisture-resistant gown, and mask.[3]

After treatment, areas of intact skin should be dried with a towel. Open areas may be left open to the air, patted with a sterile gauze sponge, or covered with a sterile towel. The clinician should perform any debridement or measurements prior to bandaging the wound.

Alternative Interventions

Alternative interventions to wound irrigation may include soaking the wound with saline-moistened gauze, whirlpool, and pulsed lavage. See Box 8–2 for a summary of wound irrigation.

BOX 8–2 **Wound Irrigation**

Purpose/Effects

- Removes loosely adhered debris, bacteria, exudate, dressing residue, topical agents
- Facilitates debridement
- Promotes moist wound healing

Indications	**Contraindications**
• All wound types	• Wounds with active, profuse bleeding

Advantages	**Disadvantages**
• Simple	• Messy
• Quick	• May not use adequate amount of irrigant
• Inexpensive	
• Effective	
• Can be used for any wound location	
• Can be used in any setting	

Method

- Irrigation pressure of 4–15 psi
- 35-mL syringe and a 19-gauge angiocatheter

Whirlpool

Hydrotherapy is one of the oldest forms of treatment used for wound care. Whirlpools come in many shapes and sizes, from small tanks that can hold a single extremity to large Hubbard tanks (see Figure 8–1) in which a patient lies recumbent on a stretcher. Ninety-five percent of burn units use some form of whirlpool.[17] Whirlpool is a form of nonselective mechanical debridement and has seven main purposes.[18] First, the force of moving water can help debride loosely adherent devitalized tissues, foreign debris, and surface bacteria.[5,16,19,20] Second, the whirlpool softens necrotic tissue and eschar, facilitating their removal.[3] Third, whirlpool hydrates the wound bed and promotes moist wound healing. Fourth, the whirlpool promotes circulation,[20–22] which can enhance wound healing. Fifth, the use of whirlpool treatments is associated with decreased patient pain complaint during wound care procedures.[22] Sixth, whirlpool eases range of motion for patients with burn injuries. Last, the whirlpool, without agitation, can be used to help soak off adherent wound dressings while minimizing pain and trauma to the wound bed.

Indications

Whirlpool is indicated for use on infected wounds to help reduce bacterial load, on nondraining wounds

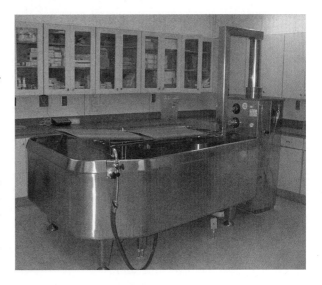

FIGURE 8–1 Hubbard tank.

to rehydrate the wound bed, on wounds with thick eschar to soften necrotic tissue, and on wounds with loosely adherent necrotic tissue or thick exudate to facilitate debridement.[5,18]

Contraindications/Precautions

Whether due to ready accessibility or lack of current knowledge on wound pathophysiology, whirlpool is one of the most overused interventions in wound management. As with any intervention, the inappropriate use of whirlpool treatments may actually prolong, or even prevent, wound closure. A recent study showed that while clinicians novice to wound care report using whirlpool for patients with open wounds up to 85%, clinicians with more advanced training on wound management utilized whirlpool about 46% of the time.[23] Therefore, it is imperative that physical therapists and physical therapist assistants are aware of the specific indications, contraindications, and precautions for whirlpool use and are prepared to educate other members of the wound management team on these points.

With few exceptions, whirlpool treatments are contraindicated for ulcers due to venous insufficiency,[18] edema, or lymphedema. It should be noted that a 25–140 mL increase in upper extremity volume has been found with the use of whirlpool baths for uninjured individuals and even larger increases noted in injured upper extremities.[24] Similarly, significant increases in lower limb volume have been noted after just 10 minutes of whirlpool therapy.[25] The dependent positioning and warm water temperature cause an increase in peripheral edema[24] that will exacerbate venous insufficiency,[20] traumatic edema, and lymphedema while the additional hydration will only increase the already heavy amounts of wound drainage.[22] Whirlpool is also contraindicated for use with patients who are incontinent of bowel and have wounds that would require submersion of the perineum. Patients who are incontinent of urine and require submersion of the perineum should have a catheter placed. However, because this increases the risk of urinary tract infection,[19] alternative interventions may need to be considered. Whirlpool is contraindicated for wounds with active, profuse bleeding. Patients who are confused and combative and patients with uncontrolled seizures should not receive whirlpool treatments because of the risk of injury and possible drowning and to protect the clinician from splash injuries. If a patient has multiple open areas and not all wounds are believed to be infected (or infected with the same organisms), whirlpool will increase the likelihood of cross-contamination and, therefore, is contraindicated. However, if the wounds occur in separate locales, such as the right and left lower extremities, it is possible to use separate whirlpools for each wound. Clinicians should be aware of the potential for cross-contamination between patients when treated using the immersion technique.[18,26] There are reports in the literature of outbreaks of certain types of infection as a result of whirlpool use.[19] Therefore, clinicians must ensure the whirlpool is properly cleaned using current infection control procedures following each patient treatment.

Whirlpool is a form of nonselective mechanical debridement. It is not indicated for clean, granulating wounds, as the force of agitation may traumatize granulation tissue and slow epithelialization.[3] Although one source suggests that whirlpool treatment should not be used with wounds that are less than 75% necrotic,[22] clinicians should weigh the possible benefits of whirlpool against the potential for traumatizing granulating and epithelializing tissues[18] for each individual wound. Tunneling wounds, wounds with significant undermining, and wounds in areas of skin folds, such as abdominal or trunk wounds in patients who are obese, will not be sufficiently irrigated using this technique and, therefore, are not indicated for whirlpool treatments. If whirlpool treatments are to be performed on patients with arterial insufficiency ulcers, the water temperature should be decreased to between 92 and 98°F to allow an increase in circulation while avoiding placing excessive metabolic demands on the tissues.[22] Additionally, clinicians should lower the force of agitation to prevent traumatizing the fragile wound bed.[20] Because whirlpool treatments hydrate treated tissues, areas of maceration may be best treated with alternative interventions to prevent an increase in maceration and the potential for enlarging the open area. Whirlpool treatments may not be appropriate for a patient with severe hydrophobia. Water temperature should be decreased if a patient who is pregnant or has multiple sclerosis is to be immersed within a Hubbard tank.[27] Patients with cardiac instability should not be fully immersed in a whirlpool unless cleared by their physician. Alternative treatment methods should be chosen for patients who exceed the weight limit of the Hubbard tank hoist. To ensure patient safety, patients should not be left unattended during whirlpool treatments.

Method

Immersion Technique

Eighty-one percent of burn units using whirlpool therapy use the immersion method.[17] Prior to whirlpool treatment, the clinician should explain the procedure to the patient. Smaller whirlpools should be filled with water between 92 and 98°F.[18,19,28] Larger whirlpools in which patients will be immersed may need to be slightly warmer, although water temperature should never exceed 102°F.[18] Enough room should be left within the tank to compensate for the added volume of the patient without overflowing. Next, the areas to be treated should be exposed. If the patient is to be treated in the Hubbard tank or other large whirlpool, a gown or pair of disposable shorts should be provided for patient modesty while allowing exposure of the affected area. Any dressings present should be removed. If necessary, adherent dressings can be soaked off in the whirlpool prior to turning on the turbine. To protect from a splash injury, the clinician must use appropriate barrier devices including gloves, protective eyewear or face shield, water-resistant gown, and mask.[3] The patient should be positioned comfortably with the affected area immersed within the whirlpool. The turbine should be adjusted to the appropriate position and force of flow to reach the desired goal. Wounds with larger amounts of granulation or epithelialization should receive indirect agitation at lower forces to protect these fragile tissues. Although there is a tendency for bacterial counts to lower as whirlpool time increases, there is no significant difference in bacterial counts of wounds treated for 5, 10, 15, or 20 minutes. After 20 minutes of treatment, wound bacterial count remains essentially unchanged.[16] Therefore, whirlpool treatments should be completed in 10–20 minutes.[16] Patients with extensive burns may require slightly longer treatment times, while shorter times may be appropriate to soften eschar or if there are any precautions, such as patients with cardiac instability. During the whirlpool treatment, patients should be encouraged to perform active range of motion exercises unless contraindicated. Active motion may decrease the potential for edema and may decrease joint stiffness or impaired range of motion.[19] With the turbine off, clinicians may assist with range of motion exercises or perform debridement during whirlpool treatments if desired.

After treatment, the turbine should be turned off and the patient removed from the whirlpool. Areas of intact skin should be dried with a towel, while open areas may be left open to the air, patted with a sterile gauze sponge, or covered with a sterile towel. Heat lamps, sterile sheets, and/or heated blankets may be used to cover patients after Hubbard tank treatments for comfort and to help prevent hypothermia. Because irrigating a wound after whirlpool treatment has been shown to remove four times as much bacteria as whirlpool alone,[15] clinicians should consider irrigating the wound after removing the patient from the whirlpool. The clinician should assess the results of the whirlpool treatment and perform any debridement or measurements prior to bandaging the wound. Patients with edema in whom the benefits of whirlpool outweigh the potential side effects of increased swelling should be positioned supine with the involved extremity elevated for 10 minutes after whirlpool treatments.[25] Ankle pumps[25] or active range of motion will further assist with, but not completely resolve, the increase in edema. The whirlpool should be drained and cleaned with a disinfectant approved by the Occupational Safety and Health Administration (OSHA) following appropriate infection control guidelines.

Whirlpool treatments are generally performed anywhere between twice daily[29] for acute burn injuries to three times per week for less severe outpatient wounds. Whirlpool should be discontinued when the wound is clean and granular[30] or when the purpose for using the whirlpool (e.g., full active hand range of motion in a patient with a partial-thickness burn injury or removal of loosely adhered debris) has been met. In many cases, one or two whirlpool sessions may be sufficient.

Showering Technique

When using the showering technique, clinicians should follow the steps for immersion technique with a few exceptions. The patient or affected area is positioned over the empty whirlpool and sprayed with water between 92 and 98°F.

Use of Chemical Additives

Many authors recommend the use of chemical additives to the whirlpool water[22,29] to reduce infection and the potential for cross-contamination. Povidone–iodine has been recommended at a dilution of four parts per million. Sodium hypochlorite (bleach) has been recommended at a dilution of 500–5,000 parts per million.[22] Chloramine-T (chlorazene), a chemical agent containing a chlorine molecule linked to a hydrogen–nitrogen bond that comes in prepackaged quantities based on whirlpool size, has also been recommended for short-term use to reduce wound bioburden[31] at a concentration of 100–200 ppm solution.[32] However, all of these chemical additives, although antimicrobial, are also cytotoxic to human cells.[33–42] Therefore, the clinician must carefully weigh the potential benefits of this method of antimicrobial application with the known risks of delayed wound healing.[3] Chemical additives are contraindicated for use on patients with chemical wounds to prevent a chemical reaction. They are also contraindicated for use with the very young, older adults, and those with sensitivities to these agents. Because chemical additives are known to be cytotoxic and increase the cost of wound care, their use is *not* recommended except in isolated cases.[32,42] For a patient with an acute animal bite, the benefits of short-term use of a chemical additive (up to three treatments) *may* outweigh the potential harm,[42] as bite wounds present with significant numbers of bacteria and foreign debris that increase the likelihood of infection. In such cases, it may be appropriate to delay granulation tissue formation and epithelialization for a few days to kill any bacteria remaining within the wound bed.

Alternative Interventions

Alternative interventions to whirlpool treatments may include wound irrigation, soaking the wound with saline-moistened gauze, and pulsed lavage. See Box 8–3 for a summary of whirlpool therapy.

Pulsed Lavage with Concurrent Suction

Lavage is the delivery of a wound irrigant under pressure by an electrically powered device. The most common irrigant is saline, followed by tap water. **Pulsed lavage** involves the regular, automatic interruption of fluid flow with a handheld device to regulate irrigation pressure (see Figure 8–2).[4] Pulsed lavage with concurrent suction applies a negative pressure to the wound bed, which removes the irrigant. Negative pressure may also facilitate the removal of pathogens and enhance granulation tissue formation, epithelialization, and local tissue perfusion.[43, 44] Although the literature comparing the efficacy of pulsed lavage with irrigation or whirlpool treatments is scarce, several studies on patients with chronic wounds found a significantly higher rate of granulation tissue formation, faster removal of necrotic tissue, better removal of fibrin, and less procedure-related pain in wounds treated with pulsed lavage.[7, 45, 46] Because of the many positive results with this intervention, pulsed lavage with suction is now considered the standard of care for wound irrigation.[18]

Indications

Pulsed lavage is indicated for cleansing or debriding wounds due to arterial insufficiency, venous insufficiency, diabetes, pressure, small burns, surgery, or trauma.[5, 26, 44, 47] Pulsed lavage is also appropriate for tunneling or undermining wounds with the use of interchangeable tips to facilitate irrigating areas of various sizes. Because pulsed lavage does not increase edema, it may be more appropriate than whirlpool for treating venous insufficiency ulcers. Pulsed lavage may be most effective during the inflammatory phase of wound healing to soften and remove necrotic tissue and exudate.[3] Pulsed lavage with concurrent suction may be beneficial during the proliferative phase of wound healing to facilitate granulation tissue formation and epithelialization.

Contraindications/Precautions

Pulsed lavage with concurrent suction is contraindicated near exposed arteries, nerves, tendons, capsules, or bones. Pulsed lavage should not be used in body cavities, for facial wounds, on recent grafts or surgical procedures, or on wounds that are actively bleeding. Because the tubing and tips of some older commercially available units contain latex, these pulsed lavage units should not be used on patients with known latex sensitivities or allergies. Pulsed lavage should be used with

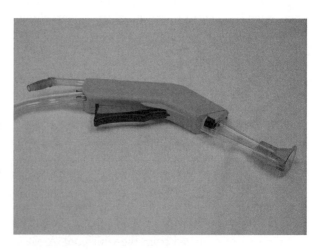

FIGURE 8–2 Pulsed lavage.

BOX 8–3   Whirlpool

Purpose/Effects

- Removes loosely adhered debris, bacteria, exudate, dressing residue, and topical agents
- Facilitates debridement
- Promotes moist wound healing
- Promotes circulation
- Decreases pain
- Makes range of motion exercises easier
- Helps remove adhered dressings without trauma

Indications

- Infected wounds
- Nondraining wounds
- Wounds with thick eschar or exudate
- Wounds with loosely adherent necrotic tissue or debris

Contraindications/Precautions

- Clean, granulating, or epithelializing wounds
- Wounds that are edematous, draining, or macerated
- Wounds with active, profuse bleeding
- Wounds that are tunneling, undermining, or in skin folds may not be effectively irrigated
- Venous insufficiency ulcers
- Wounds due to arterial insufficiency should be treated at lower temperatures
- Patients who are hydrophobic, confused, or combative
- Patients with uncontrolled seizures
- Patients who are incontinent that have wounds requiring perineal submersion
- Patients with multiple wounds with different infectious agents
- Cardiac instability
- If immersing patients who are pregnant or have cardiac instability or multiple sclerosis, water temperature should be decreased
- Chemical additives are not recommended for general use

Advantages

- Comfortable
- Promotes moist wound healing
- Available in most clinical settings
- Simple, effective

Disadvantages

- Cannot calibrate irrigation pressure
- Potential for maceration, edema, cross-contamination
- Requires time for setup/cleanup
- Expensive

Methods

- Immersion
- Showering over whirlpool or Hubbard tank

caution on patients taking anticoagulants because of the potential for hemorrhage, insensate patients to decrease the risk of unperceived trauma, and patients with deep tunneling wounds to prevent damage from the probing wound tip. Because wounds treated with high irrigation pressures have been shown to retain higher concentrations of bacteria and have increased bacterial penetration into wound tissues, irrigation with greater than 15 psi is contraindicated for wound management.[48]

Method

Prior to pulsed lavage, the clinician should explain the procedure to the patient. Next, the patient should be positioned comfortably to provide the clinician with easy access to the affected area. Any dressings present should be removed. The patient should be draped for modesty, and toweling or water-impermeable padding should be placed to absorb any irrigant runoff. In addition, all intravenous access sites or other open areas not being treated should be covered with a sheet or toweling. The patient should wear a mask due to aerosolization during treatment. To protect from a splash injury and aerosolization of pathogens, the clinician (and any other personnel in the room) must use appropriate barrier devices, including gloves, shoe coverings, hair covering over the ears, protective eyewear or face shield, moisture-resistant gown, and mask.[3,47,49] The irrigant reservoir, typically one or more bags of normal saline, should be warmed to between 102 and 106°F, if possible,[19,50] to maintain normothermia. The (warmed) irrigant should be hung from an intravenous pole or other locale within easy reach of the patient's wound. The tubing, with appropriate tip for the wound, should be attached to the irrigant reservoir and suction device if used. Depending on wound size and severity, between 1,000 and 3,000 mL of irrigant is required for thorough wound irrigation. The pump should be turned on, and the pressure adjusted according to the wound's needs, between 4 and 15 psi.[47,50] Typically, lower pressures are used initially or with tunneling and undermining wounds. Treatments generally require 15–30 minutes.[44] It is the responsibility of the clinician to read and follow the procedures outlined by the manufacturer of the specific unit. In some situations, such as the home care setting, it may be beneficial (and necessary) to perform pulsed lavage without suction. To decrease the risk of cross-contamination, the patient should be treated in a room with four walls and a door, rather than a curtained area. For inpatients, a private room is preferred.

After treatment, areas of intact skin should be dried with a towel. Open areas may be left open to the air, patted with a sterile gauze sponge, or covered with a sterile towel. The clinician should assess the result of the pulsed lavage and perform any debridement or measurements prior to bandaging the wound. The tubing should be disposed of according to facility policy for infectious waste. If a reusable handpiece is used, it should be cleaned with an OSHA-approved cleanser following appropriate infection control guidelines. The irrigant within the reservoir should be disposed of in the commode. If a plastic reservoir container is used, it should be disposed of after emptying. If a glass reservoir is used, it should be properly bagged before transport for resterilization. All horizontal surfaces that can be touched by hand should either be covered with linen before treatment and then removed or wiped down with a facility-approved topical antimicrobial after treatment.[47,49] Because improper infection control while using pulsed lavage with suction has been linked to a deadly outbreak of resistant bacterial infections, strict adherence to infection control guidelines is paramount.[49] No increase in environmental or wound contamination has been found with pulsed lavage when following infection control guidelines.[47]

Treatment frequency may be as often as twice daily for wounds that are severely infected, contain significant amounts of necrotic tissue, or have thick exudate, or as infrequently as three times per week for granular wounds.[44] Pulsed lavage should be discontinued when treatment goals have been met.

Alternative Interventions

Alternative interventions to pulsed lavage may include wound irrigation, soaking the wound with saline-moistened gauze, and whirlpool treatments. Refer to Box 8–4 for a summary of pulsed lavage.

BOX 8–4   **Pulsed Lavage**

Purpose/Effects

- Irrigates wound bed with precisely calibrated pressure
- Assists with obtaining and maintaining a moist wound environment
- Facilitates debridement
- May enhance granulation tissue formation, epithelialization, and tissue perfusion

---

BOX 8–4   *(Continued)*

Indications	Contraindications
• Wounds requiring thorough irrigation or debridement	• Wounds with exposed deep tissues • Facial wounds • Recent surgical procedures • Patients with latex allergies or sensitivities • Patients on anticoagulants—precaution • Patients with insensitivity or deep tunneling wounds—precaution

Advantages	Disadvantages
• Encourages thorough irrigation • Can be used in any setting • Quick • Less expensive than whirlpool • Low risk of cross-contamination • Can be used for any wound location • Decrease patient pain complaint • Ergonomical	• Messy • More expensive than wound irrigation • Not appropriate for large wounds

Method

- Irrigation pressure of 4–15 psi
- Handheld device with tubing attached to (warmed) irrigant reservoir (and suction device if used)

 Checkpoint Question #1

Based on the following brief wound descriptions, choose the most appropriate intervention: wound irrigation, whirlpool, or pulsed lavage. Explain your rationale.

a. Partial-thickness burn covering the dorsal foot and anterior leg.

b. Full-thickness volar forearm wound measuring 3.0 × 5.2 cm with 3.2-cm tunnel. The wound bed is 50% granular and 50% yellow slough covered with thick, purulent exudate.

c. Dehisced total knee replacement incision with open area measuring 2.0 × 0.3 cm with a depth of 0.2 cm. The wound is 100% granular and has serous drainage.

Electrical Stimulation

There is extensive research to support the use of electrical stimulation as an adjunct to enhance wound healing. Although the vast majority of research studies has employed the use of high-voltage pulsed current,[51–70] low-intensity direct current[67,71–77] and microcurrent stimulation[78–80] have also been shown to facilitate wound healing. However, some studies have shown no improvements with the use of electrical stimulation.[58,66] A recent placebo-controlled, double-blind, randomized clinical trial demonstrated that patients with chronic lower extremity ulcers treated with electrical stimulation healed twice as fast as those receiving sham treatment,[81] while a meta-analysis demonstrated a 144% increase in the rate of wound healing using electrical stimulation over standard care.[82] Therefore, future research should compare the effects of different treatment parameters, including type of electrical current, stimulation frequency, polarity, and electrode placement, as well as the effects of electrical stimulation on different types of wounds.

There are seven purported ways in which electrical stimulation is thought to facilitate wound healing: restoring the current of injury, causing galvanotaxis, stimulating cells, enhancing blood flow, combating infection, reducing edema, and enhancing autolysis.

1. **Restores the Current of Injury.** Normally, the epidermis is electronegative with respect to the dermis, creating a bioelectric field or "skin battery."[53,83] A break in skin continuity not only lowers the skin's electrical resistance, but also disrupts the skin battery, making the wound electropositive compared to the surrounding tissues.[53] It is thought that this local change in polarity, or endogenous **current of injury,** triggers the wound healing cascade.[84] This current of injury may be arrested in chronic wounds. The application of exogenous electrical stimulation may mimic the normally occurring current of injury and stimulate wound healing.[27,56,83,85–88] Similarly, wound bed desiccation impedes the current of injury,[89] retarding wound healing and further supporting the principles of moist wound healing.

2. **Causes Galvanotaxis.** Galvanotaxis is the stimulation of cells to move along an electrical gradient.[71,86,90] Electrical stimulation may attract and enhance the migration of macrophages, neutrophils,[53] fibroblasts,[63] endothelial cells,[85] and keratinocytes.[53,56,85,86,88,91] Therefore, the exogenous application of electrical stimulation has been shown to enhance all three phases of wound healing[77] by attracting the cells necessary for repair and regeneration to the affected area.

3. **Stimulates Cells.** Electrical stimulation causes a general increase in cell proliferation.[83] Macrophages, fibroblasts,[73,77,92] platelets, and endothelial cells[91] seem to be particularly susceptible to the effects of electrical stimulation. Electrical stimulation also enhances cell function, including collagen synthesis,[73,83,91,93] DNA synthesis,[83,85] granulation tissue formation,[73] and epithelialization,[73] further hastening the repair process and improving wound breaking strength.[77]

4. **Increases Blood Flow.** The application of electrical stimulation enhances blood flow to the treated area,[18,53,70,73,87,88,90,94,95] resulting in higher capillary oxygen tension[90] and tissue partial pressure of oxygen.[29,53] Electrical stimulation–mediated angiogenesis may be mediated by the activation of vascular endothelial growth factor (VEGF).[96,97] In a study on the effect of electrical stimulation on blood flow in the rat, both negative and positive stimulation increased blood flow velocity, although this effect was greater with negative stimulation.[98] Greater oxygen availability not only enhances the ability to fight infection, but also increases the body's ability to build new tissue in all three phases of wound healing.

5. **Increases Bactericidal Abilities.** Electrical stimulation has an antibacterial effect on wound tissues.[27,29,53,64,69,71,73,85,87,88] Neutrophils and macrophages appear to be attracted to both the anode (positive electrode) and cathode (negative electrode),[86] although the antibacterial effect seems to be greatest at the cathode.[99] In one animal study of full-thickness wounds inoculated with *Staphylococcus aureus*, there was a 98% mean decrease in bacterial load with electrical stimulation.[52]

6. **Reduces Edema.** Electrical stimulation is believed to reduce edema within the treated area,[18,54,73,87,94,100] possibly by reducing microvascular permeability induced by injury and inflammation.[101] However, at least one animal experiment resulted in no change in edema formation with the application of electrical stimulation.

7. **Facilitates Debridement.** Electrical stimulation, particularly negative or cathodal stimulation, is believed to facilitate autolytic debridement.[18,29,56,73,75,86,87] This may be a result of the previously listed effects of electrical stimulation or may occur by way of another, as yet unidentified, method.[102]

Indications

Electrical stimulation is indicated as an adjunct to wound healing for chronic or recalcitrant wounds that are clean or infected,[52,57,64,99] granular or necrotic.[22,73,94] When electrical stimulation in combination with standard wound care is compared with standard care alone, electrical stimulation has resulted in increased healing for wounds of various etiologies,[81] including pressure ulcers,[57,58,60–62,65,103] neuropathic ulcers,[54,55,104,105] venous ulcers,[54,68] arterial ulcers,[54] burns,[63] traumatic wounds, and surgical wounds.[88,93] The National Pressure Ulcer Advisory Panel recommends clinicians consider the use of electrical stimulation for patients with category/stage III and IV pressure ulcers and for patients with recalcitrant category/stage II ulcers.[5] Because of the research support for the use of this modality, the Centers for

Medicare and Medicaid Services cover the use of electrical stimulation in chronic wounds (category/stage III or IV pressure ulcers and ulcers due to diabetes, or arterial or venous insufficiency) that fail to respond after 30 days of standard wound management.[85, 106, 107] Electrical stimulation may also be used to improve slow-healing wounds in older adults.[108]

Contraindications/Precautions

In addition to the standard precautions for the general use of this modality,[27, 85] there are several contraindications for the use of electrical stimulation to facilitate wound healing.[81] First, electrical stimulation is not indicated for simple, uncomplicated wounds. Rather, this modality should be reserved for chronic, nonhealing wounds or for patients at risk for delayed wound healing.[85] Second, wounds with osteomyelitis should not be treated with electrical stimulation.[22] This is because electrical stimulation cannot resolve a bone infection, and facilitating wound closure for these wounds would only result in abscess formation and, therefore, is contraindicated.[85] Wounds with osteomyelitis must first be surgically debrided. Third, electrical stimulation should not be used in combination with topical agents containing heavy metal ions.[53, 85] Fourth, actively bleeding wounds should not be treated with electrical stimulation prior to the attainment of hemostasis.[22] Electrical stimulation should be used with caution on patients with sensory neuropathy to avoid excessive current intensities. When using electrical stimulation in this patient population, clinicians must not depend on patient report of a comfortable paresthesia; rather, clinicians must ensure submotor intensities and should not exceed the maximum recommended treatment intensity.

Method

The literature on the use of electrical stimulation to facilitate wound healing describes various types of stimulation and treatment parameters. The following represents a compilation of the available literature. Refer to the reference list for specific studies and further details on treatment variations. There are three techniques described in the literature for applying electrical stimulation to facilitate wound healing: direct, immersion, and periwound.

Direct Technique

Unfortunately, occlusive dressings have too great a resistance to electrical flow to be used as a conductive medium for electrical stimulation,[109] therefore, electrical

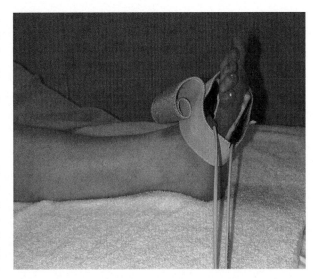

FIGURE 8–3   Direct technique for electrical stimulation.

stimulation must be applied directly to the wound bed (see Figure 8–3). This technique is the most researched method for using electrical stimulation to facilitate wound healing. After performing any necessary debridement and irrigation, a saline- or hydrogel-moistened gauze[110] is placed within the wound bed and covered with a carbon electrode.[77, 111] Alternatively, a piece of cleaned aluminum foil can be cut to the size of the wound and attached to the lead wire by way of an alligator clip. Because of the potential for maceration to develop in areas where the moist gauze contacts the surrounding intact periwound, the clinician may choose to apply a skin sealant or moisture barrier to this area prophylactically. The similarly prepared return electrode may be placed in any convenient location, usually approximately 15–20 cm proximally.[81] If the wound is on an extremity, especially on the lower leg, foot, forearm, or hand, the return electrode may be placed on the opposite body surface. The electrodes should be secured in place. The use of saline-moistened gauze rather than the typical electrical stimulation sponges may reduce the risk of cross-contamination between patients, as even after 20 minutes of disinfection, 8% of sponges tested continued to be contaminated with bacteria.[112]

After treatment, the clinician should assess the result of the treatment and perform any measurements prior to bandaging the wound. Carbon electrodes should be cleaned with an OSHA-approved disinfectant following appropriate infection control guidelines. Foil electrodes and gauze should be discarded according to facility policy for infectious waste. The clinician should monitor the effects of treatment. If there is a decline in wound status or if there is no improvement after 2 weeks of electrical stimulation, alternative interventions must be considered.

Immersion Technique

When using this technique, the wound is placed in a nonmetal basin filled with water. The treatment electrode is then placed contact side down within the basin, essentially making the entire water-filled area the treatment electrode.[54] This method may be beneficial for patients with multiple foot or hand ulcers. The major disadvantages to this technique include a lack of controlled studies using this protocol, potential maceration of the periwound and hyperhydration of the wound bed, and dependent positioning.

Periwound Technique

The periwound technique involves the application of electrodes to the intact periwound rather than the wound bed. Treatment electrodes are placed so as to straddle the wound bed.[55,111] The two advantages to this technique include the ability to keep wound dressings in place and the decreased potential for wound contamination. However, the disadvantage is the lack of research using this indirect technique.

Parameters

Stimulation frequency should be 80–125 Hz.[18,69,81,82,88,110,111] If the interpulse interval can be adjusted, it should be 50–100 microseconds.[69,81,105] Stimulation intensity should be between 75 and 200 volts[69,81,82,110] and produce a comfortable paresthesia.[111,113] In patients with decreased sensation, the intensity should be submotor and still should not exceed 200 volts.[82] Perhaps the area of most intense controversy is the treatment polarity. The most consistent results have been found using cathodal stimulation to decrease wound infection[56,61,73,111,114] and anodal stimulation to restore the normal current of injury, promote granulation tissue formation, and enhance epithelialization.[18,53,93,111] Some authors contend that initial cathodal stimulation may reduce wound bioburden even in wounds that are not clinically infected and, therefore, should be used for the first several days of treatment before changing to anodal stimulation.[61,71,73,114–116] A recent animal study compared an initial 3-day use of cathodal stimulation followed by continued treatment with anodal stimulation with the opposite polarities and a control group that was not treated with electrical stimulation. While all wounds treated with electrical stimulation healed statistically faster than control wounds, there was also a nonstatistically significant trend toward faster healing in the wounds that were initially treated with negative stimulation.[74] Less well understood is the suggestion to alternate between cathodal and anodal stimulation "when healing plateaus."[22] This suggestion appears to stem from a single study on the use of electrical stimulation on experimentally induced wounds in pigs.[117] This study found that the control group had a 7% decrease in size, the negatively stimulated wounds had a 42% decrease, and the wounds that were subjected to 3 days of negative current alternating with 3 days of positive current had an 82% decrease in wound size. However, because this study did not use high-voltage pulsed current, its findings may not be applicable. Until this result can be replicated in human studies using high-voltage stimulation, this procedure is not recommended. Treatments should be 45–60 minutes[69,74] or as little as 30 minutes if performed twice daily.[18,77,88] Inpatient treatments should be performed once or twice daily, while outpatient treatments may be as little as three times per week.[81,113]

Alternative Interventions

Although less supported by research, ultrasound and hyperbaric oxygen may be appropriate alternative adjunctive interventions to facilitate wound healing. See Box 8–5 for a summary of electrical stimulation.

Ultrasound

The research regarding the use of ultrasound as an adjunct to facilitate wound healing is less extensive and less detailed than for electrical stimulation. Much of the research to date has been conducted on animal models with acute or traumatically induced wounds, performed in vitro, sponsored by manufacturers, or contained too few subjects to adequately detect a significant treatment effect and, therefore, does not directly support its efficacy on humans with acute or chronic wounds.[118–120] There are several human studies that report no significant difference in healing between control wounds and those treated with ultrasound.[121] Two of these studies were on geriatric patients with pressure ulcers and did not control for comorbidities.[122,123] Another two studies had methodological flaws, including the application of ultrasound gel directly into the wound bed.[124,125] Despite these few studies, there appears to be sufficient evidence to support the use of this intervention to facilitate wound healing in recalcitrant wounds.[5,91,126–133]

BOX 8–5   Electrical Stimulation

Purpose/Effects

- Restores the current of injury
- Causes galvanotaxis
- Stimulates cells
- Increases blood flow
- Combats infection
- Reduces edema
- Enhances autolysis

Indications	Contraindications
• Adjunct for chronic or recalcitrant wounds	• General precautions for electrical stimulation • Untreated osteomyelitis • Should not be used in combination with topical agents containing heavy metal ions • Patients with sensory neuropathy—precaution

Advantages	Disadvantages
• Research supports efficacy • Can be used in any setting • Does not cause pain • Less setup and cleanup time than whirlpool	• More time consuming than irrigation and whirlpool • Risk of contamination • Cannot be used on extensive wounds

Methods

- Techniques
  - Direct
  - Immersion
  - Periwound
- Frequency: 80–125 Hz
- Intensity: 75–200 volts, submotor
- Polarity
  - Cathodal stimulation for infected wounds; may also be used for the first 3 days of treatment to help reduce wound bioburden
  - Anodal stimulation to promote granulation tissue formation and epithelialization
- 45–60 minutes 3–7 days per week or 30 minutes twice a day

Ultrasound has been purported to enhance all three phases of wound healing. Some authors report that pulsed ultrasound stimulates the release of chemoattractants by fibroblasts,[134] mast cells, and macrophages, thereby reducing the inflammatory phase.[18,20,22,27,91,130] During the proliferative phase, ultrasound may stimulate fibroblast proliferation, resulting in greater collagen deposition,[96,128,129,134,135] enhanced granulation tissue formation, increased angiogenesis,[96,135] and hastened wound contraction.[18,22,130,136,137] Ultrasound may also facilitate angiogenesis.[18,20,22,27,68,96,130] While ultrasound is purported to enhance epithelialization of wounds,[136] this appears to be due to ultrasound's effect on the extracellular matrix rather than direct stimulation of epithelial cells.[138] During the later phases of wound healing, ultrasound increases wound tensile strength.[22, 128, 129, 134, 139] Ultrasound performed during the maturation and remodeling phase may yield a stronger and more pliable scar.[22, 27, 130, 140, 141] The therapeutic effects of ultrasound on wound healing are believed to result from changes in cell membrane permeability due to the nonthermal processes of cavitation and microstreaming.[27, 68, 92, 142] However, there is currently no conclusive evidence to support this theory.[143] Recent studies appear to support the use of low frequency (25–40 kHz) ultrasound in combination with saline mist to assist with debridement of adherent fibrin and to decrease bioburden within chronic wounds.[142, 144, 145] Further controlled studies are needed to determine the most effective treatment parameters, best method of application, and specific wound or patient characteristics that may influence treatment outcomes.[133]

Indications

Ultrasound is indicated as an adjunct to wound healing for chronic or recalcitrant wounds that are clean or infected. Noncontact low-frequency ultrasound combined with saline mist may be most appropriate to assist with the debridement of fibrin within chronic wound beds.[5, 142, 144, 145] Studies to date have shown that ultrasound facilitates wound healing in wounds due to pressure, venous insufficiency, acute trauma, and recent surgery.

Contraindications/Precautions

In addition to the standard precautions for the general use of this modality,[27, 118] contraindications for the use of ultrasound as an adjunct to wound healing include the presence of osteomyelitis, active profuse bleeding, severe arterial insufficiency, and acute deep vein thrombosis. Clinicians should not use ultrasound on untreated acute wound infections. Although there is no scientific evidence to support or refute the use of high-frequency ultrasound over highly necrotic wounds, it would seem logical that eschar may block ultrasound transmission to the underlying tissues. When using ultrasound to treat wounds with large amounts of necrosis or fibrous tissue, noncontact, low-frequency ultrasound parameters should be followed. Like electrical stimulation, ultrasound is not indicated for simple, uncomplicated wounds.[146]

Method

The literature on the use of ultrasound to facilitate wound healing provides significant variability in both treatment technique and parameters. The following represents a compilation of the available literature. Refer to the reference list for specific study details. There are three techniques described in the literature for applying ultrasound to facilitate wound healing: direct, periwound, and immersion. Alternatively, noncontact low-frequency ultrasound combined with a saline mist is also described.

Direct Technique

This technique is the most researched method for using ultrasound to facilitate wound healing and involves applying ultrasound directly to the wound bed (see Figure 8–4).[27] After determining the need for ultrasound as an adjunct for wound healing, choosing the most appropriate method of application, and selecting treatment parameters, the clinician should explain the procedure to the patient. Next, the patient should be positioned comfortably to provide the clinician with easy access to the affected area. The patient should be draped for modesty as needed. Any dressings present should be removed. The wound should be irrigated and the clinician should perform any debridement necessary prior to initiating the ultrasound treatment.

Deep wounds should be filled with an amorphous hydrogel or normal saline to allow the transmission of

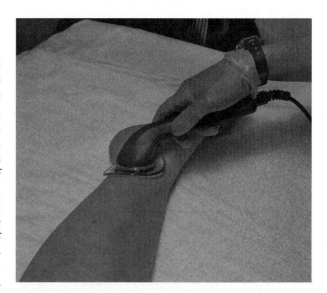

FIGURE 8–4 Direct technique for ultrasound.

energy into the wound bed. The wound must be covered with a barrier to prevent contamination from the conductive gel. Several types of barriers have been suggested in the literature, including semipermeable films, sheet hydrogels, and a glove or condom filled with saline or ultrasound gel. Unfortunately, the ability of these products to transmit ultrasound energy is highly variable, even within a particular class of wound dressings.[147] In general, sheet hydrogels appear to transmit the greatest amount of ultrasound energy; therefore, these should be considered the best barrier for this technique.[147,148] However, at this time the most effective dosage of ultrasound to facilitate wound healing is unknown, and this recommendation is based solely on the assumption that receiving the highest percentage of applied ultrasound energy will lead to superior results. Perhaps more important, clinicians should be discouraged from alternating between various types of barriers to ensure a consistent treatment dosage. Recently, bacteriostatic gel pads have been marketed specifically for use on wounds. They may be equivalent, or superior to, sheet hydrogels. If the wound is 100% granular and a sheet hydrogel is used for bandaging, the clinician may choose to leave the dressing in place for several days and perform ultrasound over the dressing without removal and irrigation.[147] After selecting a wound barrier, ultrasound gel is applied over the barrier as a coupling medium. Because scars have intact skin barrier function, a barrier is not used when applying ultrasound to assist with scar remodeling. Rather, ultrasound gel is applied directly to the scar. Ultrasound is then applied over the wound and periwound or scar.

After treatment, the clinician should assess the result of the ultrasound treatment and perform any measurements prior to bandaging the wound. The sound head should be cleaned with an OSHA-approved cleanser following appropriate infection control guidelines. The clinician should monitor the effects of treatment. If there is a decline in wound status or if there is no improvement after 2 weeks of ultrasound, alternative interventions must be considered.

The advantages to this technique include the ability to maintain a sterile wound environment if desired, minimal risk for wound contamination, and the assumption that treating the wound directly will enhance wound healing more than using an indirect technique. The major disadvantage to the direct technique is the increased cost for wound care supplies if the wound will not also be bandaged with the sheet hydrogel.

Periwound Technique

Ultrasound has been applied to the intact periwound tissues to facilitate wound healing. A meta-analysis of the literature on the use of ultrasound for chronic leg ulcers suggests that ultrasound applied to the periwound *may* be more effective than ultrasound delivered to the wound bed.[149] This method may be particularly beneficial for patients whose wounds are painful, tunneling, or necrotic. Additional advantages of this technique include the ability to leave the wound dressing in place and the lowered risk of wound contamination. The key perceived disadvantage to treating the periwound is the assumption that by treating the periwound *only*, the ultrasound treatment will be less effective than treatment directly over the ulcer.

Immersion Technique

This technique uses the same method as underwater ultrasound for nonwound injuries.[27,68] The affected area is exposed (in this case by removing the dressing, irrigating the wound, and performing any necessary debridement) and then placed in a nonmetal, water-filled basin. The moving sound head is kept 0.5–1.0 cm away from the surface of the wound and periwound.[83] Because the immersion technique does not involve direct contact with the wound, this technique is particularly advantageous for patients with wounds that are painful or sensitive to pressure, or wounds in bony areas such as the malleolus. The disadvantages include the need for dependent positioning, potential for contamination from the basin or sound head, potential for maceration or hyperhydration of the wound bed, and greater setup time. Because this technique is the least studied method, little guidance regarding treatment parameters is available. However, it would seem logical that ultrasound intensity should be increased by as much as 50% to accommodate for the dispersion of energy within the basin.[83]

Parameters

Superficial wounds should be treated with 3.0 MHz ultrasound. Deeper wounds should be treated with 1.0 MHz ultrasound to provide deeper tissue penetration. Because the nonthermal effects of ultrasound appear to be responsible for the beneficial effects on wound healing, ultrasound should be pulsed at 20–25% with a low intensity, around 0.5–1.0 W/cm.[130,134] One study noted wounds treated with 1 MHz and 0.5 W/cm^2 had a greater reduction in wound surface area than those treated with 1.0 W/cm^2. Similar to the use of ultrasound for nonwound care, acute wounds should be treated with lower intensities compared to chronic wounds, and treatment duration should be dependent on the size of the treatment area. The treatment area (either wound and periwound or periwound only if using the indirect technique) should be divided into zones equal to 1.5 times the area of the sound head. Each zone should be treated for 2 minutes initially, increasing in 30-second intervals until reaching 3 minutes of treatment per zone.[20,22] Acute wounds may be treated once or twice daily. Chronic wounds require less frequent treatments, anywhere from daily to three times per week.[20,92] If using ultrasound to help remodel scar tissue, reduce contractures, or improve range of motion, a thermal effect is desired. In such cases, clinicians should consider increasing ultrasound intensity up to 1.5 W/cm^2, continuous ultrasound, or both. This technique is most commonly used on burn scars. Scars that are greater than 1 year old, especially keloids, may not be responsive to ultrasound therapy.[150]

Noncontact Low-Frequency Ultrasound

This is the most recent technique cited in the literature. While low-frequency ultrasound is unlikely to have any cavitational effects, it may be able to produce changes at the protein and cellular levels due to the greater amounts of acoustic streaming.[118] Purported cellular effects that may enhance wound healing include growth factor and collagen production, increased angiogenesis and fibrinolysis, increased macrophage activity, and increased nitric oxide levels.[118,151,152] Low-frequency ultrasound assists with wound debridement and destruction of biofilms, bacteria, viruses, and fungi within the wound bed.[153] Noncontact low-frequency ultrasound has FDA approval for wound debridement and wound cleansing.[153] A noncontact ultrasound device, such as the MIST™ therapy system or the Sonoca Ultrasonic Debridement Device, operates at a frequency of 25–40 kHz. The unit is connected with tubing to a sterile saline bottle. The probe is held perpendicular to the wound surface and moved in a grid pattern slowly on, or within 15 mm above, the wound bed. Treatment time varies but 15–20 seconds per cm^2, with a minimum of 4 minutes for wounds less than 15 cm^2.[144,145] Because aerosolization of fluids and splash injury may occur, clinicians must don appropriate personal protective equipment, including gloves, shoe covers, hair cover over the ears, moisture-resistant gown, and face shield or face mask and protective eye wear.[118] A retro-spective review of the use of noncontact low-frequency ultrasound[151] noted a statistically significant increase in percentage of wounds treated with noncontact low-frequency ultrasound closed (53% vs. 32%). However, the standard care group contained wounds of a longer duration and wounds of multifactorial etiology healed faster with just standard care.

Alternative Interventions

Electrical stimulation, negative pressure wound therapy (see following section), or topical growth factors are alternative interventions that may be beneficial as adjuncts to wound healing.[154] Paraffin, soft tissue mobilization, or silicone dressings may be appropriate alternative interventions for assisting with scar tissue modulation. Other forms of debridement, such as sharp, autolytic, or enzymatic, may be used as alternative or additional interventions to noncontact low-frequency ultrasound. See Box 8–6 for a summary of ultrasound.

Negative Pressure Wound Therapy

Although less extensive than the research on hydrotherapy and electrical stimulation, there is growing evidence to support the use of **negative pressure wound therapy (NPWT)** to enhance healing in chronic, slow-healing, and acute wounds (see Figure 8–5).[155] Alternative terminology for NPWT includes topical negative pressure, sub-atmospheric pressure, and VAC because the first system available in the United States was Kinetic Concepts' **Vacuum-Assisted Closure (VAC)** unit. Currently there are more than 13 manufacturers of negative pressure wound therapy devices, with no clear advantage of any one over

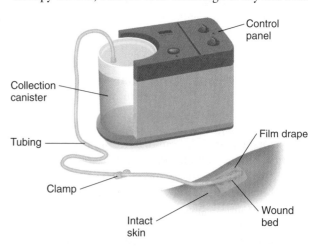

FIGURE 8–5 Negative pressure wound therapy.

BOX 8–6   Ultrasound

Purpose/Effects

- Enhances all three phases of wound healing
- Increases collagen deposition, granulation tissue formation, angiogenesis
- Enhances wound contraction
- Improves scar pliability

Indications	**Contraindications**
• Adjunct for chronic or recalcitrant wounds	• General precautions for ultrasound • Untreated osteomyelitis • Wounds with active, profuse bleeding • Severe arterial insufficiency • Deep vein thrombosis • Direct technique may not be effective with highly necrotic wounds

---

Advantages	**Disadvantages**
• Can be used in any setting • Quick • When compared to whirlpool: less setup/cleanup time, does not require dependency, does not hyperhydrate	• Less research support • Not appropriate for medium or large wounds • May be painful or difficult to apply effectively • Risk of contamination

---

Method

- Techniques
  - Direct
  - Periwound
  - Immersion
- Frequency
  - Superficial wounds: 3.0 MHz
  - Deep wounds: 1.0 MHz
- Intensity
  - Pulsed, 0.5–1.0 W/cm^2
  - Continuous, up to 1.5 W/cm^2 to assist with remodeling of closed wounds
- 2–3 minutes per zone
- Two times per day to three times per week

Method

Noncontact low-frequency ultrasound

20–60 seconds per cm^2 or a minimum of 4 minutes for wounds <16 cm^2 2–3 times per week

---

another.[156] Perhaps because of the limited manufacturers of this modality or the relative newness of the technology, much of the research on NPWT has been sponsored in part by the manufacturer. In fact, one review noted that of 28 randomized controlled trials referred to in the literature, 13 were completed, six were discontinued, six were ongoing, and the status of three were unknown.[1] A single manufacturer sponsored 68% of these studies, while the sponsorship of nine remained unclear.[1]

As with any research, clinicians should carefully review the studies to determine if clinically significant results have been demonstrated.[157] Following are five examples for the reader to consider. First, a systematic review of the literature found only four randomized controlled trials that met inclusion criteria for neuropathic (diabetic) ulcers. The review stated that NPWT can be expected to increase granulation tissue within a wound bed as well as decreasing wound healing by approximately 20%.[158] Second, a small study comparing NPWT to standard wound care on patients with neuropathic ulcers reported a 28.4% decrease in wound surface area using NPWT and only a 9.5% decrease using standard wound care.[159] Third, a larger study using NPWT on 300 wounds (chronic, subacute, and acute) reported 296 favorably responding wounds.[160] Fourth, a small study comparing NPWT and standard treatment post-surgery found that the NPWT patients had an average of 5.6 more days in the hospital (not statistically significant), had no significant difference in average wound size reduction per day, but cost an average of $2,244 more to treat.[157] Lastly, the use of NPWT has been found to be more expensive than standard wound care, with as much as a 54-fold increase in cost noted in one study without a significant improvement in wound healing.[161]

The beneficial effects of NPWT appear to be due to the negative pressure this intervention applies to the wound bed and surrounding tissues.[155,159,162–177] NPWT is believed to increase local blood flow and capillary filling and lymphatic flow, thereby enhancing tissue perfusion and oxygenation. Histological studies demonstrate cellular deformation with NPWT that appears to promote cellular proliferation, division, angiogenesis, and the release of growth factors. Other proposed reasons for the success of this intervention include improved exudate control, increased granulation tissue formation, reduced wound and periwound edema, and enhanced epithelialization. While most of the literature seems to confirm that NPWT decreased wound bioburden, two studies noted either no change or an increase in bacterial bioburden with the use of NPWT.[178,179] NPWT may also help approximate wound edges, facilitating wound contraction and closure. Additional beneficial results of NPWT may be due to the warm, moist wound healing environment obtained through the use of foam and a semi-occlusive film dressing.

Indications

At this time, the U.S. Food and Drug Administration has approved NPWT for use on chronic, acute, and traumatic wounds; partial-thickness burns; dehisced wounds; pressure ulcers; neuropathic ulcers;[180] and muscle flaps and skin grafts.[181–183] The Centers for Medicare and Medicaid Services have determined that negative pressure wound therapy is a component of active wound management and, as such, is reimbursable under Medicare guidelines.[184] Published studies report that NPWT has been successfully used with nonhealing and acute grafts and flaps,[185,186] pressure ulcers,[187,188] neuropathic (diabetic) ulcers,[189–192] acute and dehisced sternal and abdominal wounds,[193–200] traumatic wounds,[201] partial foot amputations,[180] and nonspecified chronic wounds.[155] Additional indications for NPWT include wounds due to arterial or venous insufficiency.[172] NPWT is being used more often over wounds with exposed bone,[186,202] tendon,[203] orthopedic injuries such as degloving,[204] and hardware.[205–208] One recent study even reported the successful use of NPWT over prosthetic vascular bypass grafts.[165] NPWT has also been used successfully in pediatric populations.[209]

Contraindications/Precautions

NPWT is contraindicated for use on dry wounds, necrotic wounds, in body cavities, over malignancies, and in the presence of exposed blood vessels or untreated osteomyelitis.[155,172,173,192] NPWT is associated with at least six deaths and 77 injuries from 2007 to 2009, most related to excessive bleeding.[210] Extreme caution should be used when applying NPWT to patients on anticoagulants, near vascular grafts or vasculature, and to wounds with active bleeding as the negative pressure may cause increased bleeding.[160,172] If NPWT is the modality of choice for these patients, negative pressure should be reduced so that there is no bleeding into the tubing. NPWT should not be applied immediately after an incision and drainage procedure[192] to allow for adequate wound visualization and monitoring for infection. NPWT units should not be connected to traditional wall-mounted suction devices because these devices cannot be as carefully regulated and lack pressure-sensing and alarm mechanisms that will shut off the suction force if unsafe levels are detected.[183]

Method

Prior to initiating NPWT, the wound must first be debrided so the wound bed is free of eschar, slough, and nonviable tissue.[183,192] Next, the sterile foam is cut to the wound size and placed in the wound bed. The manufacturer recommends the black (polyurethane, or PU) foam be used to enhance granulation tissue formation and wound contraction. The softer white (polyviny alcohol, or PVA) foam is used to enhance epithelialization or when the denser foam is uncomfortable to the patient.[155] PVA foam is hydrophilic and should be moistened with saline prior to use.[183] Any areas of undermining or tunneling should also be lightly filled with appropriately sized foam pieces. If multiple pieces of foam are used, they must be in contact with each other to ensure equal distribution of suction.[172] The collection canister should then be connected to the pump and the free end of the tubing should be placed within the hole in the wound dressing to lie within the wound bed. In addition to using a skin sealant, it may be wise to pad the periwound area where the tube exists with a hydrocolloid or sheet hydrogel to prevent excessive pressure from the tubing. The wound is then covered with a film drape, with adequate overlap of the intact periwound tissue to ensure an airtight seal. The tube clamps are opened and the pump turned on to allow wound fluid and bacteria to travel into the 300–1,000 mL collection canister in minutes (see Figure 8–6). The dressing is left in place up to 48–72 hours.[155] If used on an infected wound, the dressing should be changed every 12–24 hours.[155] The pump is battery powered to allow patient mobility but can also be plugged into a conventional wall electrical outlet. The estimated cost of the pump and supplies is $100 per dressing change.[175] To remove the dressing, the clamps are closed, the pump is turned off, and the tubing disconnected. The film drape and drainage tube are removed. The foam pieces are soaked with normal saline to facilitate trauma-free removal. The wound is then thoroughly irrigated and reassessed, and a new dressing is applied.

Parameters

There is not yet consensus in the literature regarding pump parameters. The negative pump pressure is adjustable between 50 and 175 mm Hg.[172] However, because the maximal increase in blood flow appears to occur with 125 mm Hg, most studies have been performed at this pressure.[173] Pressure may need to be increased gradually to this level for patient comfort.[155] The pump may be run continuously or intermittently, with the continuous mode recommmended for flaps, grafts, painful or highly exudating wounds, tunneling or undermining wounds, and wounds in which the dressing application was difficult.[155] At least one author reports that intermittent pressure yields superior results.[175] Intermittent interval therapy, in which negative pressure is applied for 2.5–3.0 hours daily, has also been recommended.[211]

Alternative Interventions

Because there is more extensive research supporting the use of electrical stimulation, unless contraindicated, clinicians would be wise to perform a trial of high-voltage pulsed current prior to initiating NPWT.[171] Small wounds may be treated more cost effectively with standard interventions.[161, 183] As with any wound intervention, treatment effectiveness should be reassessed regularly and at least every 2 weeks. See Box 8–7 for a summary of negative pressure wound therapy.

Hyperbaric Oxygen
Contributions from Lam Le, MD, CWSP, FACHM, FAPWCA

Hyperbaric oxygen therapy (HBO) is defined as the administration of 100% medical-grade oxygen at greater than 1.5 atmospheres absolute pressure. Oxygen reaches a wound bed by being attached to hemoglobin molecules. Under normal atmospheric pressure, hemoglobin is 97% saturated with oxygen. However, under the high pressures of HBO, oxygen dissolved within the plasma is increased by about a factor of 14.[212] HBO is carried out by a specially trained nurse and under the direct supervision of a qualified physician. HBO can be administered in monoplace or multiplace chambers for various conditions, including wound healing. Tissue partial pressures of oxygen must be greater than 40 mm Hg for normal healing.[213,214]

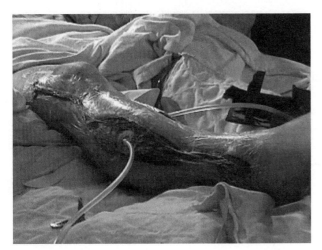

FIGURE 8–6   Negative pressure wound therapy.

BOX 8–7   Negative Pressure Wound Therapy

Purpose/Effects

- Increase local blood flow
- Decrease wound/periwound edema
- Increase granulation tissue formation
- Increase angiogenesis
- Increase epithelialization
- Decrease wound bioburden
- Promote cellular proliferation
- Maintain moist, warm wound environment

Indications

- Adjunct for chronic wounds
- Post-surgical wounds and grafts

Contraindications

- Necrotic wounds
- Body cavity wounds
- Untreated osteomyelitis
- Exposed blood vessels
- Caution with patients on anticoagulants

Advantages

- May cost less over time than standard care for small wounds
- Can be used in any setting
- Maintains warm, moist wound environment

Disadvantages

- No standard for use
- Pain with treatment and dressing changes
  - May be ameliorated with use of medications, lower pressures, PVA foam, or continuous setting
- Noisy
- May hinder patient mobility
- Can be difficult to obtain air-tight seal with drape
- May cause skin damage
- May increase wound care costs

Method

- Irrigate and debride wound bed if needed
- Cut foam pieces to size of wound and place within wound bed
- Protect periwound with hydrocolloid or skin sealant
- Place tubing within wound bed and connect to canister
- Cover with semipermeable film drape; ensure air-tight seal
- Unclamp tubing and turn pump on

Parameters

- Negative pressure: 50–175 mm Hg
- Constant or intermittent
- Treatment time: 12–72 hours

Any injury increases the demand for oxygen while simultaneously causing damage to the microvasculature in the area, increasing the distance oxygen must diffuse across. Additionally, ischemia may be part of wound etiology, as with arterial insufficiency ulcers. HBO *may* enhance wound healing in several ways (see Box 8–8).[18, 187, 212, 213, 215–224] First, HBO therapy increases the concentration gradient for oxygen. This improves oxygen's ability to diffuse into the affected area and hemoglobin's ability to carry oxygen, ultimately providing more oxygen for cell metabolism. The increased oxygen concentrations may also help eliminate oxygen-free radicals. Second, HBO may increase the ability of white blood cells to kill bacteria by providing an oxidative burst to help reduce bacterial growth. Third, HBO may stimulate angiogenesis, collagen synthesis, granulation tissue formation, epithelialization, and wound contraction. Last, the pressure of HBO and patient positioning for treatment may help reduce edema.

BOX 8–8   Hyperbaric Oxygen Therapy

Purpose/Effects

- Increases oxygen concentration gradient
- May reduce bacterial growth
- May enhance angiogenesis, collagen synthesis, granulation tissue formation, epithelialization, and wound contraction
- May reduce edema

Indications*

- Gas gangrene
- Acute traumatic peripheral ischemia
- Acute peripheral arterial insufficiency
- Crush injury
- Grade 3 or worse lower extremity diabetic wounds
- Progressive necrotizing infection
- Chronic refractory osteomyelitis
- Osteoradionecrosis
- Soft tissue radionecrosis
- Preparation and preservation of compromised grafts and flaps

Contraindications

- DVT
- CHF
- Claustrophobia—relative
- COPD—relative
- Pregnancy—relative
- Severe arterial insufficiency

Advantages

- TCOM test can help predict treatment efficacy
- May prevent loss of limb

Disadvantages

- Extremely high cost[†]
- Requires extensive treatment time

Method**

- Patient placed in a chamber breathing 100% oxygen at 1.5–2.5 Atm
- Treatment time: 90–120 minutes
- Treatment frequency: two times per day to three times per week
- Treatment length: 10–60 sessions

*Centers for Medicare and Medicaid Services approved indications for HBO in wound management.

[†]The average patient will require 37 treatments at an overall cost of more than $75,000

**Systemic hyperbaric oxygen is performed by specially trained nurses or respiratory therapists and not by physical therapy personnel.

It should be noted that significant controversy exists in the literature as to the effectiveness of HBO. A recent literature review on the use of systemic HBO as an adjunct for healing diabetic foot ulcers found few well-controlled studies and none that controlled for comorbidities and their effect on wound healing.[225] The following cursory information on systemic HBO is presented in the hopes that future studies will provide further insights as to the efficacy of topical and systemic HBO on wounds of various etiologies.

Indications

Systemic HBO is indicated for several types of chronic or slow-healing hypoxic wounds. **Transcutaneous oxygen monitoring (TCOM)** can be used to detect periwound hypoxia, to determine if a wound is capable of healing without additional interventions such as revascularization or HBO, and to determine the level of amputation if necessary. To perform an oxygen challenge test using transcutaneous oxygen monitoring, an oxygen sensor warmed to 44°C is placed centrally at the chest as a reference point and a second sensor is placed in the periwound. Tissue oxygen levels are recorded while the patient breathes room air at sea level and then repeated with the patient breathing 100% oxygen at sea level.[221,226] If periwound hypoxia is present with TCOM testing on room air and increases at least 10–15 mm Hg when the patient breathes 100% oxygen,[226] the wound is likely to respond to HBO treatments.[18,221,222] However, wounds with significant hypoxia (i.e., periwound oxygen tensions below 30 mm Hg) are unlikely to heal even with HBO therapy.[222,227] HBO has been used successfully on the following types of wounds: thermal burns,[93,228,229] skin grafts and musculocutaneous flaps,[93,216] osteomyelitis,[215,228] pyoderma gangrenosum,[228] necrotizing fasciitis,[228] refractory leg ulcers,[214,228,230] pressure ulcers,[216] acute crush injuries,[216] surgical wounds,[187] and wounds due to radiation tissue damage.[215,231] However, the best candidates for HBO appear to be patients with neuropathic foot ulcers.[213,216,227,228,232–234] In this patient population, systemic HBO has been shown to improve the chance of wound closure and reduce the risk of amputation.[217]

Contraindications/Precautions

Systemic HBO should only be used on patients with wounds that demonstrate improvement in transcutaneous hypoxia with TCOM testing.[221] HBO is contraindicated for use with patients with certain types of metallic or electrical implants as well as certain wound dressings (such as those containing heavy metals). To minimize the risk of embolism, HBO is contraindicated in patients with a deep vein thrombosis. Due to the potential for systemic fluid overload during treatment, HBO is also contraindicated in patients with uncontrolled congestive heart failure.[222] Patients with severe claustrophobia should be treated with extreme caution[222] and may benefit from the use of anxiolytics or mild sedation. Relative contraindications to (systemic) HBO include patients with chronic obstructive pulmonary disease (COPD) and patients who are pregnant.[93] HBO, like electrical stimulation, is not indicated for simple, uncomplicated wounds or for patients with hypoxic wounds who are able to undergo a revascularization procedure.[235] Topical hyperbaric oxygen was historically performed by physical therapists and physical therapist assistants. There is little to no evidence that topical hyperbaric oxygen is effective in accelerating wound healing and it is rarely performed at this time.

Method

Because physical therapy personnel generally do not perform systemic HBO therapy, only cursory procedures are provided. Systemic HBO involves the application of oxygen in a pressurized chamber, typically 2.0–2.5 Atm.[93,217] The patient breathes 100% oxygen in this environment for 90–120 minutes (see Figure 8–7).[217,234] Treatment frequency varies from twice daily to three times per week.[216,222] Patients typically require anywhere between 10 and 60 treatments,[228] with an average of between 37 and 44 treatments.[223,235] It may be

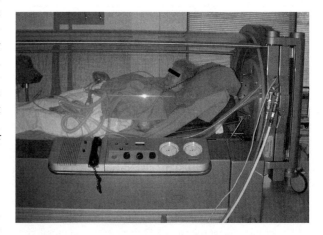

FIGURE 8–7   Patient in a systemic hyperbaric oxygen chamber.

possible to stop treatments sooner once the wound is satisfactorily granulating and improvements in follow-up transcutaneous oximetry demonstrate resolution of peri-wound hypoxia.[235] If a 50% reduction in wound surface area is not noted after 10 HBO treatment sessions, the wound is unlikely to respond to this modality and alternative interventions should be considered.[221]

Alternative Interventions

Prior to considering HBO therapy, the potential for revascularization must first be considered.[235] In addition, electrical stimulation is a less expensive, better researched intervention that may be beneficial as an adjunct to wound healing.

 ## Checkpoint Question #2

You have been working with a home health patient with a leg ulcer for the past month. Initially the wound was necrotic and heavily draining. After 1 week of debridement you were able to achieve a 100% granular wound bed with mild serous drainage. However, the wound size has failed to decrease for the past 3 weeks. You believe the wound may respond to electrical stimulation as an adjunct for wound healing. Describe the parameters you would choose.

Other Promising Modalities to Enhance Wound Healing

Recent research studies in the United States and Europe using additional modalities to enhance wound healing have shown promising results. This section provides a brief overview of the use of monochromatic ultraviolet, low-intensity laser, and infrared energy.

Ultraviolet

Ultraviolet light (UV) has a bandwidth of 200–400 nm.[96] UVA and UVB (280–400 nm) have been used to treat psoriasis and dermatitis for many years.[236] More recent studies have examined the effect of UVC (200–290 nm) on chronic wound healing. The beneficial effects of UVC therapy on wound healing are believed to be due to its ability to increase epithelial cell turnover, enhance cell proliferation, promote growth factor release, stimulate granulation tissue formation, enhance capillary blood flow, and increase vascular permeability.[91,96,126,236,237] In addition, ultraviolet therapy appears to have a bactericidal effect, presumably by altering bacterial DNA structure.[91,126,236,237] Ultraviolet light has been shown to facilitate wound healing in patients with ulcers due to venous insufficiency,[238,239] arterial insufficiency, pressure, and diabetes.[236] The National Pressure Ulcer Advisory Panel suggests that the short-term use of UV-C may be considered to reduce wound bioburden in critically colonized category/stage III/IV pressure ulcers.[5] However, because there are few controlled studies documenting the ability of ultraviolet light to facilitate wound healing, this modality is not currently a standard treatment modality and is not reimbursed by Medicare and Medicaid services. Future research should be directed toward comparing standard wound care procedures with standard care combined with ultraviolet therapy in specific wound types.

Laser Therapy

Laser—light amplification by stimulated emission of radiation—therapy shows promise as a means to stimulate wound healing.[240] **Low-intensity laser therapy** using helium–neon (HeNe, 632.8 nm), gallium–aluminum–arsenide (GaAlAs 830 nm laser), or gallium–arsenide (GaAs, 904 nm) lasers has been used successfully to treat venous insufficiency, pressure, and neuropathic ulcers.[134,241,242] Box 8–9 lists the purported effects of laser on wound healing.

While some studies support the use of laser therapy, much controversy exists. First, while some authors purport laser therapy to be effective due to an increase in blood flow, no such increase has been found when using Doppler probes to assess local circulation changes.[243,244] Second, when comparing the effect of laser therapy to electrical stimulation in acute wound healing, electrical stimulation was found to be more effective.[77] Third, a blind, randomized controlled trial demonstrated no benefit of laser therapy over standard care in the management of category/stage III pressure ulcers.[245] Last, additional studies, including a comprehensive review of

---

BOX 8–9   Purported Effects of Laser Therapy*

- Increased cell proliferation
  - Keratinocytes
  - Fibroblasts
  - Monocytes
- Simulated mitochondria
- Decreased inflammation
- Bacteriocidal
- Stimulated growth factor production and release
- Increased collagen synthesis, organization, and maturation
- Increased angiogenesis
- Increased granulation tissue formation
- Increased epithelialization
- Faster wound contraction
- Higher wound tensile strength

*Majority of research has been conducted in vitro or in animal models.[134,243,249–266]

---

the literature on the use of laser therapy on venous insufficiency ulcers,[30,246,247] found low-intensity laser therapy to have no effect on wound healing. Because there are few well-designed studies to support the use of lasers in accelerating wound healing (and very few that involve human subjects), laser therapy is considered to be experimental and not a recommended intervention.[5,248] Laser is not currently reimbursed by Medicare.

Monochromatic Infrared Energy

Monochromatic infrared energy, or MIRE, involves the delivery of near-infrared energy at 890 nm wavelength to the skin by way of flexible diode pads.[153,267] MIRE therapy is purported to improve blood flow to the treated area by up to 400%.[268] The resulting increased tissue perfusion and oxygenation are believed to result in enhanced wound healing, increased nitric oxide formation, and improved cell proliferation.[267–270] While MIRE therapy has been used in patients with pressure ulcers, arterial insufficiency ulcers, and venous insufficiency ulcers,[269] wound healing seems to be facilitated most in patients with neuropathic ulcers.[268] Patients with diabetic peripheral neuropathy who received MIRE therapy for 30 minutes 3 days per week were found to have improved light touch sensation compared to those receiving sham treatment[271] and to have a lower incidence of subsequent diabetic foot ulcers.[272]

In addition, treated patients reported a 25% decrease in neuropathic pain and an improved sense of balance.[271] However, while these patients were able to detect 10 grams of force (5.07 Semmes–Weinstein monofilament) in a statistically significant number of sites, they continued to lack protective sensation.[268,272,273] It should be noted that nearly all of the research on monochromatic infrared energy has been sponsored by the manufacturer. The National Pressure Ulcer Advisory Panel states there is insufficient evidence at this time to recommend the use of infrared technology for pressure ulcer management.[5] Infrared technology currently has FDA approval only to improve circulation and decrease pain despite the manufacturers' promotion of effectiveness in wound healing and resolution of peripheral neuropathy.[274] As of June 2010, the Centers for Medicare and Medicaid Services have determined that the use of infrared and MIRE are not reasonable and necessary and, therefore, are not covered interventions.[275] Clinicians should check for the most updated local and national (non)coverage decisions prior to seeking reimbursement for the use of MIRE technology. Further research is required before the use of this modality should be considered for the enhancement of wound healing.

CLINICAL DECISION MAKING

Before choosing a modality, the clinician must first assess the patient and the patient's wound(s) to determine appropriate wound management goals with the patient and/or caregiver. Table 8–1 provides a decision grid for intervention options for chronic or slow-healing wounds. Note that there may be several options based on wound description. The clinician must then take into account other factors, such as patient characteristics, wound location, wound etiology, wound size, treatment setting, and equipment availability, before choosing the best intervention. Next, the clinician must determine the wound's needs and the proposed purposes and effects of each intervention, determine if a given procedure is indicated or contraindicated, and carefully weigh the advantages and disadvantages of each procedure before selecting the modality with the greatest chance of enhancing wound healing and the lowest risk of adverse effects. The clinician must then explain the procedure to the patient and/or caregiver, including the rationale, method, risks, benefits, and expected outcome(s).

After the procedure, it is important to assess and document the effect of treatment. Once the expected

TABLE 8–1   Adjunctive Intervention Decision Grid for Chronic or Slow-Healing Wounds Based on Wound Description

Wound Description	Acceptable Adjunctive Intervention Options	Sample Procedural Goal
Granular, nondraining	Pulsed lavage with suction Electrical stimulation Ultrasound (US) Hyperbaric oxygen*	Decrease wound surface area by 20% in 1 week using electrical stimulation and standard wound care.
Granular, draining	Pulsed lavage with suction Whirlpool Electrical stimulation Ultrasound Low-frequency US Hyperbaric oxygen*	Decrease the signs and symptoms of infection within 5 days using electrical stimulation and bandaging with topical antimicrobial agents.
Necrotic, nondraining	Whirlpool Pulsed lavage with suction Electrical stimulation Low-frequency US Hyperbaric oxygen	Softening of eschar with daily whirlpool to allow debridement of all devitalized tissue within 3 days.
Necrotic, draining	Whirlpool Pulsed lavage with suction Electrical stimulation Ultrasound to periwound Low-frequency US Hyperbaric oxygen*	Wound will be 100% granular and have minimal serous drainage within 1 week of initiating pulsed lavage with suction.
Closed wound with red, raised scar limiting range of motion	Continuous ultrasound	Normal scar mobility to allow full active range of motion within 2 weeks of initiating ultrasound and scar tissue mobilization.

*If wound is hypoxic, responds to oxygen test, and at least one adjunctive intervention has failed to assist with wound healing.

goals for a given intervention are met, the procedure should be discontinued. Likewise, if there is no appreciable change in wound status after 2 weeks of appropriate standard wound care and properly performed adjunctive therapy, the intervention should be discontinued,[43] and the patient and patient's wound should be reassessed. If any adverse effects of treatment are identified, the treatment procedure should be reassessed. Any procedural errors found should be corrected, and the treatment should be attempted again. If no procedural errors have been noted, the intervention

should be discontinued immediately. Too often, clinicians forget to assess the effect of a given intervention or fail to modify treatment once treatment goals are met or when wound status changes. For example, although whirlpool therapy may have been initially indicated for a necrotic ulcer with thick, purulent exudate, once the wound becomes granular and the exudate controlled, continued whirlpool treatments will likely retard, rather than enhance, wound healing. In this case, the wound would be best managed with gentle irrigation during each dressing change.

CHAPTER SUMMARY

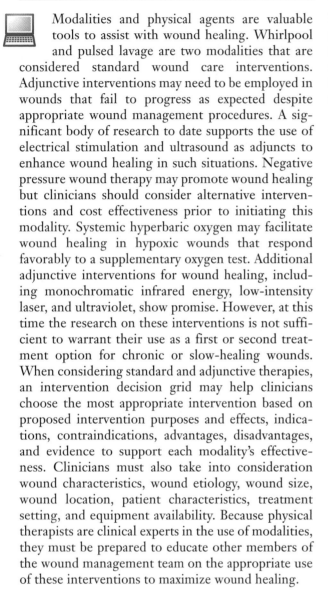

Modalities and physical agents are valuable tools to assist with wound healing. Whirlpool and pulsed lavage are two modalities that are considered standard wound care interventions. Adjunctive interventions may need to be employed in wounds that fail to progress as expected despite appropriate wound management procedures. A significant body of research to date supports the use of electrical stimulation and ultrasound as adjuncts to enhance wound healing in such situations. Negative pressure wound therapy may promote wound healing but clinicians should consider alternative interventions and cost effectiveness prior to initiating this modality. Systemic hyperbaric oxygen may facilitate wound healing in hypoxic wounds that respond favorably to a supplementary oxygen test. Additional adjunctive interventions for wound healing, including monochromatic infrared energy, low-intensity laser, and ultraviolet, show promise. However, at this time the research on these interventions is not sufficient to warrant their use as a first or second treatment option for chronic or slow-healing wounds. When considering standard and adjunctive therapies, an intervention decision grid may help clinicians choose the most appropriate intervention based on proposed intervention purposes and effects, indications, contraindications, advantages, disadvantages, and evidence to support each modality's effectiveness. Clinicians must also take into consideration wound characteristics, wound etiology, wound size, wound location, patient characteristics, treatment setting, and equipment availability. Because physical therapists are clinical experts in the use of modalities, they must be prepared to educate other members of the wound management team on the appropriate use of these interventions to maximize wound healing.

REVIEW QUESTIONS

You are a physical therapist in a nursing home and are trying to prepare for a new patient with a pressure ulcer. The staff member who called to make the referral for physical therapy stated the patient's wound has failed to respond to standard care and describes the wound as necrotic and heavily draining.

1. What alternative intervention options may be indicated?

2. After reviewing the patient's chart, you find the patient has a nonhealing pressure ulcer over her sacral area, which apparently occurred after she sustained an embolic stroke 2 months ago. A wound culture performed 5 days ago was found to be positive for *Escherichia coli* and *Staphylococcus aureus* and sensitive to Keflex. The patient is incontinent and dependent in bed mobility but is cognitively intact. The patient is on the following medications: Zoloft, Lasix, Keflex, and Coumadin. How does this new information change your list of adjunctive intervention options and why?

3. When examining the wound you find it contains 90% yellow adherent, stringy eschar, and 10% granulation tissue with moderate drainage. The wound measures 11.0 × 8.0 cm. You are unable to determine wound depth because of eschar. The periwound has a 0.2-cm border of slight erythema and appears macerated. Based on this new information, choose the most appropriate adjunctive intervention option and provide your rationale.

4. Describe the method and parameters you would use to apply your chosen intervention.

5. Describe the local wound care procedures you would use with this patient.

6. What additional interventions would be appropriate for this patient?

PEARSON
myhealthprofessionskit

Use this address to access the Companion Website created for this textbook. Simply select "Physical Therapy" from the choice of disciplines. Find this book and log in using your username and password to access images, video clips, and additional learning tools.

REFERENCES

Go to myhealthprofessionskit.com to view this chapter's references.

Holistic Management of Patients with Wounds

Chapter Objectives

After reading this chapter, learners will be able to:

1. Describe the role water, protein, carbohydrates, fats, vitamins, and minerals play in wound healing.
2. Describe the components of a nutritional screening for patients with open wounds.
3. Perform a nutritional screening to identify patients in need of an in-depth nutritional assessment.
4. Interpret laboratory tests used to assess nutritional status.
5. Describe nutritional interventions that can facilitate wound healing.
6. Identify potential barriers and methods to facilitate patient adherence.
7. Describe three key components to an interdisciplinary approach to patient management.

Key Terms

Adherence	Negative nitrogen balance	Serum transferrin
Albumin	Positive nitrogen balance	Total lymphocyte count (TLC)
Creatinine	Prealbumin	Urea

INTRODUCTION

Some wounds will heal uneventfully regardless of the interventions provided. The same cannot be said for chronic and slow-healing wounds. These wounds require close attention to every potential cause of impaired wound healing. Clinicians actively engaged in the care of patients with open wounds are generally able to identify and address wound characteristics, such as necrosis or maceration, that may adversely affect healing. However, only the astute clinician is able to recognize and attend to the more global factors that can impact wound healing. This holistic chapter provides a broad view of wound management by examining the vital roles of nutrition, adherence, and interdisciplinary care. The chapter begins with a discussion of the specific functions various nutrients play in wound healing. Next, the key components of nutritional assessments and interventions are presented. This is followed by a presentation of the barriers to patient adherence and clinician strategies to resolve these issues. The chapter concludes with a discussion of interdisciplinary wound management and a detailed case study emphasizing the importance of achieving a coordinated and comprehensive approach to patient care.

NUTRITION AND WOUND HEALING

Clinical and subclinical malnutrition can impair all aspects of wound healing, and remediation of dietary deficiencies can facilitate wound healing.[1] Although patients with noncomplicated wounds successfully achieve wound closure without specific attention to nutritional status, the same is not necessarily true of patients with chronic wounds. This section describes the role of various nutrients in wound healing, the key aspects of a nutritional assessment, and interventions that can help improve a patient's nutritional status to enhance wound healing.

Nutrients

Sufficient amounts of water, protein, carbohydrates, fat, vitamins, and minerals are required for homeostasis, repair, and regeneration. Deficiencies in one or more nutrients can lead to impaired wound healing.

Water

A healthy male is approximately 60% water while a healthy female is approximately 50% water. Water is absolutely vital to wound healing. In the absence of other nutritional deficiencies, dehydration will still result in impaired wound healing[2] and increased risk for pressure ulcer development[1] because a fluid environment is vital to all cell functions. Clinically, dehydration is defined as a 1% decrease in body weight due to fluid loss.[3] If severe, dehydration can lead to hypovolemic shock and even death. Signs of dehydration include decreased urine output, dark-colored urine, rapid decrease in body weight, and decreased skin turgor.[4] When performing a dressing change on a patient with a chronic wound who is also dehydrated, the clinician may notice a dry wound bed or increased necrotic tissue and eschar.

Healthy individuals without open wounds should consume 30–35 mL of fluid per kilogram of body weight every day.[5] Women and men with open wounds should consume roughly 2.7–3.7 liters[6,7] of water per day. Patients with heavily draining wounds or large surface area wounds, such as burn injuries, may need to significantly increase this amount to counteract the fluid lost through evaporation and drainage.[8] Patients

on air-fluidized beds, specialty beds for patients with severe pressure ulcers, require up to 40–60 mL of water per kilogram of body weight to counteract the dehydrating effect of the bed.[2,7] Ideally, this fluid should be water; however, other noncaffeinated, nonalcoholic beverages may also be appropriate. Because attaining and maintaining proper fluid balance is so important and many patients may be clinically or subclinically dehydrated, clinicians should instruct patients with open wounds to try to meet this recommendation to enhance wound healing. Patients with swallowing difficulties, patients on fluid restrictions, and patients who are NPO for more than a few days should be referred to a registered dietitian for assessment.

Protein

Amino acids are the building blocks of proteins. There are 22 amino acids, nine of which are essential and cannot be made by the body.[6] Therefore, these must be obtained through the diet. Protein is required for tissue repair and regeneration.[9] Protein energy malnutrition increases the risk of pressure ulcer development.[1] Deficiency also impairs all three phases of wound healing.[5,8] Without adequate protein stores, collagen synthesis, granulation tissue formation, angiogenesis, and remodeling are all significantly impaired.[10,11] Normal immune function, such as phagocytosis and antibody response time, are also hindered by low protein levels.[6] Protein deficiency alters osmotic pressure, allowing fluid to move from within the vasculature into the interstitium.[6] This impairs healing in two ways. First, edema decreases oxygen's ability to diffuse into the affected area.[11] Second, the pressure created by edema can restrict blood flow within the affected area, further decreasing the availability of oxygen and allowing the accumulation of metabolic waste products.[12]

Although the key cause of protein deficiency is inadequate protein intake, patients may lose a significant amount of protein through wound drainage.[7,11] This is particularly relevant to patients with heavily draining wounds and patients with large surface area burns. Because protein is required throughout the wound healing process, it is imperative that patients with open wounds have sufficient protein intake until satisfactory wound closure has been achieved.[7] Because proteins consist of 16% nitrogen,[13] nitrogen excretion can be used as an indicator of protein intake. If the amount of nitrogen excreted is equal to the amount of nitrogen ingested, the patient is said to be in nitrogen balance.[6,14] If more nitrogen is excreted than is ingested in the form of protein, the patient is said to have a **negative nitrogen balance.**[6,14] This occurs when the body turns to stored proteins as a source of energy. It is desirable for patients to maintain a **positive nitrogen balance** to enhance wound healing. There is some evidence to suggest that a high-protein diet may enhance the healing of burns[15] and pressure ulcers.[4,16] However, the National Pressure Ulcer Advisory Panel currently recommends patients (with pressure ulcers) take in 1.25–1.5 grams of protein/kg of body weight per day to maintain a positive nitrogen balance, when compatible with the patient's overall treatment plan.[4]

Carbohydrates

Carbohydrates, primarily in the form of glucose, provide the energy needed to power the repair and regeneration process.[8] Glucose is also needed for normal phagocytosis.[11] Carbohydrates have a protein-sparing effect.[6] If sufficient energy is not attained from a patient's diet, the body will convert fat and protein to energy.[6] Although this strategy resolves the energy deficit crisis, if protein stores are not replaced, the patient will develop protein deficiency, retarding healing. Therefore, adequate carbohydrate intake is imperative to maximize wound healing. The current recommendation is that patients take in 30–35 kilocalories/kg body weight per day.[4]

Fats

Although generally perceived as a negative factor by laypeople, fat is essential to the healing process. Most important, fat provides a needed energy source to fuel cellular processes when carbohydrate sources have been depleted.[6] Fat is required to carry fat-soluble vitamins, including vitamins A, E, and K,[6] needed for wound healing[15] and helps with thermoregulation by providing insulation. Fats, in the form of free fatty acids, are vital components of cell membranes and are required for the synthesis of new cells.[17]

Vitamins

Vitamins are organic compounds that are needed in small amounts to build new tissue, to maintain tissue health, and to aid in normal immune function.[14] Vitamins A, C, E, and K and the B complex vitamins are especially important for wound healing. The general recommendation is for patients to consume a balanced diet and to use supplementation when dietary intake is inadequate or deficiencies have been confirmed or suspected.[4] Fat-soluble vitamin supplementation must be initiated with caution as, unlike water-soluble vitamins, they can accumulate within the body and become toxic.

Vitamin A

Vitamin A, or retinol, is a fat-soluble vitamin that helps maintain healthy skin and epithelial integrity.[6,14] Vitamin A is required for collagen synthesis,[7] promotes granulation tissue formation,[18] and facilitates epithelialization.[2,8, 11, 19] It may also enhance macrophage function.[6] Vitamin A plays an important role in cellular differentiation, both in epithelial cells and the immune system.[6] Vitamin A may be particularly important for individuals taking corticosteroids, such as patients with chronic inflammatory conditions.[20] Supplementation may reverse the inhibitory effects of long-term corticosteroid therapy, including decreased collagen synthesis, granulation tissue formation, and wound contraction.[10] Vitamin A supplementation may also increase wound tensile strength and decrease the risk of wound dehiscence in these patients.[21] It is believed that vitamin A may enhance wound healing that is retarded by diabetes mellitus, radiation treatment, and stress.[21] Both topical and systemic supplementation are effective. However, because systemic supplementation may counteract the effects of prescribed steroids, systemic supplementation is not recommended.[21] Vitamin A gelcaps may be applied directly to granulating wounds or new scar tissue to enhance healing without risk of side effects or systemic drug interactions.

Vitamin C

Vitamin C, or ascorbic acid, is needed to build[17] and maintain tissues.[14] Overt or subclinical deficiencies will delay wound healing.[14] Vitamin C helps the body absorb iron[14] and is required for collagen synthesis.[1, 6, 18] Deficiencies result in altered capillary integrity, decreased wound tensile strength,[6, 8] and an increased risk of wound dehiscence.[11] Vitamin C may help control infection by activating white blood cells and enhancing their ability to migrate into the wound region.[1, 18, 22, 23] It is also an antioxidant and, therefore, may limit the damaging effects of free radicals.[6]

Vitamin C supplementation may enhance wound healing in malnourished patients[16] and patients with pressure ulcers. In one study, patients with pressure ulcers received standard care or standard care in addition to 500 mg of vitamin C two times per day. The average decrease in wound size for the supplementation group was 84%, whereas wounds of the standard care group decreased only 43%.[24] Pretreatment of irradiated skin with topical vitamin C may delay the onset, decrease the severity, and improve the healing time of radiation skin reactions.[25,26] Although only prolonged and severe vitamin C deficiencies will result in scurvy, subclinical deficiencies may be common.[2] If a vitamin C deficiency is suspected, supplementation should be considered.

Vitamin K

Vitamin K is a fat-soluble vitamin that is essential for blood clotting.[6,14] Due to its effect on clotting factors, deficiencies may lengthen the inflammatory phase of wound healing and cause wounds to bleed readily. Patients on anticoagulants should not initiate vitamin K supplementation without prior clearance and explicit dosage recommendations from their physicians.

B Complex

The B complex vitamins are a group of eight water-soluble vitamins that are required for normal immune function and energy metabolism.[6] B complex vitamins aid in white blood cell function, antibody formation, and resistance to infection.[11,19] They also facilitate normal fibroblast function and collagen synthesis, improving wound tensile strength.[9] Thiamine (B1), riboflavin (B2), and niacin are important coenzymes for the metabolism of proteins, carbohydrates, and fats into energy.[6] Folate and B_{12} (cobalamin) facilitate normal blood formation and red blood cell maturation.[11,23]

Vitamin E

Vitamin E is a fat-soluble antioxidant that helps prevent free radical–related cellular damage.[6] Vitamin E decreases the inflammatory phase of wound healing, enhances immune function, and decreases platelet adhesion.[22]

Minerals

The microminerals zinc, iron, copper, and magnesium as well as the macrominerals calcium, phosphorous, and selenium are also important for the wound healing process.

Zinc

The skin contains 20% of the body's stores of the mineral zinc. Zinc is vital to many cellular processes, including collagen and protein synthesis, cell proliferation,

epithelialization, and normal immune function.[1,6,7,18] Zinc, like vitamins C and E, is an antioxidant and may enhance wound healing by reducing the number of free radicals.[1,14]

Research on zinc supplementation is inconclusive.[27] However, because studies have shown that providing zinc supplements enhances wound healing in zinc-deficient animals[2] and may facilitate wound healing in malnourished humans,[16] zinc supplementation should be considered if serum levels are deficient.[1,9,11]

Iron

Iron-deficiency anemia is the most common cause of anemia.[7] Iron deficiencies can occur due to excess iron loss (e.g., excessive blood loss due to severe trauma or a gastrointestinal ulcer), decreased iron absorption by the gastrointestinal system, reallocation of iron stores to assist with production of other molecules—such as macrophages in the case of chronic infection, rather than red blood cells—or inadequate dietary iron intake compared to the body's metabolic iron demands.[7] Iron is an essential component of hemoglobin and is required for oxygen transport.[6,14] It is also required for antibody production and normal immune function.[23] Iron is a cofactor in many enzyme systems and is required for collagen and DNA synthesis.[6,28] Iron-deficiency anemia may lead to tissue hypoxia, decreased immune function, decreased cell replication, and decreased wound tensile strength.[28]

Copper

The mineral copper is required for hemoglobin synthesis and iron absorption and transport.[6,14] Because copper is a cofactor in the production of collagen and elastin,[6] it helps increase wound tensile strength.[1] Copper deficiencies may lead to poor wound healing and decreased immune function.[6]

Magnesium

Magnesium is important in bone formation, protein synthesis, repair, and is a critical cofactor to more than 300 enzyme systems.[6] Magnesium deficiency is often found in patients with diabetes mellitus, alcoholism, chronic diarrhea, or dehydration.[6,23] Inadequate stores of this mineral lead to hypertension and vasoconstriction.[6]

Calcium

Calcium is vital to bone formation, bone remodeling, and muscle contraction.[6] Calcium is required for fibrin synthesis and, therefore, is important for blood clotting.[14] Calcium is an important neurotransmitter and assists with cellular membrane stability. Together, calcium and phosphorus account for over half of all minerals in the body.[6] Hyperparathyroidism, skeletal tumors, and drug toxicity can cause hypercalcemia. In contrast, hypocalcemia may be caused by inadequate calcium dietary intake, vitamin D deficiency, or excessive phosphate intake.[7]

Phosphorus

In addition to being required for bone formation, phosphorus is needed for normal metabolism, fluid balance, and is an essential component of many enzyme systems.[6] Phosphate homeostasis is primarily controlled by the kidneys. Hypophosphatemia may be caused by vitamin D deficiency, prolonged respiratory alkalosis, gastrointestinal malabsorption, or excessive use of (phosphate-binding) antacids.[7]

Selenium

Selenium is required for the synthesis of up to 30 proteins and assists with normal immune function.[6]

However, because both too little and too much selenium can compromise a patient's ability to fight infection,[6] regular supplementation is not recommended.

Nutritional Assessment

Malnourished patients have higher rates of surgical complications[18] and wound dehiscence.[7,10] Severe malnutrition not only increases a patient's length of stay, but also increases the risk of infection, sepsis, and even death.[2] Therefore, clinicians should routinely perform a nutritional screening on every patient[7] with an open wound just as they would perform wound measurements or a vascular assessment. The clinician should report any positive findings on the screening to the physician, request additional laboratory tests to verify suspicions, and request a consult with a registered dietitian for medical nutrition therapy.

Nutritional Screening

To perform a nutritional screening, the clinician must consider patient characteristics, recent dietary history, wound characteristics, and patient comorbidities (see Figure 9–1). Patient characteristics suggestive of malnutrition include the following physical signs: emaciation, petechiae, transparent skin, pallor, dull or

NUTRITIONAL SCREENING			
Patient Characteristics	Recent Dietary History	Wound Characteristics	Patient Comorbidities
• Cachexia • Emaciation • Petechiae • Transparent skin • Pallor • Dull or thinning hair • Pale eye membranes • Missing or poor dentition • Redness or swelling of the mouth • Swollen gums that bleed easily • Mouth sores • Brittle, pale, or ridged nails	• Significant weight loss • Grossly inadequate intake of vital nutrients • Poor understanding of proper nutritional guidelines	• Chronic wounds • Slow-healing wounds • Repeat ulcerations • Pressure ulcers • Neuropathic ulcers • Extensive burns	• Diabetes mellitus • Cancer • Obesity • HIV/AIDS • Dysphagia • Gastrointestinal dysfunction • NPO status • Receiving parenteral nutrition

FIGURE 9–1 Practitioners should screen for the following clinical manifestations to identify individuals at risk for impaired wound healing due to malnutrition.

TABLE 9–1   Body Mass Index

Body Mass Index (kg/m^2)	Interpretation
<16.0	Underweight—Severe protein-energy malnutrition
16.0–16.9	Underweight—Moderate protein-energy malnutrition
17.0–18.4	Underweight—Mild protein-energy malnutrition
18.5–24.9	Normal Weight
25.0–29.9	Overweight
30.0–34.9	Obese—Class 1
35.0–39.9	Obese—Class 2
≥40.0	Obese—Class 3

thinning hair, pale eye membranes, missing or poor dentition, redness or swelling of the mouth, swollen gums that bleed easily, and/or mouth sores.[2,6,16] Healing is best in patients who are lean and well nourished.[8] The body mass index, or BMI, is calculated by dividing a patient's weight in kilograms by his or her height in meters squared. Clinicians should compare the patient's BMI to normative values (refer to Table 9–1),[1,6,20,29,30] Easy reference tables and BMI calculators are available in both metric and standard units.

Clinicians should identify any recent changes in body weight. Significant weight loss is defined as a decrease of 1–2% of body weight per week, 5% per month, 7.5% in 3 months, or 10% in 6 months.[1,22,31] Although clinicians generally recognize that patients who are severely underweight are at risk for impaired healing, they must also understand that patients who are obese are also at risk. In one study of patients with pressure ulcers, 53% were obese.[32] In addition, obese patients were 23% more likely to get an infection than patients whose body weight was within recommended limits.[8] Obtaining a recent diet history may also help elucidate nutritional problems.[7] From this information, wound care practitioners should be able to identify grossly inadequate fluid or caloric intake or a patient's lack of understanding of proper nutritional guidelines, such as the need of a patient with type 2 diabetes mellitus to limit the intake of fats and simple sugars. Wound characteristics that may represent impaired nutritional status include chronic wounds, slow-healing wounds, repeat ulcerations, pressure ulcers,[16] neuropathic ulcers, and extensive burns.[2] Comorbidities that may represent impaired nutritional status include diabetes mellitus, cancer, obesity, HIV/AIDS, dysphagia, and gastrointestinal dysfunction such as malabsorption. Patients who have had prolonged NPO status and patients receiving parenteral nutrition are also at risk for malnutrition. Table 9–2 describes the clinical manifestations of possible nutrient deficiencies.

Laboratory Testing

After identifying a patient who is at risk for malnutrition, the physician will order laboratory tests to obtain a more clear picture of the patient's nutritional status. As with other tests and measures, laboratory values should be considered a piece of the overall clinical picture of a patient's status, along with changes in body weight, daily food and fluid intake and output, diagnoses, and medications.[2] The five most commonly performed diagnostic tests to determine the presence of malnutrition include creatinine, serum albumin, prealbumin, serum transferrin, blood urea nitrogen, and total lymphocyte count (see Table 9–3).[7] Patients with known or suspected diabetes mellitus should also have blood glucose levels assessed.

TABLE 9–2   Clinical Manifestations of Possible Nutrient Deficiencies

Nutrient	Clinical Manifestations of Possible Deficiency
Water	• Dry skin, hair, and mucous membranes • Poor skin turgor • Increased heart rate and respirations • Orthostatic hypotension • Confusion • Sunken eyeballs
Protein	• Dull, dry hair • Pallor • Peripheral edema • Pressure ulcers, especially multiple or repeat ulcerations
Carbohydrates/energy	• Decline in body weight • Pallor • Extremely poor dentition
Fats	• Emaciated • Epidermal flaking • Fissuring of the skin • Large flakes of dandruff
Vitamin A	• Night blindness • Difficulty adapting to changes in light intensity • Scleral changes and dry eyes • Gingivitis • Pigment changes • Dry skin
Vitamin C	• Swollen gums that bleed readily • Transparent skin quality • Weakness • Delayed wound healing
Vitamin K	• Petechiae • Wound bleeds readily

(Continued)

TABLE 9–2   Continued

Nutrient	Clinical Manifestations of Possible Deficiency
B complex vitamins	• Pallor • Pale eye membranes • Hyperpigmentation • Redness or swelling of the mouth • Mouth sores • Purple discoloration of the tongue with loss of villi • Swollen gums that bleed readily • Confusion • Muscle cramps • Anemia
Zinc	• Decreased sense of taste • Dull, dry, or thinning hair • Seborrhea-like dryness and redness of the face
Iron	• Pallor • Yellow discoloration of the skin • Soft, spoon-shaped nails • Easily fatigued • Dyspnea • Anemia
Copper	• Thinning of hair • May have pigmentation changes
Magnesium	• Dehydration • Neuromuscular hyperexcitability • Confusion
Calcium	• Acute: neuromuscular hyperexcitability, dysrhythmias • Skeletal deformities such as kyphoscoliosis • Idiopathic and compression fractures • Bone pain • Dry scaling skin and hair • Brittle nails
Phosphorus	• Skeletal deformities • Idiopathic fractures • Bone pain
Selenium	• Decreased ability to fight infection • Muscle pain • Muscle wasting

TABLE 9–3   Laboratory Values to Identify Malnutrition

Test	Normal Value
• Creatinine	0.8–1.5 mg/dL
• Serum albumin	3.5–5.5 g/dL
• Serum prealbumin	16–40 mg/dL
• Serum transferrin	>170 mg/dL
• BUN	5–25 mg/dL
• Total lymphocyte count (TLC)	>1,800 cells/mm³
• Blood glucose	70–110 mg/dL

Creatinine

Creatinine is a measure of kidney function and protein status.[22] Normal creatinine levels are 0.8–1.5 mg/dL.[33] Malnutrition decreases creatinine levels.[31]

Serum Albumin

Albumin is a plasma protein produced by the liver that accounts for over half of all plasma proteins.[34] Normal serum albumin levels are at least 3.5 g/dL.[5,16,34,35] Albumin levels fall rapidly with protein deficiency and malnutrition.[5,8] Decreases in serum albumin levels below 3.2 mg/dL are associated with longer hospitalization and increased complications.[22] There is also a positive correlation between low serum albumin and pressure ulcer severity.[32] A decrease in serum albumin will result in a drop in plasma oncotic pressure, leading to tissue edema.[9,34,35] Dehydration will elevate serum albumin levels.[2,5,31]

Prealbumin

Prealbumin is a major transport protein whose normal value is 16 to 40 mg/dL.[5] Deficiencies in prealbumin status are classified as mildly low (13.6–17.9 mg/dL), moderately low (10–13.5 mg/dL), and severe depletion (less than 8 mg/dL).[5,36] Mortality risk increases as prealbumin levels drop.[5] Although serum albumin is a marker for nutritional status, its long half-life (20 days)[5] and high prevalence do not allow this measurement to respond to short-term changes in nutritional status that would be expected after initiating an education or supplementation program.[8, 11, 22, 35]

In contrast, prealbumin has a relatively short half-life of 2–4 days,[2,8] making it a better indicator of the effect of nutritional interventions.[35,37] Unfortunately, prealbumin levels, as well as albumin levels, can be reduced by metabolic stress and inflammation and, contrary to previously thought, prealbumin levels may be maintained at normal levels during states of malnutrition.[2]

Serum Transferrin

Serum transferrin levels are a sensitive indicator of protein status that, like prealbumin levels, are responsive to short-term change.[31] Serum transferrin levels will increase with iron deficiency and decrease with protein deficiency.[8] Serum transferrin levels less than 170 mg/dL indicate malnutrition.[11]

BUN (Blood Urea Nitrogen)

Urea is a by-product of protein metabolism and is excreted by the kidney. BUN is an indicator of renal function. Normal BUN levels are 5–25 mg/dL.[17] Elevated BUN levels are associated with a decrease in wound healing.[5]

Total Lymphocyte Count (TLC)

Total lymphocyte count (TLC) is an indirect measure of nutritional status and immune function.[22] TLC can be calculated using the following equation: TLC = white blood cell count × percent lymphocytes. Normal TLC is greater than or equal to 1,800/mm³. Decreased TLC is associated with delayed wound healing[38] and increased mortality.[2,31] TLC less than 1,500/mm³ indicates immunocompromise[22]; TLC less than 1,200/mm³ indicates protein deficiency.[11] In one study, the presence of normal serum albumin and TLC successfully predicted healing of patients with lower extremity amputations with 75% sensitivity and 90% specificity.[18]

Blood Glucose

Normal blood glucose levels are 70–110 mg/dL.[6] Increased blood sugar levels are associated with an increased risk of ulceration, infection, and impaired wound healing.[28,39,40] The higher a patient's blood sugar, the greater the risk.[41] Refer to Chapter 13 for further details on the adverse effects of poor glycemic control.

Nutritional Interventions

To facilitate wound healing, nutritional status must be maximized.[42,43] Three main causes of malnutrition are lack of knowledge, poverty, and health problems.[8] Therefore, education is crucial. Physical therapists should instruct patients and caregivers in proper nutritional guidelines and ways to effectively meet these requirements within their financial constraints. Patients whose nutritional status fails to improve or who are severely ill, such as a patient receiving chemotherapy with excessive weight changes or a patient receiving parenteral nutrition, should be referred to a registered dietitian for more individualized and thorough nutritional interventions. Patients who fail to recognize the importance of proper nutrition and follow recommended guidelines upon discharge from medical care are likely to have recurrent ulcerations.

Many patients require assistance or encouragement to increase their food intake to satisfactory levels. For example, a patient in an extended care facility recovering from a left-sided cerebrovascular accident may require physical assistance or adaptive utensils and equipment because he is unable to use his dominant extremity for feeding. Therefore, an aide may be necessary to assist the patient during meal times. Likewise, the patient's sense of taste may be altered, or he may find the food choices available in the facility unfamiliar. In this situation, encouraging the patient to eat a certain percentage of each meal or providing more appealing food items may be beneficial.

Some patients may require short- or long-term nutritional supplementation to alleviate nutritional deficiencies.[1] Patients with chronic wounds may require greater than the U.S. recommended daily allowance (RDA) of protein to maximize wound healing.[9] It is suggested that patients consume 30–35 calories per kilogram of body weight per day and 1.25–1.50 grams of protein per kilogram of body weight per day to maintain a positive nitrogen balance.[1] Patients who are unable to meet these requirements should receive appropriate supplementation. Because even clinically inapparent nutritional deficiencies, particularly vitamin and mineral deficiencies, can impair wound healing, patients with any known or suspected vitamin or mineral deficiencies should be given appropriate supplementation. Patients who receive nutritional supplementation to reach adequate levels generally have better wound healing than those who do not receive supplementation.[18] Total parenteral nutrition (TPN) should be considered if a patient's gastrointestinal system is not functioning

normally and healing is consistent with the patient's overall treatment goals.[16,31] In addition to reassessing laboratory values, a complete nutritional assessment should be performed by a registered dietitian every 3 months in all patients who are malnourished or at risk for becoming so (see Figure 9–2).

An all too common scenario in the United States today is not inadequate food intake, but rather consumption of food with little or no nutritional value. Thanks to multibillion-dollar marketing campaigns and its omnipresence, the fast-food industry has changed Americans' eating habits. What was once a monthly treat has for some become a daily stop for breakfast, lunch, dinner, or more. Out-of-proportion serving sizes; high-fat "main courses"; carbonated beverages, which are cheaper than water; and the ever-present suggestive selling—"Would you like fries with that?"—are all too commonplace in the American diet. Even once relatively nutritionally benign beverages, like coffee, are now regularly infused with fat and sugar. Prepared meals, such as the old stand-by "TV dinner," may be the most "home cooking" a person eats in a week. While nutritional information is required on grocery items, such as frozen dinners, only a few regions now require restaurants and fast-food chains to make nutrition information available. Marketing ploys such as so-called "healthy option" salads loaded with cheese, meat, and a dressing that combined contain nearly three times the recommended daily amount of fat and sodium further confuse and malnourish the average consumer. The clinician must help patients and caregivers navigate past the fat-laden, nutrition-starved streets and onto the road of nutrient-dense food choices while staying within their budget, time constraints, and taste preferences.

Special Situations

Certain patient populations, including patients with pressure ulcers, neuropathic ulcers, and burn wounds, require particularly close attention to nutritional status to maximize wound healing. Pressure ulcer formation is associated with protein-calorie deficiency,[44] and pressure ulcer severity is correlated with the severity of malnutrition.[16,18] Neuropathic ulcerations are more prevalent in patients with poor glycemic control, and improvements in glycemic control are correlated with improvements in wound healing.[41,45] Extensive burn wound injuries increase the patient's metabolic rate. A high-calorie, high-protein, high-carbohydrate, and low-fat diet can help maximize the patient's recovery.[15] These patients should also take a

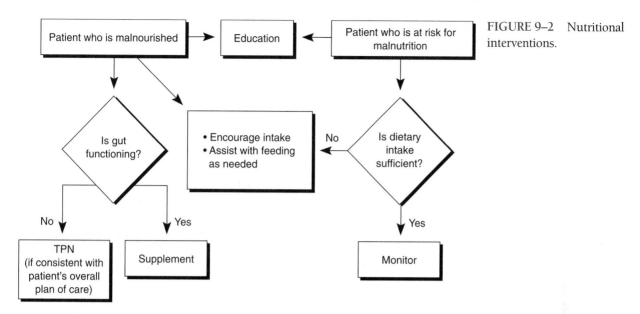

FIGURE 9–2   Nutritional interventions.

multivitamin daily in addition to supplements of vitamin A, vitamin C, and zinc. Patients with burn injuries covering more than 20% of total body surface area and patients who require prolonged ventilatory support may require supplemental external nutrition,[15] including tube feedings or total parenteral nutrition. Refer to Section III for details on the examination and management of pressure ulcers, neuropathic ulcers, and burns.

In summary, wound care practitioners should be aware of the role various nutrients play in normal wound healing. Clinicians must be able to perform a nutritional screening to identify patients at risk for malnutrition. Laboratory tests should be used to confirm suspected cases of malnutrition and a registered dietitian should be consulted to help correct nutritional deficiencies. Nutritional assessment and support can vastly improve wound healing.[10,42]

 ## *Checkpoint Question #1*

Since more than half of the patients with pressure ulcers in one study were found to be obese and obesity is associated with impaired wound healing, explain why it may be imprudent to place a patient with a pressure ulcer who is obese on a very-low-calorie diet.

PATIENT ADHERENCE

The terms *adherence* and *compliance* are often incorrectly used interchangeably. Compliance implies a one-way interaction in which the omniscient clinician directs the patient to follow certain procedures.[46] The patient complies solely because the clinician said to do so. In contrast, **adherence** implies the patient freely chooses to follow suggested guidelines.[46] Because patients have the freedom to act, or not act, upon clinician suggestions, adherence is the more appropriate term. Patient adherence, or lack thereof, is not just an issue for clinicians

involved in wound care, but affects all areas of clinical practice. For instance, initial patient adherence to suggested exercise programs after a myocardial infarction ranges from 80% to 100%.[47-49] However, there is a steady decline in adherence with the passage of time, to as little as 20% after 1 year.[49] Adherence with antibiotic regimens has been documented to be 95% initially, decreasing to a mere 30% after 5 days.[50] Perhaps more applicable to wound care providers, patient adherence to diabetic regimens has been shown to be as low as 10–20%.[51] While it has been estimated that diabetes-related foot complications can be reduced between 49%

and 85% with appropriate preventive strategies such as patient education and self-care, 64% of patients with diabetes surveyed reported not inspecting their shoes prior to donning, and 23% reported never performing foot skin checks.[52] One study found that patients with chronic wounds of various etiologies who were adherent, defined as those who did not miss more than three consecutive appointments and followed home bandaging instructions, healed faster than nonadherent patients. All adherent patients went on to achieve wound closure.[53] Because patient adherence is critical to timely wound healing and prevention, clinicians must answer two critical questions: Why do some patients fail to follow clinical recommendations, and how can clinicians facilitate patient adherence?

Understanding and Enhancing Adherence

Understanding the factors affecting adherence is the first step toward improving patient adherence. In order to understand and address these factors better, clinicians should think of them in relation to the following: patient, task, and clinician. It may be helpful to relate some of the potential problems with adherence to a communication model in which the patient is the receiver of information, the task is the message, and the clinician is the sender. Inherent in this model is the acknowledgment that messages are never unambiguous and senders are never fully in control of the message. For example, the clinician may tell the patient, "You need to keep the wound covered to prevent dirt and bacteria from entering the wound" in an attempt to instill in the patient the importance of not leaving the wound unbandaged. However, the patient's interpretation of this message may be that the dressing should not be removed *at all* until the next clinic visit. When the patient returns to the clinic 1 week later with the same wound dressing on, the clinician is exasperated by the patient's *apparent* nonadherence, the patient is irritated by the inconvenience of not having been able to bathe for a week, and both are frustrated because the wound has deteriorated. Nonadherence may be unintentional,[54] due to a misunderstanding, as described in the example above, or poor eyesight limiting skin inspection, or just plain forgetfulness. In contrast, nonadherence may be intentional, that is, a patient may make a rational decision not to adhere to suggested recommendations because of real or perceived barriers.[54] For example, a patient may choose not to wear recommended protective footwear during

wound healing because it is not cosmetically appealing to him or her.[55] This section describes patient, task, and clinician characteristics that can detract from patient adherence in addition to clinician strategies to foster adherence.

Patient Characteristics

Patients' prior experiences can have a profound effect on their current actions. Consider a patient with diabetes who is referred to physical therapy for an ulcer on the plantar aspect of his great toe. The patient was seen 1 year ago for an ulcer in the same location that healed after 2 months of physical therapy. The patient may believe that, since the previous ulcer healed uneventfully, there is no reason to change his current behaviors, such as walking 54 holes of golf per week and frequently snacking on high-sugar, high-fat foods. Alternatively, consider a patient with arterial insufficiency who was adherent to clinician recommendations but went on to have a below-knee amputation due to the severity of her disease process. Six months later, the same patient is again referred to physical therapy for an ulcer on the remaining foot. This patient may be nonadherent because she perceives that regardless of her actions, this wound will also fail to heal.[56] To facilitate patient adherence, the clinician should emphasize that past experience does not dictate future outcomes. Rather, the clinician should highlight the control the patient has over the current situation and specifically how action, or lack of action, can affect outcomes.[57] Self-efficacy, or a patient's confidence in his or her abilities to perform a given task or behavior, is associated with adherence.[54,56]

Patient support systems and lifestyle choices can have an effect on adherence. Individuals who perceived less support from others were less adherent to suggested regimens.[58] Clinicians should encourage caregiver involvement to increase patient adherence.[57,59] Obesity and lifestyle choices, such as smoking, may be correlated with poor adherence.[57] Clinicians should nonjudgmentally inform patients of the potential risks of nonadherence and the expected benefits of adherence. In addition, clinicians should set mutually agreed-upon, low-risk solutions.[59,60] For example, smoking is known to be addictive and to impair wound healing.[39] Rather than demanding a two-pack-a-day smoker to quit smoking, a more realistic goal might be for the patient to decrease to one pack per day in a given period of time. Patients with less education or poor motivation may be less adherent because they choose a more passive approach in which it is the clinician's job to effect a cure. By emphasizing a cooperative effort and clearly defining both patient and caregiver role expectations, adherence may be increased.[60]

Patients may be nonadherent because they do not know what to do or what is expected of them.[61] For example, the patient may know that his bandage is to be changed three times per day, but does not recall the exact procedure. In addition, the patient may lack the understanding as to why it is important to follow suggested guidelines. The clinician must provide the patient and caregiver with the knowledge to make informed decisions to help control the patient's disease process[62] and improve the patient's healing potential. Simply telling a patient to follow a procedure is insufficient.[54] The patient should be told why, for example, it is important to change the dressing this frequently (because the antimicrobial is ineffective after 8 hours) or what the potential consequences of nonadherence are (delayed wound closure, infection, sepsis, etc.). The patient should be educated as to how to reach this goal (step-by-step instructions). Individuals who perceive their situation to be serious[55] or report fear of complications[63] are more likely to be adherent. It is the clinician's responsibility to provide the patient with a link between knowledge and action,[54,64] thereby increasing adherence.

Task Characteristics

Clinicians should help patients identify and remove barriers to task performance.[54] Patients may be nonadherent because the involved task is too complex.[65] By concisely communicating expected patient behavior and providing clear written instructions, adherence and proper performance may be enhanced.[66,67] Patients may perceive that they are unable to perform suggested procedures.[57] By having the patient or caregiver demonstrate the task,[68] such as bandaging an open wound, all parties can be certain the task is understood and manageable.[69] Many times, suggested regimens may be aversive. For example, performing range of motion exercises after a severe burn injury is likely to evoke pain. Adherence may be increased by ensuring appropriately timed pain medication, setting limits for the procedure (reaching a certain range), and educating the patient on the importance of task performance.[58] The clinician should emphasize both the short- and long-term effects of task performance. Using the previous example, a session goal may be to increase range of motion 5 degrees while a long-term goal may be to increase range of motion to allow ambulation without deviation. This strategy is particularly important for prevention programs and regimens that require long-term adherence.

The extent to which task recommendations coincide with patients' previous behaviors and lifestyles affects adherence.[55,64] Patients report changes in diet and exercise behaviors to be the most difficult to follow and adherence of patients with diabetes to recommended exercise plans may be as low as 21%.[70] For example, Mr. Rodriguez, a mail carrier and avid athlete with a neuropathic ulcer on his plantar first phalanx, may have a difficult time adhering to the recommendation of limited weight bearing. By providing him with safe alternative exercise choices, such as an upper body ergometer, adherence may be enhanced. Patients who are able to establish a routine for recommended behaviors, such as exercise or taking medication, are more likely to be adherent.[63] Consider Mrs. Jackson, a sedentary computer programmer with a similar ulcer, who is requested to perform aerobic exercise to help control her elevated blood sugars, high cholesterol, hypertension, and obesity. Problem solving with Mrs. Jackson to find a safe, convenient activity, such as nonforefoot weight-bearing stationary cycling at her apartment complex's exercise room while watching the morning news prior to going to work, may enhance adherence.

Clinician Characteristics

Because patients who have poor relationships with their health care providers are less likely to be adherent, clinicians should strive to develop a therapeutic partnership with their patients.[60] Clinicians should demonstrate concern for their patients' well-being, express empathy,[60] and use good listening skills when interacting with patients. Patients should be encouraged to voice their concerns.[66] In one study, 61–66% of patients diagnosed with breast cancer did not discuss their problems of pain, range of motion loss, or lymphedema with their physicians.[71] The clinician should then restate these concerns to ensure the messages were accurately received and to emphasize that the patients' input matters. Clinicians should encourage patients and reinforce desired behaviors.[31,65] The simple act of a physician checking protective sensation in a patient with diabetes was a significant predictor of patient follow-through with self-care behaviors.[52] If patients are nonadherent, clinicians should be nonjudgmental; they should recognize that a relapse into previous behaviors is to be expected, but encourage patients to break bad habits. Although most researchers and clinicians define an adherent patient as one who follows at least 80% of recommended procedures,[72] clinicians must be oriented toward the facilitation of perfect patient adherence. Clinician inertia, or failure to act in response to patient nonadherence or changes in patient status, is associated with poorer outcomes.[73] For example, if a clinician suspects or knows that a patient has been nonadherent (the patient has not been bandaging his or her wound), it is important to provide the patient with objective evidence of nonadherence (the presence of dog hair and dirt within the wound bed), state the ramifications of this behavior (delayed wound healing and infection), and restate the intended behavior (keep the wound covered at all times except for dressing changes).[57,60] Having the patient complete a log to track performance of intended behaviors or sign a contract agreeing to mutually determined goals may facilitate adherence.[60] Because some wounds may require significant time to heal, clinicians should reassure the patient that he or she is progressing,[69] if indeed this is true, by providing specific examples: "The wound is now one-third of its previous size" or "You are now able to get in and out of bed without assistance whereas previously you required assistance." By providing concrete evidence of intervention success, adherence can be increased. Finally, because poor continuity of care, such as frequent changes in health care providers or inconsistent approaches to healing, detracts from patient adherence, clinicians should strive for a coordinated, consistent, interdisciplinary approach to patient care.

 Checkpoint Question #2

Give three reasons why it may be difficult for a patient with type 2 diabetes to adhere to a diet that is low in simple sugars and low in fat.

Interdisciplinary Wound Management

A 4-year retrospective study demonstrated that an interdisciplinary, therapy-based approach to chronic wound management resulted in more effective and efficient wound healing than wound healing rates previously described in the literature using less holistic approaches.[53] The development of an interdisciplinary team specific to each patient's individual needs is part of the best practice recommendations for management of pressure ulcers.[74] An interdisciplinary approach to the management of patients with chronic venous insufficiency ulcers,[75] chronic neuropathic ulcers,[76] and chronic wounds of mixed etiologies[77,78] resulted in significantly shorter wound healing times, a lower rate of wound-related complications, and fewer amputations than standard care. The "collective wisdom"[79] of an interdisciplinary approach to the management of patients with chronic or extensive wounds is paramount for successful outcomes. The three key components to a successful interdisciplinary approach are cooperation, communication, and commitment.[79]

Wounds cannot be treated in isolation of the patient as a whole. Rather, clinicians must work together to identify and address any underlying wound etiologies, such as peripheral vascular disease or diabetes mellitus. Risk factors and impairments that contribute to delayed wound healing, such as decreased mobility or patient/caregiver lack of knowledge about a disease process, must also be identified and addressed. Successful cooperation requires that all members of the wound management team work synergistically with respect for one another's knowledge and expertise. It may be necessary to clarify each team member's role, especially in areas where scopes of practice overlap.

Seamless communication is imperative when different disciplines work together with the patient and caregiver to facilitate wound healing. All team members must provide consistent information in a timely fashion to the patient and caregiver. The flow of information can be improved through the use of interdisciplinary documentation systems, frequent team meetings, and, in some settings, patient rounds or conferences. Disciplines can provide in-servicing to other team members to enhance understanding about individual areas of expertise or recently attended continuing education courses and conferences.[79] Team members can also bring case studies to review for brainstorming sessions and to identify areas to improve upon within the wound management team. Even informal encounters between team members can provide an opportunity to collaborate and improve patient care.

Health care providers can have difficulty adhering to recommended practices, just as patients do. For example, adherence of health care providers to evidence-based practice recommendations range from 17% for providing nutritional support to malnourished patients, 20% for repositioning patients with pressure ulcers, 59% for avoiding cytoxic agents in wound and skin care, to 77% for off-loading strategies to manage neuropathic foot ulcerations.[80] The biggest barriers to health care provider adherence appear to be lack of current information, insufficient time, poor habits, and lack of access to appropriate supplies. Health care provider education programs, like patient education programs, have proven successful. For example, pressure ulcer incidence decreased from 7.14% to 0% after an interdisciplinary education program was implemented.[81] Team members must be committed to the patient and to the interdisciplinary goals set with the patient and caregivers. This commitment helps reinforce the importance of the many interventions that may be part of a patient's overall plan of care and continually emphasizes the behaviors expected of the patient/caregiver, ultimately increasing patient adherence.

A Team Approach

The following scenario is meant to better illuminate the benefits of a holistic approach to patient care. Mrs. H is a 68-year-old retired teacher with a history of hypertension, peripheral vascular disease, and type 2 diabetes. On admission, Mrs. H's blood pressure was 198/62 and her blood glucose was 220 mg/dL. Mrs. H. sustained a myocardial infarction 7 days ago and had a triple bypass performed that same day. Her post-surgical course was significant for sternotomy dehiscence with a *Pseudomonas aeruginosa* infection, resolving bilateral basilar lung infiltrates, a partial-thickness right posterior heel pressure ulcer, and prolonged ventilation, as she was extubated on post-operative day 6. On post-operative day 7, the patient's level of alertness improved enough to allow participation in mobility; however, the nursing staff reports the patient required a maximum assist of two people to move from supine to sitting at the edge of the bed and was unable to sit unsupported. Mrs. H lives with her 71-year-old retired husband in a two-story home. Her goal is to return to independent living with her husband.

Table 9–4 outlines one possible interdisciplinary approach to maximize successful outcomes for Mrs. H's care. Many of the disciplines assisting with Mrs. H's care have overlapping scopes of practice. For example, both registered dietitians and diabetic educators are knowledgeable about dietary methods to improve glycemic control and both disciplines are essential to Mrs. H's care. The diabetic educator is less familiar with instructing patients in diets low in fat and cholesterol and maximizing protein intake to assist with wound healing. Likewise, the registered dietitian is not adept at educating patients in the peak action time of oral or injectable hypoglycemic agents and precautions for neuropathic changes that can accompany diabetes. Similarly, pulmonary hygiene, activities of daily living, bed mobility, and strengthening are all within the physical therapist's scope of care. However, by using the expertise of other disciplines, the patient is able to receive additional benefits, such as more rehabilitation, management of comorbidities, more in-depth information, and reinforcement of instructions and interventions.

Within this particular scenario, each discipline's primary roles are clearly defined and no "turf wars" exist. All are directed toward the common goal of Mrs. H's return to independent living with her husband. Each discipline must also reinforce, whenever possible, the smaller goals of the other disciplines. For example, although in Mrs. H's situation the physical therapist is not primarily responsible for working with the patient on bed mobility, the physical therapist can reinforce the goals of occupational therapy by having the patient assist with bed mobility to get in position to initiate transfer training.

Formal communication between disciplines is achieved in several ways. First, physicians and nursing staff participate in daily rounds. Second, the patient's chart consists of multidisciplinary flow sheets in which it is possible to follow the interventions and effects of each discipline's care. Third, a dry erase board within the patient's room is used to facilitate communication with the patient and caregiver. Fourth, weekly conferences are held with the husband, physical

TABLE 9–4   Example of Interdisciplinary Responsibilities for Assisting with Mrs. H's Care

Team Member	Primary Responsibilities
Patient/caregiver	• Participates actively in rehabilitation program • Asks questions to clarify any areas of concern or uncertainty
Attending physician	• Manages peripheral vascular disease and infection • Directs rehabilitation team • Provides patient/caregiver with information about overall medical status
Cardiologist	• Manages cardiac status, hypertension
Endocrinologist	• Manages glycemic control
Pharmacist	• Ensures therapeutic drug dosages • Monitors for possible drug interactions or toxicities
Diabetic educator	• Instructs patient/caregiver in methods to improve glycemic control
Registered dietitian	• Assists with maximizing nutrition • Educates patient/caregiver on healthy diet after discharge to help control hypertension, diabetes, and cholesterol
Respiratory therapist	• Assists with pulmonary hygiene
Occupational therapist	• Assists patient in returning to previous level of function within sternotomy precautions, including activities of daily living, bed mobility, sitting balance, and upper extremity motion/strength
Certified occupational therapist assistant	• Assists occupational therapist as allowed by law
Physical therapist	• Directs wound management • Designs positioning protocol for team members to follow • Assists patient in returning to previous level of function within sternotomy precautions, including lower extremity strengthening, transfers, and gait
Physical therapist assistant	• Assists physical therapist as allowed by law
Nurse	• Serves as primary contact for interdisciplinary team regarding patient's overall care • Follows through with medication orders • Assists with the positioning and mobility protocol defined by the physical and occupational therapist • Assists with pulmonary hygiene
Medical social worker	• Assists with discharge planning • Assists with obtaining any necessary durable medical equipment

therapist, occupational therapist, medical social worker, nurse, and attending physician. Informal communication oc-curs spontaneously as each discipline interacts within the intensive care unit. Because of this multifaceted approach to patient management, Mrs. H is able to return to independent living with her husband. Clear role delineation between the varied health care providers, multiple lines of communication, and a cooperative approach toward common goals are vital to the success of an interdisciplinary team.

☑️ *Checkpoint Question #3*

You are a physical therapist working with Mr. B, a patient with a diabetic ulcer. How can you reinforce the teachings of the patient's diabetic educator?

CHAPTER SUMMARY

In order to attain successful outcomes, patients with chronic or slow-healing wounds require a holistic approach. Clinicians should routinely perform a nutritional screening on all patients with open wounds to identify potential impediments to wound healing. Patients deemed at risk for malnutrition should be referred to the attending physician and a registered dietitian for a formal assessment and appropriate interventions. Clinicians must be able to identify and remove barriers to patient adherence to maximize wound healing. An interdisciplinary approach, using the collective wisdom of various health care providers, can also facilitate wound healing. The three components to successful interdisciplinary care are cooperation, open lines of communication, and commitment to mutually defined goals.

REVIEW QUESTIONS

You are a physical therapist working with Miss W, a 7-year-old inpatient with partial-thickness burns to bilateral upper extremities and anterior trunk sustained 2 days ago. Miss W is receiving physical therapy twice daily for wound management. The patient is reluctant to move because of pain and fear. She screams if you attempt sharp debridement of burn eschar and will allow only minimal active assisted range of motion. Miss W is also in occupational therapy once daily for hand range of motion and night-splinting to reduce finger flexion deformities.

1. Explain how Miss W's injuries may affect her nutritional status.

2. How might you limit the potential for nutritional deficiencies?

3. Describe three things you can do prior to the physical therapy treatment session to increase Miss W's participation in therapy.

4. What clinician characteristics will likely enhance patient participation?

5. Describe three things you can do during the physical therapy treatment session to increase Miss W's participation in therapy.

6. Describe how you might reinforce the occupational therapy goals of improved hand range of motion during Miss W's physical therapy session.

PEARSON myhealthprofessionskit™

Use this address to access the Companion Website created for this textbook. Simply select "Physical Therapy" from the choice of disciplines. Find this book and log in using your username and password to access images, video clips, and additional learning tools.

REFERENCES

Go to myhealthprofessionskit.com to view this chapter's references.

SECTION III

Wound Types

Wound Types

10

Arterial Insufficiency Ulcers

Chapter Objectives

After reading this chapter, learners will be able to:

1. Differentiate the etiology of arterial insufficiency ulcers from other types of open wounds.
2. Explain the risk factors contributing to arterial insufficiency ulceration.
3. Describe and choose appropriate physical therapy tests and measures to assess patients with arterial insufficiency.
4. Assess the typical characteristics of arterial insufficiency ulcers.
5. Design an interdisciplinary approach in the management of patients with arterial insufficiency ulcers.
6. Apply basic foot care guidelines and protective principles for patients with arterial insufficiency ulcers.
7. Describe precautions clinicians should be aware of when working with patients with arterial insufficiency ulcers.
8. Integrate the keys to local wound care for patients with arterial insufficiency ulcers.
9. Select physical therapy procedural interventions for patients with arterial insufficiency ulcers, including integumentary repair and protective techniques, therapeutic exercise, and devices and equipment.
10. Discuss possible medical and surgical interventions for patients with arterial insufficiency ulcers.

Key Terms

Ankle-brachial index (ABI)	Duplex scanning	Segmental pressure measurements
Arterial insufficiency	Gangrene	Toe pressures
Arteriography	Intermittent claudication	Transcutaneous oxygen
Arteriosclerosis	Intimal layer	monitoring (TCOM
Atherosclerosis	Ischemic rest pain	or $TcPO_2$)
Capillary refill	Ischemic ulcers	Tunica externa
Doppler ultrasound	Plethysmography	Tunica media
	Rubor of dependency	Venous filling time

INTRODUCTION

The prevalence of lower extremity ulcers in the general population is estimated to be between 0.6% and 5.0%.[1–4] Lower extremity ulcers are the most common chronic wounds. From 5% to 10% of all lower extremity ulcerations are due to arterial insufficiency, or lack of adequate blood supply. Arterial insufficiency affects an estimated 8–12 million Americans[5–7] or up to 23% of those over 55 years of age.[8] While 40% of these cases are asymptomatic,[7] peripheral arterial disease is a causative factor in 5% of all amputations.[9] The estimated cost of peripheral arterial disease–related treatment is $4.37 billion, with the majority of these costs going toward surgical interventions.[6] The first priority of wound management is to identify the causative and contributing factors to integumentary impairment.[10] More than 80% of patients with peripheral arterial disease are current or former smokers.[11] Once identified, these factors must be corrected or controlled as much as possible to restore the skin's structure and function. Patients with advanced arterial insufficiency have impaired tissue oxygenation as part of the disease process. Because the amount of oxygen required to promote wound healing is significantly greater than that needed to maintain tissue quality, once tissue damage has occurred, arterial ulcers are likely to progress without holistic and meticulous interventions.

This chapter provides a brief overview of the arterial system, followed by a review of the etiology of arteriosclerosis and arterial insufficiency–related tissue damage. Next, the classification and characteristics of arterial ulcers are outlined along with physical therapy tests and measures commonly used to identify arterial ulcers. Finally, the chapter presents a thorough description of physical therapy, medical, and surgical interventions.

ARTERIAL SYSTEM OVERVIEW

To understand the pathophysiology of arterial insufficiency, one must first review the normal anatomy of the circulatory system. The arterial system is the high-pressure system of vessels that carries blood from the left ventricle of the heart, through the aorta, and into body tissues. Arteries have three layers: the tunica externa, the tunica media, and the intimal layer (see Figure 10–1). The **tunica externa,** or adventitia, is the protective, outer layer.[12] Composed of connective tissue along with collagen and elastin fibers, the tunica externa provides support to the vessel walls. The **tunica media,** or middle layer, is made of thick smooth muscle

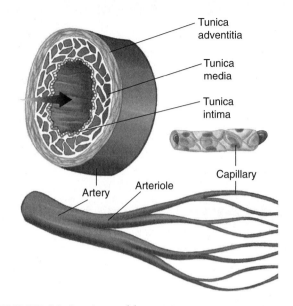

FIGURE 10–1   Arterial layers.

Source: Paramedic Care: Principles & Practice—Trauma Emergencies by Bledsoe/Porter/Cherry.

and some collagen and elastin fibers.[12] Innervated by the sympathetic nervous system, this muscular layer has the ability to modulate vessel diameter between 1.0 and 2.5 cm according to body and tissue demands.[12] The inner **intimal layer** is a single layer of endothelial cells in direct contact with circulating blood.[12] The intima is very fragile and may be easily traumatized.

Arteries vary in diameter and in the makeup of these three layers. Elastic arteries, such as the aorta and its branches, are large vessels whose elasticity helps to maintain blood pressure by expanding during heart contraction and rebounding to normal during diastole.[12] To protect the delicate endothelial cells against the high pressures within these arteries, the middle layer of elastic arteries is relatively thick. Muscular arteries, such as the femoral and brachial arteries, are also known as distributing arteries. These vessels have a thicker tunica media and a smaller lumen ranging from 1.0 cm to 0.3 mm.[12] An increase in sympathetic output causes the smooth muscles within the tunica media to contract. This vasoconstriction decreases the artery's lumen and, therefore, limits the amount of blood flowing through the vessel. Arterioles are the smallest type of artery, ranging from 0.3 mm to 10 μm.[12] Similar to the larger muscular arteries, arterioles have significant sympathetic innervation and may play a role in maintaining blood pressure. Pressure within the arterial system is normally 90–100 mm Hg in the larger vessels and decreases to 25–35 mm Hg when reaching the arterioles.[12]

Capillaries are the simplest type of vessel, composed of a single layer of endothelial cells resting on a thin basement membrane.[13, 14] Capillaries are only 1 mm in length and 8–10 μm and are wide enough for a single red blood cell to squeeze through at a time.[12] Small channels between capillary endothelial cells allow oxygen and nutrients from the blood to diffuse along their concentration gradients into the tissues. Carbon dioxide and metabolic wastes diffuse in the opposite direction, moving from the tissues into the capillaries. Most tissues are only 0.1 mm away from the nearest capillary.[15] From the capillaries, blood returns to the heart via the venous system. As blood flows through the capillaries, pressure drops from 25 to 35 mm Hg on the arteriole side to about 15 mm Hg on the venous side.[12] Blood pressure decreases to almost 0 mm Hg upon reaching the right atrium.[15] Refer to Chapter 11 for further details on the anatomy of the venous system.

ETIOLOGY OF ARTERIAL INSUFFICIENCY AND ARTERIAL INSUFFICIENCY–RELATED TISSUE DAMAGE

Arterial ulcers are caused by a decrease in arterial blood supply, also known as **arterial insufficiency.** There are many potential causes of arterial insufficiency, including trauma and acute embolism. Rheumatoid arthritis and diabetes mellitus commonly cause microvascular disease, which may also impair tissue blood supply.[16, 17] Thromboangiitis, or Buerger's disease, causes arterial insufficiency and is most often seen in young adults who smoke heavily.[16] The primary cause of arterial insufficiency, however, is arteriosclerosis.[16]

Arteriosclerosis is a general term for the thickening and hardening of arterial walls.[18] The most common form of arteriosclerosis, and the leading cause of arterial insufficiency ulcers in the United States, is atherosclerosis.[19–21] **Atherosclerosis** is a systemic, degenerative process in which the arterial lumen is gradually and progressively encroached upon. Atherosclerosis begins when circulating cholesterol is deposited on vessel walls, causing fatty streaks or plaques (see Figure 10–2).[18] Generally, this first occurs where arteries bifurcate, or branch.[22, 23] High-density lipoproteins (HDLs) and low-density lipoproteins (LDLs) carry cholesterol through the bloodstream. High levels of LDLs enhance cholesterol deposition, whereas HDLs seem to serve a protective function.[24] Cholesterol deposition appears to trigger biochemical changes and intimal cell injury.[15, 23] The body attempts to repair damaged endothelial cells, resulting in a buildup of blood products, such as platelets, and fibrous scarring. Lipids, calcium deposits, and scar tissue accumulating on the damaged intimal

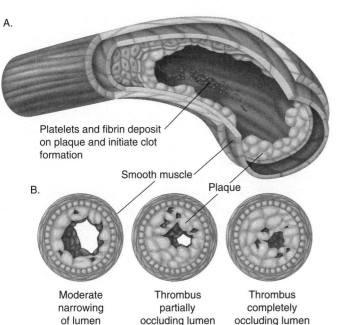

FIGURE 10–2   Atherosclerosis (plaque) development.

Source: Human Diseases: A Systematic Approach 6/e Mulvihill/Selman/Holdaway/Tompary/Raymond.

layer bulge into the lumen, causing progressive vessel stenosis, or narrowing. Arterial stenosis leads to increased resistance to blood flow and decreased blood flow distal to the obstruction.[13] In addition to stenosis, atherosclerosis is thought to lead to a thickening of the capillary basement membrane,[3, 25] further decreasing the exchange of oxygen and nutrients to affected tissues.

Vessel stenosis progresses gradually in most cases, slowly decreasing the amount of oxygen and nutrients delivered to tissues perfused by the affected vessels. This decreased blood supply may no longer be able to meet tissue demands. In fact, one of the first signs of arterial insufficiency is intermittent claudication.[7, 26] **Intermittent claudication** is activity-specific discomfort due to local ischemia,[11, 27] which stops within 1 to 5 minutes of ceasing the provocative activity.[28] For example, imagine a patient develops an atherosclerotic plaque at the bifurcation of the popliteal and anterior tibial arteries of the leg. This leads to decreased blood flow to the affected calf and foot. While the patient is at rest, even though there is less blood flowing into the lower leg, it is still enough to meet tissue demands. However, if the patient ambulates, the working calf and foot muscles require more oxygen and nutrients. Patients generally have at least 50% vessel stenosis if they are experiencing intermittent claudication.[16, 22] Approximately one-third of patients with arterial insufficiency experience claudication.[29] The body may accommodate for increased tissue demands immediately by decreasing the sympathetic output, thereby causing vasodilation. However, once there is about 70% vessel occlusion[10] or tissue demands are large enough, even maximal vasodilation does not provide sufficient circulation, and the tissue distal to the occlusion becomes ischemic and painful. At this point, the patient complains of foot or calf pain when the delicate balance between blood supply and tissue demand is upset by the increased oxygen demands of ambulation (see Figure 10–3).

The pain of intermittent claudication is sometimes described as cramping, burning, or fatigue.[28] Pain location is typically distal to the site of arterial occlusion. Obstruction of the iliofemoral arteries typically results in buttock, thigh, or calf pain, whereas obstruction of the infrapopliteal arteries results primarily in foot pain.[28] Within minutes of stopping ambulating, the patient's pain abates. The pain of intermittent claudication is repeatable and predictable at the same workload.[28] That is, the onset of pain will consistently occur after the patient has walked X number of feet or Y number of minutes. The body may be able to improve circulation by forming collateral circulation to bypass the occluded vessel section,[12] thus allowing the patient to ambulate longer or farther before the onset of symptoms. However, it takes time to develop new vessels and the potential for improved circulation is limited.[14] Additionally, the rate of plaque progression may exceed the rate of angiogenesis.

As atherosclerosis progresses and the vessel becomes more stenosed, circulation distal to the occlusion will eventually be unable to meet the demands of even nonexercising tissues. **Ischemic rest pain** represents more significant arterial disease than intermittent claudication[26] and is frequently characterized as a burning pain that is exacerbated at night or with elevation, and is relieved by dependency.[5, 30] At this point, circulation is so poor that gravity has a significant effect on tissue perfusion.[22] For example, a patient with ischemic rest pain would have an increased pain complaint if his leg is elevated up on a pillow because this position requires blood to flow against gravity to reach the foot. In contrast, lowering the leg off the edge of the bed decreases his pain complaint as this position allows blood to flow more freely into the foot because it is assisted by gravity. As occlusion progresses, even positioning the affected extremity in a dependent position may not alter blood flow or the patient's pain complaint. Arterial insufficiency ulcerations, sometimes called **ischemic ulcers,** are most commonly seen after the disease has progressed from intermittent claudication to ischemic rest pain (see Figure 10–4).[31] Biopsies of ischemic skin showed increased extracellular matrix turnover rates, which may be the cause of insidious arterial insufficiency ulcerations.[32] Although it is possible to have spontaneous skin breakdown and ulceration due to arterial insufficiency, it is probably more common for ulcers to result from some sort of trauma on an already ischemic limb. Anything increasing tissue oxygen demand has the potential to fatally upset the balance between oxygen supply and tissue demand, resulting in ulceration.[33]

The prevalence of asymptomatic arterial insufficiency is greater than that of symptomatic disease (e.g., intermittent claudication).[5] The prevalence of

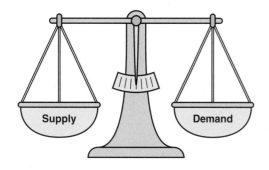

FIGURE 10–3   Balance of supply and demand.

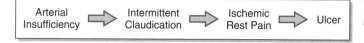

FIGURE 10–4   The progression of atherosclerotic pain.

symptomatic disease, in turn, is greater than that of ulceration.[5, 23] Ulceration and gangrene ultimately result when local tissue oxygen requirements exceed perfusion.[14] The term dry **gangrene** can be used to describe dead tissue that is dry, dark, cold, and contracted when compared to similar areas or the contralateral side (see color image 13). Oxygen is vital not only for homeostasis but also, as discussed in Chapter 2, for each phase of wound healing. Therefore, even a small abrasion from bumping into a table corner or increased pressure due to ill-fitting shoes may result in ulceration. These normally benign forms of trauma may be just enough of an overload on the failing circulatory system to initiate a negative spiral of tissue breakdown. Arterial ulcerations represent potential limb loss if not managed appropriately. Unfortunately, despite appropriate conservative interventions, amputation may sometimes still be necessary.

Risk Factors Contributing to Arterial Ulceration

There are several risk factors contributing to arterial insufficiency ulcerations, including hyperlipidemia, elevated cholesterol, smoking, diabetes, hypertension, trauma, and advanced age (see Figure 10–5).[20, 22, 23, 28, 34, 35] Because even the best wound management cannot overcome a lack of blood supply to bring about tissue repair and regeneration, the potential for successful outcomes for patients with ischemic ulcers is enhanced if risk factors are identified and corrected or controlled as much as possible.[3, 36]

Hyperlipidemia and Elevated LDL

As discussed earlier in the chapter, high cholesterol plays an important role in the development of arterial insufficiency.[10, 15] High cholesterol, particularly elevated LDLs, enhances cholesterol deposition within vessel walls and, therefore, increases the rate of atherosclerosis. High triglyceride levels are also thought to promote atherosclerotic plaque growth.[23] Because atherosclerosis is a systemic process, individuals with coronary artery disease (CAD) have an increased risk of developing peripheral arterial insufficiency compared to individuals without CAD.[23]

Smoking

Smoking is the number one modifiable risk factor for peripheral vascular disease[15, 37] and can contribute to

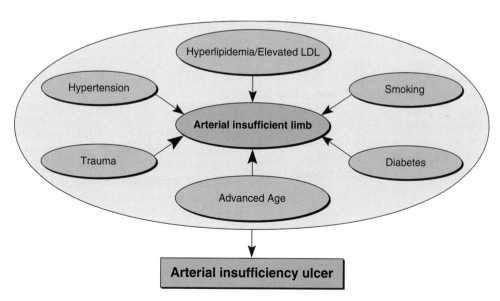

FIGURE 10–5   Confluence of factors leading to arterial insufficiency ulcers.

arterial ulceration in several ways.[7, 10, 11] First, nicotine causes vasoconstriction, thus decreasing tissue perfusion. Second, smoking decreases the availability of oxygen by increasing the amount of nonfunctioning hemoglobin. Smoking just one cigarette decreases wound and tissue oxygen saturation by 30% for 1 hour in healthy individuals.[38] Individuals with healthy circulatory systems have the reserves to compensate for this decrease in blood flow. Unfortunately, individuals with arterial insufficiency have little or no remaining reserves. Third, smoking increases the rate of clot formation[39] and blood viscosity, thereby decreasing tissue perfusion. Fourth, nicotine enhances cholesterol deposition within vessel walls, thus hastening the atherosclerotic process and further impairing circulation. Last, smoking causes a greater mismatch between oxygen delivery and oxygen demand. Even when comparing patients with the same ankle-brachial index, smokers will have lower oxygen saturation rates, lower maximal calf blood flow, and less distance walked prior to claudication than nonsmokers.[11]

Diabetes

People with diabetes have an increased prevalence of calcific arterial insufficiency;[28, 40, 41] that is, their vessel walls tend to accumulate calcium. This calcification of the tunica media and basement membrane can even be seen on an x-ray. Presumably, calcium deposits both adversely affect vessel lumen diameter and interfere with the exchange of oxygen and nutrients. Diabetes also is associated with an increased prevalence of microvascular disease.[42] Sustained hyperglycemia decreases all three phases of wound healing. High blood sugar levels decrease collagen synthesis, angiogenesis, and fibroblast proliferation and reduce the tensile strength of wounds.[43] In addition, high blood sugar levels impair the body's ability to fight infection.[42, 44] Unfortunately, arterial insufficiency may be easily overlooked as a cause of ulceration in individuals with diabetes because they often have coexisting sensory neuropathy, making them unable to sense the pain of ischemia.[42] See Chapter 13 for more details about the adverse effects of diabetes on wound healing.

Hypertension

The intimal layer of arteries is very fragile and easily traumatized. The increased force of blood flow that occurs with hypertension is thought to both initiate and perpetuate endothelial cell injury, thereby augmenting the atherosclerotic process.[7, 12] Systolic hypertension appears to be more damaging to blood vessels than diastolic hypertension.[12] Although the reason for this is unclear, the repetitive waves of higher pressures generated during cardiac contraction may be more traumatic to endothelial cells than sustained levels of lower pressure. In addition, arteries respond to sustained hypertension by thickening the layer of smooth muscle within the tunica media and increasing production of vasoconstrictive agents. These two reactions to chronic hypertension result in greater contact of blood components with the intimal layer, increasing the risk of trauma as blood flows through affected vessels.

Trauma

Although arterial ulcers can develop spontaneously due to decreased perfusion, trauma is a common precipitating factor.[22] Many individuals with arterial insufficiency never develop an ulceration. However, the increased metabolic demand of tissues resulting from minor trauma may be enough to disrupt the delicate balance between tissue repair and tissue breakdown. Initiating trauma may be mechanical, thermal, or chemical in nature.[23] Mechanical trauma due to excessive pressure from ill-fitting shoes or stubbing a toe may be the most common event preceding arterial ulceration. Forms of chemical trauma that may trigger an ulcer include the use of over-the-counter chemical agents. For example, using a simple corn remover or topical home remedies to manage skin and nail conditions may damage the skin, causing an ulcer. Perhaps the most overlooked direct precipitating cause of arterial ulcers is thermal injury. Patients with arterial insufficiency frequently complain of cold feet and legs and may attempt to warm themselves with heating pads or by soaking their feet in hot water. Unfortunately, the heat may be too much for their circulation to dissipate, and this may cause tissue damage.

Advanced Age

Age-related changes make the body less able to adapt to changes in the metabolic demands of tissues by vasodilating or vasoconstricting. It is estimated that 29% of older adults have arterial insufficiency and 5% of older adults experience intermittent claudication.[7] The rate of arterial insufficiency increases with age, and individuals with ulcers due to arterial insufficiency are generally older than individuals without ulcers.[2, 4, 28] The increased rate of coexisting medical problems may put older persons at increased risk of integumentary injury due to trauma. For example, presbyopia or impaired balance may cause older individuals to bump into objects, causing skin tears or other integumentary trauma. As discussed in Chapter 3, anatomical and functional changes occurring over the normal course of aging adversely affect wound healing: the immune response is slowed, the inflammatory response is decreased, and the epidermis and dermis are more susceptible to trauma.[45-47] Therefore, once an older person sustains an injury, the healing potential is less than that of a younger individual. To decrease the risk of integumentary damage and to improve outcomes once a wound has occurred, comorbidities should be continually assessed and addressed.

CASE STUDY: Mr. Vahrm Gupta

This case study is referenced throughout the chapter.

PART 1

History

Vahrm Gupta is a 55-year-old East Indian male seen this morning in outpatient physical therapy for wound management. His primary language is English. He lives alone in a fifth-floor apartment with an elevator. Mr. Gupta is an electrical engineer whose job involves sitting at a computer or working on circuit boards.

Wound History: Mr. Gupta reports his wound began 2 months ago after being scratched by his dog. The wound initially increased in size, but has not changed in the last month since he began rinsing it nightly with hydrogen peroxide and covering it with a large Band-Aid.

Past Medical History: Mr. Gupta has a history of coronary artery disease with a stent and a demand-style pacemaker placed 2 years ago after a myocardial infarction, HTN, high cholesterol, and high triglycerides. He was diagnosed with rheumatoid arthritis 5 years ago. He has used a cane for the past year due to left lower extremity pain with walking. He reports a family history of cardiac disease and cerebral vascular disease. He has no allergies.

General Health Status: Mr. Gupta reports he is in relatively good health despite his multiple medical problems. He has minimal hand stiffness and soreness that is most evident in the mornings. He reports no problems with work-related tasks but fatigues quickly when cleaning his apartment. He reports left calf cramping that occasionally wakes him at night and left calf pain that limits his ability to walk through the grocery store.

Current Medications: Trichlormethiazide, aspirin, naproxen, simvastatin

Other Available Data: Most recent fasting laboratory values available from his primary care physician: hematocrit = 46%, white blood cell count = 9,000/mm^3, platelets = 160,000/mm^3, albumin = 5.2 g/dL, blood glucose 85 mg/dL, cholesterol 410 mg/dL, high-density lipoproteins 25 mg/dL.

Systems Review

Cardiovascular/Pulmonary System: Heart rate 62 bpm, blood pressure 125/88 mm Hg, respiratory rate 14 bpm, no lower extremity edema noted.

Musculoskeletal System: No deficits noted in gross assessment of range of motion and strength. Note minimal hand deformities consistent with RA. Height: 5 feet 9 inches (1.75 m). Body weight: 165 pounds (75 kg). Body mass index (BMI) = 24.5 kg/m^2.

Neuromuscular System: No gross deficits noted in gross coordinated movement or motor control. Mr. Gupta uses a straight cane in his right upper extremity while ambulating.

Gastrointestinal System: No problems noted.

Urogenital System: No problems noted.

Integumentary System: Open wound left distal lateral calf, skin is anhydrous, there is minimal hair growth noted below the knee bilaterally, callus noted plantar 2nd MTP joints bilaterally, toenails adequately trimmed and have normal color and structure.

Communication, Cognition, Language, and Learning Style: No deficits noted. Mr. Gupta reports he learns best by listening to new information. He demonstrates an understanding of his situation and a willingness to participate in wound management interventions.

☑ *Checkpoint Question #1*

Your patient, Mr. H, is a 72-year-old overweight male who presents to physical therapy with the following diagnosis: arterial insufficiency ulcer near his lateral malleolus. Mr. H's history includes the following: appendectomy age 12, CABG × 4 1998, high cholesterol—last measured at 260 mg/dL, left THR 1999, HTN-BP in the clinic measured at 170/85, DM with blood sugars measured daily and averaging 190 mg/dL, two-pack-per-day smoker for 20 years. Mr. H's vision is corrected with the use of bifocals and he lives with his 68-year-old wife. Current medications: Lortab 2–3 times per day, Lasix, insulin, Coumadin, and Zocor.

a. List the patient's nonmodifiable risk factors for arterial insufficiency and arterial insufficiency–related ulcers.

b. List the patient's modifiable or controllable risk factors for arterial insufficiency and arterial insufficiency–related ulcers.

c. What additional resources or services might be beneficial for this patient?

PHYSICAL THERAPY TESTS AND MEASURES FOR ARTERIAL INSUFFICIENCY

Clinicians may perform various tests and measures to assess for arterial insufficiency and identify changes in patient status. In addition to the routine tests and measures clinicians should perform on all patients with open wounds (see Chapter 4), there are several tests that are specific to the diagnosis of arterial insufficiency. It is critical that the clinician identify the presence and severity of circulatory compromise in order to make a prognosis for wound healing and to develop an appropriate plan of care including consultation with, or referral to, other health care providers.[7, 48] This section details six of the more common clinical tests and measures used to assess individuals with arterial insufficiency: pulses, Doppler ultrasound, ankle-brachial index (ABI), segmental pressures, rubor of dependency, and venous filling time.

Pulses

Peripheral pulses should be assessed for all extremity wounds.[49] However, since decreased arterial circulation is the underlying pathology of arterial insufficiency ulcers, it is particularly important for the clinician to assess pulses in both the involved and uninvolved extremity. The vast majority of arterial insufficiency ulcers occur in the lower extremity. Refer to other sources for a description of anatomical landmarks for the palpation of upper extremity pulses.[12, 50]

Clinicians should assess the pulses of the femoral, popliteal, dorsalis pedis, and posterior tibial arteries (see Figure 10–6). The femoral artery is easily palpated within the femoral triangle, just inferior to the inguinal ligament and midway between the anterior inferior iliac spine and the pubic tubercle. Diminished femoral pulses may be the result of an occlusion of the more proximally located common iliac or external iliac arteries.[12, 22] The femoral artery provides most of the blood supply to the lower extremity. The bifurcation of the common femoral artery into the superficial and deep femoral arteries is the most common site for occlusion.[5, 51] The popliteal artery is a direct continuation of the superficial femoral artery located centrally within the popliteal fossa. The popliteal artery is best palpated by holding the relaxed extremity with the knee semiflexed to decrease overlying soft tissue tension.[21] However, because of its depth within the fossa, the popliteal artery is sometimes difficult to palpate despite sufficient circulation.[50] The posterior tibial artery is the main blood supply to the foot. It is located between the tendons of the flexor digitorum longus and flexor hallucis longus. The pulse in this artery may be difficult to find and is easily occluded by excessive examiner force. To facilitate identifying the pulse, the posterior tibial artery can be lightly compressed against the posterior-medial portion of the distal tibia just superior to the medial malleolus. The dorsalis pedis artery provides blood supply to the dorsal foot and is located superficially on the dorsum of the foot. It is usually found over the second ray between the tendons of the extensor hallucis longus and the extensor digitorum longus but may be absent up to 15% of the time.[50] Diminished or absent pedal pulses likely represent more proximal arterial occlusion.[21, 26, 51, 52]

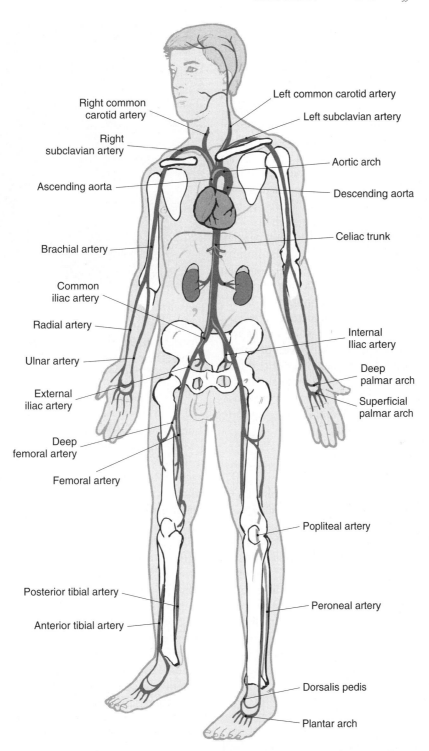

Right common carotid artery

Right subclavian artery

Ascending aorta

Brachial artery

Common iliac artery

Radial artery

Ulnar artery

External iliac artery

Deep femoral artery

Femoral artery

Posterior tibial artery

Anterior tibial artery

Left common carotid artery

Left subclavian artery

Aortic arch

Descending aorta

Celiac trunk

Internal Iliac artery

Deep palmar arch

Superficial palmar arch

Popliteal artery

Peroneal artery

Dorsalis pedis

Plantar arch

FIGURE 10–6   Arterial system.

Source: Medical Terminology, A Living Language 3/e, by Fremgen/Frucht.

Pulses should be assessed with the patient resting supine and are graded on a 0–3+ scale ranging from absent to accentuated (see Table 4–9).[30, 53] Palpating pulses requires skill and practice. While lack of a posterior tibial artery pulse is more sensitive and specific than a nonpalpable dorsalis pedis pulse,[54] absence of a palpable pulse in both pedal arteries is evidence of peripheral arterial disease.[26, 55, 56] Unfortunately, normal pedal pulses and arterial insufficiency are not mutually exclusive: there is a possibility of both false positives and false negatives. False-positive tests are possible when arterial disease primarily affects the microvasculature, as in a thickening of the basement membrane. In such cases, the problem is distal to the site of palpable pulses, making assessment through palpation impossible. False-positive tests can also occur when clinicians are unskilled or when pulse pressures are weak. Pulses are generally palpable if the pulse pressure is greater than 80 mm Hg.[57] Pulses may also be difficult to palpate in the presence of edema or excessive overlying soft tissue. It is estimated that when using palpable pulses as the determinant of arterial sufficiency, 20% of patients with critical peripheral arterial disease will be missed.[58] Therefore, the absence of palpable pulses should be followed up with more sensitive testing devices, such as a Doppler ultrasound, to more accurately assess perfusion.[26, 55]

Doppler Ultrasound

When peripheral pulses are not easily palpable, a **Doppler ultrasound** may be helpful in further assessing arterial patency.[58] A Doppler ultrasound is a hand-held probe that produces an audible signal when placed over moving fluid (the Doppler effect). To perform a Doppler examination, first place ultrasound coupling gel over the area in which the artery to be assessed is normally located. While holding the Doppler probe at a 45-degree angle to the skin directed proximally, the pulse can be heard as a swooshing noise.[58, 59] Lack of an audible signal indicates no fluid movement, that is, no perfusion. Note that this procedure can also be used to assess venous perfusion (see Chapter 11).

Ankle-Brachial Index

The **ankle-brachial index (ABI)** is a reliable[60] and fairly sensitive indirect and noninvasive measure of peripheral tissue perfusion (see Figure 10–7).[7, 61–64] Lower values correlate with increased severity of atherosclerosis and coronary artery disease.[65, 66] The ABI is 89–97% sensitive and 95–100% specific for diagnosing peripheral arterial disease.[8, 51, 58, 62, 64, 67, 68]

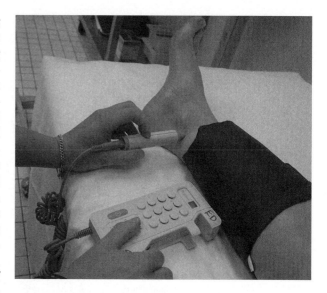

FIGURE 10–7 Measuring the ankle-brachial index. A Doppler ultrasound is used to identify the pulse at the posterior tibial artery. Next, the sphygmomanometer around the patient's distal calf is inflated, and the systolic pressure of the artery is measured and used to calculate the ABI.

The lower the ABI, the more likely a patient with an arterial insufficiency ulcer would undergo a revascularization procedure or amputation.[7, 69] In addition, lower ABI values are associated with decreased patient function and mobility.[7, 67, 70, 71] If arterial insufficiency is suspected or if pulses are not readily palpable, the ABI should be calculated to provide a better indicator of healing potential.[5, 58, 72] This test provides a ratio of the systolic blood pressure of the lower extremity compared with the upper extremity. First, with the patient supine, place a blood pressure cuff around the upper arm. Palpate the brachial artery within the cubital fossa, then place ultrasound gel over this site. Holding the Doppler probe at a 45-degree angle to the skin directed proximally,[58] the pulse can be heard as a swooshing noise. Inflate the cuff at least 20 mm Hg above the point at which the swooshing stops. Release the cuff and record the pressure measured at the time the swooshing of the pulse returns. Repeat the same procedure on the contralateral upper extremity, using the higher value to calculate the ABI.[62] Next, place the cuff just proximal to the medial malleolus and repeat the procedure on the posterior tibial artery and record the systolic pressure.[64, 73]

To calculate the ABI, divide the systolic pressure of the lower extremity by the systolic pressure of the upper extremity (see Box 10–1). A normal ABI measurement

TABLE 10–1   Interpretation of the Ankle-Brachial Index

ABI	Interpretation	Possible Vascular Interventions
1.1–1.3	Vessel calcification	ABI is not a valid measure of tissue perfusion
0.9–1.1	Normal	None needed
0.7–0.9	Mild to moderate arterial insufficiency	Conservative interventions normally provide satisfactory wound healing
0.5–0.7	Moderate arterial insufficiency, intermittent claudication	May perform trial of conservative care, physician may consider revascularization
<0.5	Severe arterial insufficiency, rest pain	Wound is unlikely to heal without revascularization, limb-threatening arterial insufficiency
<0.3	Rest pain and gangrene	Revascularization or amputation

BOX 10–1   Calculation of the Ankle-Brachial Index

$$ABI = \frac{\text{Systolic Pressure of the Lower Extremity}}{\text{Systolic Pressure of the Upper Extremity}}$$

---

is 0.9–1.1. Table 10–1 provides an interpretation of differing ABI values.[5, 7, 17, 23, 37, 51, 53, 62, 65, 74–79] Systolic ankle pressures of less than 60–80 mm Hg have been associated with poor healing potential.[76, 80] However, because of the prevalence of hypertension in patients with arterial insufficiency, ankle pressures in patients with arterial insufficiency ulcers are quite variable, ranging from as low as 0 mm Hg to as high as 130 mm Hg.[81] ABI testing can also be used to identify claudication by taking measurements before and after a treadmill or walking test.[7] A drop of more than 15% from the resting value is considered abnormal and consistent with arterial insufficiency.[7, 58] To rule out potentially critical changes in patient circulatory status, clinicians should repeat ABI testing if a wound that was initially improving is no longer progressing or worsens.[78, 82]

A drop of more than 0.15 on repeat ABI testing is indicative of peripheral arterial obstructive disease progression.[58, 65, 83]

Unfortunately, vessel calcification makes arterial walls abnormally stiff.[74] The pressure required to compress and collapse a calcified vessel is greater than the actual blood pressure within the vessel's lumen. Therefore, vessel calcification can cause misleadingly high ABI measurements.[21, 58, 79] An ABI greater than 1.1 denotes vessel calcification and is not a valid indicator of peripheral perfusion.[30] Clinicians should consider that ABI values within the normal range *may* be artificially inflated by arterial calcification, particularly in patients with diabetes, as these individuals have an increased risk of vessel calcification. In the presence of vessel calcification, a physician may order more direct or invasive measurements of arterial perfusion, such as a transcutaneous oxygen measurement or an arteriogram, to more accurately determine healing potential.[84, 85] Even though an ABI cannot account for collateral circulation that may have developed over time, this test still correlates well with transcutaneous oxygen measurements.[85] ABI values will be lower if the patient smoked on the day of measurement.[11, 65]

 Checkpoint Question #2

Your patient's resting heart rate is 72 bpm, respiration rate is 15, right brachial blood pressure is 120/80 mm Hg, right posterior tibial blood pressure is 70/50 mm Hg.

a. Calculate the patient's ABI.

b. What is your interpretation of this value?

Other potential courses of error in ABI measurements may occur in patients who cannot lay supine or patients with elevated blood pressure due to anxiety or pain.[63] Despite these shortcomings, the ABI can provide critically important information for the evaluation and ongoing reassessment of patients with peripheral vascular disease.

Segmental Pressure Measurements

Segmental pressure measurements can help localize areas of decreased arterial blood flow.[5, 16] Maintaining a Doppler probe over the dorsalis pedis or posterior tibial artery, systolic pressures are measured and recorded with the cuff placed above the malleoli, below the knee, and around the thigh. A pressure drop of greater than 20 mm Hg in adjacent segments is indicative of significant arterial occlusion in the interim segment.[5, 23, 65, 76, 79] Segmental pressure measurements are best at identifying distal arterial occlusion or stenosis rather than proximal.[86]

Capillary Refill

The **capillary refill** test is a reliable indicator of surface arterial blood flow.[48, 87] To perform the test, first observe the color of the patient's toes. Then push against the distal tip of the toe to be examined with enough pressure to blanch the skin and hold for 3 seconds, thereby emptying surface vessels of blood. Capillary refill time is recorded as the amount of time required for toe surface color to return to normal after the removal of pressure.[53] Normal capillary refill time is less than 3 seconds.[45, 88, 89] Patients with arterial insufficiency will have delayed capillary refill.[20, 26] Although uncommon, false-negative test results (e.g., capillary refill time of less than 3 seconds despite poor circulation) due to retrograde arterial filling have been reported.[23] Some studies have shown capillary refill is not predictive of peripheral arterial disease or impaired healing.[90]

Rubor of Dependency

The **rubor of dependency** test is a noninvasive test that can be used to indirectly assess arterial flow in the lower extremity (see Table 10–2).[7, 22, 23, 53, 56] With the patient in the supine position, note the color of the plantar aspect of the patient's foot. Next, elevate the lower extremity to be assessed approximately 60 degrees for 1 minute. Again, note the color of the plantar surface of the patient's foot. Patients with normal arterial flow will exhibit little or no color change with elevation, whereas arterial insufficient limbs will become pale because of decreased blood flow against gravity in this position.[76] Return the extremity to the support surface, and record how long it takes for the extremity to return to its original color.[91] Individuals with normal arterial supply will have a return to normal color in the tested foot within 15–20 seconds,[76] and the color will be light red or pink. In individuals with moderate arterial insufficiency, pallor usually occurs within 30 seconds of elevation. Pallor usually develops within 45–60 seconds in those with mild arterial insufficiency. Pallor occurring within 25 seconds of elevation and a bright red color with dependency, or dependent rubor,[92] usually indicate severe arterial insufficiency.[30] Dependent rubor results from the two-step process of reactive hyperemia.[12] First, elevating an arterial insufficient limb further deprives tissues of blood supply, causing arterioles to vasodilate to try to improve perfusion. Next, when the limb is placed in a more dependent position, blood flow increases significantly through the now maximally vasodilated vessels, giving the skin a reddened appearance.

TABLE 10–2   Rubor of Dependency Test

Test Result	**Interpretation**
Pallor after 45–60 seconds of elevation	Mild arterial insufficiency
Pallor after 30–45 seconds of elevation	Moderate arterial insufficiency
Pallor within 25 seconds of elevation, dependent rubor	Severe arterial insufficiency

TABLE 10–3   Interpretation of Venous Filling Time

Venous Filling Time	Interpretation
<5 seconds	Venous insufficiency
5–15 seconds	Normal
>20 seconds	Arterial insufficiency

Venous Filling Time

Prolonged **venous filling time** is predictive of arterial insufficiency (see Table 10–3).[22, 23] To perform this test, first place the patient supine and observe the superficial veins on the patient's dorsal foot. Then, elevate the limb approximately 60 degrees for about a minute or until the veins have been drained by gravity. Next, place the limb in the dependent position, and record the time it takes for the superficial veins to refill. Normal venous filling time is 5–15 seconds. Venous filling times greater than 20 seconds generally indicate severe arterial insufficiency.[23] In patients with venous insufficiency, veins refill almost immediately.

See Table 10–4 for a summary of physical therapy tests and measures used to assess individuals with arterial insufficiency.

TABLE 10–4   Clinical Guideline for Physical Therapy Tests and Measures for Arterial Insufficiency

Test	Indications
Pulse examination	• All open wounds located on the extremities
Doppler ultrasound and ankle-brachial index	• Decreased or absent pulses • Signs and symptoms of arterial insufficiency • History of peripheral vascular disease
Segmental pressure measurements	• Suspected arterial insufficiency in an ulcer proximal to the ankle • Decreased or absent proximal pulses
Capillary refill	• Digital ulcer • Abnormal Doppler ultrasound or ABI
Rubor of dependency	• Unable to tolerate ABI • ABI > 1.1 • History of diabetes or vessel calcification
Venous filling time	• Unable to tolerate ABI • ABI > 1.1 • History of diabetes or vessel calcification • Suspect concomitant venous insufficiency

 Checkpoint Question #3

Your patient presents with an ulcer near his lateral malleolus that is covered with adherent yellow slough. Pedal pulses are absent on the affected side. You are unable to perform an ABI because the patient complains of severe pain when the cuff is inflated more than 30 mm Hg.

a. Why is performing the ABI painful?

b. What other tests and measures might you perform to assist in your examination? Why?

CLASSIFICATION AND CHARACTERISTICS OF ARTERIAL ULCERS

Classification

After identifying the etiology of a wound, it is important to classify the wound into one of the five integumentary preferred practice patterns. The practice patterns in the *Guide to Physical Therapist Practice* provide physical therapists with valuable patient management information for general wound care. These practice patterns describe components of the examination, evaluation, diagnosis, prognosis, and interventions for patients who have an increased risk for integumentary disorders or who have impaired skin integrity. Patients with arterial insufficiency ulcers can readily be placed into the appropriate classification system based on the depth of tissue involved. It is not uncommon for patients with severe vascular compromise to present with full-thickness ulcers or ulcers extending into fascia, tendon, joint capsule, or bone.

Characteristics

To facilitate identification of ulcer similarities and differences, typical characteristics of various types of ulcers are described using the "5PT" method: pain, position, presentation, periwound, pulses, and temperature (see Box 10–2). Color images 3 and 14 are examples of arterial insufficiency ulcers.

Pain

Individuals with arterial insufficiency ulcers commonly report severe pain.[23, 74, 93] Patients may describe this pain as cramping, aching, or fatigue.[28] The cause of pain is tissue ischemia. This pain may increase during activities that increase tissue metabolism, such as ambulation.[28] Positions that further compromise tissue perfusion, such as leg elevation, may also increase their pain complaint.[49] Individuals with arterial insufficiency often report difficulty sleeping secondary to leg or foot pain and may even hang their foot off the edge of the bed to relieve this pain complaint. Uninformed health care workers or family members may aggravate the

BOX 10–2	Typical Characteristics of Arterial Insufficiency Ulcers
Pain	• Severe* • Increased with elevation
Position	• Distal toes • Dorsal foot • Areas of trauma
Wound presentation	• Regular appearance • May conform to precipitating trauma • Pale granulation tissue if present • Black eschar • Gangrene • Little or no drainage
Periwound and structural changes	• Thin, shiny, anhydrous skin • Loss of hair growth • Thickened, yellow nails • Pale, dusky, or cyanotic skin
Pulses	• Decreased or absent pedal pulses
Temperature	• Decreased
*Pain may be masked in individuals with sensory neuropathy.	

situation by insisting the patient keep the leg elevated. Although this is a common and useful strategy for most soft tissue injuries, such as strains and sprains, and even for other types of wounds, such as venous insufficiency ulcers, elevating an arterial insufficient limb only exacerbates the condition and pain complaint by further compromising circulation. Because of the progressive nature of atherosclerosis, the relative severity of arterial occlusion can be assessed by the characteristics of the patient's pain complaint. Generally speaking, patients with rest pain have more severe occlusive disease than those with intermittent claudication. However, the pain of arterial insufficiency may be masked in individuals with diabetic neuropathy, and the absence of claudication pain does not rule out arterial insufficiency.[28]

Position

Arterial ulcers are almost always located in the lower extremities because of the increased distance blood must travel to reach this area.[76] Arterial insufficiency ulcers are rarely found above the knee,[81] presumably because there is sufficient collateral circulation in this region compared to below the knee. Arterial ulcers are commonly located on the toes,[20] either dorsally or distally.[5] In fact, ulcers located on the distal, nonplantar aspect of the foot should be considered ischemic in nature unless proven otherwise.[72] Ulcerations may be seen by the lateral malleolus[81] or anterior leg[81] because of the decreased arterial supply in these regions.[5, 17] Trauma is a leading precipitating factor in arterial ulcer development. Therefore, ulcers located in aberrant positions should be assessed for potential causes of trauma. For example, a wound on the lateral border of the foot may be due to ill-fitting shoes. An ulcer on the anterior shin may be caused by bumping into objects.

Wound Presentation

Arterial ulcers generally begin as small, shallow wounds that gradually increase in size and depth. Ulcers are normally round and regular in appearance[20] or conform to precipitating trauma.[74] Granulation tissue, if present in the wound bed, is pale[5] or gray in color because of decreased oxygen supply. Necrotic tissue is generally desiccated, black eschar but may be yellow if the wound is bandaged in a way that maintains tissue hydration.[30] Gangrene may be present with more advanced disease.[34, 79] Because of diminished circulation, there is minimal or no wound drainage,[5] even in the presence of infection, and only minimal bleeding takes place with wound debridement. There is usually little evidence of progression through the phases of wound healing such as active granulation tissue formation or epithelialization.

Periwound and Structural Changes

Patients with chronic arterial insufficiency ulcers usually show signs of decreased perfusion.[94] When blood supply distal to the occlusion becomes inadequate, trophic changes occur. The epidermis becomes thinned, shiny, and anhydrous, and there is loss of hair growth.[5, 7, 95] Poor tissue oxygenation increases the risk of fungal infections, making nails become yellow, thickened, and fragile.[10, 26] Prolonged, severe ischemia may cause muscle atrophy.[30, 54, 70] Color changes may be evident, with the affected limb(s) appearing pale, dusky,[20] or cyanotic in color,[30] especially with elevation.[7, 10, 94] The limb may have dependent rubor.[7, 26] Edema is unusual with arterial insufficiency,[5] but if present, may represent concomitant venous insufficiency or congestive heart failure.[30] Patients with arterial insufficiency may try to reduce ischemic pain by prolonged dependent positioning, which may result in minimal edema or exacerbate concomitant venous insufficiency.

Pulses

Pulses at the dorsalis pedis artery and the posterior tibial artery are likely decreased or absent in the case of lower extremity arterial insufficiency.[7, 93] In severe cases, popliteal artery and femoral artery pulses may also be altered. If pulses are not readily palpable, more sensitive measures of circulation such as a Doppler ultrasound, ABI, or toe pressure measurements (refer to Medical Interventions section later in this chapter) should be performed.

Temperature

Ischemic digits or limbs will be cool or cold to the touch because of decreased blood supply.[7, 76] Since the dorsum of the hand is more sensitive to temperature changes than the fingertips, skin surface temperature can easily be assessed by lightly palpating with the back of the hand after allowing the patient to rest supine with shoes and socks removed for at least 5 minutes prior to testing. The temperature of the patient's foot should be compared with more proximal body segments such as the trunk. Palpation of temperature differences is a qualitative assessment of peripheral circulation and should be recorded as such. Clinicians may attempt to quantify temperature differences; however, quantification does not alter the plan of care or interventions to be provided.

Checkpoint Question #4

Your patient presents with ulcers on the dorsal aspect of his left fourth and fifth toes. The ulcers are dry with a pale base. On examining his lower leg, you notice the skin is pale and fragile and there is a loss of hair growth.

a. Is this patient's presentation consistent with an arterial insufficiency ulcer? Why or why not?

b. Describe at least three additional pieces of information you would like to gather to more accurately assess the etiology of this patient's wound.

PROGNOSIS FOR ARTERIAL INSUFFICIENCY ULCER HEALING

As with all chronic wounds, there is great variability in arterial insufficiency wound healing. Because many factors can contribute to delayed wound healing, the clinician must always consider local and systemic factors as well as wound characteristics when determining a patient's prognosis for wound healing. Given the etiology of arterial insufficiency ulcers, in addition to wound size and depth, local tissue perfusion must be considered when determining wound healing prognosis.[96] Unfortunately, there is little research specific to arterial insufficiency ulcer healing prognosis to guide clinicians, perhaps because they are far less common than venous insufficiency ulcers. Suggested benchmarks for ability to heal a wound in a patient with arterial insufficiency include having an ABI over 0.5, toe pressure of at least 50 mm Hg, and transcutaneous oxygen levels over 30 mm Hg.[57]

In general, wounds that are deeper or involve a greater amount of tissue loss will take longer to heal than wounds that are more superficial or smaller in size.[97–108] Research on nonarterial insufficiency ulcers suggests that a 20–40% decrease in wound surface area within 2–4 weeks of initiating treatment is a good indicator that a wound is responding to current interventions and full closure will follow.[102, 104, 108] If a wound does not decrease in size or show evidence of healing within 2 weeks, the clinician should reassess the patient and modify the plan of care or make appropriate referrals.[104, 108, 109] A rapid decline in wound status warrants immediate reassessment and referral.

CASE STUDY: Mr. Vahrm Gupta

PART 2

Tests and Measures

Integumentary Integrity: Position: L lateral distal calf wound 5 cm proximal to the lateral malleolus. Presentation: full-thickness wound: 3.2 cm length × 2.9 cm width (wound surface area 9.28 cm^2). Depth 0.5 cm—unable to determine exact depth due to presence of necrotic tissue. Wound bed contains 15% black eschar and 85% yellow adherent slough. There is no evidence of epithelial edge advancement or scar formation.

Wound drainage: minimal, thin, serosanguinous. No wound odor is present. Periwound skin is very thin and anhydrous skin. Temperature: periwound skin temperature appears equal to R distal calf as well as B thighs.

Sensory Integrity: patient is able to identify 4.17 monofilament B feet and lower legs.

Circulation: Pulses: dorsalis pedis L 0/R 1+, tibialis posterior L 0/R+, popliteal and femoral B 2+. Capillary refill: 5" L/3" R. Doppler ultrasound: audible signal in all pedal arteries. Ankle-brachial index

(ABI): LUE 122 mm Hg/RUE 125 mm Hg, LLE 84 mm Hg/RLE 105 mm Hg. ABI LLE 0.67/RLE 0.84. Segmental pressures: systolic pressure measured at the L posterior tibial artery with cuff just proximal to ankle = 84 mm Hg, with cuff at proximal calf; 90 mm Hg, with cuff at thigh 115 mm Hg. Rubor of dependency and venous filling time: not performed given several other positive tests for peripheral arterial occlusive disease.

Gait, Locomotion, Balance: Mr. Gupta is independent ambulating on level surfaces with a straight cane on the right. During a treadmill assessment using bilateral handrails at self-selected pace of 2.0 mph, he reports left calf cramping begins after 2 minutes of walking. After 8 minutes, he is unable to continue walking due to 7/10 left calf pain. LLE systolic pressure immediately after stopping ambulation: 63 mm Hg for an LLE ABI = 0.50. Mr. Gupta reports his left calf symptoms resolve after 2 minutes of sitting.

Pain: none at rest, 7/10 L calf pain at worst with walking for shopping causing him to stop the activity.

Evaluation and Diagnosis

Mr. Gupta has a full-thickness left lateral lower extremity ulcer consistent with Integumentary Preferred Practice Pattern D: Impaired Integumentary Integrity Associated with Full-Thickness Skin Involvement and Scar Formation. Mr. Gupta has several risk factors for arterial insufficiency including a history of coronary artery disease, hypertension, high cholesterol, low HDL levels, and rheumatoid arthritis. The lack of both left lower extremity pulses is evidence of arterial insufficiency. His ABI values are consistent with moderate arterial insufficiency in his left lower extremity and mild to moderate arterial insufficiency in his right lower extremity. He has intermittent claudication, consistent with at least 50% arterial occlusion, that limits his functional mobility. Since a 20% decline in ABI values with ambulation is consistent with arterial insufficiency, the 25% decrease noted in Mr. Gupta's left lower extremity ABI is also consistent with these findings. Segmental blood pressure measurements reveal a 25 mm Hg drop between his thigh and proximal calf. Because more than a 20 mm Hg drop is indicative of significant occlusion, Mr. Gupta appears to have a significant occlusion of his left femoral artery, likely at the bifurcation into the superficial and deep branches.

Prognosis and Plan of Care

While Mr. Gupta is a relatively young nonsmoker with protective sensation and no history of diabetes, his wound healing will be limited due to moderate LLE arterial insufficiency. Additionally, research on arterial insufficiency ulcers suggests that systolic ankle pressures less than 60–80 mm Hg are associated with poor wound healing. The wound shows no signs or symptoms of infection but has a high percentage of devitalized tissue. Mr. Gupta and his physician would like to see if the wound will improve with a trial of physical therapy interventions.

The following functional goals have been discussed and mutually agreed upon:

1. Mr. Gupta's left calf pain will be reduced to allow him to walk through the grocery store with a cart in 8 weeks.
2. Mr. Gupta's integumentary integrity will be fully restored in 10 weeks.

The following wound-related component goals have been discussed and mutually agreed upon:

1. The wound will be ≥80% granular over the next 2–3 weeks.
2. Wound surface area will be decreased by at least 20% (to ≤7.42 cm^2) over the next 2–3 weeks.
3. Mr. Gupta will verbalize an understanding of skin care protection techniques and methods to enhance wound healing in 2 weeks.

Mr. Gupta will be seen three times per week for a 2- to 3-week trial of physical therapy. If satisfactory progress is not made toward wound-related component goals, he will be referred back to his physician or a vascular surgeon for alternate medical and surgical interventions. Physical therapy interventions will include coordination, communication, and documentation; patient/client-related instruction; integumentary repair and protective techniques; and therapeutic exercises.

PHYSICAL THERAPY INTERVENTIONS

Coordination, Communication, and Documentation

As with all other patients, physical therapy services for patients with arterial ulcers must be coordinated with the patient, caregivers, and other disciplines to maximize outcomes. In addition to the physician, physical therapist, and physical therapist assistant, health care team members for the management of patients with arterial ulcers may include a registered dietitian, counselor, vascular surgeon, general surgeon, and prosthetist.

A registered dietitian can provide invaluable advice to patients and caregivers on dietary methods to improve blood pressure and blood sugar levels. Tighter control of hypertension and diabetes can decelerate the rate of atherosclerosis and improve the body's ability to heal. Dietitians can also ensure patients' diets include adequate hydration to decrease blood viscosity and improve tissue perfusion.[23] Eliminating or minimizing caffeine intake can also improve tissue perfusion by decreasing peripheral vasoconstriction.[23] Patients with open wounds require more nutrients for tissue repair and regeneration than individuals without open wounds. Appropriate nutrition provides the patient with the correct combination of protein, vitamins, and minerals needed for healing. Refer to Chapter 9 for more details regarding nutrition and wound healing.

A counselor or behavioral psychologist can assist patients who smoke with smoking cessation alternatives[93] including individual and group therapy.[7] Because smoking cessation alone can improve tissue perfusion,[79] it is vital that patients with arterial insufficiency ulcers are counseled on the significant risks of smoking and the many benefits of quitting.[7, 29] An often overlooked treatment strategy in the management of patients with arterial ulcers is the use of counseling for stress management and support. Because physical and emotional stress activates the sympathetic nervous system in increasing vasoconstriction, such interventions may improve circulation and wound healing.[23] All team members must provide consistent and ongoing feedback to patients and caregivers regarding risk factor modification in order to effect a change in patient behaviors. By addressing these controllable risk factors, patients' healing potential can be greatly enhanced.

Patients presenting with low ABIs or wounds failing to respond to conservative treatment should be referred to a vascular surgeon for consultation[48] regarding the feasibility of revascularization versus amputation. It is imperative that the physical therapist remember that the etiology of arterial insufficiency ulcers is a lack of adequate oxygen and nutrition to the region. Regardless of clinician skill and knowledge levels, some wounds will be unresponsive to physical therapy interventions. This should not be regarded as a failure of the clinician to select and follow an appropriate treatment plan, nor of the patient to adhere with the recommended treatment plan. Failure of the physical therapist to refer patients in a timely fashion will prolong patient recovery, risk limb loss, and cause potentially life-threatening complications due to gangrene and sepsis.

If amputation is performed, unless the amputation site is left to close by secondary intention, the primary focus of physical therapy interventions shifts from wound healing to effecting a functional recovery. This may include education and performance of range of motion exercises, strengthening exercises, and mobility training. Depending on the surgical technique used and the status of the patient's residual limb, a prosthetist may provide a temporary prosthesis immediately after surgery or after allowing the amputation site adequate time to regain tissue integrity and strength. Timely and ongoing communication with the prosthetist can improve patient mobility and prevent additional skin trauma by ensuring appropriate prosthesis design and fit.

Patient/Client-Related Instruction

Individuals with arterial insufficiency must be provided with the knowledge and resources to increase their control over the disease process. Patients must be advised of ways to modify risk factors for arterial insufficiency and methods to protect at-risk limbs from ulceration and reulceration.[53, 78] They should know that by controlling their smoking, high blood pressure, diabetes, and high cholesterol they can not only improve wound healing potential,[7, 20, 92, 110] but also reduce the risk of significant life-threatening cardiovascular events, such as heart attack and stroke.[22]

Because patients with arterial insufficiency are at increased risk for skin breakdown resulting from even minor trauma, clinicians should instruct patients in injury prevention techniques and proper foot care guidelines[78, 92, 93] (see Box 10–3). They should teach patients how to protect themselves from mechanical, thermal, and chemical trauma. Many, but not all, types of mechanical trauma can be prevented by a

BOX 10–3	Foot Care Guidelines for Patients with Arterial Ulcers

Protect Your Feet and Legs From Trauma

- Inspect your feet and legs daily for signs of trauma or irritation.
- Wash and dry feet carefully.
- Trim nails straight across and file gently, or have a podiatrist do so.
- Wear clean socks with smooth seams or without seams.
- Always wear shoes that fit properly, are comfortable, and are easy to get on and off.
- Avoid constrictive clothing.
- Avoid unnecessary leg elevation.

Protect Your Feet and Legs From Chemicals

- Do not use home remedies or chemicals, such as corn removers, unless directed to do so by a clinician.

Protect Lour Leet and Legs Lrom Lxcessive Leat and Cold

- Do not use hot water bottles or heating pads.
- Do not soak your feet in hot water.
- Use heavy socks and/or insulated boots to protect feet from the cold.
- Test bath water with your elbow or a thermometer.

Protect any Open Wounds

- Wear bandages as instructed.
- Do not put pressure on open areas when walking.

Live Healthy

- Follow your physician's instructions regarding medication.
- Control medical conditions such as diabetes, high blood pressure, and high cholesterol as much as possible.
- Eat a balanced diet.
- Exercise regularly.
- If you smoke, quit.

Call Your Clinician if:

- You notice your wound is getting larger, is draining more, or has a foul odor.
- You have increased pain or swelling.
- You detect a new wound.

careful home assessment. For example, clinicians should ensure walkways are clear of clutter and wide enough to allow patient thoroughfare without tripping or bumping into table ends or other furniture. Clinicians should direct patients to wash and moisturize their feet and legs daily and to perform daily skin checks,[5] reporting any new lesions to their physician or therapist immediately. Patients should be instructed to perform a hand check of their shoes to identify and remove any foreign objects before donning. Patients should be told to dry thoroughly between their toes and to wear white socks to allow easier identification of blood or wound drainage. Because patients with arterial insufficiency tend to complain of cold feet due to poor circulation, many will try to warm themselves with heating pads or hot water soaks. Unfortunately, many times their circulation is not sufficient to diffuse this added heat, resulting in skin burns. Rather than directly heating cold limbs, patients should be encouraged to don heavy socks and wear warm, insulated boots in cold weather. If an ulcer is already present, patients should be instructed in a means of mobility that does not put pressure on the injured area.

 Checkpoint Question #5

Your patient with arterial insufficiency complains that her feet are cold and asks if she should use a heating pad to warm them. What is your response and why?

Procedural Interventions

Precautions

Compression and compression dressings should be avoided in patients with arterial insufficiency ulcers because this further impedes circulation to the affected area.[11, 74] Physical therapy interventions for wound care will be of limited value in patients who have low ABIs without prior revascularization.[48] Although a trial of conservative interventions, including physical therapy, may be indicated, wounds that regress or fail to improve mandate referral to the physician of record or a vascular surgeon on a timely basis to prevent more extensive tissue destruction. A general guideline for wound management suggests that if wound healing does not significantly progress within 2–6 weeks of treatment,[94] the plan of care must be reassessed.

Sharp debridement should not be performed on dry, eschar-covered, uninfected arterial ulcers with low ABIs (certainly wounds with ABIs less than 0.3, and possibly less than 0.5) prior to surgical intervention.[5, 20] Without revascularization, circulation is likely inadequate to heal the larger wound created by debridement.[111] Some authors suggest that wounds of this nature should be covered with a dry gauze dressing and observed.[23] Gangrenous wounds also should not be debrided by physical therapists or physical therapist assistants. Gangrenous tissue must be removed surgically (see Box 10–4).

Peripheral arterial disease is a predictor for coronary artery disease: patients with PAD have a threefold increase in risk of death and a sixfold increase in risk of cardiovascular-related deaths.[7] Therefore, caution must be used when prescribing therapeutic exercises for this patient population.

Integumentary Repair and Protective Techniques

Request for Further Medical Testing

Patients with invalid ABI measurements (e.g., greater than 1.1) and wounds that fail to progress as expected require further medical testing and/or intervention. Additional medical tests may include noninvasive measurements, such as tissue oxygen levels and toe pressures, or invasive procedures, such as arteriograms. An order for a wound culture and sensitivity should be requested if the patient presents with the signs and symptoms of infection. Unfortunately, the signs and symptoms of infection in arterial ulcers can be subtle. This is because circulation is sometimes so poor that the body is unable to mount the normal inflammatory and immune response to microorganisms. Ischemic ulcers that present with increasing pain and necrosis, a faint halo or erythema around the wound, and a fluctance of periwound tissues should be assessed for infection.[23] If infected, the physician should initiate appropriate antibiotic therapy immediately. Because of the increased risk of osteomyelitis, an order for a bone scan or x-ray should be requested in wounds presenting with exposed capsule or bone. If osteomyelitis is present, the infected bone, or the infected portions of the

> **BOX 10–4   Wound Care Precautions for Patients with Arterial Insufficiency**
>
> - Avoid compression and compression dressings.
> - Avoid sharp debridement of dry, eschar-covered, uninfected ulcers in patients with low ABIs.
> - Gangrenous tissue must be removed surgically.

bone, must be promptly surgically removed prior to allowing the wound to close.[112]

Local Wound Care

Highlights of local wound care specific to patients with arterial insufficiency ulcers are included here and in Box 10–5. Refer to Section II of the text for more detail. Moisturizing lotions should be applied daily to protect anhydrous skin, keep it pliable, and decrease the risk of skin breakdown due to friction or shearing.[5, 92] Cotton, toe spacers, or toe caps should be placed between toes as needed to provide padding and reduce friction between adjacent toes. Necrotic tissue should be debrided unless circulation is severely limited.[5] Because arterial ulcers are typically dry, occlusive dressings or amorphous hydrogels can be used to promote a moist wound healing environment.[5, 78] The use of strong adhesives should be avoided to prevent further integumentary trauma. The ischemic limb should be protected from further trauma,[92] and unnecessary elevation should be avoided. Modalities such as negative pressure wound therapy and hyperbaric oxygen may be helpful adjuncts in wounds that are slow to heal (see Chapter 8).[84]

BOX 10–5   Keys to Local Wound Care for Patients with Arterial Insufficiency

Protect surrounding skin
- Moisturize dry skin.
- Avoid adhesives.
- Reduce friction between toes.
- Provide padding to protect ischemic tissues.

Address wound bed
- Choose dressings to moisten wound bed.
- Debride necrotic tissue if appropriate.

Maximize circulation
- Avoid compression.
- Choose footwear to accommodate for bandages and decrease stress to wound.

Educate patient/caregivers
- Wound etiology.
- Intervention strategies.
- Risk factor modification.
- Foot care guidelines.

 ## Checkpoint Question #6

Your patient presents with an arterial insufficiency ulcer on his left foot. The ulcer has a pale, granular base and measures 0.8 × 0.6 × 0.2 cm. There is no wound drainage. The surrounding tissue is anhydrous, mildly pale, slightly cool to the touch, and edematous. Pedal pulses are decreased and his ABI is 0.6. The patient has been dressing the wound with a moisture-retentive dressing and an elastic compression bandage. Given your examination findings, do you agree with the current dressing? Why or why not?

Therapeutic Exercise

Gait and Mobility Training

Physical therapists and physical therapist assistants must instruct patients with arterial ulcers in mobility that protects healing tissues. Patients must not be allowed to bear weight on open wounds. Appropriate assistive devices should be chosen to off-load affected areas. An additional benefit of assistive devices is that they may help reduce the pain of ambulation associated with arterial insufficiency. In addition, many patients with peripheral arterial disease exhibit lower extremity strength deficits, which are associated with a functional decline in mobility including decreased walking distance, time, and pace.[70, 71] Appropriately titrated mobility exercises have been shown to result in functional gains.[113]

Patient Positioning

ABIs are increased with foot dependency and decreased with hip and knee flexion.[65] Therefore, it would seem appropriate to counsel patients with arterial insufficiency to periodically dangle their legs to improve blood flow and to avoid extreme hip and knee flexion.[92]

Aerobic Exercise

The pain of intermittent claudication and the muscle atrophy that can accompany arterial insufficiency generally lead to profound debilitation. Aerobic exercise can have many positive results in patients with arterial insufficiency.[29] Toe pressures and TBIs have been shown to increase in patients with peripheral arterial disease after a brief exercise session.[114] A graded exercise program can stimulate collateral vessel formation over time,[92] improving perfusion distal to the occlusion. Several controlled trials have demonstrated that a progressive walking program can improve symptom-free walking distance and maximum walking distance.[21, 113] One trial even found exercise to be superior to, and less expensive than, vascular surgery in improving symptom-free walking distance.[7, 21] Although no studies have examined the effect of aerobic exercise on wound healing, theoretically an increase in collateral vessels will enhance healing. In addition, this new vasculature can enable a patient to ambulate farther or longer prior to the onset of pain.[29] Aerobic exercise promotes weight loss, improves blood sugar control,[79] and raises HDL levels,[15] all of which ultimately enhance wound healing potential.[79] However, *excessive* exercise of lower extremity muscles can divert already limited blood supply to exercising muscles and away from the wounded area, thus delaying wound healing. In addition, because 60–90% of patients with arterial insufficiency have evidence of coronary artery disease,[37, 51, 115] clinicians should judiciously prescribe and carefully monitor aerobic exercise.[22]

Resistive Exercises

While the effect of strength training on arterial ulcer healing is not known, patients with peripheral arterial disease who performed resistive exercise training had significant improvements in walking time, walking distance, stair climbing ability, knee extension strength, and several quality of life indices.[113] Clinicians should particularly emphasize exercises for plantarflexors, quadriceps, and hip extensors.

Flexibility Exercises

Patients with arterial insufficiency may develop adaptive shortening of connective tissue because of immobility or pain. For example, decreased ankle flexibility, specifically reduced dorsiflexion and gastrocnemius length, is commonly seen in less ambulatory patients. This loss of flexibility causes increased tissue stress on the plantar aspect of the foot during ambulation. Because of the already precarious blood supply to the foot, increased plantar pressure may be just enough stress to cause skin breakdown by upsetting the balance between blood supply and tissue demand. Flexibility exercises targeting areas such as limited dorsiflexion and gastrocnemius length may prevent new ulcers from forming or, in the case of a plantar wound, decrease the risk of ulcer recurrence.

Buerger's Exercises

Buerger's exercises consist of cyclic leg elevation until blanching, followed by leg lowering until reactive hyperemia occurs. It was once thought that such a regimen would help "exercise" diseased vasculature, ultimately making it more responsive to tissue demands.[116] However, researchers now believe it is doubtful that Buerger's exercises are effective.[17]

Prescription, Application, and Fabrication of Devices and Equipment

Temporary Footwear

Because patients with arterial ulcers frequently present with dorsal or distal digit ulcerations, clinicians should ensure appropriate footwear[5, 22] is used both during the healing phase and long term. Walking shoes or cast shoes generally serve as ideal temporary footwear because they allow adequate space for bandages, have a high toe box to prevent excessive pressure on the dorsal digits, and are of sufficient length to prevent pressure on the distal toes. Additional features that may be helpful are a rocker-bottom sole to facilitate a more normal gait pattern and an enclosed shoe (vs. a sandal-type shoe) to better protect the foot from foreign objects and cold temperatures.

Permanent Footwear

Permanent footwear for patients with arterial insufficiency should include many of the same features as temporary footwear: extra-depth toe box, adequate length, and sufficient space for heavy socks during cooler weather. Shoes should be made of soft, flexible material to prevent undue pressure on the foot. Patients with severe foot deformities or amputations should be referred to a skilled shoemaker or orthotist for more customized footwear.

Physical Agents and Mechanical Modalities: Therapeutic Heat

Cold temperature further inhibits tissue perfusion in an ischemic limb by causing vasoconstriction. A logical corollary to preventing ischemic limbs from becoming too cold is that gentle warming of the affected region would improve perfusion.[23, 38] There are several key biological responses to heat. Heat causes vasodilation, enhancing tissue perfusion. Increased temperature also increases tissue oxygen saturation by decreasing hemoglobin's affinity for oxygen. Greater tissue oxygen levels enhance processes in all three phases of wound healing, including phagocytosis, resistance to infection, granulation tissue formation, wound contraction, epithelialization, and scar tissue formation.[38, 117, 118]

The phrase *gentle warming* is key because ischemic tissues cannot dissipate excessive heat and will sustain a thermal injury if it is applied directly to ischemic regions. Therapeutic heat can be as simple as placing a properly prepared hot pack to the femoral triangle or lumbar paraspinals.[119] Heat applied to the femoral triangle causes the femoral artery passing within the triangle to vasodilate. As the femoral artery provides the main blood flow to the lower extremity, the assumption is that increasing blood flow proximally will also improve blood flow distally. Heat applied to the lumbar region is thought to enhance lower extremity circulation by causing reflex vasodilation by affecting the lumbar sympathetic innervation.

Simply applying a wound dressing helps to decrease heat loss through an open wound. Because wound temperature decreases with each dressing change, minimizing the frequency of dressing changes may also assist with maintaining wound normothermia.

Case Study: Mr. Vahrm Gupta

PART 3

Interventions

The following highlights some of the key procedural interventions that will be incorporated into Mr. Gupta's plan of care.

Coordination, Communication, and Documentation: Mr. Gupta's physician has been contacted regarding his examination findings of moderate left lower extremity arterial insufficiency and mild to moderate right lower extremity arterial insufficiency. As a result of this communication, the physician prescribed cilostazol for Mr. Gupta in an attempt to improve his circulation and increased the dosage of his cholesterol medication. If Mr. Gupta's cholesterol and triglyceride levels do not improve, his physician stated he would make a referral to a registered dietician. Because there is no local, proximal, superficial artery, a nitroglycerin patch was believed to be of no additional benefit. The physician concurred with the physical therapist's decision to initiate sharp debridement in combination with autolytic debridement because of the large percentage of devitalized tissue within the wound bed, Mr. Gupta's arterial insufficiency, and an ABI > 0.5.

Patient/Client-Related Instruction: Mr. Gupta will be instructed in the importance of skin protection techniques and maximizing peripheral circulation. Mr. Gupta will be instructed to wear socks along with hard-soled shoes or slippers at all times and avoid the use of heat or ice below his thigh to decrease the risk of integumentary damage. He will be instructed to decrease the risk of skin trauma by performing a home safety check to identify and remove any clutter or environmental barriers that might increase his risk of falling or bumping his legs, such as narrow passageways between his coffee table and couch. He will be instructed to avoid constrictive clothing, particularly tight socks, pant legs with elastic cuffs, and tight elastic leg bands to his undergarments. He will be instructed in proper positioning to maximize his lower extremity circulation including not propping his legs up at night and avoiding extremes of hip and knee flexion. He will be instructed to inspect his legs and feet thoroughly twice daily and to attend to any areas of redness or trauma so minor problems are less likely to progress. He will be instructed to apply a moisturizer to his feet and legs twice daily to improve skin hydration. In an attempt to increase lower extremity circulation, Mr. Gupta was instructed to apply a heating pad set on low to his left femoral triangle for 20 minutes twice daily.

Procedural Interventions:

- Local wound management will consist of pulsed lavage with suction to irrigate the wound and assist with the removal of adherent slough. Sharp debridement was chosen because it has the fastest results and was determined to be safe for Mr. Gupta. Any remaining nonviable tissue will be crosshatched. The wound will be dressed with a skin sealant to the periwound, a small amount of amorphous hydrogel will be applied to the wound to add moisture to the wound bed,

CASE STUDY   Continued

and the wound will be covered with a nonadherent semipermeable foam. A wide roll gauze will be used to secure the foam. This dressing will protect the fragile epithelium from maceration and adhesives, promote autolytic debridement between sessions, and maintain a warm wound environment.

- Therapeutic exercises will include a progressive walking program to attempt to increase Mr. Gupta's symptom-free and maximum ambulation. While aerobic exercise, such as an upper body ergometer, may assist with raising Mr. Gupta's HDL levels, this was deferred during the initial physical therapy trial.
- Negative pressure wound therapy and noncontact normothermic wound therapy were not recommended due to Mr. Gupta's poor skin quality and the potential for the adhesive to create new

skin trauma. Because of his demand-style pacemaker, electrical stimulation is contraindicated without further examination and careful monitoring by his cardiologist.

Reassessment

After 2 weeks of physical therapy, Mr. Gupta's wound has not changed in size and there is no evidence of epithelial edge advancement. The wound bed is now 50% adherent yellow slough and 50% pale granulation tissue. Mr. Gupta reports his left calf symptoms appear to occur sooner and he must sit for at least 5 minutes before they resolve. His left lower extremity ABI is now 0.50 at rest, indicating significant progression of his peripheral arterial occlusive disease. The physical therapist requests an immediate consult with Mr. Gupta's physician and referral to a vascular surgeon.

MEDICAL AND SURGICAL INTERVENTIONS

Ischemic tissue is easily infected and heals poorly if at all.[38] Additional medical tests, such as transcutaneous oxygen measurements, toe pressures, and arteriography, are employed to more accurately assess the potential for wound healing in ischemic limbs. Key medical and surgical interventions for arterial insufficiency ulcers are aimed at trying to improve circulation to the affected area. If this is not possible, amputation may be required. Although medical and surgical interventions are clearly beyond the scope of physical therapy, they are presented here to provide a better understanding of the valuable roles these disciplines play in the management of patients with arterial insufficiency ulcerations.

Medical Interventions

Physicians play a vital role in the management of patients with arterial ulcerations by selecting appropriate medical testing, managing risk factors, providing pharmacological interventions to decrease pain and improve circulation, and performing sympathetic blocks. Clinicians need to be aware of these options in case standard measures fail to yield the desired results.

Medical Testing

Diagnostic studies are sometimes used to confirm clinical impressions regarding wound etiology. Plethysmography, duplex scanning, transcutaneous oxygen monitoring, toe pressures, and arteriography may be performed on patients with arterial insufficiency ulcers.

Plethysmography and Duplex Scanning

Plethysmography and **duplex scanning** are two noninvasive methods of assessing regional blood flow.[53] A variety of different plethysmography methods exist, including electrical impedance, photo, and air, although the latter two are currently used more frequently. To perform this test, a cuff connected to a force transducer is placed around the extremity or digit to be assessed. The pulsatile nature of blood flow causes pressure changes within the cuff that are picked up by the transducer and recorded graphically. Because it measures volume changes, plethysmography provides a better assessment of regional blood flow in patients with vessel calcification who cannot otherwise be accurately assessed with an ABI. Duplex scanning combines a directional Doppler probe with a scanner. This scan provides information about blood flow, velocity, and turbulence in arteries and veins.[120]

Transcutaneous Oxygen Monitoring

Transcutaneous oxygen monitoring (TCOM, also called **TcPO$_2$)** studies are used to evaluate slow-healing wounds and to assess the severity of peripheral vascular disease.[85, 121] The test uses a series of electrodes adjacent to the patient's wound to measure the oxygen tension in periwound tissues. Because TCOM measures tissue oxygen content, it is able to detect both macrovascular and microvascular perfusion (or lack thereof) and more objectively quantify healing potential.[53] Normal periwound tissue oxygen tension levels exceed 50 mm Hg. Values of 35 mm Hg and higher are considered sufficient to support wound healing in chronic ischemic wounds.[65, 75] However, periwound tissue oxygen tension levels less than 30 mm Hg are unlikely to heal without surgical intervention.[30] TCOM studies are commonly used to document the level of wound hypoxia, determine if additional interventions may be required to aid wound healing, or map perfusion levels prior to amputation.

Toe Pressure

Toe pressures are similar to ankle and brachial pressure measurements used to calculate an ABI.[7] However, because the equipment required—a digital pneumatic cuff and photoplethysmograph—is quite expensive and highly specialized, most testing is performed by vascular surgeons or in research settings. In spite of the increased cost, toe pressure measurements have several advantages over ABI measurements.[58, 80, 122] First, because the ABI only assesses circulation proximal to the foot, it provides a misleading representation of actual tissue perfusion of the digits and foot.[52] For example, a patient may present with a normal ABI even though there is significant microvascular disease. Second, ABI measurements may be falsely elevated because of arterial calcification. Toe pressure measurements are not subject to this type of error.[51] A toe pressure of greater than 30 mm Hg is indicative of good healing potential.[57, 69, 76]

Arteriography

Arteriography is a procedure in which radiopaque dye is injected into an artery to better visualize blood flow within the vessel.[7, 30] Because arteriography is an invasive procedure with inherent risks, it is usually performed only if surgical revascularization is being considered as a treatment option.[7, 79]

Management of Risk Factors

By identifying and controlling risk factors for arterial ulcers, physicians can lessen arterial insufficiency[51] and significantly enhance wound healing.[7, 53] Cholesterol, triglycerides, and blood pressure levels must be controlled.[28] Maintaining blood sugars as close to normal as possible greatly improves healing potential in patients with diabetes.[79] For every 1% increase in glycosolated hemoglobin A1c, there is a 26% increase in PAD.[7] Patients having difficulty attaining or maintaining the ideal levels presented in Table 10–5 may benefit from medical nutrition therapy and, if necessary, pharmacological management.

Patients with arterial insufficiency ulcers can improve with smoking cessation alone.[79] Therefore, physicians must stress the importance of abstaining from tobacco products and may refer patients who smoke to supervised smoking cessation programs. Physicians may suggest the use of transdermal patches to provide a gradual reduction in nicotine exposure. Physicians may also prescribe bupropion hydrochloride (Zyban or Wellbutrin), a drug commonly used in the treatment of depression.[7] This non-nicotine drug has shown promising results in assisting individuals with smoking cessation by reducing the craving for nicotine.[123]

Pharmacological Interventions for Pain and Circulation

Because ischemic ulcers are often severely painful, pain management is an important part of the overall care of patients with arterial insufficiency.[124, 125] Physicians may prescribe pain medications to help patients with arterial ulcers for two reasons. First, controlling pain obviously makes patients feel better and improves their

TABLE 10–5   Ideal Values for Decreasing the Risk of Arterial Insufficiency Ulceration and Enhancing Wound Healing

Measurement	Ideal Value
Total cholesterol	<200 mg/dL
LDL/HDL	≤3.0
Triglycerides	<150 mg/dL
Blood pressure	<130/85
Blood sugar	70–110 mg/dL

sense of well-being. Second, pain management indirectly improves circulation by reducing patient anxiety and sympathetic nervous system stimulation.[38]

Pharmacological interventions can also be used to enhance circulation.[7, 22] Transdermal patches, such as nitroglycerin and clonidine, have been shown to improve local circulation.[38, 52, 126] Physicians should try to minimize the use of vasoconstrictive agents because they adversely affect tissue perfusion.[30] Pentoxifylline (Trental) and cilostazol may be prescribed to enhance circulation.[7, 27, 29, 51, 127–130] The mechanisms by which these medications work are not entirely clear. However, they seem to decrease blood viscosity, decrease platelet aggregation,[130] increase red blood cell flexibility, and have a vasodilatory effect,[130] resulting in improved tissue perfusion.[19, 30, 127] In addition to improving wound healing, cilostazol may reduce or even abolish ischemic pain.[37, 130] Low-dose aspirin may be prescribed to decrease blood viscosity.[19, 131] While the effect on arterial insufficiency and arterial insufficiency–related wounds is not known, this drug has been shown to substantially reduce the risk of heart attack and stroke.[131] Physical therapists should review the patient's current medications during the initial examination. If a patient does not have adequate pain control or is on vasoconstrictive agents, the physical therapist should consult with the physician.

Sympathetic Block

Patients who are not revascularization candidates may benefit from a lumbar sympathetectomy, or block.[38, 79] This procedure eliminates central nervous system control over vasoconstriction, yielding maximally vasodilated lower extremity arteries.[19, 30] This may improve circulation to the affected limb and increase wound healing potential.

Surgical Interventions

Sometimes patients with arterial ulcers require surgical intervention. Surgeons may perform debridement, revascularization, or angioplasty.[22, 52] In cases of severe arterial insufficiency, amputation may be required.

Debridement

The primary goals of surgical debridement are to rid the wound of debris and nonviable tissue and to produce a wound bed that is conducive to healing. This type of debridement may include a combination of cleansing and excision of both necrotic and unwanted viable tissue, such as hypergranular tissue. Surgical debridement has several advantages over debridement by physical therapists and physical therapist assistants. First, surgical debridement is performed in a sterile surgical suite, which may reduce the risk of infection. Second, surgical debridement may be more efficient than repeated bouts of debridement performed in physical therapy, allowing a one-time removal of all devitalized tissue present. It is not unusual for surgical debridement to include a wide margin of healthy tissue to ensure a viable wound bed. This type of surgical excision requires the knowledge and skill of a surgeon for successful patient outcomes.

Revascularization

A vascular assessment should be recommended if a patient presents with night pain, rest pain, slow-healing wounds with coexisting diabetes, or an ABI less than 0.8.[17, 48] Vascular surgery is generally indicated, if feasible, in patients with ABIs less than 0.7.[48] Failure of a borderline wound to respond to conservative interventions mandates revascularization.[23] The basic concept of revascularization involves first identifying the most distal segment with normal blood flow and the occluded artery segment, then choosing a new conduit, or bypass, to replace the diseased segment. Commonly used bypass material includes the patient's own greater or lesser saphenous veins or prosthetic graft material such as Gortex or Dacron.[21] Revascularization restores adequate blood flow to the ischemic limb, with ABIs averaging as much as 1.0 after surgery.[81] Therefore, the potential for, and the rate of, wound healing is greatly improved.[5] Graft patency and restoration of pedal pulses after bypass surgery are predictors of wound healing.[52] Bypass surgery is not without risks, given a 10–15% patient morbidity and mortality after surgery.[5] In addition, graft patency rates may be as low as 40% 4 years after surgery.[5] However, more recent studies have shown 5-year patency rates of 66% for femoral–popliteal vein grafts, 50% for femoral–tibial vein grafts.[28] Patency rates appear to be significantly less when using prosthetic materials at this time.[28]

Percutaneous Balloon Angioplasty

Nonvascularization candidates with significant arterial insufficiency may undergo percutaneous balloon angioplasty, a procedure in which a balloon-tipped catheter is expanded at the site of stenosis, compressing any plaque

Case Study: Mr. Vahrm Gupta

PART 4

Medical and Surgical Interventions

The following highlights changes in Mr. Gupta's plan of care as a result of the lack of improvement with physical therapy interventions.

- The physician ordered electrical impedance plethysmography, which confirmed the physical therapist's ABI results. An arteriogram was then performed, which showed a localized obstruction at the bifurcation of the femoral artery with 70% arterial occlusion. Although HBO may improve wound healing in patients with arterial insufficiency, the vascular surgeon thought that Mr. Gupta was an excellent surgical candidate due to his localized and progressive obstruction. Given Mr. Gupta's relatively young age, the surgeon chose to perform a prosthetic bypass graft rather than a stent placement due to the potential for stent reocclusion over time. During the vascular procedure, the surgeon debrided the remaining slough within the wound bed.

- After surgery, physical therapy was restarted. Reexamination findings included normal left pedal pulses and capillary refill. An ABI was not performed to protect the graft. Mr. Gupta reported incisional pain but no longer noticed left calf cramping or pain with ambulation. Physical therapy interventions at this time included reinforcing previous education information, local wound care, and resumption of therapeutic exercise. The wound dressing was changed to an amorphous hydrogel, impregnated gauze, gauze square, and wide roll gauze to allow daily inspection of the wound during the early post-operative period.

---

formations that are obstructing blood flow against the vessel wall.[17, 30] This procedure works best with larger arteries and when the length of stenosis is short and clearly identified.[21] Sometimes a stent, a small metallic device, is placed within the diseased artery segment to maintain lumen integrity by preventing elastic recoil of the artery.[21, 30] If successful, angioplasty and stent placement increase the potential for wound healing by enhancing circulation distal to the procedure. Unfortunately, these procedures rarely improve circulation to the same extent as revascularization, and plaques are likely to recur over time. Researchers have recently created a stent coating that appears to help prevent or delay plaque recurrence.[132]

Amputation

The treatment of choice for gangrene and severe ischemia is usually amputation.[5, 21] Amputation for severe ischemia is usually preceded by attempts at revascularization.[133] The level of amputation is determined by the most distal satisfactorily perfused arteries and the patient's future mobility.[21, 30] For example, if patient X has a gangrenous toe with adequate circulation in the remainder of the foot, the surgeon will likely amputate only the gangrenous digit. In contrast, if patient Y has a gangrenous toe with an ABI of 0.3, poor capillary refill, and an arteriogram showing poor perfusion distal to the popliteal artery, the surgeon will likely perform a transfemoral amputation. Although a transfemoral amputation requires greater energy expenditure than a transtibial amputation,[5] it would provide the patient with superior mobility with a prosthesis than disarticulation at the knee or a short residual limb below the knee.[133]

CHAPTER SUMMARY

Atherosclerosis is the leading cause of arterial insufficiency ulcers. There are many risk factors contributing to arterial insufficiency and arterial insufficiency ulcerations, including hyperlipidemia, elevated cholesterol, smoking, diabetes, hypertension, trauma, and advanced age. Identifying and controlling, or correcting, these risk factors enhance the potential for wound healing. Physical therapy tests and measures, including pulses, Doppler ultrasound, ankle-brachial index (ABI), segmental pressures, rubor of dependency, and venous filling time, should be performed to estimate the degree of circulatory compromise and the potential for wound healing.

Physical therapy interventions for patients with arterial ulcerations should emphasize patient/client-related instruction, risk factor modification, local wound care, and protection from further trauma. Procedural interventions may include debridement, dressing selection and application, therapeutic exercise, and modalities. Clinicians have the obligation to refer patients not responding to conservative interventions for further medical evaluation.

REVIEW QUESTIONS

1. You are a physical therapist working in a nursing home. Your patient presents with an arterial ulcer on the anterior aspect of her shin. The ulcer began as a result of bumping her leg against the leg rest of her wheelchair. On initial physical therapy examination, the wound measured 2.0 × 2.5 cm, pedal pulses were 1+, ABI was 0.6, capillary refill time was 5 seconds, and there was a positive rubor of dependency test with pallor after 27 seconds of elevation and dependent rubor. After 2 weeks of physical therapy, the wound now measures 2.5 × 3.6 cm. Describe and defend your course of action.

2. Your patient presents with arterial ulcers on the tip of his left second toe and on the dorsum of his left third toe. The wounds are dry and covered with eschar. The affected leg has no palpable pedal pulses, but they are present using a Doppler probe. The ABI is 0.7.

   a. Should physical therapy interventions include debridement for this patient? Why or why not?

   b. Describe two topical agents that might be used on this patient's wounds.

   c. Describe two methods you might use to bandage this patient's wounds.

   d. What footwear would you consider for this patient and why?

3. Use the wound in color image 15 to answer the following series of questions.

   Your patient, Mrs. Y, is a 65-year-old who presents for an initial physical therapy examination with an ulcer near her left medial malleolus. Mrs. Y states the ulcer began 4 months ago as a small hole, which has slowly increased in size. Her daughter was treating the wound at home with daily wet-to-dry dressings. Five days ago, Mrs. Y began applying a heating pad to the wound to try to decrease the pain and warm her foot. Since that time, the wound has significantly increased in size. Mrs. Y's past medical history includes a right transfemoral amputation 13 months ago, which she states was due to poor circulation and diabetes, with her most recent blood sugar level 190 mg/dL. She has been a two-pack-per-day smoker for the past 20 years. Mrs. Y lives with her daughter in a one-story home. She uses a manual wheelchair independently for mobility and requires moderate assistance for transfers.

   a. What tests and measures would you perform on Mrs. Y?

   b. Document wound and periwound characteristics as you would in the patient's chart.

   c. Should you debride this wound? Why or why not?

   d. Describe how you might bandage Mrs. Y's wound.

   e. Describe other physical therapy interventions you would include in your plan of care.

PEARSON myhealthprofessionskit™

Use this address to access the Companion Website created for this textbook. Simply select "Physical Therapy" from the choice of disciplines. Find this book and log in using your username and password to access images, video clips, and additional learning tools.

REFERENCES

Go to myhealthprofessionskit.com to view this chapter's references.

11

Venous Insufficiency Ulcers

Chapter Objectives

After reading this chapter, learners will be able to:

1. Differentiate the etiology of venous insufficiency ulcers from other types of open wounds.
2. Explain the risk factors contributing to venous insufficiency ulcers.
3. Describe and choose physical therapy tests and measures to assess patients with venous insufficiency.
4. Assess the typical characteristics of venous insufficiency ulcers.
5. Assess the typical characteristics of venous and arterial insufficiency ulcers.
6. Design an interdisciplinary approach in the management of patients with venous insufficiency ulcers.
7. Apply basic guidelines and protective principles for patients with venous insufficiency ulcers.
8. Describe precautions clinicians should be aware of when working with patients with venous insufficiency ulcers.
9. Integrate the keys to local wound care for patients with venous insufficiency ulcers.
10. Select physical therapy procedural interventions for patients with venous insufficiency ulcers, including integumentary repair and protective techniques, physical agents and modalities, and therapeutic exercise.
11. Describe the therapeutic effects and contraindications for compression therapy in patients with venous insufficiency ulcers.
12. Select appropriate compression therapy for patients with venous insufficiency ulcers.
13. Discuss possible medical and surgical interventions for patients with venous insufficiency ulcers.

Key Terms

Calf muscle pump
Cellulitis
Compression garment
Deep veins
Dermatitis
Fibrin cuff theory
Hemosiderin deposition
Homans' sign
Laplace's law
Ligation
Lipodermatosclerosis

Multilayer compression bandage
Paste bandage
Percutaneous ablation of perforators (PAPS)
Perforating veins
Pruritus
Respiratory pump
Sclerotherapy
SEPS procedure
Short-stretch compression wrap

Superficial veins
Trendelenburg test
Tubular bandage
Varicosity
Vasopneumatic compression device
Vein stripping
Venography
Venous hypertension
Venous stasis ulcer
White blood cell trapping theory

INTRODUCTION

The prevalence of chronic venous insufficiency, also known as postphlebitic syndrome, may be as high as 9.4%.[1] One percent of the adult population has a venous insufficiency ulcer; this increases up to 3.6% for people over 65 years of age.[2] The severity of this problem is further compounded by the fact that the majority of patients with venous ulcerations have had their ulcers for over a year.[3] The cost of treating chronic venous insufficiency ulcers in the United States is estimated to be between $750 million to $1 billion per year.[2,4] Venous insufficiency ulcers are the most common type of leg ulcer,[5] accounting for 70–90% of all ulcers.[6–9] Of the remaining ulcers, an estimated 6–15% are due to combined venous and arterial insufficiency.[8,10,11] Women are three times more likely than men to have a venous insufficiency ulcer.[6,7,12] The risk of ulceration is 7.5 times greater in individuals over the age of 65,[13] and the prevalence of ulceration on admission to long-term care facilities is as high as 2.5%.[14] Fortunately, up to 91% of venous ulcers can be resolved through conservative measures.[15] However, the recurrence rate of venous ulcers ranges from as low as 13% to as high as 81%.[6,16–18] Nonadherence is correlated with ulcer recurrence.[17,19,20] To successfully manage patients with venous ulcers, it is imperative to understand the etiology of venous insufficiency, identify concomitant diseases, such as arterial insufficiency,[21] correct or control contributing factors,[22] and provide appropriate interventions.[6]

This chapter provides a brief anatomical overview of the venous system and a discussion of the etiology of venous insufficiency and venous insufficiency–related tissue damage. Next, the classification and characteristics of venous insufficiency ulcers are outlined along with physical therapy tests and measures commonly used to identify venous insufficiency. This is followed by a detailed presentation of physical therapy management of patients with venous insufficiency ulcers. The chapter concludes with a brief review of medical and surgical interventions that may be required for the management of venous insufficiency ulcers.

VENOUS SYSTEM OVERVIEW

A brief review of the normal anatomy of the venous system will provide a better understanding of the pathophysiology of venous insufficiency ulcers (see Figure 11–1). In contrast to the high-pressure arterial system, the peripheral venous system is a low-pressure system that carries blood high in carbon dioxide and metabolic wastes from the tissue capillaries to the heart. While blood pressure within the arterioles is 25–35 mm Hg, pressure generally drops to around 15 mm Hg as it leaves the capillaries and enters the venous system.[23] Blood pressure decreases to almost 0 mm Hg upon reaching the right atrium via the vena cava.[24]

The anatomy of the venous system is similar to the arterial system. Veins are comprised of the same three layers: an outer tunica externa, a middle tunica media, and an inner intimal layer. Unlike the arterial structure, these layers are thinner, containing smaller amounts of smooth muscle and less connective tissue support.[23] This makes veins more extensible than arteries and able to accommodate greater volumes of blood. At any one time, the venous system stores approximately 65–80% of the total blood volume.[23,25] The intimal layer of veins produces enzymes that help reduce clot formation.

The venous system has three types of veins: deep, superficial, and perforating.[13,26] The **deep veins,** including the femoral, popliteal, and tibial veins, are located within the muscles and roughly parallel the arterial system.[27] The deep veins have a greater pressure than the superficial veins and carry 80–90% of blood back to the heart. The **superficial veins,** including the greater and lesser saphenous veins, carry the remaining blood and are located within the subcutaneous tissues.[13,27] The two major functions of the superficial veins are to drain the skin and subcutaneous tissues and to assist with temperature regulation.[23] By increasing blood flow through the superficial vasculature, the body is able to dissipate heat. The thinner tunica externa and superficial location of superficial veins provide less connective tissue support and make these vessels more vulnerable to trauma. **Perforating veins,** so named because they pierce, or perforate, the fascia, connect the deep and superficial vein systems throughout the lower leg.[28] There are 60–100 perforating veins in each leg.[29] Medium and large veins have bicuspid valves that allow only unidirectional blood flow toward the heart.[23] Because the venous system is a low-pressure system, and venous blood must travel against gravity in upright postures, these valves are especially important in preventing retrograde venous blood flow, thereby preventing in-creased venous pressures (see Figure 11–2). Perforating veins also contain valves that allow unidirectional blood flow from the superficial veins to the deep veins.[28]

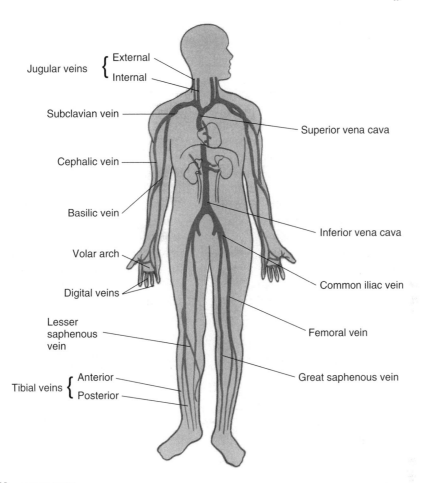

FIGURE 11–1   Venous system.
Source: Medical Terminology, An Anatomy and Physiology Systems Approach, 2/e by Fremgen/Frucht.

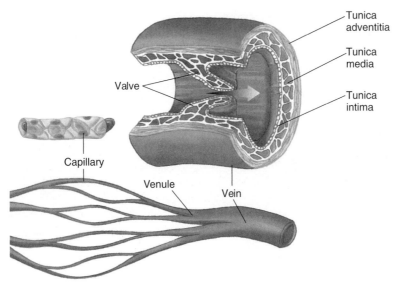

FIGURE 11–2   Close-up of lower extremity veins.
Source: Paramedic Care: Principles & Practice—Trauma Emergencies by Bledsoe/Porter/Cherry.

After blood leaves the capillaries, very little pressure from the ventricle's contraction remains to assist the blood in returning to the heart. During quiet standing, instead of the 10 mm Hg of proximally directed pressure within the venous system,[24] gravity creates up to 90 mm Hg of downward pressure on the column of blood within the veins of the lower extremity (see Figure 11–2).[30,31] Therefore, the proximal flow of venous blood relies on alternative pumps: the respiratory pump and the calf muscle pump (see Figure 11–3). The **respiratory pump** is powered by the pressure changes that occur with breathing.[23] During inspiration, the diaphragm descends, causing a decrease in thoracic pressure and a concomitant increase in abdominal pressure. This creates a pressure gradient pushing blood from the higher pressure abdominal veins to the lower pressure thoracic veins and into the right atrium.[32] The greater the inspiration, the greater the pressure gradient, and the greater the effect on venous blood flow.[23] More pertinent to the etiology of venous insufficiency ulcers is the mechanism behind the **calf muscle pump.**[33] The deep veins are located within the calf musculature and surrounded by fascia. As the calf muscles contract, they become shorter and thicker, compressing the deep veins within them. This dramatically increases the pressure within the deep veins, forcing blood proximally up the leg.[33] The thick fascia surrounding the muscles enhances this pressure increase during calf muscle contraction by acting as a rigid surrounding wall against which the calf muscles push. When the calf muscles relax, venous pressure is decreased. In a healthy state, the valves prevent retrograde blood flow, thereby preventing increased venous backpressure, also known as **venous hypertension.**[6,28]

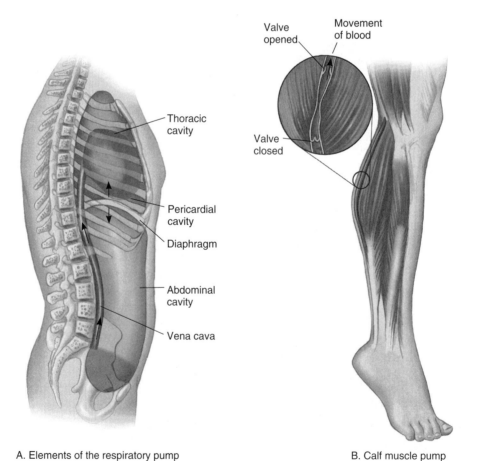

A. Elements of the respiratory pump

B. Calf muscle pump

FIGURE 11–3   *A.* Respiratory and *B.* calf muscle pump.
Source: Paramedic Care: Princilples & Practice—Trauma Emergencies by Bledsoe/Porter/Cherry.

☑ *Checkpoint Question #1*

Based on your present knowledge of venous blood flow, describe two types of therapeutic exercises that can enhance venous return.

ETIOLOGY OF VENOUS INSUFFICIENCY AND VENOUS INSUFFICIENCY–RELATED TISSUE DAMAGE

Venous insufficiency and venous insufficiency–related tissue damage take time to develop (see Figure 11–4).[34] It is generally agreed that sustained venous hypertension is required for the development of venous insufficiency ulcerations.[6,7,28,35] The most common causes of venous hypertension are vein dysfunction,[28] calf muscle pump failure,[6] or a combination of the two.[1,36] While the majority of venous insufficiency appears to be caused by reflux, venous hypertension may also occur due to obstructions to venous outflow, such as stenosis or thrombosis.[37] What is not agreed upon is the mechanism by which venous hypertension causes

tissue damage. There are two main theories as to the etiology of venous insufficiency ulcers: the fibrin cuff theory and the white blood cell trapping theory.[18,32,38]

Venous hypertension leads to vein distention. Increased venous pressure is also transmitted to the capillaries, causing a similar increase in pressure and distention.[17] According to the **fibrin cuff theory,** vessel hypertension and distention cause an increase in vascular permeability.[39] As a result, fluid and proteins are allowed to move from within these vessels into the interstitial tissues, causing peripheral edema.[28] Once within the interstitium, the protein fibrinogen is converted into fibrin.[17] Fibrin adheres to capillary walls, forming a "cuff."[40,41] This cuff is thought to pose a barrier to the exchange of oxygen and nutrients,[38] causing local hypoxia and malnutrition and, ultimately, cell death and ulceration.[13,42] Limited oxygen and nutrition may predispose the individual to ulceration from minor trauma by diminishing the body's capacity to respond to any increase in cellular demand.[43,44] The fibrin cuff theory is supported by studies showing increased vascular permeability to fibrinogen and fibrin cuffs in some patients with venous insufficiency ulcers. However, if the fibrin cuff theory is correct, one would expect to find a decrease in transcutaneous oxygen levels within affected areas. This has not been found.[35] Therefore, although the fibrin cuffs likely play a role in the development of venous insufficiency–related tissue damage, they are not the sole cause of ulceration.

According to the **white blood cell trapping theory,** venous hypertension and distention cause congestion.[39,41,42,45] Decreased blood flow through the veins and capillaries causes margination of white blood cells. As this process progresses, white blood cells adhere to the vessel walls, further impeding circulation. Once adhered, or "trapped," white blood cells become activated, beginning the inflammatory process.[28,35,41] White blood cells then move into the interstitium, releasing proteolytic enzymes, free radicals, and other inflammatory substances, which further contribute to endothelial cell damage.[17,34,35,41] According to this theory, ulceration results from local hypoxia due to venous congestion, white blood cell trapping, and the increased demands placed on

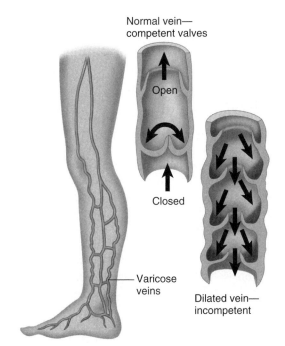

FIGURE 11–4   Venous insufficiency.

Source: Human Diseases: A Systematic Approach, 6/e by Mulvihill/Zelman/Holdaway/Tompary/Raymond.

affected tissues by the ensuing inflammatory response.[40] This is why venous insufficiency ulcers are sometimes called **venous stasis ulcers.** The white blood cell trapping theory is supported by research finding decreased circulating white blood cells after experimentally induced venous hypertension and evidence of white blood cell degranulation.[35] Most likely, venous insufficiency ulcers are a result of a combination of both fibrin cuff formation and white blood cell trapping.[34, 46] Both theories agree that the cause of skin and tissue breakdown is hypoxia secondary to venous hypertension.[40, 47]

RISK FACTORS CONTRIBUTING TO VENOUS ULCERATION

Anything that results in sustained venous hypertension has the potential to cause venous insufficiency–related tissue damage.[35, 39, 42] The subsequent list of risk factors for venous insufficiency ulcers is roughly divided into the following categories: vein dysfunction, calf muscle pump failure, trauma, previous venous insufficiency ulcer, advanced age, and diabetes mellitus.

Vein Dysfunction

Venous insufficiency ulcers are associated with incompetent superficial and perforating veins.[28, 29, 48] However, patients with deep vein insufficiency are more likely to experience a recurrent venous insufficiency ulcer.[19] The bicuspid valves of veins are delicate flaps that close to prevent retrograde flow.[23] Failure of these valves to close completely results in venous hypertension,[23] increasing the risk of venous ulceration.[44, 49] Valves may fail to close snugly for a variety of reasons. First, the valves themselves may degenerate, becoming stiff and unable to close completely. Second, the valves may become damaged or scarred because of endothelial cell trauma or the resulting inflammatory process, thereby impairing normal function.[40] Valvular damage may also be the sequelae of a thrombosis, or blood clot,[40, 50] as many patients with venous insufficiency ulcers have a history of deep vein thrombosis.[7, 51, 52] Third, the valves may close completely but fail to prevent retrograde flow due to venous distention.[13, 50] Distended veins have an increased vessel diameter, allowing some blood to flow backward through the closed, but not overlapping, valve leaflets[40, 46]

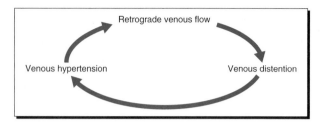

FIGURE 11–5   Cycle of venous hypertension.

Retrograde flow, in turn, exacerbates venous distention, and a vicious cycle of venous hypertension begins (see Figure 11–5).[40]

Primary venous distention may be caused by an inherent weakness within the vein itself, or **varicosity.**[40, 53] Varicosities, or varicose veins, are dilated veins characterized by an increase in length and tortuosity.[31, 34] Varicose veins may be present for years prior to ulceration.[34] Peripheral edema produced by congestive heart failure, pregnancy, obesity,[28] and constrictive clothing may result in secondary venous distention by decreasing venous return.[26, 53]

Valve dysfunction also adversely affects the calf muscle pump.[50] Incompetent deep vein valves decrease the pump's effectiveness by allowing retrograde flow while incompetent perforating valves transmit the pressures generated by the pump to the superficial vasculature.[34, 49] Because the superficial vessels lack the connective tissue support typical of deep veins, this increased pressure can lead to varicosities, venous hypertension, endothelial trauma, and, ultimately, skin breakdown.[34, 40]

Calf Muscle Pump Failure

The calf muscle pump is vital to normal venous blood flow.[54] Without the pressure gradient caused by calf muscle contraction, there is an increased risk of venous hypertension.[6] Therefore, anything that alters the effectiveness of this pump increases the risk of developing venous insufficiency ulcers.[47] Calf muscle weakness or paralysis precludes the compression of deep veins that propels blood up the leg, as does arthritis or decreased mobility.[28, 34, 39] Individuals with occupations requiring prolonged standing, such as teachers and bank tellers, are at increased risk of developing a venous insufficiency ulcer because prolonged static standing essentially eliminates the pumping effect of the calf musculature.[34] Incompetent valves also decrease calf muscle pump effectiveness.

Trauma

Venous insufficiency results in pooling of fluid within the leg along with local hypoxia and malnutrition.[9] Even relatively benign trauma to an area of venous insufficiency, such as brushing against a thorn bush or scratching an itchy and dry leg, may be just enough of an overload on an already taxed system to result in ulceration.[43] Clinically, chronic venous insufficiency ulcers are thought to be initiated by minor trauma to an edematous leg.[9,15,43] The presence of edema increases the diffusion distance for oxygen and nutrients.[55] Once a break in skin integrity occurs, the likelihood of delayed wound healing is increased in the presence of venous insufficiency because oxygen is critical to each phase of wound healing.

Previous Venous Insufficiency Ulcer

Individuals with prior venous insufficiency ulcers are at increased risk of reulceration.[53] Venous ulcer recurrence rates are as high as 81%.[16,39] Repeat ulcerations commonly occur in the same location as previous ulcers. There are three plausible reasons for this. First, repeat ulceration may be due to the same cause as the first ulcer: local hypoxia and malnutrition. The location of the ulcer is likely the least oxygenated and least nourished region of the leg and, therefore, is at the greatest risk of ulceration and reulceration. Second, the scar tissue resulting from previous ulceration has less tensile strength and elasticity than the original, healthy tissues,[56] thereby increasing the risk of skin breakdown. Third, and perhaps most important, venous insufficiency ulcers will recur if the precipitating factors are not addressed. If interventions are directed solely toward the venous ulcer without regard for wound etiology, recurrence is to be expected.

Advanced Age

The risk of venous insufficiency ulceration increases with age.[3,7,12,51] Recall from Chapter 3 that advanced age causes a variety of anatomical and functional changes that adversely affect wound healing, including decreased inflammatory response, slowed immune response, decreased collagen synthesis and tensile strength, epidermal and dermal atrophy, and an increased number of comorbidities.[57–59] Specific to the development of venous insufficiency ulcers, the aging process may cause valve degeneration.[53] This degeneration may explain the sevenfold increase in venous insufficiency in individuals over the age of 65.[13]

Diabetes

Patients with diabetes have an increased risk of microvascular disease and an impaired immune response.[5,60] Diabetes impairs all three phases of wound healing in all types of open wounds. The poorer the control over blood sugar levels, the more sustained the hyperglycemia and the greater the adverse effect on wound healing.[61] See Chapter 13 for more details about the adverse effects of diabetes on wound healing.

PHYSICAL THERAPY TESTS AND MEASURES FOR VENOUS INSUFFICIENCY

Clinicians may perform various tests and measures to assess for venous insufficiency, make a prognosis for wound healing, and identify changes in patient status. In addition to the routine tests and measures clinicians should perform on all patients with open wounds (see Chapter 4), there are several tests that are specific to the diagnosis of venous insufficiency. This section details five of the more common clinical tests and measures used to assess individuals with venous insufficiency: clinical assessment for deep vein thrombosis, ankle-brachial index (ABI), Trendelenburg's test, Doppler ultrasound, and venous filling time.

Clinical Assessment for Deep Vein Thrombosis

A life-threatening complication of a deep vein thrombosis (DVT) is a pulmonary embolism. While less than 20% of distal (below the knee) DVTs will embolize if left untreated, roughly 50% of proximal DVTs will result in a pulmonary embolism.[62] Therefore, it is

CASE STUDY: Mrs. Jessica Gibbons

This case study is referenced throughout the chapter.

PART 1

History

Jessica Gibbons is a 68-year-old white female seen this morning in outpatient physical therapy for wound management. Her primary language is English. She lives with her daughter in a one-level home. Mrs. Gibbons works 32 hours per week as a secretary primarily answering phones.

Wound History: Mrs. Gibbons reports her wound began 3 months ago, although she does not recall any specific injury. She notes that she heals slowly, for example, she cut her leg on a rose bush and it took about a month to heal. She has been washing her wound daily during her shower then covering it with an adhesive telfa dressing. She changes the dressing two to three times per day due to the amount of wound drainage. She reports her right lower leg is itchy.

Past Medical History: Mrs. Gibbons has a history of basal cell carcinomas removed from her right ear and right forearm 4 years ago, right distal tibia fracture with open reduction and internal fixation 2 years ago, right lower extremity blood clot found 2 days after tibial surgery, asthma, and depression.

General Health Status: Mrs. Gibbons believes she is in good health. She reports she walks more slowly since her fracture and that her right leg swells as the day progresses, making her shoe feel too tight by the end of the day. She reports she has not been able to walk her dog to the park since her ankle fracture due to right ankle pain and fatigue.

Current Medications: Albuterol as needed, amitriptyline.

Systems Review

Cardiovascular/Pulmonary System: Heart rate: 76 bpm, blood pressure 138/85 mm Hg, respiratory rate 12 bpm, minimal right lower extremity edema noted.

Musculoskeletal System: Gross assessment of range of motion and strength reveals deficits in right/left ankle dorsiflexion, gastrocnemius length, and plantar flexor strength. Height: 5 feet 2 inches (1.57 m). Body weight: 195 pounds (88.6 kg). Body mass index (BMI) = 36 kg/m^2.

Neuromuscular System: No gross deficits noted in gross coordinated movement or motor control.

Gastrointestinal System: No problems noted.

Urogenital System: No problems noted.

Integumentary System: Open wound right distal lateral calf, skin is anhydrous with minimal hemosiderin deposition, superficial varicosities B, mild erythema and excoriation noted near wound, toenails adequately trimmed and have normal color and structure.

Communication, Cognition, Language, and Learning Style: No deficits noted. Mrs. Gibbons reports she learns best by reviewing written information. She demonstrates an understanding of her situation and a willingness to participate in wound management interventions.

imperative that clinicians are able to identify this potentially devastating condition. The gold standard for identifying a DVT is a venogram.[63, 64] However, this test is expensive, invasive, and uses a dye that is a potential allergen to patients and may actually cause a DVT up to 5% of the time.[65] Ultrasonagraphy is a noninvasive exam that is noted to be 95% sensitive and 95% specific for identifying a DVT.[62] However, it still requires expensive equipment and training to interpret the results, making it inappropriate for a clinical screening exam.

The **Homans' sign** was intended to identify the presence of a DVT. To perform the test, the patient's ankle is passively dorsiflexed with the knee extended. Discomfort with this test movement or with deep palpation of the gastrocnemius muscle belly are positive test results.[66] Because the Homans' sign is quick and noninvasive, it has historically been used as a routine screening test for deep vein thrombosis. However, patients with many alternative diagnoses, such as a gastrocnemius strain, would most likely have a positive Homans' sign. Because the Homans' sign has a sensitivity as low as 33% and a specificity as low as 21%,[67] it is an inaccurate, unreliable, and insufficient screening tool.

Alternatively, a clinical prediction guideline has been used that incorporates risk factors for the development of a DVT as well as alternative diagnoses that may produce a false-positive diagnosis of a DVT (see Table 11–1).[65] According to this guideline (sometimes referred to as the Wells and Colleagues prediction guidelines based on the work of Anand, Wells, and Riddle), patients scoring ≥3 should be considered to have a high probability of DVT and further medical assessment, such as a diagnostic ultrasound, should be requested.

Ankle-Brachial Index (ABI)

Coexisting arterial and venous insufficiency occurs in 15–25% of all lower extremity ulcers.[7, 46] Until proven otherwise, arterial insufficiency should be suspected in all chronic lower extremity ulcerations.[6] It is critical to identify or rule out concomitant arterial insufficiency not only because of the frequency with which this occurs, but also because the presence of arterial insufficiency precludes, or at best modifies, the most effective treatment for venous insufficiency ulcers: compression.[21, 68] Therefore, clinicians should perform an ABI on all patients with suspected arterial or venous insufficiency.[11,18,69–73] It is theorized that performing an ABI may dislodge a DVT. Therefore, patients with a high probability of having a

DVT should *not* be tested until cleared.[68] While an ABI should never be the sole source of consideration for treatment decisions,[38] patients with venous insufficiency ulcers and an ABI less than 0.7 should not be managed with compression due to coexisting arterial insufficiency.[74] Low compression levels, 25–30 mm Hg, have been used successfully on patients with combined arterial and venous insufficiency ulcers and ABIs as low as 0.50,[33, 75] but this should not be undertaken without careful consideration, ongoing consultation with the physician of record, and close monitoring of patient status. To rule out potentially critical changes in patient circulatory status, clinicians should repeat ABI testing if a wound that was initially improving with compression is no longer progressing or worsens.[18,69,71,76] Over a 3-month period of time, 9% of patients with CVI had a decline in their ABIs from normal to less than 0.8.[33] After a year, 29% of these patients had ABIs less than 0.8.[33] Therefore, ABI measurements should be repeated regularly, perhaps every 3 months, to ensure the appropriateness of ongoing interventions. Refer to Chapter 10 for detailed information on how to perform and interpret an ABI.

Trendelenburg Test

The **Trendelenburg test** is used to identify vein incompetence.[28, 49] To perform the test, position the patient supine with the leg to be tested elevated approximately 45 degrees for about 1 minute. Note

TABLE 11–1   Clinical Assessment Guideline for Deep Vein Thrombosis

Clinical Parameter	Score
• Active cancer (or within the previous 6 months)	1
• Paralysis, paresis, or recent cast immobilization of the lower extremities	1
• Recently bedridden for >3 days or major surgery within 1 month	1
• Localized tenderness along the distribution of the deep venous system	1
• Entire leg swelling	1
• Calf swelling by >3 cm (measured 10 cm below tibial tuberosity)	1
• Pitting edema (greater in symptomatic leg)	1
• Collateral superficial veins (nonvaricose)	1
• Alternative diagnosis as likely or more likely than that of DVT	−2

Scoring: Hold treatment and consult with physician if score is 3 or higher.

Adapted from Anand SS, Wells PS, Hunt D, et al. Does this patient have a deep vein thrombosis? *JAMA.* 1998;279(14):1094–1099; Wells PS, Anderson DR, Bormanis J, et al. Value assessment of pretest probability of deep-vein thrombosis in clinical management. *Lancet.* 1997;350:1795–1798.

TABLE 11–2   Interpretation of the Trendelenburg Test

Tourniquet	Time to Venous Distention (sec)	Suggested Pathology
On	<20 sec	Deep or perforator vein incompetence
Removed	<10 sec	Superficial vein incompetence

the amount of superficial venous distention present. Secure a tourniquet, such as those used for drawing blood, around the distal thigh. Have the patient stand upright for up to one minute and watch for superficial venous distention. Record the time when superficial venous distention occurs. Venous distention occurring in less than 20 seconds indicates deep or perforator vein incompetence.[77] Next, release the tourniquet and repeat the same procedure. Venous distention occurring shortly after the tourniquet is released is an indicator of superficial vein incompetence (see Table 11–2).[11] With the increased availability and accuracy of ultrasonography, the reliance on this test has decreased.[28]

Doppler Ultrasound

Doppler ultrasonography is the gold standard for evaluating the venous system.[1, 7, 47] A Doppler ultrasound examination of the venous system is more subjective than the Doppler examination of the arterial system. When performing an arterial Doppler examination, the clinician must identify the presence or absence of sound. When performing a venous Doppler examination, the clinician must also interpret changes in the sound's intensity. The examination consists of three parts: a resting test, an augmentation test, and a reflux test.[26] With the patient supine, place coupling gel over the large vein to be tested and position the probe at a 45-degree angle.[78] Normally, veins should have spontaneous sounds. If these are not present, it may indicate an obstruction in venous flow. For the augmentation test, apply pressure in the form of a quick squeeze distal to the probe placement. In healthy veins, this should enhance the Doppler signal. If this does not occur, it may indicate a partial venous obstruction. To perform the reflux test, apply a similar pressure proximal to the probe placement. In healthy veins, this compression should make the signal disappear. When the compression is released, the resting signal returns. If compression proximal to the probe enhances the signal, it may indicate valve incompetence (see Table 11–3).[79]

Venous Filling Time

This test is performed in the same manner when testing for either arterial or venous insufficiency. First, position the patient supine and observe the superficial veins on the patient's dorsal foot. Then, elevate the limb approximately 60 degrees for about a minute or until the veins have been drained by gravity. Next, place the limb in the dependent position and record the time it takes for the superficial veins to refill.[11, 80, 81] Normal venous filling time is 5–15 seconds. Immediate venous filling is predictive of venous insufficiency. Recall from Chapter 10 (see Table 10–4) that venous filling times greater than 20 seconds generally indicate severe arterial insufficiency.[81] Refer to

TABLE 11–3   Interpretation of Venous Doppler Examination

Test	Location of Pressure	Signal	Suggested Pathology
Resting	None	• Spontaneous • No spontaneous signal	• None • Venous obstruction
Augmentation	Distal to probe	• Enhanced • Not enhanced	• None • Partial venous obstruction
Reflux	Proximal to probe	• Decreased/abolished • Enhanced	• None • Valve incompetence

TABLE 11–4   Clinical Guideline for Physical Therapy Tests and Measures for Venous Insufficiency

Test	Indications
Clinical assessment for vein thrombosis	• Lower leg ulcer • Lower leg edema • Suspected venous insufficiency
Ankle-brachial index	• Decreased or absent pulses • Signs and symptoms of arterial or venous insufficiency • History of peripheral vascular disease
Trendelenburg test	• To differentiate deep or perforating vein incompetence from superficial vein incompetence
Doppler ultrasound	• To differentiate normal venous flow from vein incompetence or obstruction
Venous filling time	• Unable to tolerate ABI • ABI > 1.1 • History of diabetes or vessel calcification • Suspect concomitant arterial insufficiency

Table 11–4 for a summary of clinical tests and measures used to assess individuals with venous insufficiency.

CLASSIFICATION AND CHARACTERISTICS OF VENOUS ULCERS

Classification

The practice patterns for the integumentary system in the *Guide to Physical Therapist Practice* provide physical therapists with valuable patient management information for general wound care. These practice patterns describe components of the examination, evaluation, diagnosis, prognosis, and interventions for patients who have an increased risk for integumentary disorders or who have impaired skin integrity. Patients with venous insufficiency ulcers can readily be placed into the appropriate classification system based on the depth of tissue involved. Although usually superficial, venous insufficiency ulcers may be full thickness or extend into fascia, muscle, or bone.[82]

The Clinical–Etiology–Anatomy–Pathphysiology (CEAP) classification system for chronic venous disease is commonly used by physicians and surgeons to describe venous disease (Table 11–5).

Characteristics

To facilitate identification of ulcer similarities and differences, typical characteristics of venous ulcers are described using the "5PT" method: pain, position, presentation, periwound, pulses, and temperature (Table 11–6). Color image 16 is an example of a patient with a venous insufficiency ulcer, while color

TABLE 11–5   Clinical–Etiology–Anatomy–Physiology Classification System for Chronic Venous Insufficiency

Classification	Description
C0	Asymptomatic
C1	Telangiactasias or spider veins <3 mm
C2	Varicose veins >/= 3 mm
C3	Leg edema
C4	Skin and subcutaneous tissue changes • C4A: Hemosideran deposition • C4B: Lipodermatosclerosis
C5	Healed venous ulcer
C6	Current venous ulcer

TABLE 11–6   Comparison of Typical Characteristics of Venous and Arterial Insufficiency Ulcers

Characteristic	Venous Insufficiency Ulcers	Arterial Insufficiency Ulcers
Pain	• Mild to moderate*	• Severe*
	• Decreased with elevation or compression	• Increased with elevation
Position	• Medial malleolus	• Distal toes
	• Medial lower leg	• Dorsal foot
	• Areas of trauma	• Areas of trauma
Wound presentation	• Irregular shape	• Regular appearance
	• Red or ruddy wound bed	• May conform to precipitating trauma
	• Fibrous yellow or glossy coating over wound bed	• Pale granulation tissue if present
	• Copious drainage	• Black eschar
		• Gangrene
		• Little or no drainage
Periwound and structural changes	• Edema	• Thin, shiny, anhydrous skin
	• Cellulitis, dermatitis	• Loss of hair growth
	• Hemosiderin deposition	• Thickened, yellow nails
	• Lipodermatosclerosis	• Pale, dusky, or cyanotic
Pulses	• Normal or decreased due to edema or coexisting arterial disease	• Decreased or absent pedal pulses
Temperature	• Normal to mild warmth	• Decreased

*Pain may be masked in individuals with sensory neuropathy.

image 3 provides an example of a patient with an arterial insufficiency ulcer.

Pain

Individuals with venous insufficiency and venous insufficiency ulcers commonly complain of dull, aching leg pain or "heaviness."[83] The cause of this pain is venous hypertension and the resulting peripheral edema. The pain is usually increased with dependency and relieved by elevation or compression.[83] Patients typically report a decrease in pain at night, due to the gravity-lessened position in bed, and first thing in the morning, due to edema reduction overnight. Many patients report increasing leg heaviness and aching as the day progresses and that their shoes feel tight by the end of the day. This results from prolonged dependent positioning, such as sitting or standing. Pain may be severe in the presence of infection or concomitant arterial insufficiency.[13] Clinicians should be aware that

patients with diabetic neuropathy are unlikely to complain of pain associated with their wounds.[84]

Position

Venous insufficiency ulcers are most usually located on the medial aspect of the lower leg or medial malleolus,[1, 85] although it is not uncommon to find venous ulcers in areas exposed to trauma, such as the anterior shin.[82] Venous ulcerations do not occur on the plantar aspect of the foot and rarely occur above the knee.[34]

Wound Presentation

Venous insufficiency ulcers are generally superficial, irregular in shape, and have moderate to high amounts of drainage.[7, 34, 86] If the dressing does not absorb enough wound drainage, the wound edges will be white and fragile because of maceration.[87] The wound bed contains beefy red granulation tissue but may take on a ruddy appearance.[82] A thin, yellow fibrous coating may cover the wound bed, giving it a glossy look.[47] Undermining is not uncommon.[13] Although there may be evidence of epithelialization at the wound margins, this often fails to progress without skilled interventions because edema stops or delays epithelialization by making the wound bed three-dimensional, rather than a flat surface for keratinocytes to move across.[15]

Periwound and Structural Changes

Venous insufficiency is often associated with **dermatitis**[6, 83] and dry, scaling skin,[18] which may cause **pruritus.**[7] **Cellulitis** is not uncommon.[34] Superficial varicosities[6] and evidence of previous ulceration may be present.[49, 88] Lower extremity edema is to be expected[18, 86] and may be pitting, especially at the end of the day, after prolonged dependent positioning,[7] or with severe venous insufficiency.[77] In cases of long-standing venous insufficiency, the edema may become firm or indurated.[85] Initially, skin changes may include a subtle erythema.[40] With chronic venous insufficiency, the skin becomes stained and more darkly pigmented due to stimulated melanin and **hemosiderin deposition.**[83] Hemosiderin is a by-product of the breakdown of red blood cells forced into the interstitium by venous hypertension.[13, 34] The term **lipodermatosclerosis** is used to describe the hyperpigmentation and accompanying erythema, induration, and plaque-like structural changes that occur due to long-standing venous insufficiency.[6, 18, 47, 53, 83, 85] The skin and subcutaneous tissues are more fibrotic and less elastic than healthy tissue. It is important to note this condition because it is associated with lower wound healing rates.[89]

Pulses

Pedal pulses are generally present and normal in patients with venous ulcers. Although the etiology of venous insufficiency ulcers does not directly affect the arterial blood flow, patients with venous ulcers may have decreased pulses for two reasons. First, peripheral edema resulting from venous insufficiency may make pedal pulses difficult to palpate.[82] Second, it is not unusual to have concomitant arterial disease, which may decrease pedal pulses. An ABI should be performed to assess for arterial insufficiency.[7, 83]

Temperature

It is not uncommon for cellulitis or edema from venous hypertension to cause a mild increase in skin temperature of the affected extremity.[90] Local warmth may also be the result of ulcer infection.

Prognosis for Venous Insufficiency Ulcer Healing

As with all chronic wounds, there is great variability in venous insufficiency wound healing rates,[91] which makes prediction of time to healing difficult at best. Because many factors can contribute to delayed wound healing, the clinician must always consider local and systemic factors as well as wound characteristics when determining a patient's prognosis for wound healing. After reviewing the available evidence on wound healing in patients with venous insufficiency ulcers, it is possible to make scientifically grounded judgments on wound healing prognosis. Table 11–7 includes several factors that may be used to assist with making a wound healing prognosis for this patient population. Venous ulcers of smaller size,[41, 92] that is, less than 10 cm,[2, 93] have a better wound healing prognosis than larger ulcers.[93–98] Venous ulcers existing for a shorter duration prior to the start of interventions have a better chance of expedient wound healing,[93, 94, 98] with wounds present for less than 3 months healing better than those present for a year, and those present for a year healing better than those present for 3 years.[97] Most importantly, venous ulcers treated with compression are more likely to heal and heal faster than those that are not treated with compression.[92, 99] There is some evidence to support that patients will heal faster using a combination of compression and pentoxifylene.[99] However, some studies have shown that even with appropriate interventions about 6% of ulcers will not heal.[41] These refractory ulcers are more likely to be recurrent ulcers or of mixed etiology, combined arterial and venous insufficiency.[41]

Venous insufficiency ulcers that have an initial decrease in wound area after the first 2–4 weeks of interventions have a better prognosis than those that do not decrease in size and those that initially increase in size.[91, 92, 96, 99–103] The average time to healing for full-thickness venous insufficiency ulcers is 8 weeks of appropriate interventions,[96, 97, 104, 105] with smaller ulcers healing in 5–7 weeks[96, 97] and larger ulcers healing in 10–16 weeks.[95, 106, 107] A 20–40% decrease in venous insufficiency ulcer surface area within 2 to 3 weeks of initiating treatment is a good indicator that the wound is responding to wound management interventions.[96, 97, 101] If this reduction is not seen, clinicians

TABLE 11–7   Predicting Chronic Venous Insufficiency Ulcer Healing

Predictors of CVI Ulcer Healing	Predictors of Poor CVI Ulcer Healing	Not Predictors of CVI Ulcer Healing
Smaller ulcer size	Larger ulcer size	Gender
Ulcer present for shorter duration	Ulcer present for longer than 3 months prior to interventions	Race
A decrease in ulcer size during the first 2–3 weeks of interventions	An increase in wound size over 4 weeks of interventions	Skin condition
No deep vein involvement	Concomitant arterial insufficiency	Presence of infection
Adherence with prescribed compression therapy	Older age	
	High body mass index	

should reassess the patient and modify the plan of care or make appropriate referrals. Thirty to 60 percent of patients treated with compression will heal within 3 months.[99]

Adherence with prescribed compression therapy is significantly related to wound healing.[97] While deep vein involvement[98] or concomitant arterial insufficiency[94, 95] are predictors of poor venous insufficiency ulcer healing potential, gender, race, skin condition, and the presence of infection at initial presentation do not appear to be predictive of venous insufficiency ulcer healing.[97] The effect of body mass index and age on venous insufficiency ulcer healing potential is less clear cut,[95, 97] however, it appears that patients with high body mass indices and patients who are elderly have a poorer prognosis.[94, 98]

CASE STUDY: Mrs. Jessica Gibbons

PART 2

Tests and Measures

Integumentary Integrity: Position: R medial distal calf wound 3 cm superior to the medial malleolus. Presentation: full-thickness wound: 6.0 cm length × 4.7 cm width (wound surface area 28.2 cm²), 0.3 cm depth. Wound bed contains 25% slough-covered, fibrous coating over remaining wound bed. Wound drainage: moderate, thin, serosanguineous. No wound odor is present. Periwound: minimal periwound maceration, superficial varicosities B, minimal hemosiderin deposition right lower leg, mild erythema and excoriation noted near wound. Circumferential measurements (cm): smallest ankle L 20.5/R 22.5, 10 cm inferior to tibial tuberosity L 31.2/R 33.3, 15 cm proximal to knee joint line L 41.4/R 41.6. Temperature: left lower leg is slightly warmer than right to palpation.

Sensory Integrity: Patient is able to identify 4.17 monofilament B feet.

Circulation: Pulses: dorsalis pedis and tibialis posterior L + 1/R + 2. Capillary refill: 2 seconds B. Ankle-brachial index (ABI): LUE 138 mm Hg/RUE 138 mm Hg, LLE 124 mm Hg/RLE 117 mm Hg. ABI: LLE 0.90/RLE 0.85. Clinical assessment for a deep vein thrombosis: 2 points: 1 point for calf swelling >3 cm, 1 point for collateral superficial veins. Trendelenburg test: venous distention occurs within 15 seconds of standing.

Gait, Locomotion, Balance: Mrs. Gibbons is independent on level surfaces. She demonstrates an early right heel off and decreased stance time on the right. She reports 3/10 right ankle pain with ambulation.

CASE STUDY   Continued

Muscle Performance: Right tibialis anterior 4/5, she is unable to perform a unilateral heel raise on her right lower extremity even with assistance for balance. She accepts moderate manual resistance to right ankle plantaflexion.

Pain: Patient reports 2/10 right ankle pain with transfers. Mrs. Gibbons reports her left leg is achy at the end of the day. She reports 6/10 pain with dressing changes or if her wound is touched.

Range of Motion: Ankle dorsiflexion L + 8°/R0°, gastrocnemius length L + 5°/R lacks 5° from neutral.

Evaluation and Diagnosis

Mrs. Gibbons has a full-thickness ulcer consistent with Integumentary Preferred Practice Pattern D: Impaired Integumentary Integrity Associated with Full-Thickness Skin involvement and scar formation. Mrs. Gibbons has three key risk factors for venous insufficiency, including a history of a deep vein thrombosis, advanced age, and calf muscle pump failure due to limited dorsiflexion range of motion and plantar flexor weakness. Her integumentary presentation is consistent with chronic venous insufficiency with minimal inflammation, possibly due to pruritis. Her decreased right pedal pulse is likely due to the presence of edema rather than significant arterial insufficiency. Her ABI values are consistent with minimal arterial insufficiency in her right lower extremity. Following the clinical prediction guideline, it is unlikely that Mrs. Gibbons has a deep vein thrombosis. The results of the Trendelenburg test are suggestive of deep or perforating vein incompetence, which is consistent with her history of a deep vein thrombosis. Her BMI places Mrs. Gibbons in class 2 obesity. She is limited in her leisure activities.

Prognosis and Plan of Care

The following factors are associated with delayed wound healing and a worse prognosis: large full-thickness chronic venous insufficiency ulcer size (>10 cm^2), mild arterial insufficiency, deep vein involvement, and advanced age. Mrs. Gibbons's obesity, sedentary job, and ankle pain with mobility will also detract from her wound healing prognosis. However, because the wound has been present for less than 1 year, her calf muscle pump function may be improved with therapeutic interventions, and she is motivated to adhere to the use of compression therapy, her overall prognosis is good. Because she rarely requires her inhaler, Mrs. Gibbons's asthma is not thought to be a factor in her wound healing prognosis.

The following functional goals have been discussed and mutually agreed upon:

1. Mrs. Gibbons will be able to walk her dog to the park and return after a 10-minute seated rest in 10–13 weeks.
2. Mrs. Gibbons's integumentary integrity will be fully restored in 10–13 weeks.
3. Mrs. Gibbons will be independent with managing her chronic venous insufficiency and decrease the risk of recurrence with the use of a 20–30 mm Hg knee-high compression garment.

The following wound-related component goals have been discussed and mutually agreed upon:

1. Periwound maceration, erythema, and escoriation will be resolved within 2 weeks.
2. The wound will be ≥95% granular in 2–3 weeks.
3. Wound surface area will be decreased by at least 20% (to ≤22.6 cm^2) over the next 2–3 weeks.
4. Wound drainage will be controlled so that Mrs. Gibbons will not need to change the dressing during her work day in two visits.
5. Mrs. Gibbons will verbalize an understanding of skin care protection techniques and methods to enhance wound healing in 2 weeks.
6. Right ankle dorsiflexion +5° and right gastrocnemius length +5° in 2 weeks to assist with calf muscle pump function.

Mrs. Gibbons will be seen two times per week for 10–13 weeks. Physical therapy interventions will include coordination, communication, and documentation; patient/client-related instruction; integumentary repair and protective techniques; electrotherapeutic modalities, physical agents, and mechanical modalities; therapeutic exercises; manual therapy techniques; and functional training.

PHYSICAL THERAPY INTERVENTIONS

Coordination, Communication, and Documentation

Interdisciplinary teams can be advantageous when working with patients with venous insufficiency ulcers[69] because they ensure a more holistic approach to patient care. To maximize effectiveness, physical therapy services must be coordinated with the patient, caregivers, and other disciplines. In addition to the physician, team members may include a plastic or general surgeon, a vascular surgeon, and a nurse specializing in wound care. At times the help of other specialists such as a registered dietitian or infectious disease specialist may be beneficial.

A surgeon's role within the wound care team may include performing more invasive and diagnostic testing to better direct patient care for individuals with problem-prone or chronic wounds. In addition, the skills of a surgeon are invaluable when patients require extensive debridement, skin grafting, or vascular procedures. A nurse or nurse practitioner specializing in wound care can assist with patient and caregiver education, dressing changes, debridement where allowed by law, and the monitoring of wound progress in patients who do not require ongoing physical therapy. A registered dietitian can assist patients and caregivers with controlling comorbidities that adversely affect wound healing, such as diabetes and obesity. An infectious disease specialist may be helpful in directing medical interventions to resolve infections in patients with venous insufficiency ulcers.

Patient/Client-Related Instruction

Venous insufficiency ulcers are the most common type of leg ulcer, and the vast majority of these ulcers can be successfully managed through conservative measures.[15] However, venous ulcers have a recurrence rate as high as 81%,[16] and recurrence is associated with nonadherence with compression therapy and wound management interventions. Patients with venous insufficiency ulcers involved in an education program were more active, followed positioning recommendations more closely, and had significantly fewer ulcer recurrences than those who did not receive this information.[108] Clinicians should take several steps to improve patient/caregiver adherence both to enhance wound healing and to decrease the risk of ulcer recurrence.[11, 109] First, clinicians must educate patients and caregivers about the etiology of venous insufficiency and venous insufficiency–related tissue damage. It is important to use terminology that is at a level appropriate for each individual and to question the patients' understanding of the information provided. Second, clinicians must provide the link between the disease process and interventions used for wound healing and maintaining integumentary integrity. Third, clinicians must educate patients and caregivers about the risk factors for reulceration and methods to control these.[69, 71] Last, clinicians should identify patients' beliefs and attitudes toward treatment and work collaboratively to maximize both adherence and outcomes.[110] Patients are more likely to adhere to suggested regimens if they are knowledgeable about their condition, actively participate in treatment, have a good relationship with the health care workers involved in their care, and possess a positive attitude toward their rehabilitation.[111] There appears to be a relation between lack of patient adherence, social isolation, and poor venous ulcer healing.[112] In addition to providing patient education, incorporating caregiver and significant others or a support group into intervention plans may enhance overall outcomes.

To better appreciate a patient's perspective on following suggested interventions, consider the following patient example. Mrs. B presents to physical therapy with a recurrent venous insufficiency ulcer 5 months after her previous ulcer had closed. Her previous ulcer was in the same location and resolved with physical therapy and a compression dressing. After the first ulcer healed, Mrs. B was fitted for a compression garment and discharged from physical therapy. She discontinued wearing the garment 4 months after discharge from therapy, stating: "The wound was healed. Besides, that sock was too hot to wear when I went to Florida for the winter and didn't go well with my clothes." At the time of her previous discharge from physical therapy, Mrs. B should have been informed that, although her wound was closed, the cause of her wound, venous insufficiency, remained. She should have been educated on the rationale for wearing the garment, as well as the risks of discontinuing compression. Another means of increasing Mrs. B's adherence would have been for the clinician to involve Mrs. B in the garment selection process. Had this occurred, a lighter weight garment and a color or style that was more amenable to the patient might have been selected.

Clinicians must also provide patients with basic guidelines for caring for their ulcers (see Box 11–1). They must instruct patients or caregivers in effective wound care and bandaging techniques if home dressing changes are required. This is especially important if compression dressings are used, as improper application will not only limit the effectiveness of treatment, but may also cause further tissue damage. Clinicians should inform patients of methods to care for skin affected by

venous insufficiency.[86] They must educate patients in proper positioning and exercise to enhance venous return,[4, 54, 71, 86] and they must advise patients of ways to protect at-risk extremities.[69]

Procedural Interventions

Precautions

Clinicians should be aware of three precautions when working with patients with venous insufficiency ulcers: concomitant arterial disease, sensitization and allergic reactions, and the inappropriate use of whirlpool treatments (see Box 11–2). Clinicians should not assume patients presenting with the signs and symptoms of venous insufficiency do not have coexisting arterial disease. Clinicians must always assess patients for concomitant arterial insufficiency.[69] In one study, over half of the patients presenting with the typical signs and symptoms of venous insufficiency had ABIs less than 0.9, indicating at least mild arterial insufficiency.[72] Because the standard of care for venous insufficiency ulcers is compression,[86, 113] failure to identify concomitant arterial insufficiency can have tragic results. Applying compression to an arterial insufficient limb will further compromise circulation and may cause limb-threatening ischemia.[114] Compression should not be used to treat patients with an ABI less than 0.7.

Sensitization and allergic reactions can also be a major problem in patients with venous insufficiency.[69, 71, 115] Local allergic reactions to preservatives, emulsifiers, and/or dressing components are common.[116] Over half of the patients with venous insufficiency ulcers have been found to be allergic to lanolin and some topical antimicrobials.[40] These reactions cause erythema and pruritus,[89] increasing patient discomfort and perpetuating the inflammatory process. Topical agents should be chosen with specific goals in mind and used with caution.[69] Because natural cotton fibers tend to be less offensive than synthetics, clinicians should consider using

---

BOX 11–1   Guidelines for Patients with Venous Insufficiency Ulcers

Control swelling

- Follow your clinician's guidelines for using compression.
- Elevate your legs above your heart when resting and sleeping.
- Exercise your legs. Keep your legs moving by walking, pumping your ankles, or shifting your weight from foot to foot.
- Avoid constrictive clothing.

Protect your feet and legs

- Wear bandages as instructed.
- Do not scratch or rub your leg even if it itches. Instead, apply moisturizing lotion or medicated cream as directed by your clinician.
- Always wear shoes that are properly fitted, comfortable, and easy to get on and off.
- Wear clean socks with smooth seams or without seams.
- Inspect your feet and legs daily for signs of trauma or irritation.

Live healthy

- Follow your physician's instructions regarding medication.
- Control medical conditions.
- Eat a balanced diet.
- Exercise regularly.
- If you smoke, quit.

Call your clinician if:

- You notice your wound is getting larger, draining more, or has a foul odor.
- You have increased pain or swelling.
- You detect a new wound.

BOX 11–2   Precautions for Patients with Venous Insufficiency

- Concomitant arterial disease
- Allergic reactions and sensitization
- Inappropriate whirlpool use

garments and contact layers of compressive wraps with a higher cotton content to decrease the risk of an allergic reaction.[117]

Whirlpool treatments are likely to exacerbate venous insufficiency and slow venous ulcer healing for three reasons.[9] First, whirlpool use requires dependent positioning of the extremity, which exacerbates edema and venous hypertension. Second, warm water temperature will further encourage superficial vein dilation and increased edema. Third, whirlpool treatments add moisture to an already highly exudating venous insufficiency wound, thus adding to the problem of providing and maintaining a moist, and not wet, wound environment. If used in the management of venous insufficiency ulcers, whirlpool treatments should be short in duration, less than 10 minutes per session, and should avoid high water temperature to discourage increasing edema. Even with these precautions, the clinician should be aware of the limited value and potential harm that whirlpool treatments can cause when used with this patient population. Alternative interventions, such as pulsatile lavage or debridement, provide a more advantageous means of removing devitalized tissue. Physical therapists who receive inappropriate wound management orders must take the opportunity to educate other members of the health care team on the safe and effective use of modalities and physical agents to enhance wound healing.

Integumentary Repair and Protective Techniques

Request for Further Medical Testing

Due to the probability for a deep vein thrombosis and the potentially devastating consequences of a pulmonary embolism, patients scoring a 3 or more on the DVT clinical prediction guideline should be referred to a physician for further assessment. As with other types of wounds, if healing does not progress despite appropriate interventions and follow-through, further medical testing should be requested. Wounds presenting with the signs and symptoms of infection should be cultured, and the physician should initiate appropriate antibiotic therapy immediately. Wounds probing to bone should be assessed for the presence of osteomyelitis. Although uncommon, clinicians should be aware that other pathologies may mimic venous insufficiency ulcers or coexist with venous insufficiency,

such as pyoderma gangrenosum and skin cancers (see Chapter 16).[118] Fortunately, these can be readily diagnosed by biopsy.[77] Wounds that fail to progress after 3–4 weeks of appropriate conservative interventions, or that do not present with the typical characteristics of venous ulcerations, should be referred for further medical assessment.

Local Wound Care

Highlights of local wound care specific to patients with venous insufficiency ulcers are included here. Refer to Section II for more details on general wound care. There are four keys to local wound care for patients with venous ulcers: protect the surrounding skin, absorb drainage, enhance venous return, and patient/caregiver education (see Box 11–3). Moisturizers should be applied to dry, scaling skin. If the skin is inflamed or weeping, topical steroids, such as cortisone, may be employed. At times, oral steroids or local steroid injections may be required to control inflammation in the surrounding skin.[26, 34] Topical agents should be used prudently because of the tendency for local allergic reactions and sensitization.[71, 116] Venous ulcers

---

BOX 11–3   Keys to Local Wound Care for Patients with Venous Insufficiency Ulcers

Protect the surrounding skin

- Moisturize dry, scaling skin.
- Use topical steroids to decrease inflammation or weeping.
- Use topical agents prudently to avoid sensitization.

Absorb drainage

- Choose absorptive dressings.
- Use skin sealants.

Enhance venous return

- Apply compression if appropriate.
- Instruct patients in methods to decrease edema.

Educate patient/caregivers

- Wound etiology.
- Intervention strategies.
- Risk factor modification.
- Guidelines for patients with venous insufficiency ulcers.

typically drain significantly. Dressings should be chosen based on their ability to absorb drainage and the length of time desired between dressing changes.[71, 83] To date, no one type or class of dressing has proven to be superior to any other.[4, 119, 120] A skin sealant should be used to protect surrounding tissues from excessive drainage. After ruling out significant arterial disease, compression should be applied to manage edema and enhance venous return.[1, 83] Compression wraps, devices, and garments are discussed in detail in the following section. After compression therapy is initiated, wound drainage normally decreases because of improved venous return. One study of 40 patients with venous insufficiency ulcers found that, as long as compression therapy was instituted, the class of primary dressing used (alginate, semipermeable foam, hydrocolloid, etc.) did not affect wound outcomes.[121]

As with other wounds, debridement of necrotic tissue should be performed as needed,[1, 83] and the wound should be monitored for signs of infection. While topical lidocaine compounds such as Eutectic Mixture of Local Anaesthetics (EMLA) cream have been found to assist with wound care–related pain in patients with venous insufficiency ulcers[54] without incidence of sensitivity, their effect on the rate of wound healing is unknown.[122] Venous ulcers that are recalcitrant to conservative management may benefit from the use of biological dressings[123] including growth factors, such as Oasis, and skin substitutes, such as Apligraf or Dermagraft (see Chapter 7).[77] Negative pressure wound therapy, also known as vacuum-assisted wound closure (see Chapter 9), may also enhance the healing of chronic venous insufficiency ulcers.

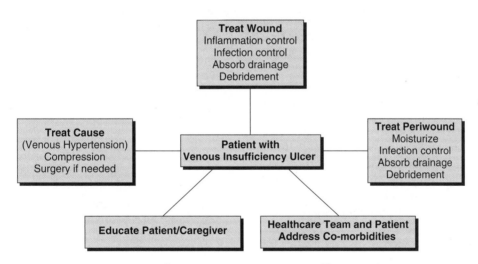

FIGURE 11–6   Integrated interventions for patients with venous insufficiency ulcers.

☑ *Checkpoint Question #2*

Local wound care for your patient with a venous insufficiency ulcer consists of once-weekly application of moisturizing lotion to the intact skin, an amorphous hydrogel, and gauze covered with a compression wrap. You notice the edges of his wound are white and friable, causing a slight increase in wound size. What is your response and why?

Physical Agents and Mechanical Modalities

Venous insufficiency ulcers result from sustained venous hypertension. If interventions are not directed toward resolving venous hypertension, there will be little or no progression of wound healing.[31, 124] Applying a compressive force around the limb can enhance the functioning of incompetent venous valves and the calf muscle pump, two key factors in the development of venous hypertension. Compression therapy also improves tissue oxygen levels during standing.[54, 85] Therefore, compression is the standard of care for venous insufficiency and venous insufficiency ulcers (provided arterial insufficiency is not present).[18, 33, 44, 71, 83, 99, 113, 125] Compression therapy appears to reduce the levels of MMPs and chronic inflammation in the affected region.[28, 31, 126]

Historically, compression has been applied using elastic and nonelastic bandages. Elasticity refers to the ability of a bandage to resist extension and return to its original length.[127] A nonelastic bandage does not yield to the force exerted by the calf musculature.[127] By resisting deformation, a nonelastic compression bandage establishes a fixed-volume compartment around the lower leg,[15] mimicking the effect of the deep fascia. When the calf muscles contract, becoming thicker and shorter, they meet the resistance of the nonelastic bandage. The deep veins are compressed between the calf muscles and the nonelastic bandage, forcing venous blood to move proximally. In contrast, bandages that are highly elastic are not appropriate for managing venous insufficiency for two reasons. First, elastic bandages have a high resting pressure,[99] which may limit circulation while the patient is stationary. Second, elastic bandages increase in length when force is applied. As the calf muscles contract and press against the elastic bandage, it yields, precluding an increase in deep vein pressure.[13] Therefore, highly elastic bandages, such as the typical Ace-type bandage, do *not* enhance the effectiveness of the calf muscle pump and have *not* been found to be effective in the management of venous insufficiency ulcers.[115, 127]

The application of compression to limbs with venous insufficiency has many positive effects (see Box 11–4). In addition to enhancing calf muscle pump effectiveness,[127, 128] compression helps shift blood from the distended superficial vasculature to the deep veins of the leg, thus enhancing venous return.[127] Compression decreases peripheral edema and venous volume, thereby decreasing superficial and deep vein distension as well as restoring the competency of

---

BOX 11–4   Therapeutic Effects of Compression for Patients with Venous Insufficiency Ulcers

- Enhances calf muscle pump
- Improves venous return
- Decreases peripheral edema
- Reduces venous distention
- Increases tissue oxygenation
- Softens lipodermatosclerosis and fibrosis
- Protects the limb from trauma
- Limits the need for bed rest or prolonged elevation

---

healthy valves. By controlling edema, compression improves tissue oxygenation and decreases wound drainage.[40] Compression has also been shown to soften lipodermatosclerosis,[127] possibly reducing the potential for ulcer recurrence by rendering the skin more pliable and resilient. All methods of compression provide the limb with some protection from trauma and environmental pathogens. Most important for the patient, compression relieves the pain of venous insufficiency without requiring prolonged periods of elevation or bed rest. If compression increases rather than decreases a patient's pain complaint, the clinician should suspect concomitant arterial insufficiency, and further assessment should be performed.

To be effective, compression must exceed venous intralumen pressure.[13] Compression should be graduated with the most compression applied distally. While there is little research to support specific compression levels, general recommendations for mild to moderate venous insufficiency are for 30–40 mm Hg at the ankle,[125] decreasing to 10 mm Hg at the infrapatellar notch.[121] For severe venous insufficiency, distal pressures of 40–50 mm Hg may be required. Compression is contraindicated in some instances (see Box 11–5). Patients with arterial insufficiency and an ABI of 0.8 may be treated with compression cautiously while being

---

BOX 11–5   Contraindications to Compression Therapy for Patients with Venous Insufficiency

- Arterial insufficiency with an ABI <0.7
- Acute infection
- Pulmonary edema
- Uncontrolled or severe congestive heart failure
- Active deep vein thrombosis
- Claustrophobia (relative contraindication)

closely monitored,[83] whereas patients with an ABI less than 0.7 should not be treated with compression because of the danger of exacerbating ischemia, which is already present.[89] While at least one author recommends judiciously reduced compression on patients with ABIs ranging from 0.5 to 0.7,[33] this action should be discussed with and cleared by the physician of record and carefully monitored. To limit the spread of infection, compression should be withheld until acute infection has been resolved. Patients with pulmonary edema or acute congestive heart failure are unable to accommodate the increased fluid return associated with applying compression to an edematous limb and, therefore, should not be treated with compression. Compression is also contraindicated in the presence of an active DVT for fear that the clot may be dislodged and travel to the lungs[128] unless a filter is in place.

There are several methods for achieving therapeutic compression for venous insufficiency ulcers and for maintaining skin integrity after wound healing, including paste bandages, short-stretch bandages, multilayer compression bandage systems, CircAid, tubular bandages, compression garments, and vasopneumatic compression devices.

Paste Bandages

A **paste bandage,** such as Unna's boot, is a nonelastic compression bandage that is proven to be effective in the treatment of venous insufficiency ulcers (see Figure 11–7).[7, 15, 17, 40, 127, 128] Paste bandages are gauze,

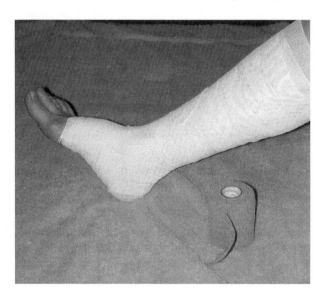

FIGURE 11–7   Paste bandage applied to patient with a venous insufficiency ulcer. The outer adhesive wrap has not yet been applied.

cloth roll bandages that are typically impregnated with zinc oxide, calamine, glycerin, and gelatin. When dry, the dressing hardens into a semirigid support. Studies seem to indicate that it is the nonelastic nature of the paste bandage that provides the most therapeutic response rather than the dressing's components.[40] Paste bandages may help patients who are nonadherent with other interventions because they stay on for several days and do not require additional attention by patients or caregivers.[128] A paste bandage has the greatest effect on ambulatory patients because it provides support against which the calf muscle pump can push during ambulation. Immobile or nonambulatory patients may be best served by simply elevating the extremity with an appropriate primary dressing.[42] Patients should be provided with instructions on how to care for their limb while the bandage is in place.

Despite the overall effectiveness of paste bandages as part of a treatment plan for the management of venous insufficiency ulcers, there are several disadvantages to this dressing. First, because the dressing remains in place for up to 1 week, patients may complain of an odor, especially if drainage is not properly controlled.[26] Second, some patients oppose the idea of not being able to shower or get the dressing wet. Third, a paste bandage requires the skill of a clinician to apply, and clinicians may find the dressing difficult to apply correctly at first.[127] Even when applied correctly, patients may report pruritus or may become sensitized to the dressing's components.[116] Fourth, paste bandages should not be used in areas of high humidity due to the increased chance of fungal infections. Finally, the inelastic nature of the paste bandage makes it unable to accommodate changes in limb size.[7] Therefore, as edema decreases, a new dressing must be applied. See Boxes 11–6 and 11–7 for instructions on applying a paste bandage and instructions for patients.

Short-Stretch Compression Wraps

Short-stretch compression wraps, such as Comprilan, have both elastic and nonelastic qualities and are the mainstay of treatment for venous insufficiency ulcers in most of Europe.[77, 129] Short-stretch compression wraps have a low resting pressure, which provides some compression at rest, but does not restrict blood flow.[4, 99] In addition, short-stretch compression bandages have little distensibility, making them capable of enhancing the effect of the calf muscle pump by creating a fixed-volume container similar to paste bandages.[17] Although short-stretch compression wraps can be used on nonambulatory patients,

BOX 11–6   **Application of Paste Bandage**

1. Prepare the wound.
   * Irrigate and debride the wound as needed.
   * Apply a skin sealant.
   * Apply an absorptive primary wound dressing, such as a hydrocolloid or semipermeable foam.
2. Protect the skin.
   * Apply moisturizing lotion to intact or anhydrous skin.
   * Glucocorticoid ointments may be used to decrease local erythema and pruritus.
3. Apply the paste bandage.
   * Position the patient in full dorsiflexion.
   * Apply in a spiral fashion from the metatarsal heads to the tibial tuberosity.
   * Wrinkles in the bandage should be avoided by cutting or pleating as needed.
   * Care should be taken to ensure all areas from the base of the toes to the bend of the knee are covered to prevent localized swelling.
4. Apply a self-adherent elastic wrap, such as Coban, over the paste bandage to increase compression.
5. Provide patient education.
6. Change dressing once or twice a week pending wound drainage.

BOX 11–7   **Instructions for Patients with a Paste Bandage**

Keep your legs moving

* The healing effects of your dressing are increased by walking regularly and pumping your ankles up and down while sitting.

Elevate your legs

* When sitting for prolonged periods of time or when sleeping, elevate your legs above the level of your heart or as much as feasible.

Keep your dressing clean and dry

* Contact your physician or therapist if your dressing becomes wet.

Protect your leg

* Do not scratch your leg.
* Do not place anything inside the dressing.

Report adverse effects

Contact your physician or therapist if you notice any of the following:

* Increased pain or swelling.
* Excessive drainage or odor.
* Color changes in your foot or toes.
* Numbness.

simple elevation may be sufficient. There are two key disadvantages of short-stretch compression wraps. First, short-stretch compression wraps are prone to slippage and must be rewrapped often.[130] Second, adequate patient/caregiver training must be performed to ensure correct wrapping technique. Improper wrapping can cause a tourniquet effect, further decreasing venous return and potentially reducing arterial blood flow.

The amount of compression exerted by a compression wrap can be expressed by **Laplace's law** (see Figure 11–8).[33] This is of prime importance to clinicians because applied compression must be enough to provide a therapeutic reduction in edema and increase in venous return without causing ischemia. According to Laplace's law, compression can be increased by applying additional bandage layers[131] or by using a narrower bandage. If all else is held constant, compression is greater at smaller limb circumferences, such as the ankle, than at larger limb circumferences, such as the calf. Therefore, the normal cone shape of a limb, narrower ankle and thicker calf, provides a graduated increase in compression. Patients presenting with limbs that do not increase in girth from ankle to knee may benefit from additional padding proximally to make the limb cone shaped. In addition to limb size affecting compression, greater pressure has been found in limb regions with the sharpest curves, such as the malleolus. To protect

$$\text{Bandage Compression} = \frac{(\text{tension})(\text{layers applied})(\text{constant})}{(\text{limb girth})(\text{bandage width})}$$

FIGURE 11–8   Laplace's law.

against undue tension, clinicians should provide padding around sharp, bony prominences.[132] Similar sub-bandage pressures have been found with using either a spiral technique or figure-of-eight technique for applying short-stretch bandages.[131] The last variable affecting bandage compression is the amount of tension used to apply the wrap. Bandages applied with greater tension will provide greater compression than those applied with less tension.[131] Clinically, the tension with which a compression wrap is applied is difficult to gauge.[131] Clinicians are encouraged to follow product-specific directions on the amount of tension to use when applying compression bandages. Some manufacturers direct the clinician to extend the bandage 150% of its original length and then make one turn around the limb, repeating this procedure with each turn. Some bandages are marked with rectangles that change to squares when sufficient tension is applied.[133] However, at least one study found the latter method of ensuring adequate compression to be inaccurate and potentially dangerous. See Boxes 11–8 and 11–9 for instructions on applying a short-stretch compression wrap and instructions for patients.

BOX 11–8   Application of Short-Stretch Compression Wrap

1. Prepare the wound.
   - Irrigate and debride the wound as needed.
   - Apply a skin sealant.
   - Apply an absorptive primary wound dressing, such as a hydrocolloid or semipermeable foam.
2. Protect the skin.
   - Apply moisturizing lotion to intact or anhydrous skin.
   - Glucocorticoid ointments may be used to decrease local erythema and pruritus.
   - Apply a hypoallergenic cotton liner extending from the base of the toes to just below the knee.
3. Apply the short-stretch compression wrap.
   - Position the patient in full dorsiflexion.
   - Follow the manufacturer's guidelines regarding the amount of tension to use when applying the wrap.
   - Anchor a 10-cm bandage at the metatarsal heads.
   - Wrap the ankle using two figure-of-eight turns around the ankle and foot. Continue up the leg in a spiral fashion and tape in place.
   - Anchor a 15-cm bandage just above the ankle and wrap proximally in a spiral fashion overlapping 50% to the tibial tuberosity and tape in place.
   - Wrinkles in the bandage should be avoided.
   - Care should be taken to ensure all areas from the base of the toes to the bend of the knee are covered to prevent localized edema.
4. The compression wrap should be worn 24 hours a day but may be removed for wound care bathing.
5. Provide patient education.
6. Bandage should be rewrapped every 24–72 hours, or if it becomes loose or slides.

BOX 11–9   Instructions for Patients Using Short-Stretch Compression Wraps or Multilayer Bandage Systems

Keep your legs moving
- The healing effects of your bandage are increased by walking regularly and pumping your ankles up and down while sitting.

Elevate your legs
- When sitting for prolonged periods of time or when sleeping, elevate your legs above the level of your heart or as much as feasible.

Monitor your bandage
- If your bandage becomes loose or wet, rewrap as instructed by your clinician. If you have not been shown how to rewrap your bandage, contact your clinician.

Protect your leg
- Do not scratch your leg.
- Do not place anything inside the bandage.

Report adverse effects
- Remove your bandage and contact your clinician if you notice increased pain, swelling, drainage, or odor.
- If you experience color changes or numbness in your foot or toes, and have been shown how to rewrap your bandage, do so. If these problems are not resolved, contact your clinician.

☑ *Checkpoint Question #3*

Which bandage will provide the greatest amount of compression: an 8-cm, 10-cm, or 15-cm short-stretch compression wrap? Why?

Multilayer Compression Bandage Systems

Multilayer bandage systems, such as Profore, incorporate short-stretch compression bandages into a **multilayer compression bandage** system (see Figure 11–9).[47, 129] The first layer absorbs excess wound drainage and provides padding to better distribute pressure around sharp curves, such as the malleoli.[130] The second layer also absorbs drainage. The third and fourth layers provide higher compression. Four-layer bandage systems have been shown to produce graduated compression from 30 to 40 mm Hg at the ankle[134] to 12–17 mm Hg below the knee.[135] This four-layer system should be modified for ankles measuring less than 18 cm in circumference either by placing additional padding distally or eliminating the third bandage layer to avoid excessive compression in the case of concomitant arterial insufficiency.[92] Ankles greater than 26 cm require an additional compression bandage layer

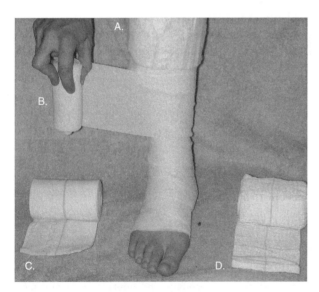

FIGURE 11–9   Multilayer compression bandage applied to patient with a venous insufficiency ulcer. The first layer has already been applied, while the second layer is being wrapped. The outer two layers have not yet been applied. *A.* Padding layer. *B.* Light conformable bandage. *C.* Light compression bandage. *D.* Flexible cohesive bandage.

to reach therapeutic compression levels.[77] Like short-stretch compression wraps, multilayer compression bandage systems are reusable and able to accommodate for unusually shaped limbs. Two advantages of multilayer compression bandage systems are that they stay in place better and maintain therapeutic compression longer than short-stretch compression wraps alone.[130] Results with multilayer compression bandage systems seem to be comparable to, or exceed, those achieved with paste bandages.[17] Comparisons of four-layer compression bandage systems with short-stretch compression bandages have found no significant difference in healing times.[106, 129, 135, 136] However, supply costs may be lower with multilayer compression bandages.[106, 136] The key disadvantage of multilayer compression bandage systems is the bulkiness of the additional layers, which often precludes patients from wearing their usual footwear.[130] See Box 11–10 and Table 11–8 for instructions on applying multilayer compression bandage systems[40] and instructions for patients.

CircAid

CircAid is a removable, semirigid orthotic compression device.[47, 127] CircAid consists of rows of nonelastic Velcro straps that are secured to provide sustained compression of the lower leg. The device is made of reusable, nondeformable fabric, which does not stretch out over time. Studies suggest CircAid provides similar outcomes to the previously mentioned compression methods.[127] One study found a clinically small, but statistically significant, improvement in weekly healing rate with CircAid compared to a multilayer compression bandage system but no difference in percent of closed wounds.[137] Because of its ease of application by patients and caregivers, CircAid may be more desirable than other forms of compression therapy. However, two disadvantages of CircAid include the high one-time cost and the need for patient adherence with the wearing schedule of the easily removable device.

Tubular Bandages

Tubular bandages, such as Tubigrip, are off-the-shelf sleeves available in several widths and compressions.

BOX 11–10 **Application of Multilayer Compression Bandage Systems***

1. Prepare the wound.
   - Irrigate and debride the wound as needed.
   - Apply a skin sealant.
   - Apply an absorptive primary wound dressing, such as a hydrocolloid or semipermeable foam.
2. Protect the skin.
   - Apply moisturizing lotion to intact or anhydrous skin.
   - Glucocorticoid ointments may be used to decrease local erythema and pruritus.
3. Apply padding layer.[†]
   - Position the patient in full dorsiflexion.
   - Wrap without tension from metatarsal heads to below the knee in spiral fashion with 50% overlap.
   - Care should be taken to ensure all areas from the base of the toes to the bend of the knee are covered to prevent localized swelling.
   - Wrinkles in the bandage should be avoided.
4. Apply second layer (light conformable bandage).
   - Use the same technique as the padding layer.
   - Follow manufacturer's guidelines for the amount of tension to apply.
   - Tape in place.
5. Apply third layer (light compression bandage) using the same technique as the second layer.[†,‡] For additional compression, this layer may be applied in a figure-of-eight fashion.
6. Apply fourth layer (flexible cohesive bandage) using the same technique as the second layer.
7. Provide patient education.
8. Bandage should be changed once or twice a week pending wound drainage, but may be removed for bathing rewrapped as needed.

*Instructions for a four-layer system; follow manufacturer's instructions for specific products.

†Patients with ankles measuring <18 cm should have extra padding or the third bandage layer should not be applied.

‡Patients with ankles measuring >26cm should use an additional third bandage layer.

compression with ease of application over a thin primary wound dressing and have been demonstrated to assist with venous ulcer healing.[138] There are two main disadvantages to tubular bandages. First, because of their rather generic shape and limited sizes, tubular bandages are not appropriate for many patients. Second, tubular bandages lose their ability to maintain therapeutic compression in a very short amount of time, usually within a week or so, which may prove costly in the long run.

Compression Garments

Long-term management of venous insufficiency usually requires the use of graduated **compression garments,** or stockings (see Figure 11–10).[7, 39, 69, 71, 83] These garments help maintain edema reduction and control venous hypertension, thereby decreasing the risk of ulcer recurrence to as low as 4%.[4] Patients should be measured for garments after edema has been reduced as much as possible.[127] It is best to measure patients shortly after they get out of bed, but if necessary, patients may be measured after resting for 10 minutes with their feet elevated above the heart.[39, 139] Fitting patients for compression garments requires obtaining a series of circumferential measurements and one or more measures of limb length. Although various manufacturers require different measurements, fitting for most off-the-shelf garments typically involves obtaining circumferential measurements of the narrowest portion of the ankle and the widest portion of the calf as well as the length from the floor to the fibular head. Fitting for a custom garment typically involves obtaining circumferential measurements every inch and a half or two inches for the length of the garment.

Garments are available in a wide variety of sizes, styles, colors, and compressions. Although the majority of patients do well with off-the-shelf garments, morbidly obese patients and patients with disproportionate extremities will likely require custom-made garments. When choosing a garment for a patient, clinicians should be aware that prices may range from as little as $25 for a pair of knee-high off-the-shelf garments to as high as $250 for a single custom garment. Compression garments may be made of a variety of different materials including cotton, nylon, polyester, latex, and synthetic elastomers such as spandex, Lycra, and Elastone. Since patients with venous insufficiency have a tendency to develop allergic reactions, clinicians should choose garments with higher cotton contents because cotton is less sensitizing than synthetics.[117] Compression garments are available in below-knee, thigh-high, stockings, and

Whereas a straight sleeve would provide the greatest compression at the widest part of the leg (the calf), restricting venous return, a tubular bandage allows for a more graduated compression from the ankle to the calf.[138] These bandages combine therapeutic

TABLE 11–8 Lower Extremity Compression Standards

Compression Level	Compression Class*	Indications
<20 mm Hg	Class 0	• Nonambulatory patients
20–30 mm Hg	Class 1	• Mild venous insufficiency
		• Venous insufficiency with mild arterial insufficiency
30–40 mm Hg	Class 2	• Moderate venous insufficiency
40–50 mm Hg	Class 3	• Severe venous insufficiency
>50 mm Hg	Class 4	• Severe venous insufficiency†

*Compression class standards vary based on country of origin and manufacturer. To ensure appropriate compression, it is recommended that the clinician prescribe compression garments using the numerical value of compression desired rather than stating a compression class.
†Rarely required.

maternity styles. Patient-reported disadvantages of compression garments are that the garments are too warm, not aesthetically pleasing, or difficult to don. A few garments are available with a zipper for ease of donning. Patients with thigh-high styles particularly complain about the garment sliding down, and adherence with

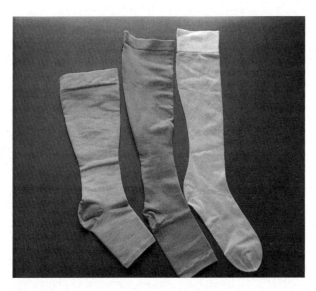

FIGURE 11–10 Two types of off-the-shelf, knee-high compression garments. The garment on the left is designed to create 40 mm Hg compression and is generally worn only if the skin is intact. The remaining two sleeves are designed to be used together along with a thin wound dressing to assist with ulcer healing. The inner liner (far right) creates approximately 10 mm Hg while the outer layer (middle) provides an additional 30 mm Hg.

this style tends to be lower than for below-knee garments. Since there is no evidence to support the need for above-knee garments for venous insufficiency unless there is proximal (iliac) venous insufficiency,[127] to increase adherence, the majority of patients with venous insufficiency should be fitted for knee-high garments.[34]

Clinicians must choose the amount of compression desired for each patient. Antiembolus stockings, such as TED hose, do not provide sufficient compression to reduce venous hypertension in nonrecumbent patients.[8] Additionally, the elastic cuff at the proximal thigh may decrease superficial venous return, potentially exacerbating venous insufficiency. For these reasons, antiembolus stockings should be used only in the case of nonambulatory patients. By convention, garment compression is termed by the highest compression at the ankle, with most garments ranging from 20 to 55 mm Hg.[39] Some manufacturers and clinicians describe compression in terms of compression class 0–4. However, because compression classes are not standardized within all countries and all manufacturers,[8] clinicians are advised to prescribe garments by the actual compression level required (e.g., mm Hg) rather than utilizing class terminology. Although limited, current research demonstrates no increase in the rate of ulcer recurrence when comparing medium and high compression levels.[140] Since patient compliance may be better with medium compression garments,[140] clinicians should prescribe the lowest effective level of compression possible (see Table 11–8).[11, 26, 33, 125, 127]

Once fitted for a compression garment, patients and caregivers must be instructed in proper wear and care of the garment. Donning garments can be difficult for patients with limited flexibility, such as those unable to reach their feet comfortably, and for individuals with limited dexterity or strength. Garments with higher compression are more difficult to don than those with lower compression.[39] Also, custom-made garments may be more difficult to don because of their more precise fit. Patients or caregivers may benefit from several aids available to assist in donning garments, including frames, socklets, or rubber dish gloves.[117] Some garments are available with zippers for ease of application. Patients should be instructed to wear their garments at all times except when bathing or sleeping. Most garments are machine washable and must be replaced every 3–6 months.[39, 117]

The Jobst UlcerCare garment is an off-the-shelf knee-high compression garment used to aid in healing venous insufficiency ulcers. This garment provides about 40 mm Hg compression at the ankle and consists of two separate layers: an inner liner that provides approximately 10 mm Hg of compression, and an outer garment that provides an additional 30 mm Hg of compression. A primary wound dressing is required under the liner. The liner is worn at all times except bandage changes and bathing, while the outer garment is worn only when the patient is awake. The UlcerCare garment is easy to don over a wound dressing or fragile skin because of the low-compression liner and the zipper on the outer, higher compression garment. The two layers allow for the compression to be modulated according to patient needs: increased compression when the patient's leg is in a more dependent position, and less compression at night when the limb is elevated on the bed. Although most patients report the UlcerCare garment is easy to use and comfortable, some have difficulty donning the outer layer.

See Table 11–9 for a comparison of the compression interventions for venous insufficiency.

TABLE 11–9   Comparison of Compression Interventions for Venous Insufficiency

Feature	Paste Bandage	Short-Stretch	Multilayer	CircAid	Tubular	Garment
Easy to don	No	Cond*	Cond*	Yes	Yes	Cond[†]
Removable by patient	No	Yes	Yes	Yes	Yes	Yes
Bulky	No	No	Yes	Yes	No	No
One-time cost	Low	Low	Low	High	Low	High
Reusable	No	Yes	Yes[‡]	Yes	Yes	Yes
Lifetime	3–7 d	2 mo	2 mo[‡]	18 mo	<1 wk	3–6 mo
Lifetime cost	Mod	Mod	Mod	Low	High	High
Sensitizing agents	Yes	No	No	No	No	No
Accommodates for change in limb size	No	Yes	Yes	Yes	Min	Min
Accommodates for unusual limb shape	Yes	Yes	Yes	No	No	Custom only
Graduated compression	Yes	Yes	Yes	Yes	Yes	Yes
Common use	H	H	H	H	H	H, M

Note: Short stretch = short stretch compression bandage; Multilayer, multilayer compression bandage system; Tubular, tubular bandage; Garment, off-the-shelf or custom-made compression garment; Cond, conditional; H, healing ulcer; M, maintaining skin integrity.

*Requires training and, commonly, caregiver assistance.

[†]Requires dexterity, some flexibility and strength, minimal training.

[‡]Outer layers may last up to 2 months; inner layers must be replaced more often.

☑ *Checkpoint Question #4*

You have been treating a patient with a venous insufficiency ulcer with a paste bandage weekly for 2 weeks. There has been a minimal decrease in wound size as well as edema. The patient's calf is warmer, redder, and itchy. What is your response and why?

Vasopneumatic Compression Devices

Vasopneumatic compression devices consist of a bilayered sleeve that slides over the patient's extremity and attaches to a pneumatic pump.[47] The pump fills the sleeve with air, compressing the leg to a preset level. Sleeves may be single- or multichambered. Single-chamber sleeves have been shown to compress the proximal veins prior to distal veins and are, therefore, not effective in increasing venous return.[141, 142] Multichamber sleeves fill and release sequentially from distal to proximal, providing a peristalsis-like wave of compression that effectively milks fluid from the limb.[26] Some studies have shown that multichamber compression enhances venous ulcer healing[142] while others report no improvement.[143, 144] Protocols for the use of pneumatic pumps vary greatly, and there is little clinical evidence to support one method over another.[141, 144] Patients are generally instructed to use the pump one to two sessions per day, each session lasting for 1–2 hours.[13] After each session, edema reduction must be maintained by using another form of compression, such as short-stretch compression wraps or a tubular bandage. Because of the high cost and extreme time commitment of this system, vasopneumatic compression devices are seldom used in current clinical practice and have been replaced by more recent advances in compression therapy.

Therapeutic Exercise

Range of Motion Exercise

Patients should be instructed to perform heel raises or active ankle pumps when sedentary and throughout the day to improve the ability of the calf muscle pump to increase venous return.[18, 54] Therapeutic exercises that target the ankle plantar flexors have been shown to improve not only calf muscle strength but also calf muscle pump effectiveness.[145] Patients using compression garments or devices will receive the greatest benefit by performing these exercises while wearing their compression garments or devices. Because suboptimal ankle dorsiflexion range of motion impairs calf muscle pump efficiency[36] and the risk of venous insufficiency ulcer recurrence is lower if full ankle motion is present,[108] patients should be instructed in gastrocnemius and soleus stretching exercises.[11]

Aerobic Exercise

Aerobic exercise can be of benefit to patients with venous insufficiency ulcers[86] for three reasons. First, aerobic exercise enhances the effect of the respiratory pump by increasing the rate and depth of respiration. Second, aerobic activities, such as biking, walking, and cross-country skiing, increase the performance of the calf muscle pump.[28, 36, 54] Third, aerobic exercise can assist with weight loss in patients who are obese and with blood sugar control in patients with diabetes, thereby improving patients' potential for wound healing. Patients with leg ulcers are typically deconditioned, physically inactive, and may have high fear-avoidance beliefs,[109] making patient/caregiver education critical to patient adherence.

Gait and Mobility Training

Up to 72% of patients with venous insufficiency ulcers stated they had difficulty walking.[18, 146] In addition to therapeutic exercise to increase lower extremity endurance and/or strength, patients with venous insufficiency ulcers may benefit from gait or mobility training. Not only will this enhance patient perception of mobility, but improved mobility can have a positive influence on both the calf muscle and respiratory pumps, weight loss, and blood sugar control. In addition, many patients with venous insufficiency ulcers report a decreased quality of life and feelings of depression.[18] Improvements in mobility may enhance a patient's sense of well-being and psychological health.

CASE STUDY: Mrs. Jessica Gibbons

PART 3

Interventions

The following highlights some of the key procedural interventions that will be incorporated into Mrs. Gibbons's plan of care.

Coordination, Communication, and Documentation: Mrs. Gibbons's physician has been contacted regarding her examination findings of mixed vascular disease including mild right lower extremity arterial insufficiency. The physician concurred with the physical therapist's decision to initiate compression therapy given that the predominant wound presentation and examination findings are of chronic venous insufficiency. A request for a prescription for EMLA cream to decrease pain with wound interventions was granted, and the physician also prescribed topical 1.0% hydrocortisone cream to decrease periwound inflammation and pruritus. A consult with a registered dietitian to assist with weight loss was also requested.

Patient/Client-Related Instruction: Mrs. Gibbons will be instructed in the etiology of chronic venous insufficiency and the implications of her prior deep vein thrombosis and other risk factors. Mrs. Gibbons will be instructed in the importance of skin protection techniques, avoidance of scratching her limb, exercise, limiting dependent limb positioning and static standing, and attaining and maintaining a more ideal body weight. She will be instructed to avoid constrictive clothing, particularly tight socks and pant legs with elastic cuffs. She will be instructed to apply a moisturizer to her feet and legs twice daily to improve skin hydration. She will be instructed to remove her compression bandage and notify her clinician immediately if her right foot or toes become cold, tingling, numb, or blue or white in color.

Procedural Interventions
- Local wound management will consist of pulsed lavage with suction to irrigate the wound and assist with the removal of slough. Sharp debridement of remaining slough will be performed after the use of EMLA cream. One percent hydrocortisone cream will be applied to intact skin in the areas of pruritus and erythema. A moisturizer without lanolin or perfumes will be used on intact, nonerythematous skin. The wound will be dressed with a skin sealant to the periwound, a hydrocolloid, and three layers of a four-layer compression bandage. A postop or cast-type shoe with a rocker-bottom will be issued to accommodate for the bandages and decrease the amount of dorsiflexion required for ambulation. The multilayer bandage was chosen over just short-stretch bandages because it was thought that the padding layer may assist with the distribution of compression and be tolerated better. A paste bandage was not chosen due to the presence of erythema and pruritus. A compression garment, such as an Ulcer-care garment, was not chosen because its high compression (40 mm Hg) cannot be modulated and Mrs. Gibbons's ABI indicates she has mild arterial insufficiency. In addition, as her edema decreases, the garment size may no longer be appropriate.
- Therapeutic exercises will include gastrocnemius and soleus stretches and strengthening exercises. Aerobic exercise, such as a stationary bicycle, may assist with venous return, weight loss, and serve as a warm-up exercise prior to ankle stretching.
- Manual therapy may include talocrural and/or tibiofibular joint mobilizations if therapeutic exercise alone is not enough to regain dorsiflexion.
- Functional training will include gait training with a cane to unload Mrs. Gibbons's ankle and improve her stability while ambulating with a rocker-bottom shoe.

Reassessment

Mrs. Gibbons's response to interventions will be monitored at all times. Her wound will be formally reassessed weekly and plan of care modified if there are any adverse effects or if no improvements are noted after 2 weeks of treatment.

MEDICAL AND SURGICAL INTERVENTIONS

Although medical and surgical interventions are clearly outside the scope of physical therapy, they are presented here to provide a better understanding of the valuable roles these disciplines play in the management of patients with venous insufficiency ulcers.

Medical Interventions

Physicians play a key role in the management of patients with venous insufficiency ulcers by selecting additional medical testing, managing risk factors, and prescribing pharmacological interventions. Physician involvement is critical in patients with wounds that fail to improve or are slow to heal. Health care workers must be aware of these diagnostic and intervention options and be able to determine when the services of a physician should be employed to assist in the overall care of patients with venous insufficiency ulcers.

Medical Testing

Diagnostic studies are sometimes used to confirm clinical impressions regarding wound etiology. Duplex ultrasonography is a noninvasive tool used to confirm the diagnosis of venous insufficiency and can identify the location(s) of insuffiency—superficial, perforator, deep, or a combination of these—as well as identify any concomitant arterial insufficiency that might alter intervention strategies.[1] **Venography** is the most accurate method of assessing venous flow. Venograms are up to 100% sensitive and 100% specific for identifying deep vein thromboses.[11, 35] This test involves injecting a radiopaque dye into the veins to provide a radiographic image of the venous system.[26] Because of the invasive nature of venography and the risk of allergic reactions to the contrast media, noninvasive tests are generally preferred and are performed more frequently. Doppler studies and air and plethysmography are noninvasive tests used to assess venous flow, vascular volume, and valve competency.[11, 26]

Management of Risk Factors

By managing risk factors and controlling underlying conditions, such as cardiovascular disease, obesity, and diabetes, physicians can decrease peripheral edema and increase the healing potential of patients with venous insufficiency.[11, 26] While clinicians may be called upon to assist in such management through controlled, progressive aerobic exercise programs, sometimes patients require medical or pharmaceutical assistance to lower blood pressure, lose weight, and control blood sugars.

Pharmacological Interventions

Pharmacological management with fibrinolytics, such as pentoxifylline (Trental), has been shown to enhance venous ulcer healing in patients with venous insufficiency both with[34, 47] and without coexisting arterial insufficiency.[4, 7, 69, 99, 147] Because of the adverse effects on wound healing, physicians should limit systemic steroid use if at all possible.[13] Topical antimicrobials should not be used wantonly or routinely without the empiric support of a wound culture or biopsy. This is particularly important for patients with venous ulcers because topical antimicrobials, most notably neomycin, may cause sensitization in patients with venous insufficiency.[116] If an increase in erythema or pruritus occurs while using a topical agent, clinicians should suspect patient sensitization. The offending agent should be stopped and the reaction reported to the physician for modification of topical treatment. When infection is present, physicians should initiate appropriate antibiotic therapy immediately to manage bacterial load.[83] Cellulitis requires systemic antibiotics.[89]

Surgical Interventions

Health care providers should be aware of some of the surgical interventions that may be available to patients with venous insufficiency ulcers if conservative treatment options fail. These include surgical debridement, skin grafting, and vein surgeries.

Debridement

As with other wound types, debridement of eschar and nonviable tissue facilitates wound healing.[1, 7] Clinicians should request a surgical consult for patients with venous insufficiency ulcers that contain large amounts of necrotic tissue or that are exceptionally painful to debridement without anesthesia.

Skin Grafting and Skin Substitutes

Surgeons may perform skin grafting or apply skin substitutes to provide better quality skin over large or multiple venous insufficiency ulcers.[7, 18] These procedures generally require less time to close than healing by secondary intention. Patients presenting with exceptionally slow wound healing rates or with large or multiple ulcers may benefit from a surgical consult.[18] However, if the underlying etiology of venous insufficiency is not addressed, the ulcer will likely recur.[7] The high rate of ulcer recurrence after split or full-thickness skin grafting, up to 20%,[13] may be attributed to this lack of attention to causative factors. So, to improve graft take and decrease the risk of ulcer recurrence, it is important for clinicians to address the underlying venous hypertension with some form of compression therapy after grafting.[148]

Vein Surgery

Patients not responding to compression therapy may benefit from surgical interventions.[28] Unlike arteries, veins are rarely reconstructed or replaced due to the high morbidity and reocclusion rate.[149] Several surgical alternatives available are vein ligation,[150] vein stripping,[150] sclerotherapy, and stenting. **Ligation,** or tying off, of perforating veins reduces hypertension in the superficial veins around the ulcer, providing a greater chance of wound healing and decreasing the risk of ulcer recurrence.[1] **Vein stripping** is the surgical resection of superficial varicosities and incompetent perforating veins.[1, 31] **Sclerotherapy,** the injection of an agent to fibrose dysfunctional veins, may also be performed to eliminate venous hypertension in the superficial and perforating systems.[28, 31] Recent advances in medical technology have led to endoscopic vein surgery such as the **SEPS procedure,** subfascial endoscopic interruption of perforating veins, to successfully manage chronic venous insufficiency and assist with venous insufficiency ulcer healing.[1, 28, 29, 48, 150, 151] The procedure has been shown to improve venous reflux as well as secondary skin changes of lipodermatosclerosis.[48] SEPS procedure requires general anesthesia and has a wound site complication rate of about 6%, far less than previously used open techniques.[1] This procedure is indicated for patients with active or healed venous insufficiency ulcers.[48] **Percutaneous ablation of perforators (PAPS)** is an alternative surgical procedure that uses ultrasound-guided percutaneous access, thus avoiding incisional wound healing complications, to inject a sclerosing agent into the vein. PAPS requires only local anesthesia, causes less post-operative pain, and can be repeated if needed.[1] Both SEPS and PAPS are technically demanding surgeries that must be performed by a skilled surgeon. Patients with more than a 50% obstruction to venous outflow appear to benefit from venous stenting.[37]

Unlike surgical debridement or skin grafting, vein surgery has a direct effect on the cause of venous insufficiency, which may help reduce recurrence rates[19] but does not seem to affect healing rates.[28] Unfortunately, vein surgery is not appropriate for all patients and may provide only a temporary cure, as new collateral veins will develop over time.[40] Patients should be encouraged to wear compression garments long term as the combination of surgery and long-term compression therapy has led to faster healing and fewer recurrences.[29]

CHAPTER SUMMARY

Venous insufficiency ulcers are the most common type of leg ulcer. Venous ulcers pose a particular challenge to health care workers because the majority of ulcers has been present for greater than 1 year, and those that have healed have a high rate of recurrence. There are several risk factors for venous ulceration: vein dysfunction, calf muscle pump failure, trauma, previous ulceration, advanced age, and diabetes. Several physical therapy tests and measures are available to identify venous insufficiency and possible coexisting arterial insufficiency including a clinical assessment guideline for identifying deep vein thromboses, ankle-brachial index, Trendelenburg test, Doppler ultrasound, and venous filling time. Keys to physical therapy interventions for patients with venous insufficiency ulcers are patient/client-related instruction, local wound care to absorb drainage and protect the surrounding tissue, and the use of compression to control venous hypertension. Patients with slow-healing wounds should be assessed for infection. If infection is present, the physician should initiate appropriate antibiotic treatment. Those not responding to conservative treatment options should be referred to a physician for further medical testing, more intensive medical management of risk factors, and possible surgical interventions.

REVIEW QUESTIONS

1. Your patient presents with a venous insufficiency ulcer on his medial lower leg. The patient's ABI is 0.9 and his pedal pulses on the affected side are mildly decreased. The limb is edematous below the knee and hemosiderin deposition is evident. The wound bed is 100% granular. The wound has

a foul odor after normal saline irrigation. There is copious wound drainage, which makes the old bandages appear neon green.

a. What medical test might you suggest to the attending physician?

b. Does the patient have arterial insufficiency?

c. Should this patient's wound be treated with compression?

d. Describe how you might bandage this patient's wound. Provide your rationale.

2. Use the wound in color image 17 to answer the following series of questions.

Your patient, Mr. V, is a 45-year-old who presents for an initial physical therapy examination with an ulcer near his medial malleolus. The wound began approximately 5 months ago and has slowly increased in size. Mr. V states that he must change the dressing two times per day because it drains so much. Mr. V's past medical history includes a previous venous insufficiency ulcer in about the same location 4 years ago, and carotid artery end-arterectomy in 1999. Mr. V lives alone and works as a cashier.

a. What tests and measures would you perform on Mr. V?

b. Document wound and periwound characteristics as you would in the patient's chart.

c. Should you whirlpool this patient's wound? Why or why not?

d. Describe how you might bandage Mr. V's wound.

e. Describe other physical therapy interventions you would include in your plan of care.

f. What suggestions do you have for Mr. V regarding his job?

3. Mr. B presented to your clinic 3 weeks ago with the diagnosis of venous insufficiency ulcer. His past medical history is unremarkable with the exception of diabetes mellitus diagnosed 5 years previously, with blood sugars normally measuring around 180 mg/dL. On initial examination Mr. B's ABI was 0.8 and his pedal pulses were 1+ bilaterally. The wound measures 3.8×2.5 cm, has a moderate amount of drainage, and is 95% pale granulation tissue with 5% fibrous, yellow slough. There is a moderate amount of peripheral edema bilaterally and the periwound is characterized by hemosiderin deposition. You have been treating Mr. B's ulcer with a multilayer compression bandage system and today the wound measures 4.2×3.0 cm and continues to be 95% pale granulation tissue and 5% fibrous, yellow slough. What is your response and why?

myhealthprofessionskit™

Use this address to access the Companion Website created for this textbook. Simply select "Physical Therapy" from the choice of disciplines. Find this book and log in using your username and password to access images, video clips, and additional learning tools.

REFERENCES

Go to myhealthprofessionskit.com to view this chapter's references.

12

Pressure Ulcers

Chapter Objectives

After reading this chapter, learners will be able to:

1. Differentiate the etiology of pressure ulcers from other types of open wounds.
2. Explain the risk factors contributing to pressure ulcers.
3. Define and describe the purpose of various pressure ulcer risk assessment tools.
4. Design interdisciplinary interventions for the prevention of pressure ulcers in at-risk individuals.
5. Compare and contrast the staging system for classifying pressure ulcers with the Integumentary Preferred Practice Pattern classification system.
6. Assess the typical characteristics of pressure ulcers.
7. Define and describe the purpose of various pressure ulcer assessment instruments.
8. Design an interdisciplinary approach in the management of patients with pressure ulcers.
9. Describe basic guidelines for patients with pressure ulcers.
10. Describe precautions clinicians should be aware of when working with patients with pressure ulcers.
11. Select physical therapy procedural interventions for patients with pressure ulcers, including integumentary repair and protective techniques, therapeutic exercise, functional training, and electrotherapeutic modalities.
12. Integrate the keys to local wound care for patients with pressure ulcers.
13. Describe factors to consider when choosing support surface technology for patients with or at risk for pressure ulcers.
14. Discuss possible medical and surgical interventions for patients with pressure ulcers.

Key Terms

Air-fluidized pressure-relieving device

Alternating pressure-relieving device

Bottoming out

Capillary closing pressure

Dynamic support surface

Fluid-filled pressure-reducing device

Foam pressure-reducing device

Friction

Hand check

International NPUAP/EPUAP Pressure Ulcer Classification System

Ischemia reperfusion injury

Low-air-loss pressure-relieving device

Key Terms (*continued*)

Maceration
Musculocutaneous flap
Pressure ulcer
Pressure ulcer assessment
    instrument

Pressure ulcer risk
    assessment tool
Pressure-reducing device
Pressure-relieving device
Reactive hyperemia

Shear
Staging system
Static support surface
Tissue interface pressure

INTRODUCTION

Pressure ulcers are localized areas of tissue necrosis that develop when soft tissue is compressed between a firm surface and an underlying bony prominence or a combination of pressure and shear.[1] Pressure ulcers vary greatly in severity. Damage may be confined to the epidermis, or it may extend through the fascia to muscle, joint capsule, or bone. A one-day pressure ulcer prevalence survey within acute care hospitals in the United States found the overall prevalence of pressure ulcers to be 15%.[2] The number of patients with pressure ulcers present on admission to acute care facilities has increased over 80% in the last 13 years.[3] The even more tragic statistic is that over 95% of pressure ulcers are thought to be preventable.[4]

The three classes of patients with the greatest risk of developing a pressure ulcer are individuals with spinal cord injuries, hospitalized patients, and individuals in long-term care facilities. The incidence of pressure ulcers in patients with spinal cord injuries ranges from 7% to 39%,[5, 6] increasing to as high as 30% 5 years after spinal cord injury.[7] The average incidence of pressure ulcers in hospitalized patients is 7%[8] but ranges from 4% to 38%.[9–13] The incidence of pressure ulcers in elderly patients with acute femoral fractures is as high as 66%.[14] In home health care, the incidence of pressure ulcers has been documented to be between 10% and 17%[11, 15] increasing to as high as 38%[16] in long-term care facilities. An estimated 1.3–3 million Americans have pressure ulcers.[6] The average cost of caring for individuals with pressure ulcers is estimated to be over $43,000.[8] In the United States, the cost of adult hospital stays for patients with a diagnosis of pressure ulcers in 2006 was $11 billion.[3] More importantly, complications from pressure ulcers may be multiple and life threatening. The earlier a pressure ulcer is recognized and interventions are initiated, the better the outcome will be.[17] An interdisciplinary approach can positively impact the efficiency and effectiveness of care for patients with pressure ulcers.[1, 18, 19]

This chapter provides an overview of the etiology of pressure ulcer formation followed by a review of risk factors and measures to prevent pressure ulcer development. Next, the classification, prognosis, and characteristics of pressure ulcers are outlined along with pressure ulcer assessment instruments. This is followed by a detailed presentation of physical therapy management of patients with pressure ulcers. The chapter concludes with a brief review of medical and surgical interventions that may be required for the management of pressure ulcers. A four-part case study following the initial examination and treatment planning for a patient with a pressure ulcer has been integrated within the chapter.

ETIOLOGY OF PRESSURE ULCERS

A **pressure ulcer** is any wound caused by unrelieved pressure or a combination of pressure and shear forces.[1, 20] Historically, pressure ulcers were thought to be caused by prolonged time in bed, hence the previously used terms *bed sore* and *decubitus* (literally meaning "lying down")[21] *ulcer.*[22] It is now known that although time is a factor in the development of pressure ulcers, it need not be prolonged. In fact, pressure ulcers may develop in less than 2 hours if the proper conditions prevail.[23] Non–bed-bound patients, including patients with improperly fitting casts or splints and patients who sit for prolonged periods,[21] can also be at risk for pressure ulcers. Therefore, these previously used terms should be abandoned as misnomers and replaced by the more correct term, *pressure ulcer.*

Pressure on any bony prominence is transmitted to the underlying tissues, compressing all intervening structures between the skin and the bone. When the applied pressure is greater than the intracapillary blood pressure,[24] blood flow to soft tissue is obstructed and local tissue ischemia occurs.[20, 22, 25] The applied pressure also obstructs local lymphatic channels.[21] Restricted blood and lymph flow leads to higher concentrations of metabolic wastes and acidosis, increasing the rate of cell death and making surviving cells more vulnerable to trauma.[22] Platelets and polymorphonuclear leukocytes accumulate in the area of pressure. If pressure is maintained, capillary permeability increases, as does local edema and inflammation, exacerbating the already precarious local circulation and increasing the amount of tissue necrosis (see Figure 12–1).[25] For reasons as yet unknown, ischemia causes a decrease in fibrinolysis that results in fibrin deposits within capillaries and the interstitial space. In patients with pressure ulcers, fibrinolytic activity at the wound border is significantly less than 9 mm away.[26] Even up to 12 mm away from the ulcer, fibrinolytic activity is still significantly less than in patients without pressure ulcers.[26] This accumulation of fibrin allows microthrombi to form, further occluding vessels, exacerbating tissue necrosis, and retarding pressure ulcer healing. Continued pressure leads to chronic inflammation, tissue fibrosis, and epidermal degeneration. Frequently, ischemic tissues are invaded by bacteria. Bacteria compete with body cells for oxygen and nutrients and add to the increase in waste products within ischemic tissues.[27]

Previously, it was thought that there was a critical level of pressure, below which no ulceration would occur. Since **capillary closing pressure** was measured as 13–32 mm Hg, it was assumed that pressures less than 32 mm Hg would not cause ulceration.[28, 29] Additionally, because studies showed that intermittently applied pressures were less likely to cause tissue damage than sustained pressures,[28] it was believed that pressure needed to be sustained for 2 or more hours before an ulceration would occur.[30] Recent studies have substantiated that an inverse pressure–time relationship exists. However, it is now known that the critical pressure required before ulceration occurs varies both from individual to individual and from body location to body location.[26, 31, 32] Therefore, the previous pressure–time model has been expanded to include individual hemodynamic factors such as hematocrit, red blood cell flexibility, blood viscosity, lower temperatures, and previous ischemia–reperfusion injury, as well as capillary closing pressures, all of which affect the amount of pressure needed to cause a pressure ulcer (see Figure 12–2).[20, 26]

The site of pressure application also affects the likelihood of ulceration. Recall that pressure is defined as force per unit area. Subcutaneous tissue provides padding and redistributes forces applied to the skin over a wider area, thereby reducing pressure. Body sites with large amounts of subcutaneous tissues, such as the abdomen, are unlikely to be adversely affected by pressure. In contrast, areas overlying bony prominences, such as the posterior heel, have little padding and smaller surface areas. These areas are less likely to attenuate pressure successfully.

To add to the confusion, different tissues have differing abilities to tolerate ischemia. Muscle tissue has the highest metabolic demand and is the least tolerant to compression.[33] Muscle is more sensitive than skin to the effects of ischemia due to pressure.[30] When pressure is applied over a bony prominence (see Figure 12–3), the greatest pressure occurs in the tissue

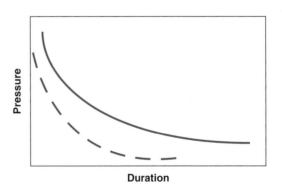

Duration

FIGURE 12–2 Note the inverse relationship of pressure and time in the formation of pressure ulcers. When higher pressure is applied, an ulceration will occur in a short period of time. In contrast, if lower pressure is applied, an ulceration will not occur unless it is maintained for a long period of time. The pressure–time curve shifts to the left (dotted line) for individuals with lower tissue tolerance to pressure due to hemodynamic changes.

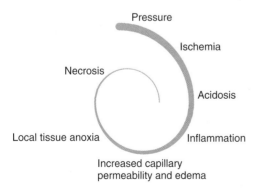

FIGURE 12–1   Etiology of pressure-related cell death.

Pressure

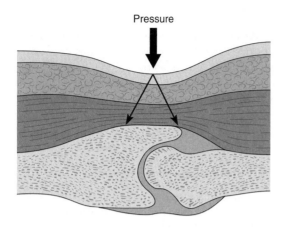

FIGURE 12–3   Pressure distribution cone.

directly over the prominence.[34] Pressure is more distributed farther away from the bony prominence (and closer to the body's surface). Therefore, when pressure is applied over a bony prominence, deeper muscle tissue overlying the bone may be suffering irreversible necrosis due to ischemia, while the overlying skin may remain unaffected.[1, 33, 35] When the destruction of these deeper tissue layers reaches a certain point, they are unable to support the health of the more superficial integument, and a break in skin integrity becomes apparent. A decline in skin integrity may also become apparent when the pressure-induced ischemia is so severe that the integument is destroyed along with the underlying tissue layers. Pressure ulcers may not develop until 2–7 days after the pressure was applied.[32, 35, 36] This means that extensive deep tissue damage may already have occurred before any clinical signs are apparent at the skin's surface.

In healthy individuals, anoxia and chemical irritation caused by pressure stimulate nerve endings, causing pain and encouraging individuals to relieve the pressure by changing position before any cell damage occurs.[22] Relief of short-term pressure is followed by **reactive hyperemia,** when ischemic tissues are flooded with blood rich in oxygen, nutrients, and vasodilatory cytokines and waste products are removed from the affected area.[37, 38] Reactive hyperemia is a localized area of blanchable erythema; that is, when digital pressure is applied to the area in question, it will turn white. As with arterial insufficiency ulcers, reactive hyperemia serves a protective role in reestablishing sufficient circulation by vasodilating local arterioles. The length of time reactive hyperemia lasts is proportional to the extent of tissue ischemia.[27, 37] If pressure is maintained, this area of erythema will become nonblanchable.[39, 40]

Individuals with paralysis, decreased sensation, or altered consciousness are unable to recognize ischemia and the damaging effects of pressure, and a pressure ulcer may result.

RISK FACTORS CONTRIBUTING TO PRESSURE ULCERS

Aside from pressure and time, there are many factors known to contribute to pressure ulcer formation. The four key factors that increase the risk of pressure ulceration are shear, excessive moisture, impaired mobility, and malnutrition.[41] Impaired sensation, advanced age, and history of pressure ulceration also increase the risk of pressure ulcers.[42 41] Several additional risk factors are believed to play a smaller role in the development of pressure ulcers. The greater the number of risk factors, the greater the risk of ulcer development.[43] Therefore, it is important for clinicians to pay close attention to a patient's medical history.

Shear

Whereas pressure occurs when a force is applied perpendicular to a body part compressing soft tissue, **shear** occurs when a force is applied parallel to the soft tissue. Shearing forces are common clinically. For example, if a patient is sitting in a hospital bed with the head of the bed elevated, there is a tendency for the patient to slide down toward the foot of the bed.[44] In this situation, the skin and superficial fascia are relatively fixed against the sheets while the skeleton and deeper fascia slide downward. This shearing force between the skin and deeper tissues leads to stretching and angulation of the vasculature,[21] compromising tissue perfusion, causing local ischemia, and paving the way for pressure ulcer development.[20, 32, 41, 45–47] Pressure ulcers with a shearing component may have a teardrop appearance and undermining is commonly present.[34] Friction is another force that is applied parallel to soft tissue. **Friction** occurs when two surfaces move across one another, such as when a patient is dragged, rather than lifted, from cart to bed. Although friction does not directly cause pressure ulcers, it can strip the stratum corneum, making the skin more susceptible to pressure ulcers.[20, 32, 45, 48]

Moisture

Excessive moisture predisposes the skin to pressure ulcers[38] by causing **maceration** and increasing shear and friction forces.[20, 41, 45, 46] Macerated skin can be identified as white, friable, overhydrated, and sometimes wrinkled skin.[49] Maceration may be caused by uncontrolled wound drainage, perspiration, or incontinence.[20] Because of the acidity of urine and the bacteria present in urine and feces, incontinence poses the most significant problem. Regardless of the cause, wet skin is more easily abraded, more permeable, and more readily colonized by microorganisms than healthy skin.[49] Wet skin is also less resistant to infection than dry skin.[20] Urinary incontinence has been shown to be significantly associated with pressure ulcers,[9, 50, 51] increasing the risk of ulceration fivefold.[21] Moreover, patients who are incontinent of bowel seem to be more at risk for the development of pressure ulcers than patients who are only incontinent of urine.[9, 52]

While excessive moisture increases the risk of pressure ulcers, anhydrous skin is also at risk[41] because it is less flexible and more vulnerable to trauma.[20]

Impaired Mobility

There is a direct correlation between impaired mobility and pressure ulcer development.[40, 41, 46, 50, 53, 54] Healthy individuals reposition themselves every 15–20 minutes, even during sleep. Individuals who are unable to reposition themselves, or who do so less than 20 times per night, are at increased risk of pressure ulcer development.[27] There are three types of factors that affect a patient's mobility.[55] First, there are factors actually affecting the ability to move, such as restricted range of motion, limited strength, infants and neonates, and the presence of mechanical devices such as oxygen and intravenous tubing. Second, there are factors that affect the desire of a patient to move or change positions, such as pain and depression. Third, there are factors that decrease the patient's ability to perceive pain, such as medications and upper or lower motor neuron damage.

The most frequently studied causes of impaired mobility with respect to pressure ulcer development are hospitalization, fracture, spinal cord injury, and infants/neonates. The declining health status that frequently accompanies hospitalization can also result in decreased mobility. Pressure ulcers are most likely to develop within the first 3 weeks of hospitalization, surgery, change in medical condition, or admission to a nursing home.[56, 57] Several studies report that patients who are bed-bound, chair-bound, or unable to ambulate without assistance have an increased risk of pressure ulcer development.[21, 43, 58] The significant association of fractures, particularly hip fractures, with pressure ulcer development[9] may be due to the acute inability of patients to independently reposition themselves because of pain, weakness, sedation from surgery or pain medications, or confinement (as with bone traction).

The combination of decreased mobility and altered sensation found in individuals with spinal cord injuries likely contributes to the 7.5% incidence of pressure ulcers in this population.[5] Among individuals with spinal cord injuries, several characteristics were found to be highly correlated with pressure ulcer development, including current age, age at the time of injury, severity of injury, education, general mobility, health motivation, social support, financial resources, access to care, and alcohol abuse.[59, 60] The best predictors of ulcer development in individuals with spinal cord injuries are current age over 40, young age at the time of injury, complete spinal cord injury, lengthy hospitalization, low education level, alcohol abuse, and history of previous ulceration.[5, 52, 59 60]

The prevalence of pressure ulcers in pediatric and neonatal intensive care units is 23%–27%.[56] Infants and neonates are at risk for pressure ulcers due to the fragility of their skin, their inability to reposition themselves, and the presence of medical tubing and devices.[56, 61] High-frequency oscillatory ventilation devices may also cause friction and shearing forces, which increase the risk for pressure ulcers.[56]

Other causes of impaired mobility that are associated with pressure ulcer development include altered mental status, spasticity, and confinement.[9, 21, 25, 27, 58, 62] Patients with altered mental statuses, such as those who are comatose, medically sedated, demented, or severely depressed, make little or no spontaneous movements, subjecting them to prolonged bouts of pressure. In addition, they are unable to sense or respond to the pain of anoxia and ischemia. Therefore, these patients are reliant on others to reposition them prior to the onset of tissue trauma. Likewise, patients who have severe spasticity or who are confined by seat belts, lap tables, or restraints are unable to freely change positions to unload areas of undue pressure.

Malnutrition

Poor nutrition,[63, 64] specifically low serum albumin levels,[9, 65] is also a risk factor for pressure ulcer development.[1, 25, 46, 51, 58, 62, 66] Hypoalbuminemia causes interstitial edema[67] and signals that the body lacks the protein stores necessary for building and repairing tissues. One study cites malnutrition as the second most common risk factor, after decreased mobility, for pressure ulcer development.[52] The majority of new patients admitted to hospitals with severe pressure ulcers was malnourished,[68] and a decrease in nutrition is associated with new ulcer development.[58] In a study of nursing home residents, all patients with pressure ulcers were classified as being "severely malnourished,"[69] which indicates the seriousness of the problem and the need to assess nutrition on a regular basis. There is also a positive correlation between low serum albumin and pressure ulcer severity.[70]

Malnutrition does not simply apply to patients who appear to be emaciated. Although many patients who are significantly underweight have low serum albumin levels, it is also possible to have low serum albumin levels and be overweight. One study found 53% of patients with pressure ulcers were, in fact, obese.[70] For this reason, it is imperative that each patient's nutrition level is assessed, regardless of body type or appearance.[41] Inadequate hydration is also associated with pressure ulcer development.[20, 62] Because poor hydration also affects body weight, albumin measurements, and overall health, patient hydration should be included as part of a nutritional assessment.[1]

Impaired Sensation

Impaired sensation precludes the ability of an individual to detect the pain of tissue damage caused by undue pressure. Without pain as an early warning signal of developing tissue ischemia, patients with impaired sensation are unlikely to shift their weight or reposition themselves to alter the distribution of pressure. Therefore, patients with conditions that alter their ability to perceive the pain of ischemia, such as spinal cord injury, spina bifida, stroke, diabetes mellitus, full-thickness burns, and peripheral neuropathy, are at increased risk of developing a pressure ulcer.[1, 24, 32, 46, 63] For example, consider Mr. H, a patient who has decreased sensation on his left side after a cerebrovascular accident 5 days earlier. While in bed, Mr. H prefers to lie in a three-fourths sidelying position on his affected side so he is able to use his unaffected arm for operating the television remote control and the call light. When assisting Mr. H with his exercises, the physical therapist notices a small area of erythema on Mr. H's left lateral malleolus. Mr. H reports the area is not painful or tender. The area does not blanch when the therapist applies pressure with her finger. The therapist concludes that Mr. H has developed a category/stage I pressure ulcer. The therapist believes that Mr. H's impaired sensation

contributed to the ulceration by not alerting him to the onset of tissue trauma and prompting him to change positions before the ulcer developed.

Advanced Age

Patients with pressure ulcers are generally older than patients without pressure ulcers.[20, 46, 52, 62–64] Of patients with pressure ulcers, more than half are over 70 years old.[10, 40] As discussed in Chapter 3, several age-related changes in the dermis and epidermis likely contribute to the increased rate of pressure ulceration that occurs with increased age,[24] including decreased elastin and collagen content, decreased tissue strength and stiffness, loss of dermal vasculature, flattening of the epidermal–dermal junction, thinning of the epidermis and dermis, decreased sebaceous gland secretion, increased skin permeability, and slower cell replacement rate.[20, 71] The ability to build new tissue and fight infection also decreases with age,[71] potentially contributing to ulcer development or severity. In addition, older individuals have an increased rate of comorbidities that may affect other known risk factors for pressure ulcer development.

Previous Pressure Ulcer

Studies have shown that a history of a previous pressure ulcer increases the risk of future ulcerations.[38, 60] Additional ulcers may develop for the same reasons as the initial ulceration, especially if the contributing factors have not been adequately controlled. Because scar tissue can only attain a maximum of 80% of the original tissue strength,[72] previous ulcerations alters local tissues' tolerance to pressure and externally applied loads.[32] Therefore, scar tissue or previous vascular insults due to pressure or shear may predispose the patient to repeat ulcerations.

Additional Risk Factors

Although less data exists to support a link between these additional risk factors and the development of pressure ulcers, these factors warrant further attention on an individual basis.

There is some evidence to support the concept of **ischemia reperfusion injuries.**[20, 32] For example, local pressure can cause tissue ischemia. The sudden reperfusion of these tissues caused by pressure relief may cause additional tissue damage. It appears that the amount of tissue injury increases with each loading–unloading cycle. In addition, unhealthy patients seem to be less able to tolerate these hemodynamic fluctuations than healthy subjects.[20]

Low diastolic blood pressure lowers capillary closing pressures. Therefore, patients with low diastolic blood pressures,[24, 73] particularly those less than 60 mm Hg,[16] may develop pressure-related tissue damage from forces lower than expected or in a shorter period of time.[41] Patients who smoke[65] or have diabetes-related microvascular changes may be at increased risk for pressure ulcer development due to a decreased hyperemic response.[37, 44, 74] Subclinical dehydration-related reductions in tissue oxygenation may increase the risk of pressure ulcer development.[75] Polypharmacy,[76] especially medications known to adversely affect mental status or mobility, may contribute to pressure ulcer development for reasons previously cited. Psychosocial factors, such as limited formal education, low financial status, and lack of a support system, may also pose an increased risk of pressure ulcer development.[59, 60] Because temperature is usually elevated where the body is in contact with a support surface,[77] and increased skin temperatures lead to a local increase in metabolism, the effect of skin temperature on pressure ulcer development warrants further consideration.[16, 31] Elevated tissue temperatures combined with pressure limiting local tissue perfusion may increase the risk for pressure ulcers.[41] Conversely, lower temperatures are thought to indicate decreased blood flow and, therefore, suboptimal tissue perfusion.[78, 79] One small study of nursing home residents demonstrated patients at greater risk for pressure ulcers according to the Braden scale had lower body temperatures and body temperatures that fluctuated less than those at less risk for pressure ulcer development.[31] Patients with Alzheimer's disease, Parkinson's disease, and rheumatoid arthritis are twice as likely to develop a pressure ulcer than those without these diagnoses.[63]

PREVENTION OF PRESSURE ULCERS

Prevention is the best intervention for pressure ulcers. By being aware of the risk factors for pressure ulcer development, assessing for changes in risk factors on an ongoing basis, and addressing risk factors, the incidence of pressure ulcers can be markedly reduced.[41, 80]

Pressure Ulcer Risk Assessment Tools

Pressure ulcer risk assessment tools are screening devices to help predict those individuals at risk for developing pressure ulcers. Risk assessments are commonly performed by nursing staff and should be performed upon admission to a service and if there is a change in patient status. In addition, it is recommended that a reassessment should be performed every visit in home health care, every 48 hours in acute care, every week for the first month in a long-term care setting, and quarterly thereafter if the patient's status is static.[11, 41] To be clinically advantageous, a risk assessment tool should have high specificity and sensitivity, be easy to use, and be linked to interventions to decrease risk.[41, 81, 82] By being able to accurately identify at-risk individuals, resources and services for pressure ulcer prevention can be more appropriately allocated to those most in need of interventions. For example, a patient who is bed-bound, unable to independently reposition him- or herself, and incontinent of urine should receive a more high-tech (and more expensive) support surface than a patient who is alert, ambulates independently, and is continent. Risk assessment tools generally consist of a series of numerically weighted subscales with descriptors to facilitate scoring. The total score indicates an individual's risk of pressure ulcer development. Several pressure ulcer risk assessment tools exist. The most widely used and researched include the Braden Scale for Predicting Pressure Sore Risk, the Norton Risk Assessment Scale, and the Gosnell Pressure Sore Risk Assessment. Of these three risk assessment tools, the Braden tool appears to be the most widely used, probably because it has the most research on a wide range of patient populations and has the best reliability and validity.[41, 83] The choice as to which risk assessment tool to use is generally a facility policy rather than an individual clinician's decision. Therefore, clinicians are encouraged to become familiar with the risk assessment tool used within their own facilities. In addition, clinicians should assess the effectiveness of their chosen risk assessment tool in preventing pressure ulcers on an ongoing basis.[41, 82] If the incidence of pressure ulcers is higher than expected, clinicians would be wise to examine both the choice of risk assessment tools and the interventions guided by these assessments.

Braden Scale for Predicting Pressure Sore Risk

The Braden Scale for Predicting Pressure Sore Risk consists of six subscales: mobility, activity, sensory perception, skin moisture, nutritional status, and friction and shear,[16, 84, 85] which have been shown to be associated with pressure ulcer risk.[1, 53, 86–89] Descriptions of each rank within each subcategory are provided to assist the clinician with scoring. Braden scale scores range from 6 to 23, with lower scores indicating greater impairment and higher risk. After a study on medical–surgical patients, a total score of 16 was considered the cutoff point at which a patient is deemed at risk for pressure ulcer development.[88] However, later studies suggest a score of less than 18 is a more accurate cutoff score for determining at-risk patients.[11, 80 87, 90, 91] In a study of patients in nursing homes, scores of less than 13 indicated high risk, 13–14 moderate risk, and 15–18 mild risk.[11] Eighty percent of patients scoring 13–15 developed pressure ulcers, although the majority of these are not severe (category/stage I).[16] In patients in the intensive care unit, all individuals scoring less than 16 had a pressure ulcer.[84] The specificity of the Braden scale has been shown to be 57–92%, while the sensitivity is 64–100%.[53, 83, 92–94] Interrater reliability is also high.[16] Of the three assessment tools, the Braden is the most well researched. The Braden scale requires less than 5 minutes to perform and has been shown to be a reliable and valid tool for the assessment of pressure ulcer risk (see Table 12–1). Pressure ulcer risk assessment for pediatric patients can be performed using the Braden Q scale.[1, 61] This assessment tool includes all of the Braden subscales as well as a tissue perfusion/oxygenation subscale. Braden Q scores range from 7 to 28, with lower scores indicating greater impairment and higher risk. A cutoff score of 16 for the Braden Q has a sensitivity of 88% and a specificity of 58% for identifying pediatric patients at risk for pressure ulcers.[95]

Norton Risk Assessment Scale

The Norton Risk Assessment Scale consists of five subscales: physical condition, mental condition, activity, mobility, and incontinence.[1, 90, 96] Each scale is rated 1–4, with lower scores indicating greater risk of pressure ulcer development. Each subscale rank contains a one- or two-word descriptor (e.g., "good" or "slightly limited") to assist the clinician with scoring. Norton scale scores range from 5 to 20, with a score of 20 being normal and indicating no risk. A total score of 16 is considered the critical cutoff score at which point a patient is deemed at risk for pressure ulcer development.[92] Individuals scoring less than 13 are deemed to be at high risk. Declining Norton scores appear to parallel decline in patient medical status.[96] The Norton scale has been criticized for its lack of descriptors and the absence of a nutrition-related subscale. However,

TABLE 12–1   Braden Scale for Predicting Pressure Ulcer Development*

Subscale	Description	Range of Scores
Mobility	Ability to change and control body position	1 = completely immobile 4 = no limitations
Activity	Degree of physical activity	1 = bedfast 4 = walks frequently
Sensory perception	Ability to meaningfully respond to pressure-related discomfort	1 = completely limited 4 = no impairment
Skin moisture	Degree to which skin is exposed to moisture	1 = constantly moist 4 = rarely moist
Nutritional status	Usual food intake	1 = very poor 4 = excellent
Friction and shear	Degree to which patient is able to move without sliding	1 = problem 3 = no apparent problem

*Adapted from Braden BJ, Bergstrom N. Clinical utility of the Braden scale for predicting pressure ulcers. *Decubitus.* 1989;2(3):45–51.

the Norton Plus Pressure Ulcer Scale, used in some institutions, contains a deductions section that accounts for malnutrition as well as other comorbidities. Using the Norton Plus scale, patients scoring less than 10 are considered to be at high risk for pressure ulcer development. The Norton scale has a sensitivity of 47–100% and a specificity of 26–89%.[83, 92, 93] Although the Norton scale compares favorably to the Braden, the Norton scale may overpredict the incidence of pressure ulcers (see Table 12–2).[84, 96, 97]

Gosnell Pressure Sore Risk Assessment

The Gosnell Pressure Sore Risk Assessment consists of five subscales: mental status, continence, mobility, activity, and nutrition. Each scale is rated 1–3, 4, or 5, with 1 being the least impaired. Total Gosnell scores range from 5 to 20, with the higher score indicating the greater risk (opposite of the Norton and Braden scales). In addition to the subscales, the Gosnell scale provides a uniform method of documenting vital signs, 24-hour fluid balance, skin appearance, medications, and interventions.[62, 98] Although the Gosnell Pressure Sore Risk Assessment includes some of the same subscales as the Braden and Norton, the weighting of these scales is different. Using a score of 16 as the critical cutoff score, a recent study found the Gosnell Pressure Score Risk Assessment to be more accurate in pressure ulcer prediction than the Braden scale, with a sensitivity of 85% and a specificity of 83%.[13] Despite this, the Gosnell tool is the least researched of the three risk assessment tools, lacking corroborating studies on standards, reliability, validity, and patient-specific populations.

Interdisciplinary Interventions for Pressure Ulcer Prevention

Once a patient is identified as being at risk for pressure ulcer development, interventions must be initiated to address and modify these risk factors.[1] As illustrated in Figure 12–4, the five arms of pressure ulcer prevention are education, positioning, mobility, nutrition, and management of incontinence. The preventive measures outlined in this section may also be required for patients who already have pressure ulcers. Although

TABLE 12–2   Norton Pressure Ulcer Scale*

Subscale	Description	Range of Scores
Physical condition	None	1 = very bad 4 = good
Mental condition	None	1 = stupor 4 = alert
Activity	None	1 = bed-bound 4 = ambulatory
Mobility	None	1 = immobile 4 = full
Incontinence	None	1 = incontinent of bowel and bladder 4 = not incontinent
Norton Plus PressureUlcer Scale Deductions†	One-point deductions for each of the following: diabetes, hypertension, low hematocrit, low hemoglobin, low albumin, fever, 5+ medications, or change in mental status over the past 24 hours	

*Norton DN. Calculating the risk: Reflections on the Norton scale. *Decubitus.* 1989;2(3):25–38.

†Norton DN, McLaren R, Exton-Smith AN. An investigation of geriatric nursing problems in hospitals. Centre for the care of old people. London, UK, 1962.

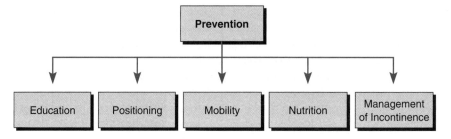

FIGURE 12–4   Interdisciplinary interventions for pressure ulcer prevention.

many of these interventions for risk factor reduction fall within the scope of physical therapy, some, such as nutrition and incontinence, do not. Some preventive measures, such as education and positioning, may be addressed by several disciplines. Therefore, an effective pressure ulcer prevention program requires a coordinated, interdisciplinary approach to patient care involving the patient, caregivers, physicians, nurses, nutrition services, and other disciplines. Interdisciplinary education and prevention programs have been shown to decrease the incidence of pressure ulcers from 7–31% to none[19, 99] and reduced the prevalence of pressure ulcers by as much as 90%.[18]

After the passage of the Deficit Reduction Act of 2005 (which was fully enacted in October 2008), health care facilities also have significant financial incentives to properly document and prevent pressure ulcers.[8] The Center for Medicare and Medicaid Services will no longer reimburse facilities at the same rate for pressure ulcers that are not clearly documented to be present on admission. One study found that health care provider adherence to evidence-based recommendations for managing tissue loads such as providing pressure relief and repositioning as infrequently as every 2 hours may be as low as 66% and 20%, respectively.[100] Barriers to implementing these changes that should be addressed by unit or facility managers include prior habits, lack of staff time, and inadequate access to needed supplies.[19] Mnemonics have been used successfully to help trigger staff memories and change habits (see Figure 12–5).[3] Having risk assessment results trigger automatic consults, streamlined documentation, and frequent brief re-training/re-education of licensed and unlicensed staff can also assist with implementing appropriate changes and interventions.[18]

Education

Education of patients, caregivers, and health care workers is key to the prevention of pressure ulcers.[27, 101] Patients should be instructed in how to perform systematic, daily skin inspections, especially of insensate skin or over bony prominences.[34] Assessments should be performed more often if erythema is noticed and

FIGURE 12–5   Mnemonics to assist with pressure ulcer prevention

Source: Ferrell VA, Artinian BM, Sessing D. The Sessing Scale for assessment of presure ulcer healing. J Am Geriatr Soc 1995;43(1):37-40.

NO ULCERS	
	Nutrition and fluid status
	Observation of skin
	Up and walking or assist with position changes
	Lift, don't drag
	Clean skin and continence care
	Elevate heels
	Risk assessment
	Support surfaces
SKIN	**S**urface selection
	Keep turning
	Incontinence management
	Nutrition

on high-risk individuals.[27] Mirrors and/or caregivers (including health care workers) should be used to assist patients as needed. Patients, caregivers, and health care workers should also be instructed in proper techniques for transfers and position changes to minimize shear by lifting, rather than dragging or sliding, the patient across support surfaces.[11] They should be instructed to manage incontinence promptly, by cleansing at-risk skin with mild soap and water, patting it dry, and using moisture barriers to protect the skin.[11, 20] Patients and caregivers should be informed that diapers are not a substitute for proper skin care. They should use talc-based powders to control excessive perspiration and moisturizing agents to keep skin adequately lubricated.[45]

Positioning

Preventing pressure ulcers may involve addressing patient position as well as the surface on which the patient is positioned.[20, 41, 102] At-risk patients should not be positioned directly on their side to prevent excessive pressure over the greater trochanter. Rather, a 30-degree lateral position should be used.[1, 26, 41, 51, 102] Pillows or foam pads should be used to prevent contact between bony prominences. The head of the bed should be kept in the lowest degree of elevation possible to decrease shear forces.[1, 11, 14, 44] Using a foot board or elevating the knees before elevating the head of the bed will reduce shear forces but not patient–surface interface pressures.[44] Bed linens should be free of wrinkles and particulate matter to avoid irritation and localized areas of increased pressure. Interface pressures between patient heels and the support surface have been measured in the ranges of 55–147 mm Hg.[103] For example, pressures over patients' sacrums have been measured as high as 60 mm Hg on emergency room gurneys and as high as 80 mm Hg on operating room tables.[48] Pillows or wedges may be used to prop heels off the bed to completely relieve pressure over these high-risk areas.[1, 32, 102] Several types of heel protectors are available on the market today, including those that reduce heel pressure with foam padding or suspend the heel above the support surface. However, because no one device has proven to be more effective in reducing the incidence of pressure ulcers, adoption of the lowest priced device would seem prudent.[103] Alternatively, the foot end of some hospital beds can be dropped to relieve heel pressure. Patients who are paralyzed or comatose are best treated by suspending or floating the heels off the support surface.[32]

However, this method is not appropriate for patients who are capable of repositioning themselves as they are likely to do so, resulting in insufficient pressure relief. Because no one position can prevent pressure ulcer development, patients must change positions often. Devices to assist patients with turning and repositioning, such as a grab bar or overhead trapeze, may be beneficial.[102] Caregivers and health care workers must assist patients who are unable to reposition themselves independently. Although many guidelines suggest patients be repositioned every 2 hours when lying down and every 15 minutes when sitting up, there is no one time frame that is acceptable for all patients.[1, 34] High-risk patients and patients who develop an area of erythema over a weight-bearing area that does not abate within 10 minutes of repositioning should be repositioned more frequently. Patients with microvascular disease, such as those with diabetes, have a blunted hyperemic response that appears to require complete pressure relief rather than pressure reduction to allow sufficient local tissue reperfusion.[32, 44] An individualized turning schedule, in combination with routine skin checks, can assist with pressure ulcer prevention.

Support surface technology, such as specialty mattresses or cushions, may also help prevent pressure ulcers.[102, 104] In addition to distributing pressure over a larger surface area, support surfaces may assist with controlling shear, moisture, and temperature.[21, 104] Donut-type devices, such as ring cushions, have been shown to increase tissue congestion, vascular occlusion, and pressure and should not be used.[1] Devices are not a substitute for changing positions or routine skin care.[1] Various support surfaces are discussed later in the chapter.

Mobility

Pressure ulcer prevention programs should encourage, rather than hinder, patient mobility.[20, 51] Intravenous tubing or other medical equipment should have sufficient length and be positioned so as not to restrict patient mobility. Likewise, bed linens should remain loose so that patient movement is not impeded. Patient mobility can be enhanced by avoiding oversedation and polypharmacy whenever possible. However, because pain can also limit patient mobility, there must be a balance between overmedication and adequate pain control. A study comparing a standard exercise program by nursing staff and bathroom cueing every 2 hours to standard care demonstrated an improvement in several pressure ulcer risk factors but not in the incidence of pressure ulcers.[105] Physical therapy may be prescribed to assist with patient mobility. Physical therapists and physical therapist assistants can improve patient mobility by instructing patients and caregivers in safe methods to change positions, get in and out of chairs, and ambulate. These clinicians may choose to instruct patients and caregivers in the use of assistive or adaptive equipment to enhance patient mobility. They may also improve patient mobility by prescribing exercises to improve patient strength, endurance, or flexibility. This more individualized approach to enhancing patient mobility may yield more substantial changes in pressure ulcer prevention.

Nutrition

Malnutrition is a significant risk factor for pressure ulcer development.[41, 54] For every gram decrease in serum albumin levels below normal, the odds of having a pressure ulcer increase fourfold.[34] In a 1991 study, no pressure ulcers developed in patients who had normal serum albumin and ideal body weight.[70] Therefore, all patients at risk for pressure ulcers should be assessed by a registered dietitian initially and reassessed at least every 3 months.[51] Healing of category/stage III and IV ulcers is related to increased protein intake[106] and adequate enteral feeding.[107] When necessary, nutritional supplementation or support should be initiated as soon as possible.[1] Refer to Chapter 9 for additional information on nutrition and wound healing.

Incontinence

Incontinence is significantly associated with pressure ulcer development.[9] It is estimated that 50% of nursing home residents are incontinent of urine.[108] Because diapers do not prevent moisture contact with the skin, the use of diapers is not a substitute for vigilance. Underpads that absorb and wick moisture away from the surface may be superior to bed linens or diapers.[87] However, moisture barriers, frequent checks for wetness, and speedy, gentle cleanup of incontinence are essential to preventing skin breakdown.[20] A prompted voiding program initiated by staff members in tertiary care units has been shown to help most patients stay dry[108] and, in combination with appropriate interventions to maintain skin dryness, such as moisture barriers and incontinence pads, significantly and dramatically reduced the incidence of pressure ulcers at a cost of just under $9.00 per resident per day.[109] Patients should be instructed to avoid foods that are known to be bladder irritants such as caffeine, alcohol, sugar substitutes, and large quantities of acidic foods such as fruits and fruit juices. Patients who are cognitively intact may benefit from neuromuscular interventions provided by physical therapists specializing in the examination and treatment of incontinence.[110] Basic patient care skills such as keeping a call light within reach, instructing patients/caregivers to alert nursing staff if linens are soiled, and posting visual reminders for staff to check patients hourly are other useful strategies.[8]

CASE STUDY: Dr. Sven Anderssen

This case study is referenced throughout the chapter.

PART 1

History

Sven Anderssen is a 71-year-old white male with a PhD in psychology seen this morning in outpatient physical therapy for wound management. Although his primary language is Swedish, he is fluent in English and lives with his 65-year-old wife who is legally blind in a two-story home. He volunteers as a lay minister 3 days a week and delivers Meals on Wheels 2 days per week.

Wound History: Dr. Anderssen reports his sacral pressure ulcer began last month during an 18-day hospitalization following an aortic valve replacement in which he was comatose for 8 days. Interventions to date include limited sitting and lying supine. According to the acute care nursing notes, initially the wound was treated with normal saline irrigation and collagenase covered with a gauze dressing secured with paper tape. This dressing was changed daily. When there was no improvement with this treatment, the dressing was modified to a skin sealant and hydrocolloid that was changed every 3 days. When measured yesterday prior to discharge from home physical therapy, no changes in wound characteristics were noted in the past 3 1/2 weeks.

Past Medical History: Aortic valve replacement 2 months ago, on 2 L/min of oxygen via nasal cannula since surgery, history of emphysema, fusion of L5–S1 without internal fixation in 1995. He was a two-pack-per-day smoker for 20 years, but quit entirely after surgery. He wears glasses and has a hearing aid for the right ear. He has no allergies.

General Health Status: Dr. Anderssen reports he is less fatigued over the past few weeks and is able to get around better, though he does get short of breath after about 5 minutes of walking with a rolling walker. He drove himself to today's physical therapy appointment. He would like to return to his previous activities and discontinue using his walker. He verbalizes frustration over his slow-healing wound and the lifestyle changes it has caused (limited sitting, sleeping on his stomach). He states he cannot see his wound and that his wife is putting the primary dressing on his wound.

Current Medications: Warfarin, digoxin, theophylline, ipratropium bromide.

Other Available Data: Laboratory values taken 2 days ago: hematocrit = 41%, white blood cell count = 6,500/mm^3, platelets = 310,000/mm^3, BUN = 9.5 mg/dL, creatinine 0.7 mg/dL, albumin = 3.2 g/dL, prealbumin 13.0 mg/dL, serum transferrin 155 mg/dL, blood glucose (random) 115 mg/dL.

Systems Review

Cardiovascular/Pulmonary System: Heart rate: 88 bpm, blood pressure 145/88 mm Hg, respiratory rate 22 bpm, resting pulse oximetry on 2 L/min of oxygen via nasal canula 93%, minimal nonpitting edema bilateral ankles and feet.

Musculoskeletal System: Gross range of motion and strength assessment reveals global lower extremity strength deficits. Stated height 6 feet (1.83 m), body weight measured 2 days ago: 133 pounds (60.5 kg). Body mass index (BMI) = 18.0 kg/m^2.

Neuromuscular System: Patient was observed seated in the waiting room while completing his intake forms demonstrating a posterior pelvic tilt, lumbar flexion, and increased kyphosis. Patient is independent with bed mobility, transfers with difficulty, and can walk short distances with his rolling walker. He is mildly short of breath walking from the waiting room into the examination room.

Gastrointestinal System: Patient and wife report he is eating about half of each meal since returning home 2 weeks ago.

Urogenital System: Patient reports no instances of incontinence of bowel or bladder, history of urinary tract infection while in critical care unit when he had an indwelling catheter. Reports his bandage sometimes becomes soiled after a bowel movement.

Integumentary System: Open wound over sacrum, closed sternal and lumbar incisions. Skin color: pale.

Communication, Cognition, Language, and Learning Style: Dr. Anderssen is able to communicate effectively in English during the examination. He demonstrates an understanding of his situation and frustration over his slow-healing wound. He reports he learns best by reviewing written information.

 Checkpoint Question #1

Why do the guidelines state that patients should change positions every 2 hours when lying down, but every 15 minutes when sitting up?

CLASSIFICATION AND CHARACTERISTICS OF PRESSURE ULCERS

Even with the most well-designed and implemented pressure ulcer prevention program, not all pressure ulcers can be prevented.[54, 64] Once a patient develops a pressure ulcer, clinicians must classify the ulcer and describe wound characteristics.

Classification

The Integumentary Preferred Practice Patterns in the *Guide to Physical Therapist Practice* described in Chapter 4 provide physical therapists with valuable patient management information for general wound care. However, other disciplines, including nurses, physicians, and insurers, use a different classification system. Since 1994, the standard definitions and treatment guidelines for pressure ulcers were known as the

staging system,[14] derived from Shea's classification system first developed in 1975.[22] In 2009 the European Pressure Ulcer Advisory Panel (EPUAP) and the National Pressure Ulcer Advisory Panel (NPUAP) published much needed updated definitions and guidelines for the classification, prevention, and treatment of pressure ulcers (see Table 12–3).[1, 41] The new categories and definitions have been quickly adopted by clinicians because of the problems with some of the previous definitions. However, the proper terminology for the classification system, the **International NPUAP/ EPUAP Pressure Ulcer Classification System,** has been slow to transition and many times in the United States continues to be referred to simply as the "staging system." Physical therapists must be familiar with the pressure ulcer classification system to effectively communicate with other disciplines regarding pressure ulcer severity (see Figure 12–6).

Several key changes include two new ulcer classifications as well as the attempt to move toward the

TABLE 12–3   International NPUAP/EPUAP Pressure Ulcer Classification System

Category/Stage	Description	Tissues Involved
Category/Stage I	Nonblanchable erythema of intact skin. In individuals with more highly pigmented skin, color may appear different from surrounding tissue. Area may be painful, warmer, cooler, firmer, softer compared to adjacent area.	May be superficial or the first sign of deeper tissue involvement. May indicate person at risk for pressure ulcer.
Category/Stage II	Superficial ulcer that presents as a shallow crater without slough or bruising. May be ruptured or intact (fluid- or blood-filled) blister.	Partial-thickness ulcer involving the epidermis, dermis, or both.
Category/Stage III	Deep ulcer that presents as a deep crater; may have undermining or tunneling.	Full-thickness skin loss involving the epidermis, dermis, and subcutaneous tissue. Bone/ tendon are not visible/palpable.
Category/Stage IV	Deep ulcer with extensive necrosis; often has undermining or sinus tracts.	Full-thickness skin loss involving the epidermis, dermis, subcutaneous tissue, fascia, and underlying structures, such as muscle, tendon, joint capsule, or bone.
Unstageable/Unclassified	A pressure ulcer should be described as unstageable if the base is obscured by eschar or slough.	Full-thickness. Will be Category III or IV.
Suspected Deep Tissue Injury	Local area of purple or maroon discoloration of intact skin or blood-filled blister. Area may have been painful, firm, mushy, boggy, or warmer or cooler than surrounding tissue. Wound may evolve and become eschar covered.	Unknown.

terminology of ulcer category versus ulcer stage. Tissue biopsies of what was previously defined as a stage I pressure ulcer have shown venous and capillary hyperemia as well as necrosis of the subcutaneous tissue.[35] For this reason, the revised category of Suspected Deep Tissue Injury is now preferred to what was previously classified as a stage I pressure ulcer.[1, 14] In the old staging system, the clinician was forced to guess the depth of an eschar-covered wound. The new classification system recognizes the inherent flaw in this by adding a new category, Unstageable/Unclassified with depth unknown, while still pointing the clinician and payors to the fact that this wound involves full-thickness skin loss. Another key change is that the new guidelines no longer recommend a particular type of support surface be used based on pressure ulcer category or severity[41] because no one support surface has proven to be superior to any other.

Benefits of the International NPUAP/EPUAP Pressure Ulcer Classification System

There are several reasons for using this classification system for pressure ulcers. First, since the system is universally understood, it promotes a uniform understanding of the depth of tissues involved. Second, the staging system and its revisions have shown to have excellent reliability.[111] Third, clinicians are required to classify or stage pressure ulcers for Medicare reimbursement.[104] Finally, the International NPUAP/EPUAP Ulcer Classification system can be used for research studies to determine the effectiveness of different interventions.

Limitations of the International NPUAP/EPUAP Pressure Ulcer Classification System

There are two main limitations to the pressure ulcer classification system. First, there are problems related to nomenclature. This system is used to classify *pressure* ulcers and does not take into account that many so-called pressure ulcers are, in fact, due to a combination of pressure with shear, moisture, or other factors.[112] This terminological error of wound etiology may decrease practitioner and caregiver understanding of the interventions necessary to heal and prevent pressure ulcers. Also, a category/stage I pressure *ulcer* is not an ulcer by definition, as the skin remains intact. Perhaps the term *preulceration* would be more appropriate for this type of lesion. Clinicians should strive to use precise terminology in their documentation and classification systems.

A second limitation of the pressure ulcer classification system is related to the staging concept. The revised guidelines attempt to address this by using Roman numerals as well as trying to shift clinicians into referring to ulcer *category* rather than *stage*. Despite the guideline's intent, the sequential numbering of this

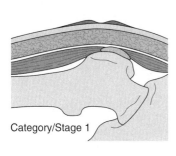

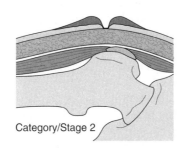

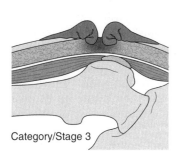

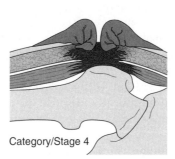

FIGURE 12–6   Schematic drawing of pressure ulcer categories/stages.

system implies both that pressure ulcers begin at the skin's surface and "progress" to involve deeper tissues and that ulcers heal in an orderly and predictable progression from one stage to the next.[112] Both of these implications are inaccurate.[113] For example, consider Mrs. D, an 82-year-old living alone who slips in the shower on Monday at 8:00 A.M., fracturing her hip. She is found on the floor by her neighbor 12 hours later. Mrs. D is admitted to an acute care hospital, and surgery is performed the same night to repair her femur. On admission to the rehabilitation floor, the patient is noted to have nonblanchable erythema without a break in skin integrity on the posterior aspect of her affected heel. The area is classified as a category/ stage I pressure ulcer and standard interventions are initiated to alleviate pressure on Mrs. D's heel(s). Two days later, the posterior aspect of Mrs. D's heel appears dark purple, it is boggy to palpation, and there is a slight drainage coming from an open area measuring 1.0 × 1.2 cm with a depth of 0.2 cm. The wound now would be classified as a category/stage III ulcer. The definitions set forth by the staging system indicate that the patient's wound has become worse while in the hospital, presumably as a result of inappropriate care. After all, the patient had no problem with her heel prior to admission to the facility. Although redness over a bony prominence is frequently the first sign of tissue damage, often there is already underlying tissue damage at the bone–tissue interface.[33] In reality, the pressure ulcer likely developed during the 12 hours the patient lay with her affected leg immobile on the hard tub surface. However, the deep tissue destruction was not detectable until the integument also became involved.[35] Moreover, this deep tissue damage can occur over the course of surgery due to positioning required despite appropriate care and vigilance and may be clinically unapparent for 2–6 days after the procedure.[35]

Clinicians using the staging system may erroneously "reverse-stage" pressure ulcers to imply the progression of wound healing. An example of reverse staging is when a wound is described as "progressing from a category/stage IV ulcer to a category/stage II pressure ulcer" when fascia, tendon, muscle, capsule, or bone is no longer exposed.[114] According to the normal wound healing model presented in Chapter 2, tissues destroyed in full-thickness wounds, such as tendon or capsule, do not regenerate. Rather, these tissues heal by scar formation. More correctly in this situation, clinicians should describe the wound as a "healing category/stage IV ulcer" or use the integumentary practice patterns. A significant problem is that patients with pressure

ulcers that are inappropriately "restaged" from a category/stage III or IV to a category/stage I or II will be denied acute or skilled care. This is because ulcers of lower severity do not generally warrant these interventions and, therefore, the interventions will not be reimbursed. As the newer nomenclature, category rather than stage, is adopted, this problem should be resolved.

Both the International NPUAP/EPUAP Ulcer Classification system and the Integumentary Practice Pattern classification systems describe the level of tissue involvement and attempt to guide appropriate intervention strategies. Physical therapists working with this patient population would be wise to use both classification systems. Since the staging system is universally accepted and understood outside of physical therapy, classification of pressure ulcers using this system will improve communication among different disciplines, assist with reimbursement, and facilitate interdisciplinary research. The practice pattern classification should also be used to assess wound progress, to assist with physical therapy research, and to guide prognosis, interventions, care plans, and outcomes. See Table 12–4 for a comparison of these two systems.

Characteristics

Determining the etiology of a pressure ulcer is generally quite simple if wound location and the patient's past and recent medical histories are known. Typical characteristics of pressure ulcers are described here using the 5PT method: pain, position, presentation, periwound, pulses, and temperature. Category/stage I pressure ulcers and suspected deep tissue injury characteristics are discussed separately. Color images 7 and 18 are examples of category/stage IV pressure ulcers.

Pain

Patients with intact sensory nerves generally complain of pain in the area of the pressure ulcer.[27] The McGill Pain Questionnaire, Visual Analog Scale, or the Faces Pain Scale are all useful for assessing pressure ulcer–related pain.[115] Obviously patients who are insensate, such as individuals with spinal cord injuries, cannot perceive pain. Patients with diabetes will seldom complain of pain if pressure ulcers are located on the heel due to peripheral neuropathy; however, more proximal ulcers will likely be perceived as painful. When working with patients with altered mental status or an inability to communicate, clinicians should assess for pain by looking for alternative signs of distress

TABLE 12–4 Comparison of the International NPUAP/EPUAP Ulcer Classification System for Pressure Ulcers with the Integumentary Preferred Practice Patterns

Category/Stage	Integumentary Preferred Practice Patterns
Category/Stage I	Pattern B: Impaired Integumentary Integrity Associated with Superficial Skin Involvement
Category/Stage II	Pattern C: Impaired Integumentary Integrity Associated with Partial-Thickness Skin Involvement and Scar Formation
Category/Stage III	Pattern D: Impaired Integumentary Integrity Associated with Full-Thickness Skin Involvement and Scar Formation
Category/Stage IV	Pattern E: Impaired Integumentary Integrity Associated with Skin Involvement Extending into Fascia, Muscle, or Bone and Scar Formation
Unstageable/Unclassified	Pattern D or E
Suspected Deep Tissue Injury	Depth of tissue involvement is unknown

such as withdrawal, moaning, or grimacing. This is especially important during local wound care.

Position

The vast majority of pressure ulcers occurs on the lower half of the body.[21] Pressure ulcers are most likely to develop over a bony prominence. Ninety-five percent of all pressure ulcers occur in five sites: sacrum, greater trochanter, ischial tuberosity, posterior calcaneus (heel), and lateral malleolus.[26] The sacrum is the most common site for pressure ulcers.[10, 52] The second most common location for pressure ulcers is the posterior calcaneous due to the large boney prominence, little subcutaneous padding, fat pad atrophy and peripheral arterial disease that occur with normal aging, and low resting skin perfusion.[32] Patients with spinal cord injuries tend to have a higher incidence of ischial pressure ulcers.[60] The occiput is the most frequent pressure ulcer location for children.[61]

The site of pressure ulcer development is generally position dependent if due to confinement or decreased mobility. Sacral ulcers are sometimes referred to as lying-down lesions, as they are more common in individuals who spend the majority of their time in bed due to the increased pressure over the sacrum in the supine or semisupine positions. Overall, patients with sacral pressure ulcers are more ill; that is, they have an increased number and severity of comorbidities compared to patients with ulcers in other locations. Likewise, ischial ulcers are sometimes referred to as sitting ulcers because of the increased pressure over these bony prominences in the sitting position.[116] The most common pressure ulcer locations by body position are illustrated in Figures 12–7 through 12–10.[21, 32, 41, 117]

Pressure ulcers may occur in other locations due to pressure from outside the body such as casts, splints, traction devices, catheter tubing, or ill-fitting shoes.[32, 61] The least susceptible locations for pressure ulcer development are areas where there is a significant amount of soft tissue between skin surface and underlying bone, such as the abdomen and thighs. The large amounts of tissue provide cushioning for tissue blood vessels so they are not compressed between externally applied pressure and the underlying bone.[17]

Wound Presentation

The International NPUAP/EPUAP Ulcer Classification System provides an excellent description of the spectrum of typical pressure ulcer presentations, ranging from nonblanchable erythema of intact skin to full-thickness destruction involving the epidermis, dermis, subcutaneous tissue, fascia, and deeper structures including tendon, muscle, joint capsule, and bone.[1] Unless previously debrided, a necrotic base is the norm.[22] Unstageable/unclassifiable ulcers commonly have a thick, black eschar that must be debrided before the clinician can accurately classify the wound. The presence

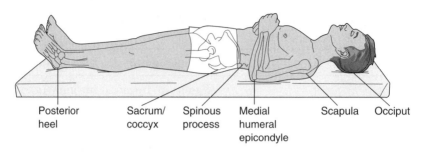

FIGURE 12–7 The most common locations for pressure ulcers while in the supine position are posterior heel, sacrum/coccyx, scapula, occiput, medial humeral epicondyle, and spinous process if emaciated.

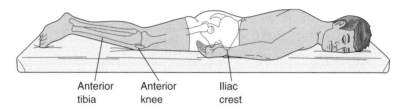

FIGURE 12–8 The most common locations for pressure ulcers while in the prone position are anterior knee, anterior tibia, and iliac crest.

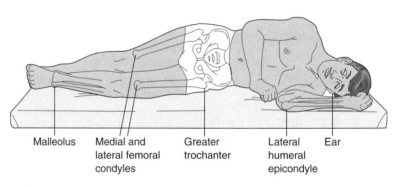

FIGURE 12–9 The most common locations for pressure ulcers while in the sidelying position are greater trochanter, malleolus, femoral condyle if emaciated, ear, and lateral humeral epicondyle.

of eschar means an ulcer is full thickness and will be a category/stage III or IV pressure ulcer once depth is known. The epidermal edge of full-thickness pressure ulcers typically thickens and rolls over the edge of the wound base, making the wound margins more distinct. If infected or heavily necrotic, deeper ulcers may drain profusely.[22] Tunneling and undermining are not uncommon with deeper ulcers.[1, 27] Intramuscular fascial planes may become more apparent because of separation by edema and fluid[22] and should not be mistaken for abscess or sinus tract formation. To ensure identification of bone, tunneling, undermining, and sinus tracts, all pressure ulcers should be thoroughly probed on initial assessment and routinely thereafter. Patients with full-thickness ulcers are more likely to have multiple ulcers[118] than patients with more superficial ulcers.

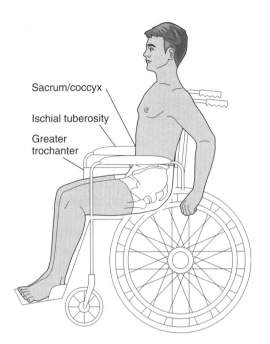

FIGURE 12–10   The most common locations for pressure ulcers while in the seated position are ischial tuberosity, greater trochanter if in a sling-like seat, and sacrum/coccyx if in a posterior pelvic tilt.

Periwound and Structural Changes

The periwound may be characterized by nonblanchable erythema or induration. The tissue may take on a mottled appearance. Typically, necrotic tissue is surrounded by a ring of inflammation.[34] Reactive fibrosis and thickening of the surrounding soft tissue is common.[22] In addition, there may be dermatitis of the surrounding skin secondary to wound etiology or location.[20] For example, dermatitis is common in incontinent patients with sacral pressure ulcers.[27, 39]

Dermatitis occurs in 5–27% of hospitalized patients and up to 73% of incontinent patients.[39] Fecal enzymes convert urea to ammonia.[51] Urine and ammonia further erode the skin and also raise the skin pH, creating an ideal environment for bacterial growth. Care must be taken to distinguish between skin damage due to dermatitis and pressure ulcers.[1]

Pulses

Because the majority of pressure ulcers occurs in the pelvic region, pulse examination is less routine with this patient population. Even with lower extremity pressure ulcers due to casts or traction devices, pulses are usually normal unless there is concomitant peripheral vascular disease.

Temperature

Areas of reactive hyperemia are typically warm to the touch, whereas necrotic or ischemic areas are cool.[31]

Category/Stage I Pressure Ulcer and Suspected Deep Tissue Injury Characteristics

It is critical to remember that both category/stage I pressure ulcers and suspected deep tissue injuries are injuries to *intact* skin. Muscle has the highest metabolic demand and is the least tolerant to compression, despite its rich vascular supply.[33] Muscle cells at the interface between bone and muscle are at greatest risk for pressure-related injury and cell death may occur in as little as one hour.[33] In contrast, skin is the last tissue layer to lose viability when subjected to pressure and can remain intact up to 14 days after losing viability.[32] Therefore, deep tissue injury may be present despite intact skin.

Category/Stage I Pressure Ulcer Characteristics

Category/stage I pressure ulcers generally present as sharply defined areas of nonblanchable erythema over a bony prominence. The clinician should assess for localized changes in skin temperature (warmer or cooler), tissue consistency (soft or firm feeling), and sensory changes (pain or pruritus) that are also characteristic of category/stage I pressure ulcers.[31, 48] Recognizing a category/stage I pressure ulcer in individuals with darkly pigmented skin may be difficult. These lesions may represent a person who is "at risk" for more significant pressure ulcers.[1] See Box 12–1 for typical characteristics of pressure ulcers.

Suspected Deep Tissue Injury Characteristics

These lesions appear as local purple or maroon discolorations of *intact* skin or a blood-filled blister.[1, 20] The area may have previously appeared to be a category/stage I pressure ulcer.[32] These lesions may also be difficult to detect in individuals with darkly pigmented skin.[32] Gradual changes may include the development of a thin blister over a darkened wound bed.[32] This may progress to a thin layer of eschar. Evolution may progress slowly or rapidly, exposing deeper tissue layers despite optimal care.[1, 32]

BOX 12–1	Typical Characteristics of Pressure Ulcers
Pain	• Tender or painful if sensory nerves are intact
Position	• Over bony prominence • Sacrum • Greater trochanter • Ischial tuberosity • Posterior calcaneus • Lateral malleolus
Wound presentation	• Deeper ulcers covered with black eschar • Deeper ulcers may have exposed tendon, muscle, capsule, and/or bone • Tunneling, undermining common • May drain profusely
Periwound and structural changes	• Surrounded by a ring of erythema • Nonblanchable erythema • Localized warmth • Fibrosis and induration • Dermatitis
Pulses	• Normal
Temperature	• Areas of hyperemia are warm to palpation • Areas of ischemia or necrosis are cool to palpation

 Checkpoint Question #2

What is the most common location for a pressure ulcer on a patient with a spinal cord injury? Why might this be so?

CASE STUDY: Dr. Sven Anderssen

PART 2

Tests and Measures

Integumentary Integrity: Full-thickness sacral wound at the superior gluteal fold 3.5 cm length × 3.0 cm width × 1.7 cm depth (wound surface area 10.5 cm²). Note wound depth is difficult to assess due to gluteus maximus muscle bulk. There is no tunneling or undermining. Wound bed is 75% yellow adherent slough covered and 25% pale granulation tissue.

Wound edges are thickened. Wound drainage: minimal, serosanguinous, thin. No wound odor is present. Periwound skin is slightly indurated to palpation. Skin temperature is within normal limits. Bates-Jensen Wound Assessment Tool (BWAT) score = 36.

Circulation: Capillary refill is 2 seconds.

Sensory Integrity: Patient is able to identify 5.07 Semmes–Weinstein monofilament in periwound, over ischial tuberosities and back.

Gait, Locomotion, Balance: Patient is independent with bed mobility, transfers relying heavily on bilateral upper extremities, and walking with a rolling walker up to 120 feet. Braden scale score = 16. Walking was limited by complaint of fatigue and shortness of breath.

Muscle Performance: Limitations noted in the following muscle groups bilaterally: knee flexion 4+/5, knee extension 4/5, gluteus maximus 3+/5, and gluteus medius 2+/5. Patient fatigues with testing and become mildly short of breath.

Pain: Patient reports 2/10 sternal pain with transfers.

Range of Motion: Grossly within functional limits.

Ventilation and Respiration/Gas Exchange: Patient is on 2 L O_2/min on nasal cannula, pulse oximeter at rest = 95%, with ambulation = 89%. Patient is an upper chest breather with hypertrophied accessory muscles of respiration.

PRESSURE ULCER ASSESSMENT INSTRUMENTS AND WOUND HEALING PROGNOSIS

Clinicians may perform various tests and measures to assess pressure ulcers, make a prognosis for wound healing, and identify changes in patient and wound status. Unlike the assessment of wounds due to vascular insufficiency or diabetes, the assessment of pressure ulcers does not require any special tests and measures in addition to the standard clinical examination outlined in Chapter 4. However, several **pressure ulcer assessment instruments** exist to describe various aspects of pressure ulcers and allow for identification of changes in wound status within a category or practice pattern. These tools are meant to measure changes in wound status, to evaluate the effectiveness of the plan of care, to document wound severity, to promote quantification of wound parameters, to standardize wound assessment, and to facilitate reimbursement.[1] Similar to pressure ulcer risk assessment tools, the choice of which pressure ulcer assessment instrument to use is generally determined at a facility level rather than by individual clinicians. Unlike pressure ulcer risk assessment tools, however, the use of pressure ulcer assessment instruments is not a standard procedure. However, the information provided by these instruments may ensure consistent and inclusive documentation of wound characteristics across disciplines. Clinicians should be familiar with the tool used by their facility and be aware of its strengths and limitations. This section describes the Sessing Scale; the Bates-Jensen Wound Assessment Tool (BWAT), formerly known as the Pressure Sore Status Tool (PSST); and the Pressure Ulcer Scale for Healing (PUSH©).

Sessing Scale

The Sessing Scale consists of a 7-point observational scale that describes wound and periwound characteristics (see Table 12–5). Higher scores represent more severe pressure ulcer status. Scores range from 0 (denoting normal skin that is at risk) to 6 (denoting purulent drainage, foul odor, necrotic tissue, and possible septic symptoms).[119] To assess changes over time, the reassessment score is subtracted from the initial score. Positive values indicate improvement, whereas negative values indicate a decline in ulcer status.[120] The Sessing Scale requires about a minute to complete after an initial half-hour training session, which may make it easier to use in the clinic than the Bates-Jensen Wound Assessment Tool (BWAT).[121] Some studies with small groups of patients and practitioners have been done to support the reliability and validity of the Sessing Scale.[120, 122] It appears to be responsive to changes in ulcer status, although further studies should be performed to confirm these initial findings.[121] The Sessing Scale is an appropriate assessment tool for use in both the clinic and research settings.

The Bates-Jensen Wound Assessment Tool (BWAT)

The Bates-Jensen Wound Assessment Tool (BWAT), formerly known as the Pressure Sore Status Tool (PSST), consists of 13 items describing wound and periwound characteristics, including size, depth, edges, undermining, necrotic tissue type and amount, exudate type and amount, skin color, tissue edema and induration, granulation tissue, and epithelialization (see Table 12–6).[123–126] Each item is rated on a 1–5 scale, with a score of 1 indicating tissue health and 5 indicating tissue degeneration. Two nonscored

TABLE 12–5   Sessing Scale

Stage	Description
0	Normal skin, but at risk
1	Skin completely closed
	May lack pigmentation or may be reddened
2	Wound edges and center are filled in
	Surrounding tissues are intact and not reddened
3	Wound bed filling with pink granulating tissue
	Slough present
	Free of necrotic tissue
	Minimum drainage and odor
4	Moderate to minimal granulating tissue
	Slough and minimal necrotic tissue
	Moderate drainage and odor
5	Presence of heavy drainage and odor, eschar, and slough
	Surrounding skin reddened or discolored
6	Breaks in skin around primary ulcer
	Purulent drainage, foul odor, necrotic tissue, and/or eschar
	May have septic symptoms

Directions:

Assign the numerical value associated with the description that most closely matches the observed pressure ulcer.

The scale is scored by calculating the change in numerical values over successive wound assessments over time. Positive scores indicate ulcer improvement and negative scores indicate worsening ulcers.

Source: Reprinted from Ferrell BA, Artinion B & Sessing D. The Sessing Scale. *Journal of American Geriatrics Society.* 1995;1(43):39.

items, wound location and wound shape, are also documented. Scores range from 13 to 65, with higher scores representing more severe pressure ulcer status.[119] Each item and scoring are adequately described in the accompanying instructions. The BWAT can be completed in about 10 minutes. Studies support the reliability and validity of the BWAT.[115, 119, 121, 124, 126, 127] However, the ability of the BWAT to respond to changes in ulcer status has not been assessed at this time.[119] The BWAT is an appropriate assessment tool for use in the clinic and in research settings.[123]

Pressure Ulcer Scale for Healing

The Pressure Ulcer Scale for Healing (PUSH), developed by the National Pressure Ulcer Advisory Panel, consists of three subscales: surface area, exudate amount, and wound appearance. Total scores range from 8 to 34, with higher scores indicating increasing pressure ulcer

severity. The PUSH requires less than 5 minutes to complete after about an hour of training initially.[119] The PUSH tool is a valid and reliable method for assessing and monitoring pressure ulcers.[115, 119, 128–131] A composite PUSH score may be used for patients with multiple pressure ulcers.[132] A PUSH healing score can be obtained by subtracting the reassessment score from the initial PUSH score: positive scores reflect improvements. The PUSH appears to be responsive to change in that lower scores paralleled wound healing,[130] but no statistical review has been performed.[121] Some clinicians feel that clinically important changes in ulcer status, such as changes in tunneling and undermining,[119] may not be detected with the PUSH tool.[129] When using the PUSH tool to monitor changes in pressure ulcers, only the surface area subscale has been shown to correlate with wound healing.[130] Therefore, it may be more advantageous to simply measure wound size rather than utilize the PUSH tool.[130]

TABLE 12–6   Bates-Jensen Wound Assessment Tool

BATES-JENSEN WOUND ASSESSMENT TOOL   NAME _____

Complete the rating sheet to assess pressure sore status. Evaluate each item by picking the response that best describes the wound and entering the score in the item score column for the appropriate data.

Location: Anatomic site. Circle, identify right (R) or left (L), and use "X" to mark site on body diagrams:

_____ Sacrum & coccyx   _____ Lateral ankle

_____ Trochanter   _____ Medial ankle

_____ Ischial tuberosity   _____ Heel   _____ Other site

Shape: Overall wound pattern; assess by observing perimeter and depth. Circle and date appropriate description:

_____ Irregular _____ Linear or elongated _____ Round/oval

_____ Bowl/boat _____ Square/rectangle _____ Butterfly _____ Other shape

Item	Data Assessment	Data Score	Data Score	Data Score
1. Size	1 = Length × width < 4 sq cm	_____		
	2 = Length × width 4–16 sq cm	_____		
	3 = Length × width 16.1–38 sq cm	_____		
	4 = Length × width 38.1–80 sq cm	_____		
	5 = Length × width > 80 sq cm	_____		
2. Depth	1 = Nonblanchable erythema on intact skin	_____		
	2 = Partial-thickness skin loss involving epidermis and/or dermis	_____		
	3 = Full-thickness skin loss involving damage or necrosis of subcutaneous tissue; may extend down to but not through underlying fascia: and/or mixed partial- and full-thickness and/or tissue layers obscured by granulation tissue	_____		
	4 = Obscured by necrosis	_____		
	5 = Full-thickness skin loss with extensive destruction, tissue necrosis, or damage to muscle, bone, or supporting structures	_____		
3. Edges	1 = Indistinct, diffuse, none clearly visible	_____		
	2 = Distinct, outline clearly visible, attached, even with wound base	_____		
	3 = Well-defined, not attached to wound base	_____		
	4 = Well-defined, not attached to base, rolled under, thickened	_____		
	5 = Well-defined, fibrotic, scarred, or hyperkeratotic	_____		

(Continued)

TABLE 12–6 Continued

Item	Data Assessment	Data Score	Data Score	Data Score
4. Undermining	1 = None present			
	2 = Undermining <2 cm in any area			
	3 = Undermining 2–4 cm involving <50% wound margins			
	4 = Undermining 2–4 cm involving >50% wound margins			
	5 = Undermining >4 cm in any area or tunneling and/or sinus tract formation			
5. Necrotic tissue type	1 = None visible			
	2 = White/gray nonvisible tissue and/or nonadherent yellow slough			
	3 = Loosely adherent yellow slough			
	4 = Adherent, soft, black eschar			
	5 = Firmly adherent, hard, black eschar			
6. Necrotic tissue amount	1 = None visible			
	2 = <25% of wound bed covered			
	3 = 25% to 50% of wound covered			
	4 = >50% and <75% of wound covered			
	5 = 75% to 100% of wound covered			
7. Exudate type	1 = None or bloody			
	2 = Serosanguinous: thin, watery, pale red/pink			
	3 = Serous: thin, watery, clear			
	4 = Purulent: thin or thick, opaque, tan/yellow			
	5 = Foul purulent: thick, opaque, yellow/green with odor			
8. Exudate amount	1 = None, dry wound			
	2 = Scant, wound moist but no observable exudate			
	3 = Small			
	4 = Moderate			
	5 = Large			
9. Skin color surrounding wound	1 = Pink or normal for ethnic group			
	2 = Bright red and/or blanches to touch			
	3 = White or gray pallor or hypopigmented			
	4 = Dark red or purple and/or nonblanchable			
	5 = Black or hyperpigmented			
10. Peripheral tissue edema	1 = No swelling or edema			
	2 = Non-pitting edema extends <4 cm around wound			
	3 = Non-pitting edema extends ≥4 cm around wound			
	4 = Pitting edema extends <4 cm around wound			
	5 = Crepitous and/or pitting edema extends ≥4 cm			

TABLE 12–6 Continued

Item	Data Assessment	Data Score	Data Score	Data Score
11. Peripheral tissue induration	1 = None present			
	2 = Induration <2 cm around wound			
	3 = Induration 2–4 cm extending <50% around wound			
	4 = Induration 2–4 cm extending ≥50% around wound			
	5 = Induration >4 cm in any area			
12. Granulation tissue	1 = Skin intact or partial-thickness wound			
	2 = Bright, beefy red; 75% to 100% of wound filled and/or tissue overgrowth			
	3 = Bright, beefy red; <75% and >25% of wound filled			
	4 = Pink, and/or dull, dusky red and/or fills ≤25% of wound			
	5 = No granulation tissue present			
13. Epithelization	1 = 100% wound covered, surface intact			
	2 = 75% to <100% wound covered and/or epithelial tissue extends >0.5 cm into wound bed			
	3 = 50% to <75% wound covered and/or epithelial tissue extends to <0.5 cm into wound bed			
	4 = 25% to <50% wound covered			
	5 = <25% wound covered			

TOTAL SCORE:

SIGNATURE:

Pressure Sore Status Continuum

1	10	13	15	20	25	30	35	40	45	50	55	60	65
Tissue Health			Wound Regeneration									Wound Degeneration	

Plot the total score on the Wound Status Continuum by putting an "X" on the line and the date beneath the line. Plot multiple scores with their dates to see-at-glance regeneration or degeneration of the wound.

Source: Harris, C, Bates-Jensen, B, Parslow, N, Raizman, R, Singh, M, Ketchen, R. Bates–Jensen Wound Assessment Tool: Pictorial guide validation project. *Journal of Wound, Ostomy and Continence Nursing.* 2010;37(3):253–259.

Prognosis

Clinicians should use pressure ulcer classification and patient and wound characteristics to make their prognosis for wound healing. Even with appropriate patient care, pressure ulcers are known to heal very slowly—slower than wounds due to trauma, neuropathy, or venous insufficiency. In contrast to biopsies from individuals without pressure ulcers, fibroblasts and epithelial cells taken from patients with pressure ulcers usually do not grow. Even after 2 weeks, the growth rate of these cells is only 70% of normal.[26] Although it is unclear why this occurs, one proposed explanation for the decreased healing rate is a decrease in fibrinolytic activity. Another hypothesis is that patients with pressure ulcers may have more comorbidities or more serious comorbidities than those without pressure ulcers,[133] although this is not a consistent finding within the literature.

After reviewing the available research on pressure ulcers, it is possible to make scientifically grounded judgments about wound healing prognosis. As with other types of wounds, wound size and the depth of tissues involved are known to affect healing time.[134] Category/stage I pressure ulcers may resolve within 1 to 3 weeks if cared for properly.[34] However, although redness over a bony prominence may be the first sign of tissue damage, frequently underlying tissue damage has already occurred, increasing healing time.[33, 98] Category/stage II pressure ulcers generally heal within days to weeks.[135, 136] While one study found the average healing time for category/stage IV pressure ulcers to be 19 weeks,[136] most studies report category/stage III and IV pressure ulcers will take an average of 8–13 weeks to reach full closure.[40, 137–139] Interestingly, although pressure ulcer category is related to healing time[57] and general health,[107] category is not associated with patient mortality.[133] Patients with better nutrition at baseline were more likely to heal or healed at a faster rate than those with poor baseline nutrition.[134] Pressure ulcer colonization is the norm rather than the exception. However, infection is less common. Full-thickness ulcers are more likely to

become infected than partial-thickness ulcers.[57] As with other wounds, infected pressure ulcers heal more slowly than uninfected ulcers.

An analysis of wound healing curves on full-thickness pressure ulcers shows that the decrease in wound size is not linear.[107, 140] Wound surface area generally increases after debridement.[107, 137] Once fully debrided, wound area decreases gradually initially, then the pace of wound closure increases during wound contraction, before slowing once again during epithelialization.[140] Pressure ulcers that progressed to healing showed about a 40–50% decrease in wound size within the first 2 weeks of treatment.[118, 140, 141] Therefore, pressure ulcers that do not decrease in size within 2 weeks should be reassessed for alternate or adjunctive interventions.[1, 118, 119, 140] In addition to this initial size reduction, pressure ulcer area should continue to decline over time. For example, one study found an 80% reduction in surface area in half of all category/stage IV pressure ulcers after 6 weeks of treatment.[140] Consequently, formal pressure ulcer reassessment should occur at regular intervals. If a wound fails to continue to improve every 2 weeks, the clinician should reassess the plan of care, its implementation, and consider the need for alternate or adjunctive interventions.[1]

CASE STUDY: Dr. Sven Anderssen

PART 3

Evaluation and Diagnosis

Dr. Anderssen has a category/stage III pressure ulcer consistent with Integumentary Preferred Practice Pattern D: Impaired Integumentary Integrity Associated with Full-Thickness Skin Involvement and Scar Formation. His BMI and laboratory data are consistent with mild protein-energy malnutrition and being underweight. Dr. Anderssen has impaired bilateral lower extremity muscle performance. In addition, he has limitations in community ambulation, decreased tissue oxygenation, and his oxygen saturation declines further with minimal activity. While wound management will be the primary focus of Dr. Anderssen's interventions at this time, his limitations in strength, respiration/gas

exchange, and mobility will also be addressed in Cardiovascular/Pulmonary Preferred Practice Pattern 6C: Impaired Ventilation, Respiration/Gas Exchange and Aerobic Capacity/Endurance Associated with Airway Clearance Dysfunction.

Prognosis and Plan of Care

Dr. Anderssen's pressure ulcer has not substantially improved in the last 3 1/2 weeks. The wound shows no signs of infection but has a high percentage of devitalized tissue despite a trial of enzymatic and autolytic debridement. His wound healing will be delayed by his decreased tissue oxygenation, malnutrition, and the normal effects of aging. In addition, his return home has led to an increase in sitting time due to fatigue with upright activities, which may place pressure on his wound.

The following functional goals have been discussed and mutually agreed upon:

1. Dr. Anderssen will be able to transfer on his first attempt without upper extremity support in four visits over the next 1–2 weeks.
2. Dr. Anderssen will be able to walk 500 feet × 2 including up and down three steps with a rail with oxygen saturation levels ≥95% while carrying 5–8 pounds to simulate his volunteer work in 12 visits over 3–4 weeks. He will manage his supplemental oxygen during ambulation and perform this task without an assistive device.
3. Dr. Anderssen's sacral ulcer will be closed and there will be no pressure-induced erythema after sitting upright with back support for 15 minutes in 31 visits over 10 weeks.

The following wound-related component goals have been discussed and mutually agreed upon:

1. The wound will be ≥90% granular in seven visits over the next 2 weeks.
2. Wound area will be decreased by 30% to ≤7.35 cm² in seven visits over the next 2 weeks.
3. Increase bilateral lower extremity strength to knee extension 4+/5, gluteus maximus 4/5, and gluteus medius 3+/5 in 10 visits over the next 3 weeks to assist with transfer ability.
4. Dr. and Mrs. Anderssen will verbalize an understanding of methods to enhance wound healing and self-manage his emphysema including a reduction in adverse mechanical forces to the wound area, maximizing tissue oxygenation, and improved nutrition.

Dr. Anderssen will be seen three times per week for 8–10 weeks to reach these goals. Interventions will include coordination, communication, and documentation; patient/client-related instruction; integumentary repair and protective techniques; electrotherapeutic modalities, physical agents, and mechanical modalities; therapeutic exercises, functional training, prescription of equipment, and airway clearance techniques.

PHYSICAL THERAPY INTERVENTIONS

It is estimated that 70–90% of pressure ulcers can be managed conservatively, that is, nonoperatively.[1, 21] Physical therapy interventions for patients with pressure ulcers consist of a tripartite approach of coordination, communication, and documentation; patient/client-related instruction; and individualized procedural interventions.[101]

Coordination, Communication, and Documentation

Physical therapy services for patients with pressure ulcers must be coordinated with the patient, caregivers, and other disciplines to maximize outcomes. In addition to the physician, physical therapist, and physical therapist assistant, health care team members for the management of patients with pressure ulcers may include occupational therapists and certified occupational therapist assistants, nursing staff, a medical social worker, and a registered dietitian. The roles of physicians and surgeons in the care of patients with pressure ulcers are discussed later in the chapter.

Physical therapists must communicate and coordinate care with occupational therapists because of the overlapping areas of expertise in terms of exercise, transfers, and wheelchair prescription. A nurse or nurse practitioner specializing in wound care may assist with patient and caregiver education, positioning, dressing changes, debridement where allowed by law, and the monitoring of wound progress in patients who do not require ongoing physical therapy. A medical social worker may be able to provide information about obtaining medical equipment and supplies in addition to assisting with discharge planning.

The association between nutrition and pressure ulcers warrants a dietary consult on all patients with pressure ulcers.[1] Because patients with good nutritional status heal significantly faster than those who are malnourished, a registered dietitian is essential to the successful management of patients with pressure ulcers. Nutrition is also an independent and significant predictor of pressure ulcer healing time.[134] Appropriate nutrition provides the patient with the correct combination of calories, protein, hydration, and vitamins and minerals needed for healing. If a patient with a pressure ulcer is malnourished, clinicians should encourage increased dietary intake or supplementation. If intake is still insufficient, nutritional support, enteral or parenteral, should be initiated (if it is consistent with the overall plan of care) to put the patient in a positive nitrogen balance.[1] Refer to Chapter 9 for more details regarding nutrition and wound healing.

In addition to communication and coordination of services, clinicians must provide appropriate documentation for insurers. Unfortunately, the incidence of pressure ulcers may be significantly underreported. A recent study reviewed the medical records of pressure ulcers in an inpatient acute care facility and found 14% of patients had documented pressure ulcers. However, upon examination, 33% of patients had a pressure ulcer.[142] Documentation of patient and pressure ulcer status is critical to ensure coverage of medically necessary support services. As discussed earlier, documentation of pressure ulcer classification is also required for reimbursement of services. Adjunctive interventions, such as electrical stimulation or ultraviolet light therapy,[1] should also be considered and will only be reimbursed if there is documentation to support the lack of wound healing with standard care.

Patient/Client-Related Instruction

Clinicians must provide patients and their caregivers with basic guidelines for caring for their ulcers, including how to cleanse and bandage the ulcer if they are to do so independently. If this is painful, patients should consider taking prescribed pain medication 20–30 minutes prior to dressing changes to allow time for the medication to take effect.[76] Clinicians should teach patients and caregivers the old adage: "You can put anything on the wound except the patient." Clinicians must educate patients and caregivers how to determine if there is a decline in ulcer status or ulcer infection, as well as how to respond to these changes. Patients and caregivers should also be informed that having a pressure ulcer does not preclude the development of additional pressure ulcers. Indeed, it increases the chance of additional pressure ulcers. Therefore, patients with pressure ulcers and their caregivers must pay careful attention to the pressure ulcer prevention guidelines outlined in Box 12–2.

Procedural Interventions

Precautions

Clinicians should be aware of two precautions when working with patients with pressure ulcers (see Box 12–3). First, clinicians must recognize the deceptive nature of pressure ulcers; that is, the depth of tissue destruction may be greater than it first appears.[21] Since the true extent of a pressure ulcer cannot be

---

BOX 12–2   Guidelines for Patients with Pressure Ulcers

Control pressure and shear forces

- Change positions or shift your weight at least every 2 hours while lying down and every 15 minutes while sitting. Do not lay on a body surface that is damaged or still red from prior positioning.
- Use positioning devices and cushions as instructed.
- Keep heels off the bed.
- Avoid pressure over bony prominences.
- Keep head of bed elevated as little as possible.
- Sit with good posture.
- When moving, avoid dragging your skin. Lift your body or have help to move instead.

Take care of your skin

- Perform daily skin checks.
- Wash with mild soap and water. Pat your skin dry.
- Protect your skin from wetness using a moisture barrier and/or incontinence pads as needed.
- Prevent dry skin with moisturizing lotion.

Take care of your ulcer

- Wear bandages as instructed.
- Cleanse your wound as instructed.
- Avoid pressure on your ulcer.

Control pain

- Take medication as prescribed.
- Consider taking prescribed pain medication 20–30 minutes before dressing changes if needed.

Eat a well-balanced diet and take supplements as directed

Notify your clinician if:

- You notice your wound is getting larger, is draining more, or has a foul odor.
- You have increased pain or swelling.
- You notice an area of redness that does not go away.
- You detect a new wound.

BOX 12–3   Precautions for Patients with Pressure Ulcers

Pressure ulcer depth can be deceptive

- Probe routinely.
- Classification may be inaccurate in the presence of eschar.

Ensure wound care goals and interventions are consistent with the overall plan of care

---

ascertained until the necrotic tissue has been removed, clinicians must use the new unstageable/unclassified category for accurate documentation. Clinicians must also understand that deep pressure ulcers may extend into body cavities, such as bowel and bladder, requiring surgical interventions. Second, and perhaps most important, clinicians must acknowledge that not all pressure ulcers can be healed and that wound closure may not be consistent with overall patient care. For example, aggressive pressure ulcer management is generally not a priority for patients with life-threatening illnesses or conditions. For this particular type of patient, the small, temporary change in skin integrity that may occur with aggressive treatment is not worth the risks of surgery, the pain of debridement, or the cost of adjunctive interventions.

Integumentary Repair and Protective Techniques

Request for Further Medical Testing

Because wound colonization is the norm rather than the exception, clinicians should not culture pressure ulcers on a routine basis.[1] Infections are uncommon in category/stage I and II ulcers.[1] Only wounds that fail to progress in a timely manner or that show signs and symptoms of infection should be cultured for infection. Wounds with exposed bone and wounds that are deep with purulent or foul-smelling drainage should be assessed for osteomyelitis.[27] Early surgical consult is advisable for patients with deep pressure ulcers.

Local Wound Care

The goal of local wound care for pressure ulcers is the same as with other types of ulcers: to create a warm, moist, granular wound bed with healthy surrounding tissue to promote wound closure.[1] Highlights of local wound care specific to patients with pressure ulcers are

included here. Refer to Section II for more details on general wound care. Note that category/stage I pressure ulcers may not require a dressing since there is no break in skin integrity. However, clinicians may choose to cover a category/stage I ulcer to decrease pressure or friction over the involved area. The topical application of balsam peru, castor oil, and trypsin to category/stage I and II pressure ulcers appears to result in clinically, but not statistically, significant improvements in wound healing time[135] presumably by increasing local tissue perfusion and maintaining a warm, moist environment conducive to healing. As outlined in Box 12–4, there are four keys to local wound care for patients with pressure ulcers: protect the surrounding tissue, address the wound bed, minimize pressure and shear forces, and educate patient and caregivers.

The tissue surrounding the ulcer should be protected from chapping or chafing, excessive moisture, and strong adhesives.[20, 54] Moisturizing ointment or lotion should be applied to protect and revitalize dry skin. Moisture barriers should be used to protect intact skin from excessive moisture due to wound drainage, perspiration, or incontinence.[106] Moisture barriers for patients with pelvic ulcers must be able to protect the skin from the chemical damage and bacterial load due

---

BOX 12–4   Keys to Local Wound Care for Patients with Pressure Ulcers

Protect the surrounding skin

- Moisturize dry skin.
- Use moisture barriers or skin sealants to protect from excessive moisture.

Address wound bed

- Choose dressings to provide a moist wound environment.
- Debride necrotic tissue if appropriate.
- Control infection.

Minimize pressure and shear forces

Educate patient and caregivers

- Wound etiology.
- Intervention strategies.
- Risk factor modification.
- Guidelines for pressure ulcers.

---

to urinary and fecal incontinence. Generally a water-repellent petroleum-based ointment works well.[49] Clinicians should read the product label carefully regarding how much barrier ointment to apply and the frequency of application. Some products are only to be used on intact skin, whereas others may be used in areas of dermatitis. In general, the barrier need not be removed if it is working, but, if desired, mineral oil or a mild soap should make barrier removal easy.[101] If it can be removed with water alone, the product is not appropriate for use as a moisture barrier.

Local wound care must address the wound bed.[47] Pressure ulcers covered with moisture-retentive dressings heal faster than those treated with dry dressings[107, 115] for several reasons. First, synthetic dressings stay in place better than gauze dressings. Some synthetic dressings are even manufactured in irregular shapes, such as the butterfly shape used for sacral ulcers, to facilitate wound coverage. Second, synthetic dressings present a continuum of absorption capabilities that can be left on for several days,[27] decreasing caregiver time, treatment cost, and patient discomfort. Third, since most pressure ulcers initially present with extensive amounts of necrotic tissue, synthetic dressings may be beneficial because they encourage autolytic debridement.[54] Although slower than surgical or mechanical debridement, autolytic debridement may be beneficial in home care and long-term care facilities as well as with patients who cannot tolerate surgery.[143] Because autolytic debridement is contraindicated for infected wounds,[143] synthetic dressings should not be used to manage infected pressure ulcers. Charcoal-containing wound dressings may assist with wound odor control by absorbing gas molecules released by bacteria.[1, 115] This may be particularly useful in patients who are not candidates for debridement to lower wound bioburden. While several studies have used topically applied growth factors, including platelet-derived growth factor, interleukin-1, interleukin-1β, and fibroblast growth factor, no significant improvements in pressure ulcer healing have been found.[1, 106]

Necrotic tissue should be actively debrided (if this is consistent with the patient's overall care plan).[1, 54, 106] In addition to autolytic debridement, clinicians may choose to use mechanical debridement or enzymes to create a granular wound bed.[1] Because of the thick eschar generally associated with pressure ulcers, sharp debridement should be performed in combination with enzyme use. Clinicians should ensure patients have adequate pain control for debridement and dressing changes.[1] Topical agents, such as EMLA cream (Eutectic Mixture of Local Anaesthetic) or lidocaine, may be helpful in reducing wound care–related pain.[115] The newest guidelines set forth by the European Pressure Ulcer Advisory Panel and the National Pressure Ulcer Advisory Panel state that stable, hard, dry, eschar-covered wounds in ischemic limbs should not be debrided.[1] These should be covered, protected from pressure and shear forces, and monitored daily for changes in status. If cracks, drainage, or signs and symptoms of infection occur, debridement is then indicated.[32] Appropriate referrals, such as a vascular or general surgeon, should be made.

Local wound care must also involve treating wound infection when present.[1] Pressure ulcers are often colonized with both aerobic and anaerobic microorganisms,[54] including *Escherichia coli, Pseudomonas aeruginosa, Proteus mirabilis, Staphylococcus aureus,* and *Streptococci.*[106] Debridement, silver-impregnated dressings, and/or a short course of appropriately diluted topical antiseptics should be considered for patients with infection or high wound bioburden that fail to progress toward healing.[1] Because infections are generally polymicrobial, treatment may require multiple drug therapy. Wounds that are slow to heal may benefit from a 2-week trial of topical broad-spectrum antimicrobial therapy or medical grade honey (if not allergic to honey, bee products, or bee stings).[1, 106] Patients not responding to this treatment should be cultured and appropriate antibiotic therapy or surgical debridement of osteomyelitis should be initiated as soon as possible.[1, 54]

Local wound care must address the cause of the ulceration in order to achieve wound healing.[26, 27] Support surface technology provides a means by which pressure to the wound, to the periwound, and over bony prominences can be minimized while the patient is in bed or sitting up. The basic premise of pressure-relieving devices is that, whereas a hard surface provides only a small amount of contact area, a soft support surface allows for a wider area of contact, thereby enveloping the body part and reducing pressure. **Tissue interface pressures** (the amount of pressure between a body part and support surface) can easily be measured. Generally, 32 mm Hg is considered to be the breakdown pressure[29, 144, 145] because it exceeds capillary closing pressure in healthy individuals.[20] Tissue interface pressures may provide a false sense of security, however, because capillary closing pressure varies with both patient and structural characteristics.[29, 31] Additionally, pressure is not the only etiological factor in the development of pressure ulcers.[31] Pressure-relieving devices are not substitutes for turning and repositioning, but may increase the interval between them without risk to skin integrity or wound healing.[1]

Support surface products are described as being either pressure reducing or pressure relieving and either static or dynamic. **Pressure-reducing devices** are devices that reduce interface pressures more than a standard hospital mattress or chair surface but do not consistently reduce pressures below 23–32 mm Hg.[145] Pressure-reducing devices are appropriate if a patient has more than one turnable surface.[145] In contrast, **pressure-relieving devices** consistently lower tissue interface pressures below the lowest measured capillary closing pressure of 23 mm Hg. Pressure-relieving devices include low-air-loss overlays and high-air-loss specialty beds.[145] **Static support surfaces** are non-moving devices that provide cushioning and pressure distribution.[146, 147] In general, a static support surface may be used if a patient can assume a variety of positions without weight bearing on an existing ulcer and without **bottoming out**.[1, 65] A **hand check** should be used to assess for bottoming out. To perform a hand check, while the patient is on the device, the clinician should place his or her hand between the support surface and the device with palm facing up. The clinician should feel 3/4 to 1 inch of thickness of support material between the patient's body and the support surface.[55] This should be assessed under existing pressure ulcers as well as under all areas at risk for pressure ulcer development. **Dynamic support surfaces** are electric devices that use currents of air or fluid to redistribute pressure across the body.[146, 147] The Centers for Medicare and Medicaid Services has three categories for support surface technology (see Table 12–7).[104] All surfaces the patient will be on—bed, commode, chair, car seat, etc.—must be considered.[51]

There are many classes of support surface products, including foam, fluid-filled, air-fluidized, low-air-loss, and alternating pressure. Choosing a product that will be successful for an individual patient can be facilitated by examining device and patient characteristics. Boxes 12–5 through 12–9 and Figures 12–11 through 12–13 provide additional information on each class of device.[51, 144–154] The updated NPUAP guidelines recommend providing a support surface that matches each individual patient's needs for pressure redistribution, shear reduction, temperature and moisture control, and mobility.[1] Patient body weight, deformities, tissue status, continence, risk for future ulcer development, ability to reposition, and transfers must also be considered. Last, product availability, reimbursement, and cost must be taken into account. A change in support surface is warranted only if clinicians have maximized holistic patient care and wound management and the wound fails to show signs of healing or is at high risk for additional ulcer formation.[1]

A randomized study comparing the effectiveness of foam mattresses and low-air-loss devices in nursing home patients with pressure ulcers found that ulcers healed three times faster for those patients using low-air-loss support surfaces.[117] A patient who has large category/stage III or IV pressure ulcers on multiple turning surfaces may benefit from an air-fluidized or low-air-loss device.[153] The low-air-loss device may be preferred because of the lower cost and ease of transfers. When combined with traditional pressure relief

---

BOX 12–5   Foam Pressure-Reducing Support Surfaces

Description: At least 4 inches of total thickness open or closed cell foam of varying densities and layers. Generally appropriate for patients at risk for pressure ulcers or with category/stage I or II ulcers.

Advantages: Inexpensive, lightweight, reduces pressure by deforming and enveloping body part, maintenance-free, ease of transfers, easy to modify or may be preformed, porosity allows moisture to diffuse, especially if used with a cover.

Disadvantages: Degrades over time, lasts about 3 years, tends to increase tissue temperature especially in hotter climates, easily soiled, only mildly effective in high-risk individuals.

TABLE 12–7   Centers for Medicare and Medicaid Services Support Surface Technology Classification

Category 1	Mattresses and mattress overlays
Category 2	Specialty mattresses
	Pressure reducing: foam, alternative air, low air loss, powered flotation, advanced pressure-reducing mattresses
Category 3	Air-fluidized beds

BOX 12–6   Fluid-Filled Pressure-Reducing Devices

Description: Multiple chambers filled with air, gel, or water

Advantages: Pressure and shear reduction, soilproof, maintain or decrease tissue temperatures, better pressure reduction through immersion than with foam, heavier patients less likely to bottom out than with foam, gel- and air-filled may be superior for sitting surfaces, moderate cost.

Disadvantages: Must monitor carefully. Gel may harden in cold weather, is heavy, and is noporous, which may allow moisture buildup. Gel may become dispersed and must be manually repositioned. Air- or water-filled devices may puncture or make transfers difficult. Air-filled devices must be properly inflated to ensure pressure reduction.

BOX 12–7   Air-Fluidized Support Surfaces

Description: Dynamic support surfaces that generally consist of silicone beads within a Gore-Tex sheet, which the patient "floats" on.

Advantages: Dynamic; allows pressure relief; controls moisture, shear, and temperature; easy for patients to reposition themselves.

Disadvantages: Expensive, may be noisy, high maintenance, high moisture-vapor transmission rate may dehydrate wound or patient, make transfers very difficult.

BOX 12–8   Low-Air-Loss Support Surfaces

Description: Dynamic support surfaces that consist of a series of air chambers or cells along with a special cover.

Advantages: Dynamic; allows pressure relief; controls moisture, temperature, and shear; head and foot of bed can be raised or lowered.

Disadvantages: Expensive, may be noisy, high maintenance, patient may slide too much during bed transfers due to low coefficient of friction.

BOX 12–9   Alternating Pressure Support Surfaces

Description: Dynamic support devices that provide pressure relief by alternately inflating and deflating multiple chambers with air.

Advantages: Dynamic, allows pressure relief, theoretically reduces frequency of repositioning, reduces shear.

Disadvantages: Expensive, may not control temperature or moisture, difficult transfers, cannot adjust head or foot of bed, high maintenance, requires frequent monitoring, patient complaint of noise/discomfort, high pressures during inflation may increase pressure ulcer incidence.

push-ups, new devices, such as special wheelchair cushions that alternate through anterior and posterior pressure relief cycles, have been shown to result in faster ulcer healing and greater percent surface area reduction when compared with a standard wheelchair cushion.[155] Because no one device is appropriate for all individuals, it is easy to become overwhelmed by the myriad classes and manufacturers of support surface technology. However, each patient will likely do well on a variety of surfaces. For patients in palliative care, pressure redistribution, support surface choices, and turning/repositioning should be replaced by patient

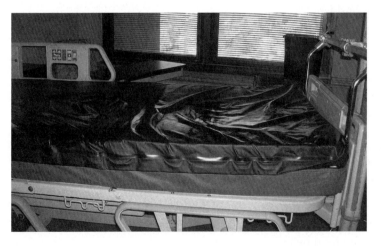

FIGURE 12–11   Foam mattress.

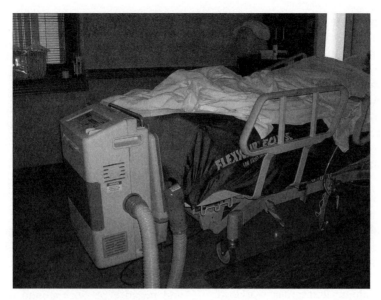

FIGURE 12–12   Low-air-loss support surfaces.

comfort and allowing the patient to adopt his or her position of choice.[64]

Therapeutic Exercise
Flexibility Exercise

Range of motion and stretching exercises should be used to prevent and minimize contractures. Contractures may increase the risk of pressure ulcer development by limiting patient mobility, making proper hygiene more difficult, and increasing pressure over bony prominences. For example, hip adductor contractures in a patient with paraplegia may lead to the development of pressure ulcers over the medial femoral epicondyles.

Strengthening Exercise

Strengthening exercises are beneficial to assist patients with bed mobility, transfers, and weight

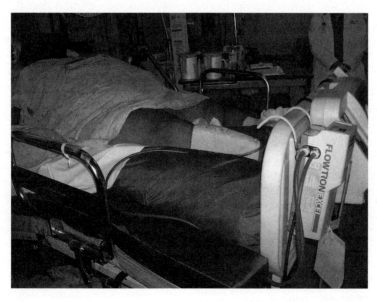

FIGURE 12–13   Low-air-loss support surfaces.

shifts.[80, 156] Improving upper extremity strength may allow patients to be more successful in rolling, moving from supine to sit, and using an assistive device for ambulation. Lower extremity strength training may help patients transfer more easily and become more ambulatory, thereby decreasing their risk of pressure ulcer development. Neuromuscular exercises to increase the strength and coordination of the pelvic floor and abdominal muscles may assist with the management of incontinence in patients who are cognitively intact.

Aerobic Exercise

Aerobic exercise can benefit patients by improving cardiovascular endurance to allow an overall increase in activity and mobility. Additionally, appropriately titrated aerobic exercise may improve tissue perfusion by increasing pulmonary volumes and cardiac workload.

Gait Training

Gait training may decrease the risk of pressure ulcer development and improve healing rates. Instructing patients in the use of canes, crutches, or walkers can improve patient mobility and decrease the need for caregiver assistance.

Functional Training

Functional training may be required to maximize patient activity and mobility.[51, 101] Training should emphasize minimizing friction and shear forces during transfers and bed mobility to protect intact skin and any existing pressure ulcers. Independent toilet transfers or transfers to a bedside commode may decrease the incidence of incontinence episodes and improve skin integrity.

Electrotherapeutic Modalities

Adjuvant interventions should be considered if a pressure ulcer does not show evidence of healing with appropriate standard care.[143] Electrical stimulation[101] is recommended for use in recalcitrant category/stage II as well as category/stage III and IV ulcers.[1] Ultraviolet, ultrasound, and negative pressure wound therapy may be helpful adjuncts to pressure ulcer healing.[1] Pressure ulcers with high wound bioburden or infection may benefit from a course of pulsatile lavage with suction or whirlpool.[1] However, these interventions may not be appropriate if wound healing is not consistent with the patient's overall plan of care. Chapter 8 presents detailed information on the use of these adjunctive interventions in wound care.

CASE STUDY: Dr. Sven Anderssen

PART 4
Interventions

The following highlights some of the key procedural interventions that will be incorporated into Dr. Anderssen's plan of care.

Coordination, Communication, and Documentation: Dr. Anderssen's physician will be contacted regarding his oxygen desaturation with mobility to determine the need for modification of his current oxygen use. A consult with a registered dietitian to assist with Dr. Anderssen's mild protein-calorie malnutrition was requested.

Patient/Client-Related Instruction: Dr. Anderssen will be instructed in the importance of limiting pressure and shear forces on his wound, which will include modifying his lifestyle short term to eliminate sitting in a posterior pelvic tilt or against seat backs as well as significantly limiting sitting and lying supine. After assessing Mrs. Anderssen's visual acuity to identify the wound and dressing location, she will be instructed in how to check the dressing to ensure it is intact between therapy sessions and how to replace the dressing if it becomes dislodged or ineffective. The Anderssens will be instructed in the importance of proper nutrition and encouraged to prepare meals that Dr. Anderssen enjoys and to have a protein drink, such as Ensure or Boost, twice daily for a high-energy snack while awaiting his consult with the registered dietitian. Dr. Anderssen will be instructed in the long-term management of his emphysema, including energy conservation strategies, the importance of continued abstinence of smoking, activity modification, and reduction of adverse effects by way of preventive strategies (e.g., flu shots, aerobic exercise, diet, sleep, stress management).

Procedural Interventions:

- Local wound management will consist of pulsed lavage with suction to irrigate the wound and assist with the removal of adherent slough. Sharp debridement will be initiated due to the lack of increase in granulation tissue with both enzymatic and autolytic debridement to date. Dr. Anderssen's wound has shown no progress in the last 3 1/2 weeks, and he has several health factors contributing to delayed wound healing, including increased age, poor tissue oxygenation, and mild protein-calorie malnutrition. Therefore, it was decided that electrical stimulation would be initiated to assist with wound healing. The following setup and parameters will be used. With Dr. Anderssen prone, saline-moistened electrodes will be applied using the direct technique with one electrode placed in the wound bed and the second electrode placed 15 cm superior. High-voltage pulsed current with an initial setting of 100 Hertz, positive polarity, and an intensity of 75–200 volts that produces a comfortable paresthesia for 45 minutes. The wound will be bandaged with a skin sealant and a hydrocolloid. This dressing was chosen despite the treatment frequency due to Dr. Anderssen's high level of mobility, wound location and potential for contamination from bowel movements, and Mrs. Anderssen's visual acuity leading to a limited ability to safely perform more complex dressing changes. If periwound skin breakdown is noted, the dressing choice or treatment frequency will be modified.
- Therapeutic exercises will focus on the large muscle groups of the lower extremities for both strengthening and endurance. Sample exercises might include mini-squats as well as standing or prone hip extension and abduction. Aerobic exercises, such as a standing upper body ergometer, walking, or stepping exercise, will be incorporated as able.
- Functional training will focus on improved transfers and gait training weaning off of the rolling walker as safety and endurance allow.
- Because Dr. Anderssen must drive due to his wife's blindness and his functional endurance is so limited, he will be prescribed a specialized seat cushion to ensure proper alignment as well as eliminate sacral pressure during limited sitting in the car and at home. A specialized mattress is not indicated due to Dr. Anderssen's mobility and because he can safely assume multiple sleep positions.
- Airway clearance techniques will include pursed breathing techniques, breath pattern training, and self-monitoring of respiratory distress using a dyspnea scale.

Reassessment

Dr. Anderssen's response to interventions will be monitored at all times. His wound will be formally reassessed weekly and plan of care modified if there are any adverse effects or if no improvements are noted after 2 weeks of treatment.

 Checkpoint Question #3

You are trying to decide upon the most appropriate wheelchair cushion for your patient, Ms. B, who has multiple sclerosis. Ms. B is obese, transfers independently but with some difficulty, and is incontinent of urine. She works 2 hours a day delivering documents, which requires her to transfer in and out of her car often. What type of wheelchair cushion do you think is most appropriate? Support your rationale.

MEDICAL AND SURGICAL INTERVENTIONS

Although medical and surgical interventions are clearly outside the scope of physical therapy, they are presented here to provide a better understanding of the valuable roles these disciplines play in the management of patients with pressure ulcers.

Medical Interventions

Physicians play a key role in the management of patients with pressure ulcers by selecting additional medical tests, managing risk factors, and prescribing pharmacological interventions. Physician involvement is critical in patients with wounds that fail to improve or are slow to heal. Surgical consultation should be considered in patients with nonhealing category/stage III and IV ulcers.[1, 101] Clinicians must be aware of these services to determine when a physician referral should be requested to assist in the overall care of patients with pressure ulcers.

Medical Testing

Unlike wounds of other etiologies, additional diagnostic studies are rarely needed to confirm clinical impressions regarding wound etiology in patients with pressure ulcers. Pressure ulcers presenting with signs and symptoms of infection should be cultured and followed up with appropriate antibiotic therapy. Deep ulcers with profuse drainage or foul odor and ulcers with exposed bone should be assessed for the presence of osteomyelitis. Patients who are septic or who have infected wounds require immediate, appropriate antibiotic coverage.[1] Because of the association between malnutrition and pressure ulcer development and healing, all patients with pressure ulcers should be assessed for septicemia and nutritional deficits. A sign of suboptimal nutrition is if body weight has changed by more than 5% in a month or 10% in 6 months.[1] If consistent with overall patient care, the National Pressure Ulcer Advisory Panel suggests nutritional supplementation or support for patients who are malnourished.[1] Patients should be reassessed at least every 3 months or if there is a change in status.[1]

Management of Risk Factors

By managing risk factors and controlling underlying conditions, such as malnutrition, anemia, and diabetes, physicians can increase the healing potential of patients with pressure ulcers.[21] Patients who are incontinent should be assessed by a urologist to identify causes for incontinence as well as intervention strategies.[80]

Pharmacological Interventions

Antibiotics should be initiated in patients with infection, advancing cellulitis, osteomyelitis, or sepsis.[1, 40] Because of the link between dementia and pressure ulcer development,[9] medication to manage dementia may decrease the risk of pressure ulcers and improve the rate of wound healing. Patients who are alert and coherent heal more quickly than those who are not.[134] Therefore, physicians should limit the amount of medication and sedation as much as medically feasible. However, physicians must try to strike a balance between oversedation and inadequate pain management.[76]

Surgical Interventions

Health care providers should be aware of some of the surgical interventions that may be available to patients with pressure ulcers if conservative treatment options fail. Although direct surgical closure and skin grafting are beneficial surgical interventions for other types of wounds, these procedures are rarely successful in patients with pressure ulcers. Pressure ulcers treated by direct closure generally dehisce because of the high tension required to bridge the wound defect. Skin grafting provides barrier protection only and neither fills the wound void nor protects the areas from future pressure.[1, 156] The blood supply to skin grafts is tenuous, increasing the risk of graft failure. Therefore, the most common surgical interventions for pressure ulcers are surgical debridement and musculocutaneous flap closure. Because of the high postoperative mortality rate in this patient population, as much as 69%, the least invasive procedure should be performed.[157]

Debridement

Surgical debridement is faster than enzymatic, autolytic, or nonsurgical debridement. In general, surgical debridement is reserved for patients with category/stage III or IV pressure ulcers that require extensive debridement.[1, 158] Surgical debridement of infected pressure ulcers of this type has been shown to improve patient survival over antibiotics alone.[27] As with other wounds, surgical excision of infected bone is required in the presence of osteomyelitis.[1, 158] Only the infected portion of the bone should be debrided, leaving a smooth, nonprominent surface to reduce pressure to the area.[158]

Musculocutaneous Flaps

The use of **musculocutaneous flaps** for surgical closure of category/stage IV pressure ulcers has dramatically increased.[159] Musculocutaneous flaps have several features that make them ideal for closing deep pressure ulcers. The muscle and its robust vasculature are transferred to the site of the pressure ulcer. This improves healing rates, decreases the risk of infection, and better supports the overlying integument.[159, 160] Muscle flaps provide greater tissue bulk to fill the wound defect and provide a degree of padding. [156, 159] This eliminates dead space within the previous wound bed, decreasing the risk of abscess and improving flap take. The padding and improved vascular supply may also help lower the risk of reulceration to some extent.[156]

Surgical debridement and musculocutaneous flaps are generally performed as one procedure.[1] Candidates for this procedure must be able to tolerate surgery and have no signs of infection. During the operation, the surgeon prepares the wound bed by removing all necrotic and scar tissue present. The muscle chosen for a flap procedure depends on the individual patient's anatomy, functional abilities, wound depth, and wound location. The gluteus maximus is most commonly used to close sacral and ischial pressure ulcers, while the tensor fascia lata is used for ulcers over the greater trochanter.[160] The borders of the muscle chosen for the flap are first outlined on the patient's skin. Then the skin and subcutaneous tissues are incised to the deep fascia. The muscle is dissected and released from the surrounding tissue. The flap is then transpositioned into the pressure ulcer cavity and sutured to the surrounding tissue. To aid in postoperative healing, flaps should not cross bony prominences.

A drain is generally placed at the time of surgery to help collapse dead space and prevent postoperative complications such as hematomas and seromas.[158, 160] An open drain, called a Penrose drain, is simply a latex-free tube with one end sutured within the wound bed and the other end extending out from the wound, allowing drainage or blood to passively flow into the dressing.[161] Alternatively, a closed or suction drain, such as a Hemovac or Jackson Pratt drain, may be used.[161] Such drains apply a negative pressure to the wound and collect drainage into a bulb measurement container. Drains must be monitored closely to ensure they remain in place and they are not blocked either

from external forces, such as kinked tubing, or internal forces, such as clot formation within the tubing.[161] Drains are generally removed once drainage is adequately controlled. Some surgeons prefer not to use postoperative drains because they may provide a pathway for bacteria to enter the surgical site.[161]

After surgery, antibiotics are used prophylactically.[160] The patient is typically placed on a low-air-loss or air-fluidized mattress for a minimum of 2 weeks (assuming pressure ulcer in the pelvic region). Splints are used to immobilize extremity grafts.[162] Drains generally stay in place for about 1 week post-surgery. Pressure and shear are strictly avoided immediately postoperatively,[158] especially during position changes.[1] Gradually, the patient is allowed to increase sitting or lying times on the affected areas to build up a tolerance to pressure. The flap must be constantly reassessed for adverse reactions to this increase in forces.[1] A healthy flap appears pink in color. If the flap is red or cyanotic, this should resolve within 10 minutes of changing positions. The temperature of the involved tissue should be approximately the same as adjacent tissues. An increase in flap temperature may signal an infection, whereas a decrease in temperature may indicate tissue ischemia. Capillary refill or Doppler ultrasound should be used to monitor flap perfusion. Flaps should also be positioned to prevent venous congestion, either by elevation or, in the case of trunk flaps, by avoiding weight bearing/dependency. Flaps should feel soft. Induration and/or a purple discoloration are signs of venous congestion and warrant a change in patient positioning or additional compression bandaging (for extremity flaps).[162] The physician should be notified if a musculocutaneous flap shows signs of infection or deterioration, such as excessive bleeding or drainage, hematoma or seroma formation, persistent color changes, increasing edema, or significant pain.[1]

Several factors, aside from surgical technique, affect flap survival. The primary reason for postoperative complications is venous congestion. However, patient adherence, particularly to positioning and weight bearing, is also critical to flap survival. Infection and hematoma/seroma formation may also compromise flap integrity. Patient characteristics, such as malnutrition, poor glycemic control, smoking, and peripheral vascular disease in the affected areas without concomitant revascularization, are known to adversely affect flap success.[162, 163] Musculocutaneous flaps are not a panacea.[156] Without careful monitoring of flap take, gradual progression of forces upon the affected area, and correction of the contributing factors that initiated the wound, there is a 38% recurrence rate.[157] Patients and caregivers must still be thoroughly instructed in measures necessary to prevent pressure ulcers.

CHAPTER SUMMARY

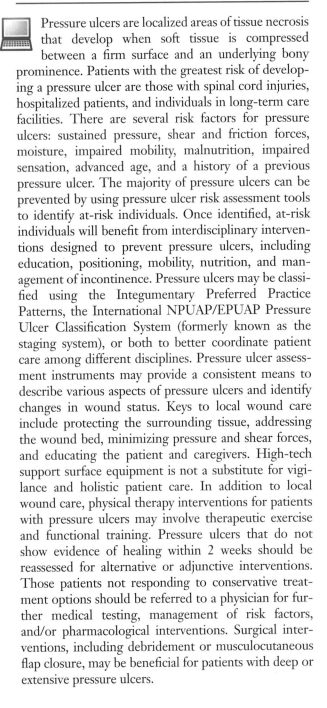

Pressure ulcers are localized areas of tissue necrosis that develop when soft tissue is compressed between a firm surface and an underlying bony prominence. Patients with the greatest risk of developing a pressure ulcer are those with spinal cord injuries, hospitalized patients, and individuals in long-term care facilities. There are several risk factors for pressure ulcers: sustained pressure, shear and friction forces, moisture, impaired mobility, malnutrition, impaired sensation, advanced age, and a history of a previous pressure ulcer. The majority of pressure ulcers can be prevented by using pressure ulcer risk assessment tools to identify at-risk individuals. Once identified, at-risk individuals will benefit from interdisciplinary interventions designed to prevent pressure ulcers, including education, positioning, mobility, nutrition, and management of incontinence. Pressure ulcers may be classified using the Integumentary Preferred Practice Patterns, the International NPUAP/EPUAP Pressure Ulcer Classification System (formerly known as the staging system), or both to better coordinate patient care among different disciplines. Pressure ulcer assessment instruments may provide a consistent means to describe various aspects of pressure ulcers and identify changes in wound status. Keys to local wound care include protecting the surrounding tissue, addressing the wound bed, minimizing pressure and shear forces, and educating the patient and caregivers. High-tech support surface equipment is not a substitute for vigilance and holistic patient care. In addition to local wound care, physical therapy interventions for patients with pressure ulcers may involve therapeutic exercise and functional training. Pressure ulcers that do not show evidence of healing within 2 weeks should be reassessed for alternative or adjunctive interventions. Those patients not responding to conservative treatment options should be referred to a physician for further medical testing, management of risk factors, and/or pharmacological interventions. Surgical interventions, including debridement or musculocutaneous flap closure, may be beneficial for patients with deep or extensive pressure ulcers.

REVIEW QUESTIONS

1. Your patient, Mrs. K., is a 34-year-old admitted to the hospital for failure to thrive. Mrs. K has chronic renal and liver failure and has multiple pressure ulcers. She has been bed-bound for the last 2 weeks because of pain and weakness. The attending physician orders a physical therapy consult for wound care. During your examination you find Mrs. K requires maximum assist to roll from side to side on her low-air-loss mattress and complains of extreme pain when doing so despite being premedicated prior to your session. She has dry, thick, black eschar-covered pressure ulcers ranging in size from 2×2 cm to 12×15 cm over her greater trochanters, heels, sacrum/coccyx, lateral malleoli, and left medial malleolus. The ulcers do not have an odor, and there is no erythema present. Bilateral lower extremities have pitting edema. During your attempts to debride the eschar at bedside the patient reports excruciating pain and sobs. You are unable to detect any granular tissue. When you call the physician, he states that the patient cannot have any more pain medication for fear of further compromising her respiratory system. In addition, the physician reports that the patient has decided to discontinue her dialysis program and that palliative care has been initiated. Provide your answers along with your rationale for the following questions.

   a. Should you debride Mrs. K's wounds?

   b. Should you refer Mrs. K for a surgical consult to manage her pressure ulcers?

   c. Is Mrs. K a candidate for electrical stimulation to assist with wound healing?

   d. What type of dressing would you use for Mrs. K?

2. Use the wound in color image 7 to answer the following series of questions.

   Your patient, Miss T, is a 68-year-old with Alzheimer's who presents for an initial physical therapy evaluation of a pressure ulcer over her left greater trochanter. The ulcer began 5 months ago and was surgically debrided to remove necrotic tissue and osteomyelitis 3 days prior to your examination. There is a moderate amount of serosanguinous drainage without odor.

   a. Document wound and periwound characteristics as you would in the patient's chart.

b. Should you debride this wound? Why or why not?

c. Describe how you might bandage Miss T's wound.

d. What positioning suggestions do you have for the nursing staff?

e. Describe other physical therapy interventions that you might include in your plan of care. Provide your rationale.

f. Are there any consults you would request for this patient? Provide your rationale.

3. You are working with a patient with a pressure ulcer over the greater trochanter. Two weeks ago the wound measured 3.4 × 4.2 cm with a depth of 0.4 cm. The wound bed contains 80% black eschar and 20% adherent yellow slough. There is a slight amount of thin yellow drainage and no odor after saline rinse. You categorize the wound as unstageable/unclassified secondary to eschar. When you reassess the patient today the wound measures 3.9 × 5.0 cm with a depth of 0.9 cm. There is 0.5 cm of undermining from the 12-o'clock position to the 6-o'clock position. The wound bed is 75% granular and 25% adherent yellow slough. There is minimal serosanguinous drainage and no odor after saline rinse. The greater trochanter is palpable with probing.

a. Classify the ulcer according to the International NPUAP/EPUAP Pressure Ulcer Classification System and the Integumentary Preferred Practice Patterns.

b. Is the wound improving or regressing? Defend your answer.

c. Is the wound infected?

REFERENCES

Go to myhealthprofessionskit.com to view this chapter's references.

13

Neuropathic Ulcers

Chapter Objectives

After reading this chapter, learners will be able to:

1. Differentiate the etiology of neuropathic ulcers from other types of open wounds.
2. Explain the risk factors contributing to neuropathic ulceration and delayed wound healing.
3. Compare and contrast the Wagner classification system for classifying neuropathic ulcers with the Integumentary Preferred Practice Pattern classification system.
4. Assess the typical characteristics of neuropathic ulcers.
5. Design an interdisciplinary approach to the management of patients with neuropathic ulcers.
6. Select physical therapy procedural interventions for patients with neuropathic ulcers, including integumentary repair and protective techniques, therapeutic exercise, devices and equipment, manual therapy techniques, and electrotherapeutic modalities.
7. Describe precautions clinicians should be aware of when working with patients with neuropathic ulcers.
8. Integrate the keys to local wound care for patients with neuropathic ulcers.
9. Discuss the purpose, indications, and contraindications for total contact casting.
10. Discuss possible medical and surgical interventions for patients with neuropathic ulcers.

Key Terms

Autonomic neuropathy	Neuropathic ulceration	Total contact cast
Charcot foot	Padded ankle-foot	Wagner classification
Incision and drainage	orthoses	system
Motor neuropathy	Sensory neuropathy	Walking splint

INTRODUCTION

Neuropathic ulcerations, also known as diabetic ulcerations, pose a serious health problem for patients with diabetes and are associated with significant morbidity, mortality, and financial burden.[1–3] More than 24 million people in the United States have diabetes.[4] While most studies report approximately 15% of individuals with diabetes have had an ulcer on the foot or ankle,[5–7] the incidence of neuropathic ulceration may be as high as 25%.[8] The age-adjusted rate of lower extremity amputations for people with diabetes is 15 times greater than it is for individuals without diabetes.[9] In the United States, diabetes is responsible for over 600,000 amputations annually,[10] with 80–85% of these following a foot ulceration.[5, 8] Half of these patients will experience a contralateral foot ulceration within 18 months of their first amputation, and more than half of these individuals will undergo a second amputation within 3 to 5 years of the first amputation.[10] Additionally, the 3-year survival rate of patients with diabetes after a lower extremity amputation is 14% after a toe amputation, 33% after a below-knee amputation, and as high as 71% after an above-knee amputation.[11] Five years after amputation, these numbers significantly increase to mortality rates of 41%, 63%, and 86%, respectively.[11] While these numbers may sound quite bleak, outcomes for patients with neuropathic ulcerations are improving. Between 1988 and 1990, only 44% of neuropathic ulcers healed, but by 2009 65% of those with good glycemic control attained wound closure.[6] Preventive care and prompt appropriate interventions are paramount in reducing these significant health problems.[6]

This chapter provides a brief review of the etiology of diabetes and of diabetes-related tissue damage, followed by a detailed account of various risk factors contributing to neuropathic ulcers and delayed wound healing. Next, the classification and characteristics of neuropathic ulcers are outlined. Finally, this chapter presents a thorough description of physical therapy, medical, and surgical interventions for patients with neuropathic ulcers to maximize positive outcomes.

ETIOLOGY OF NEUROPATHIC ULCERS

Etiology of Diabetes

Diabetes mellitus is a disorder of carbohydrate, protein, and fat metabolism related to alterations in the body's ability to produce or use insulin.[12] There are several types and subtypes of diabetes mellitus and classification is not always clear-cut.[13] However, the majority of individuals who will be seen within the physical therapy setting has type 1A or type 2 diabetes. Type 1A diabetes, formerly known as juvenile diabetes or insulin-dependent diabetes mellitus (IDDM), is typically diagnosed in children and young adults and is believed to result from an immune-mediated destruction of pancreatic beta cells.[4, 12, 13] There is a genetic predisposition for developing type 1 diabetes with a 5% chance of developing diabetes if one parent has type 1 diabetes and a 20% chance if both parents have

type 1 diabetes. In addition, researchers believe there may be an environmental trigger for the development of type 1A diabetes. Type 1B, or idiopathic, diabetes represents a fraction of individuals with type 1 diabetes and appears to be strongly hereditary.[13] Most individuals with type 1B diabetes are of African or Asian descent. The risk of ulceration due to diabetes seems to be lower in patients of Asian descent.[14] Because patients with type 1 diabetes do not produce insulin, they require exogenous insulin replacement therapy to lower blood glucose levels, to regulate metabolism of fats and protein, and to prevent ketosis.[12] Individuals with type 1 diabetes comprise approximately 5–10% of all patients with diabetes.[13, 15]

In contrast, individuals with type 2 diabetes are typically diagnosed at middle age or later and approximately 80% are overweight.[13] Because obesity causes insulin resistance, the rising obesity epidemic has led to a rise in patients with type 2 diabetes as well as an earlier onset of symptoms.[1] Native Americans and Hispanic/Latino Americans are two to three times more likely to develop diabetes than Anglo-Americans.[4, 12, 16] The lifetime risk of developing type 2 diabetes for an individual born in the United States in the year 2000 is 33% for males and 39% for females.[2] The risk for Hispanic/Latino Americans and Native Americans is nearly 50%.[2, 17] Individuals diagnosed with type 2 diabetes have a significantly shorter life expectancy (12–14 years) and lower quality of life than those without type 2 diabetes.[2] The exact cause of type 2 diabetes is unknown. Although it is not immune mediated, there is a genetic predisposition to developing type 2 diabetes.[18] Other proposed causes of type 2 diabetes are the development of insulin resistance, impaired insulin secretion, beta cell defects causing the body to make a slightly altered, less active version of insulin, and certain health behaviors such as inactivity, poor diet, obesity, and normal body weight but a high percentage of abdominal body fat.[1, 4, 12] Alarmingly, the incidence of type 2 diabetes in adolescents has increased dramatically in the past 10 years.[1] Risk factors for type 2 diabetes in children include being more than 85% percentile in body weight for age and sex, weight being more than 120% of ideal for height, having a close relative with diabetes, being of a high-risk ethnic origin, or having a mother with a history of gestational diabetes.[1] Patients with type 2 diabetes make up approximately 90–95% of all individuals with diabetes and a majority of the amputations are due to the long-term complications of diabetes (see Figure 13–1).[4, 13, 19]

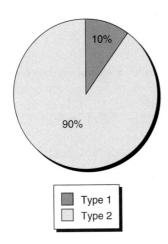

Type 1
Type 2

FIGURE 13–1   Individuals with type 1 versus type 2 diabetes.

Etiology of Diabetes-Related Tissue Damage

There are three hypotheses as to the mechanism of tissue damage due to hyperglycemia. First, the damage may be due to hemodynamic changes and the resultant increases in microvascular pressures.[20] Hyperglycemia changes red blood cells, platelets, and capillaries. Red blood cells (RBCs) become less deformable, less able to release oxygen, and more adhesive. Thus, RBCs stick to themselves and to endothelial cells lining capillary walls. Platelets also become more adhesive and stick to endothelial cells at sites of minimal injury. This causes capillary walls to become thicker[21] and less flexible. Changes to these cells and the vessel walls and the resultant decrease in lumen size alter blood flow within the vessels and increase microvascular pressure.[22]

Second, hyperglycemia causes glucose to passively bind to proteins, a process known as glycosylation. The structure of glycosylated proteins, or chemical reactions with them, may cause tissue trauma.[22, 23] The structures and functions of glycosylated proteins are vastly different from those of the original proteins. For example, low-density lipoproteins (LDLs) normally bind to LDL receptors. However, like trying to fit a square peg into a round hole, glycosylated LDLs cannot bind to these receptors. Additionally, glycosylated proteins may lead to the formation of free radicals, which are thought to cause tissue damage.[21, 24]

Third, the accumulation of sorbitol due to the breakdown of glucose through the polyol pathway may result in tissue destruction.[21–25] Some tissues use the polyol pathway to transport glucose into cells without using insulin. This pathway converts glucose into sorbitol before finally changing it into fructose. Hyperglycemia increases the rate of this conversion. Either the increase in sorbitol or by-products of this conversion may cause tissue damage.

Any one of these three mechanisms independently, in combination, or with an as yet unidentified process may be the cause of tissue damage in patients with diabetes. The severity and prevalence of the complications of diabetes appear to be directly related to the ability to maintain near normal blood glucose levels and to the number of years the patient has been diagnosed with diabetes.[1]

RISK FACTORS CONTRIBUTING TO NEUROPATHIC ULCERATION AND DELAYED WOUND HEALING

There are many risk factors that contribute to the development of neuropathic ulcers and delayed wound healing. When considered independently, each individual risk factor, other than hyperglycemia, does not pose much of a threat. However, risk factors are interrelated, making their combined impact significant. For example, poor blood sugar control can lead to a decreased immune response. Similarly, poor vision, in combination with sensory loss, severely limits a patient's ability to detect trauma to the foot.

Patients have little or no control over several risk factors, including vascular disease, ulcer characteristics, the length of time diagnosed with diabetes, and inadequate professional care. Encouragingly, other risk factors, such as neuropathy, mechanical stresses, abnormal foot function, impaired immune response, inadequate footwear, poor vision, glycemic control, and inadequate patient education, are modifiable or at least partially within the patient's control. It is imperative to minimize the number and magnitude of as many risk factors as possible[8] to successfully manage neuropathic ulcers.

Vascular Disease

Diabetes is the leading risk factor for coronary artery disease, cerebrovascular accident, and peripheral vascular disease (PVD).[1] The prevalence of peripheral arterial disease in patients with diabetes is estimated to be about 14%,[26] but may be as high as 57% in adolescents with type 2 diabetes.[27] The risk of PVD, especially below the knee, is greater in individuals with diabetes.[28]

These persons also have an accelerated rate of atherosclerosis.[29] Diabetes has been shown to cause thickening of the basement membrane,[21, 28] presumably resulting in decreased delivery of oxygen and nutrients to the tissues.[29] Whereas individuals without diabetes are more likely to undergo revascularization if circulatory problems arise, patients with diabetes are more likely to undergo amputation.[30] Smoking in patients with diabetes may accelerate the development of vascular complications[1, 31] and delay wound healing.[6]

Because of these findings, PVD was once thought to be the major contributing factor to neuropathic ulcers. However, current research does not support the theory that neuropathic ulcers are caused by decreased circulation. In fact, ischemia has been implicated as a causative factor in only 5% of all amputations.[32] It is now believed that despite these impairments in the vasculature, the major contributing factor in neuropathic ulcerations is neuropathy rather than vascular disease (see Figure 13–2).[1, 21]

Neuropathy

Neuropathy is the most common complication of diabetes mellitus, affecting 30–40% of patients with type 2 diabetes and an even higher percentage of individuals with type 1 diabetes,[21] and may be caused by neural ischemia and/or segmental demyelination. Neuropathy tends to be symmetrical and affects the distal nerves first; therefore, it has the most significant impact on the feet.[1] The incidence and severity of neuropathy increase with age and the duration of the disease.[33] Diabetic neuropathy affects the sensory, motor, and autonomic systems.

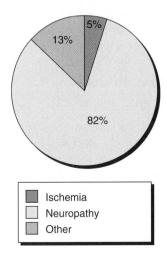

FIGURE 13–2 Causative factors for amputations in individuals with diabetes.

Sensory Neuropathy

The inability to accurately perceive trauma to the feet is arguably one of the most significant risk factors in the development of neuropathic ulcerations.[5, 22, 34, 35] Because sensory loss occurs so gradually and is painless, 50% of patients are unaware of the loss of protective sensation until the development of an ulcer or specific testing by a medical professional.[1] Eight percent of patients were found to have **sensory neuropathy** at the time they were diagnosed with type 2 diabetes, whereas 50% were found to have sensory neuropathy 25 years after initial diagnosis of any type of diabetes.[36] Fifty-seven percent of adolescents had sensory neuropathy at the time they were diagnosed with type 2 diabetes.[27] In addition to a lack of protective sensation, sensory neuropathy may also be characterized by paresthesias, such as burning pain, tingling, or aching.[1] Paresthesias are doubly problematic. First, these sensations can be quite painful and debilitating, sometimes requiring opioid management. Second, patients may erroneously believe that the presence of these sensations is evidence of accurate and intact protective sensation.

This lack of sensation equates to the lack of an early detection system to alert the patient to minor irritation or overt trauma. Two examples will help illustrate this point. A patient wearing a new pair of shoes did not perceive a blister developing in the arch of his foot and continued to walk all day. Upon removing his shoes at the end of the day, the patient was surprised to find blood on his sock because he did not feel any pain from the now open blister. Another patient walking barefoot in his house stepped on a piece of glass. Not feeling the glass, the patient continued to walk on it until the foot became noticeably red and swollen due to infection. Without the warning signal of pain, these patients did not alter their activity (change shoes or stop walking on the shard of glass) to avoid further tissue damage until more overt signs, such as an open wound or swollen foot, were present. Patients who are unable to perceive 10 grams of pressure (5.07 Semmes–Weinstein monofilament) should be considered at risk for ulceration.[1, 19]

Motor Neuropathy

Motor neuropathy leads to paralysis of the foot's intrinsic muscles. The resulting muscle atrophy may predispose patients with diabetes to plantar ulceration by increasing plantar pressures and shear forces.[5, 22] Loss of intrinsic muscle function may cause the foot to be less stable during the stance phase of gait.[22] This loss of stability may lead to excessive plantar pressures and shear forces on the second and third metatarsal heads. In addition, the muscle imbalances due to neuropathy result in hallux valgus and claw toe deformities characterized by hyperextension of the toe metatarsophalangeal joints with flexion of the interphalangeal joints.[22] This deformity makes the metatarsal heads more prominent on the plantar aspect of the foot, creating localized areas of increased pressure during weight bearing.[22, 37] Because ulcers usually occur in areas of peak plantar pressures,[38] patients with motor neuropathy should be considered at risk for ulceration.[37]

Autonomic Neuropathy

Autonomic neuropathy increases the risk of neuropathic ulceration due to disturbances in sweating mechanisms, callus formation, and blood flow.[1] Autonomic neuropathy decreases the body's ability to sweat, which may lead to dry, less elastic, and cracked skin, thus opening a pathway for microbes to enter the body as well as alterations in the ability to thermoregulate.[35, 39] Individuals with autonomic neuropathy may also have an increased rate of callus formation, resulting in up to a 26% increase in local pressure.[5, 8] Arteriovenous shunting may result in decreased perfusion of the skin and superficial structures, which reduces the skin's ability to repair.[22, 23] Finally, uncontrolled vasodilation causes an increase in blood flow to bone, which essentially leaches the bone of calcium and predisposes the bones of the foot to fracture due to osteopenia.[9] When working with patients with diabetes, clinicians must be aware that autonomic dysfunction affects almost every body system and can result in resting tachycardia, exercise intolerance, orthostatic hypotension, gastroparesis, and sexual dysfunction.[1]

Mechanical Stress

Mechanical stress due to abnormal or excessive forces predisposes individuals with diabetes to ulceration.[34, 37, 40, 41] High amounts of force, even over a very short period of time, will cause tissue failure. For example, overt trauma, such as stubbing one's toe, can lead to a break in skin integrity.

Pressure is defined as the amount of force applied per unit area. Abnormally high plantar pressures may be more common in patients with diabetes[42] because deformities like claw toes and cavus foot result in increased vertical and horizontal forces under the heel and metatarsal heads.[40] Plantar pressures are also greater in patients with limited foot mobility[43] and in patients with a history of plantar ulceration.[42] Forefoot plantar pressures have been found to be as much as 143% greater than those in the rearfoot,[38] making this area an even higher risk for skin breakdown. Static and dynamic plantar pressures can be measured directly. Unfortunately, the sophisticated laboratory equipment, increased time, and significant cost of these assessments limit their utility outside of the research setting. Clinically, patients presenting with deformities or limited joint motion should be considered at risk for ulceration because these conditions are associated with high plantar pressures and foot ulceration.[37] Ulcers are more likely to occur if high plantar pressures are coupled with sensory neuropathy.[1, 40, 43]

The potential for skin breakdown is not only a function of the amount of force and pressure applied. Tissue failure will also occur if the rate of tissue breakdown exceeds the rate of repair. Considering the inverse relationship between force and time, one can appreciate that lower amounts of pressure, if sustained or repeated over time, may lead to ulceration.[41] Think about the number of steps required to travel from one room to another, or from a parking lot into a building. This number of steps multiplied by the high plantar pressures created with each step can easily overload the tissue's ability to repair itself, resulting in a neuropathic ulceration. Conversely, with higher pressures, tissue damage can occur in less time. For example, imagine what would happen if a pebble got into a person's shoe. Due to the very small surface area, the pebble would create an area of high plantar pressure so that walking just a few steps would be enough to cause a blister or ulcer.

Abnormal Foot Function and Inadequate Footwear

Impaired motion, foot deformities, and previous ulcer or amputation adversely affect foot function, predisposing the patient with diabetes to plantar ulceration.[22, 37] Inadequate footwear, particularly when combined with abnormal foot function and sensory changes, also increases the risk of tissue damage.[40]

Impaired Range of Motion

Limited motion alone does not seem to increase the risk of ulceration for patients with diabetes. In combination with sensory neuropathy, however, decreased great toe extension, dorsiflexion, and subtalar joint motion do appear to predispose these individuals to the development of plantar ulcerations.[43–45] Restricted motion in these joints may lead to a decreased ability to attenuate the vertical pressures and horizontal shear forces created during ambulation,[46] thereby increasing the risk of ulceration.[5, 47]

Foot Deformities

Foot deformities, such as plantar flexion contractures, forefoot varus, or forefoot valgus, create increased plantar pressures at the metatarsal heads during weight bearing.[22, 34, 45, 48, 49] Similarly, neuropathic fracture and dislocation, commonly called **Charcot foot,**[9] typically result in a structural change of the foot in which the normally concave midfoot arch reverses, forming a so-called rocker-bottom foot, which also causes increased plantar pressures.[45] The presence of these deformities, in combination with sensory neuropathy, predisposes the foot to ulceration.[37, 40, 43]

Previous Ulcer or Amputation

Patients with a previous history of ulceration or amputation are more likely to have a repeat ulceration.[1, 50] The rate of ulcer recurrence after 2 years is as high as 40%,[6] with the majority of recurrences occurring in the first 6 months after wound closure. There are three plausible explanations for these findings. First, the immature cross-links and collagen bonds of newly formed connective tissue make it less able to tolerate the mechanical stress of gait even though the wound may be considered "closed." Second, scar tissue laid down during wound healing is less elastic and less mobile than its predecessor, making it less able to tolerate the shear forces created during gait. Third, those patients with histories of ulceration or amputation are more likely to have a loss of protective sensation than those without these experiences, thus increasing the likelihood of ulceration.

Inadequate Footwear

Footwear should protect the foot, decrease plantar pressures and shear forces, and accommodate foot deformities.[5, 22, 37, 40] Foot orthoses should assist with pressure relief to areas of increased plantar pressures. Although footwear should have a positive effect on preventing foot ulcers, inappropriately sized shoes and rigid orthoses may actually cause ulcerations.[51]

Impaired Healing and Immune Response

Diabetes alters the body's ability to build new tissue and fight infection.[52] Individuals with diabetes have an increased frequency of certain types of infections, including osteomyelitis, soft tissue infections, and candidal infections. Sustained hyperglycemia decreases all three phases of wound healing. High blood sugar levels decrease the rate of collagen synthesis, angiogenesis, and fibroblast proliferation and reduce the tensile strength of incisional wounds.[53] In addition, high blood sugar levels impair granulocyte chemotaxis, phagocytosis,[54] and opsonization of bacteria.[55] The risk of infection is even greater for older or obese individuals with diabetes.[53]

Poor Vision

Diabetes is the leading cause of blindness due to retinopathy, glaucoma, and cataracts.[56] Nearly all individuals with type 1 diabetes and over half of those with type 2 diabetes were found to have some degree of retinopathy 20 years after their initial diagnosis.[56] Visual dysfunction in patients with diabetes may be due to three factors.[57] First, high blood glucose levels directly damage the retina.[24] Second, the accumulation of sorbitol from the polyol pathway is known to cause eye disease in patients with diabetes. Third, vascular changes caused by diabetes lead to microaneurysms and ischemia in the retina.[24] These changes disable the blood–retinal barrier (similar to the blood–brain barrier) that controls the penetration of substances into the retina, ultimately leading to further visual dysfunction.

Impaired vision contributes to the development and progression of neuropathic ulcers[33] in two ways. First, poor vision may lead to an increase in direct trauma to the foot such as stepping on an unseen obstacle. Second, and more important, decreased vision severely hinders the ability to perform adequate foot care, including checking for signs and symptoms of trauma or infection in an insensate foot.[51]

Ulcer Characteristics

In general, ulcers that are larger, extend into deeper tissues, or have been present for longer periods of time before medical intervention take longer to heal.[58–61] The research regarding the effect that wound location has on time to wound closure is inconclusive. Some research suggests midfoot ulcerations heal faster than those on the forefoot,[61] while other studies demonstrate the reverse.[62] Unfortunately, the length of time the ulcer has been present is a confounding variable in these studies.

Disease Characteristics

Glycemic control is measured two ways. First, fasting blood sugar levels provide a snapshot in time of a patient's current blood sugar level. Second, a blood test measuring hemoglobin A1c levels (HgbA1c) is used to determine the average amount of sugar within the blood throughout the life of the red blood cell, roughly 3 months. The incidence and severity of neuropathy and foot ulcers correlate with the duration of the disease.[1, 59, 60, 63] These findings suggest that the risk of developing an ulceration increases the longer a patient has been diagnosed with diabetes. Several large-scale studies involving patients with type 1 and type 2 diabetes, such as the Diabetes Control and Complications Trial, the United Kingdom Prospective Diabetes Study Group, and the ADVANCE study, clearly demonstrate that sustained high blood sugar levels are associated with an increased risk of the long-term complications of diabetes.[64, 65] This implies an increased risk of ulceration. Encouragingly, the development and progression of many of the complications affecting wound healing, including neuropathy, retinopathy, vascular disease, and decreased ability to fight infection, can be slowed or reversed with improvements in glycemic control.[1, 24, 33, 39, 65] These benefits of tighter glycemic control (attaining and maintaining near normal HgbA1c levels) are seen regardless of patient age, sex, or duration of disease. In addition, there is a continuous relationship between glycemic control and the development of complications—that is, any reduction in hyperglycemia, no matter how small, will positively affect the development and progression of diabetic complications.[1, 64, 66] In contrast, patients with poorer long-term control of blood sugar levels, as indicated by high HgbA1c levels, healed slower and had more complications while those with more normal HgbA1c healed faster and with fewer complications.[6]

Inadequate Professional Care and Patient Education

Studies have not examined the effect of inappropriate medical care on the development and chronicity of neuropathic ulcers. However, it is easy to speculate that lack of cutting-edge knowledge about the etiology of diabetes and neuropathic ulcers can adversely affect wound care. Delayed referral to appropriate specialists or team members, the use of agents such as povidone–iodine, now known to be cytotoxic, and fear of newer techniques, such as the total contact cast, may also potentiate wound chronicity. Adherence of clinicians to evidence-based recommendations for the treatment of neuropathic ulcers is 77% for off-loading but only 23% for total contact casting.[67]

Diabetes is a chronic condition with a few, relatively minor short-term complications, such as hypoglycemia. However, there are many major long-term complications, such as ulceration, amputation, blindness, and kidney failure. Health care professionals must help patients understand the link between maintaining adequate blood sugar control and these long-term complications. With the absence of pain or any negative short-term effects, patients failing to make this link will be less likely to adhere to suggested therapeutic regimens. It is imperative that clinicians educate patients on ways to reduce or modify risk factors associated with these long-term complications and the importance of taking action.

CASE STUDY: Mr. Richard Townsend

This case study is referenced throughout the chapter.

PART 1

History

Richard Townsend is a 59-year-old white male seen in physical therapy this afternoon in an acute care hospital for wound management. Mr. Townsend has completed 2 years of college and his primary language is English. He lives with his wife in a one-level home. Mr. Townsend works 24 hours per week as a courier.

Wound History: Mr. Townsend reports his wound began 6 months ago and appears to be increasing in size. He has been washing his wound daily when he showers and covering it most days with two large Band-Aids.™ He states he has been feeling excessively fatigued for the past 3 days, getting out of bed solely to go to the bathroom for the last 2 days. He states he noticed an odor to his wound last night. He made an appointment with his primary care physician for this morning, however, he collapsed in the bathroom while getting ready for the appointment and had to be taken to the hospital by the paramedics.

Past Medical History: Mr. Townsend smoked two packs-per-day until quitting 5 years ago. He has generalized OA, HTN, CAD, type 2 DM, retinopathy, cataracts, and neuropathy. He has had two knee scopes on each leg, a right tibial osteotomy, a right total knee arthroplasty, and a left rotator cuff repair. He wears bifocals, which were revised 4 months ago. He is allergic to sulfa and adhesives.

General Health Status: Mr. Townsend believes he is in fair health. He was told to limit his walking because of his ulcer so he now uses a cart while golfing three rounds per week. He denies pain except for his right knee, which is 3/10 with golfing.

Current Medications: Home medications include naproxen, lisinopril, insulin, glyburide, metformin, and neurontin. Mr. Townsend was started on ciprofloxacin upon admission.

Other Available Data: Laboratory values available from the patient chart include hemoglobin 12 g/dL, hematocrit = 38%, white blood cell count = 14,000/mm³, platelets = 290,000/mm³, fasting blood glucose 302 mg/dL, hemoglobin A1c 12.3. Body temperature 99.2°F. Wound cultures were taken upon admission and results are pending.

Systems Review

Cardiovascular/Pulmonary System: Heart rate: 80 bpm, blood pressure 160/87 mm Hg, respiratory rate 15 bpm, pulse oximetry 97% on room air.

Musculoskeletal System: Gross assessment of range of motion and strength reveals bilateral deficits in ankle dorsiflexion, gastrocnemius length, and lower extremity strength. Height: six feet (1.83 m). Body weight: 236 pounds (107 kg). Body mass index (BMI) = 32 kg/m².

Neuromuscular System: No gross deficits noted in gross coordinated movement or motor control. He states he is normally ambulatory without an assistive device.

Gastrointestinal System: Patient reports he occasionally follows a low-calorie, low-sugar diet. He has not eaten a full meal in 2 days because of nausea.

Urogenital System: Patient reports he wakes two times per night to go to the bathroom.

Integumentary System: Open wound left plantar midfoot; bilateral Charcot deformities; clawing of the left second and third toes; skin is anhydrous with callus formation periwound, plantar right midfoot, and plantar left second metatarsal head; cracked callus bilateral heels, varicosities bilateral lower legs; bilateral great toenails are yellow, thickened, and long; OA deformities bilateral hands and knees.

Communication, Cognition, Language, and Learning Style: No deficits noted. Mr. Townsend reports he learns best by observation.

 Checkpoint Question #1

Name five tissues, aside from the integument, that are adversely affected by diabetes.

PHYSICAL THERAPY TESTS AND MEASURES FOR NEUROPATHIC ULCERS

Clinicians may perform various tests and measures to assess neuropathic ulcers, make a prognosis for wound healing, and identify changes in patient status.

In addition to the routine tests and measures clinicians should perform on all patients with open wounds (see Chapter 4), there are several tests that should be performed on patients with neuropathic ulcerations. This section provides a clinical guideline for the assessment of circulation and sensory integrity in patients with neuropathic ulcerations (see Table 13–1).

TABLE 13–1 Clinical Guideline for Physical Therapy Tests and Measures for Patients with Neuropathic Ulcerations

Test	Indications
Pulse examination	• All open wounds
Doppler ultrasound and ankle-brachial index	• Decreased or absent pulses • Signs and symptom of arterial insufficiency • History of peripheral vascular disease
Capillary refill	• Digital ulcer • Abnormal Doppler ultrasound or ABI
Sensory integrity	• All neuropathic ulcerations • All patients with diabetes • All patients with plantar foot ulcerations

Assessment of Circulation

Because of the increased risk of peripheral vascular disease in patients with diabetes, the clinician must thoroughly assess the patient's circulation.[1, 5, 8, 67] The clinician should assess pulses in all patients with neuropathic ulcers. Capillary refill should be assessed in patients with digital ulcers. Similar to patients with arterial insufficiency, clinicians should perform a Doppler ultrasound or ankle-brachial index (ABI) on patients with neuropathic ulcerations who have abnormal pulses or a history of peripheral vascular disease. Patients with ABIs less than 0.8, delayed capillary refill, or abnormal Doppler studies should be referred to a physician for further evaluation. Patients with diabetes may have artificially inflated ABI values due to vessel calcification.[1, 35] Therefore, patients who fail to respond to appropriate conservative interventions must be referred for further medical assessment. Arteriography or transcutaneous oxygen measurements may be used to provide a more accurate representation of patient circulation.[68, 69] Refer to Chapters 4 and 10 for specific details on how to perform these tests.

Assessment of Sensory Integrity

Although it may be tempting for a clinician to perform a cursory assessment of sensation using a finger or wisp of cotton or merely ask if the patient notices any loss of sensation, these methods are both inaccurate and insufficient.[70, 71] Sensory neuropathy is the leading cause of neuropathic ulcers.[72, 73] Therefore, sensory integrity must be thoroughly assessed in all patients with neuropathic ulcers.[1, 8, 40] As described in Chapter 4, Semmes–Weinstein monofilaments are the gold standard for assessing light touch sensation. Monofilaments are fast, reliable, valid, inexpensive, and clinically useful.[74, 75] Normal light touch sensation varies with anatomical location. Table 13–2 provides the normative values and interpretations for light touch sensation on the foot.[41, 63, 75–78]

To assess sensory integrity, occlude the patient's vision before applying the monofilament perpendicular to the skin with enough pressure to cause the filament to bend. Clinicians should begin with the 5.07 monofilament.[72, 73] Standard locations to be assessed at the dorsal midfoot and the plantar aspect

TABLE 13–2 Interpretation of Sensory Testing

Monofilament	Pressure Produced (grams)	Interpretation of Inability to Perceive Monofilament
4.17	1	Decreased sensation
5.07	10	Loss of protective sensation
6.10	75	Absent sensation

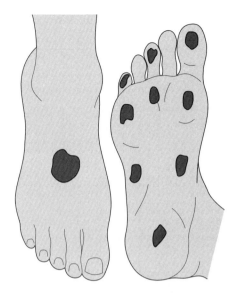

FIGURE 13–3 Locations to perform monofilament testing on the foot.

of the foot include the pulp of the first, third, and fifth digits; the first, third, and fifth metatarsal heads; the medial and lateral midfoot; and the calcaneus (see Figure 13–3).[8] Since sensory assessment over thick callous may be inaccurate,[79, 80] the clinician should attempt to assess noncallous skin when possible. If a thickly callous area is assessed, the

TABLE 13–3   Wagner Classification for Neuropathic Foot Ulcers

Wagner Grade	Ulcer Description
0	No open lesions; may have deformity or cellulitis
1	Superficial ulcer
2	Deep ulcer to tendon, capsule, or bone
3	Deep ulcer with abscess, osteomyelitis, or joint sepsis
4	Localized gangrene
5	Gangrene of the entire foot

Source: Kominsky SJ, ed. *Medical and Surgical Management of the Diabetic Foot.* St. Louis, MO: Mosby-Year Book; 1994, Table 13–3, p. 227.

clinician should document the presence and location of the callous(es) along with the test results. Each location should be tested randomly three times. Patients who are able to perceive the 5.07 monofilament should then be assessed to determine if they have normal sensation using the 4.17 monofilament. A patient who is unable to perceive the 5.07 monofilament in any portion of the test area on two or more applications has lost protective sensation and should be considered at risk for ulceration or reinjury due to insensitivity.[81] The clinician should then repeat the same procedure using the 6.10 monofilament to determine if the patient has lost all light touch sensation in the foot. If a patient fails to perceive the 6.10 monofilament on the foot, it would be wise for the clinician to continue to assess sensation more proximally to determine the extent of sensory loss.[19, 79]

CLASSIFICATION AND CHARACTERISTICS OF NEUROPATHIC ULCERS

Classification

The Integumentary Preferred Practice Patterns in the *Guide to Physical Therapist Practice* provide physical therapists with valuable patient management information for general wound care.[82] These practice patterns describe components of the examination, evaluation, diagnosis, prognosis, and interventions for patients who have an increased risk for integumentary disorders or who have impaired skin integrity. The **Wagner classification system,** used by other disciplines, including surgeons and podiatrists, is specific to neuropathic foot ulcerations (see Table 13–3).[73, 83] Both methods describe the level of tissue involvement and attempt to guide appropriate intervention strategies. The narrower scope of Wagner's system allows the classification of neuropathic ulcers to more precisely direct appropriate interventions. Physical therapists working with this patient population would be wise to use both systems to better coordinate patient care among different disciplines (see Table 13–4). It should be noted that a few clinicians utilize the University of Texas Diabetic Wound Classification System, which includes an assessment of ulcer depth, presence of infection, and circulatory status.[7, 58, 72, 83]

TABLE 13–4 Comparison of Wagner Grading System for Neuropathic Foot Ulcers with the Integumentary Preferred Practice Patterns

Wagner Grade	Integumentary Preferred Practice Patterns
Grade 0	Pattern A: Primary Prevention/ Risk Factor Reduction for Integumentary Disorders
	Pattern B: Impaired Integumentary Integrity Associated with Superficial Skin Involvement
Grade 1	Pattern C: Impaired Integumentary Integrity Associated with Partial-Thickness Skin Involvement and Scar Formation
	Pattern D: Impaired Integumentary Integrity Associated with Full-Thickness Skin Involvement and Scar Formation
Grade 2, 3, 4, or 5	Pattern E: Impaired Integumentary Integrity Associated with Skin Involvement Extending into Fascia, Muscle, or Bone and Scar Formation

Characteristics

The typical characteristics of neuropathic ulcers can be described using the 5PT method: pain, position, presentation, periwound, pulses, and temperature (see Box 13–1). Color images 2, 8, and 9 are examples of neuropathic ulcers.

Pain

Perhaps the most astonishing characteristic of neuropathic ulcers is the patient's lack of pain complaint. Because sensory neuropathy is the rule rather than the exception, most patients will continue to ambulate without even a limp despite significant tissue damage. Patients may report paresthesias,[1, 23, 84] but careful sensory assessment using Semmes–Weinstein monofilaments commonly demonstrates a lack of protective sensation.[63] These patients should be educated in basic foot care guidelines to minimize unsensed trauma to the foot.

Position

Neuropathic ulcerations tend to occur in areas of increased pressure such as the plantar aspect of the metatarsal heads. Ulcerations may occur on the plantar great toe in cases of hallux rigidus[44] or at the midfoot if a rocker-bottom deformity is present.[9, 37, 48] Claw toe deformities may lead to neuropathic ulcerations of the dorsal aspect of the toes without the use of extra-depth footwear.[50] Inappropriately sized footwear may lead to ulcers located at the tips of the toes, the lateral aspects of the fifth metatarsophalangeal joint, the medial aspect of the first metatarsophalangeal joint, or the posterior heel.[37, 85] Ulcerations may also occur under, or be obscured by, calluses.[86] Because patients with diabetes may lack protective sensation and adequate vision to perform foot checks, clinicians should thoroughly inspect all aspects of *both* feet for signs of trauma or ulceration.[1, 40]

BOX 13–1   Typical Characteristics of Neuropathic Ulcers

Pain Position

- Absent or significantly decreased
- Plantar aspect of the foot
- Areas of increased plantar pressures or shear forces such as under the metatarsal heads

Wound presentation

- Round, punched-out lesion
- Callus rim
- Little or no drainage
- Necrotic base uncommon

Periwound and structural changes

- Skin appears dry, cracked, callus
- Structural deformities such as clawing of the toes, rocker-bottom foot, or previous amputation

Pulses

- Normal

Temperature

- Normal or increased

Wound Presentation

Neuropathic ulcers commonly present as round, punched out lesions with a characteristic rim of callous indicative of increased plantar pressure and shear forces.[19, 37] Unless infected, drainage is usually minimal. Eschar or necrotic material in the base is also uncommon unless accompanied by infection or significant vascular disease.[37]

Periwound and Structural Changes

Patients with diabetes commonly have dry and cracked skin with a buildup of callus on the plantar aspect of the foot due to neuropathic changes.[5, 9] Toenails may be thickened due to coexisting fungal infections common among individuals with diabetes.[87] There may be structural deformities such as clawing of the toes or evidence of previous ulceration or amputation. Vasodilation due to autonomic neuropathy may lead to peripheral edema.[88]

Pulses

The increased risk of vascular disease associated with diabetes may yield a wide range of vascular findings. Pedal pulses may be normal. However, pulses may be decreased due to occlusive disease or accentuated due to vessel calcification.[27, 41] Abnormal pulses may require further medical testing to determine if blood flow to the involved areas is adequate for wound healing.[1]

Temperature

Autonomic neuropathy causes the foot to be hyperperfused, making even the noninfected foot of a patient with diabetes warm to the touch unless there is significant arterial insufficiency.[9, 88] Localized areas of increased temperature may be hallmarks of future ulceration or indicative of a deep space infection.[37, 89]

 ## Checkpoint Question #2

You are covering for a physical therapist who is on vacation. The assessment states that Patient Y has a grade 2 neuropathic foot ulcer. What does this mean?

PROGNOSIS FOR NEUROPATHIC ULCER HEALING

As with all chronic wounds, there is great variability in neuropathic wound healing rates, which makes prediction of time to healing difficult at best. Because many factors can contribute to delayed wound healing, the clinician must always consider local and systemic factors as well as wound characteristics when determining a patient's prognosis for wound healing. After reviewing the available evidence on wound healing in patients with neuropathic ulcers, it is possible to make scientifically grounded judgments on wound healing prognosis. Neuropathic ulcers that are smaller in size or more superficial (Wagner grade 1 or 2) have a better wound healing prognosis than larger ulcers.[60, 90, 91] Neuropathic ulcers existing for a shorter duration, particularly those present for less than 2 months prior to the start of interventions, have a better chance of expedient wound healing than those present for longer periods of time.[91] The risk for amputation is 154 times greater in patients with infected neuropathic ulcerations than in those without infection.[89] Nonsmokers with neuropathic ulcers heal significantly faster than smokers.[6] As would be expected, patients with better glycemic control healed faster than those with poor blood sugar control.[6]

Neuropathic ulcers that have an initial decrease in wound area after the first 4 weeks of interventions have a better prognosis than those that do not decrease in size. A 53% reduction in wound surface area over the first month of treatment was 91% sensitive and 58% specific in identifying grade 1 or 2 neuropathic ulcer healing at 12 weeks.[90] The average time to neuropathic ulcer healing is 12–14 weeks.[92, 93] If a 20–50% decrease in wound area is not seen after the first month of treatment, clinicians should reassess the patient and modify the plan of care or make appropriate referrals.[5, 94]

CASE STUDY: Mr. Richard Townsend

PART 2

Tests and Measures

Integumentary Integrity: Position: left plantar mid-foot. Presentation: full-thickness wound: 2.5 cm length × 2.3 cm width (wound surface area 5.75 cm²). Depth 0.3 cm. Wound bed contains friable pale granulation tissue and 10% is exposed plantar fascia. Wound drainage: minimal, thin, serosanguinous. Wound odor is present. Periwound: thick callus ring, varicosities B lower legs, minimal hemosiderin deposition B lower legs. Skin temperature: WNL.

Sensory Integrity: Patient is unable to identify 6.10 monofilament distal to the mid-calf bilaterally.

Circulation: Pulses: dorsalis pedis and tibialis posterior 2+B. Capillary refill: 2 seconds B. Ankle-brachial index (ABI): LUE 160 mm Hg/RUE 160 mm Hg, LLE 168 mm Hg, RUE 160 mm Hg, ABI LLE: 1.05. RUE: 1.0

Gait, Locomotion, Balance: Mr. Townsend ambulated with close stand-by assist for 10 feet for assessment purposes. He ambulates with a wide base of support, bilateral compensated Trendelenburg, lack of heel strike on left, excessive and prolonged pronation bilaterally.

Muscle Performance: BLE 4/5 except—left tibialis anterior 4–/5, bilateral hip abduction 2+/5, and trace volitional intrinsic foot muscles.

Pain: Mr. Townsend denies wound-related pain. He reports 3/10 right knee pain with golfing.

Range of Motion: Ankle dorsiflexion L 0°/R 4°, gastrocnemius length L lacks 9° from neutral/R lacks 3° from neutral. Knee extension lacks 8° from neutral on left/lacks 16° on right. Great toe extension L 50°/R 62°.

Assistive and Adaptive Devices: Patient brought his usual walking shoes to the hospital—a tennis-style shoe with significant wearing medially and medial counter breakdown bilaterally.

Evaluation and Diagnosis

Mr. Townsend has a Wagner grade 2 ulcer consistent with Pattern E: Impaired Integumentary Integrity Associated with Skin Involvement Extending into Fascia, Muscle, or Bone and Scar Formation. His examination findings suggest his wound is infected with chronic venous insufficiency. Mr. Townsend's ABI is normal, however, this may be artificially elevated due to arterial vessel calcification. He lacks protective sensation as well as light touch sensation distal to his mid-calf bilaterally. He has impaired great toe extension, ankle dorsiflexion, knee extension, and gastrocnemius length. He has impaired bilateral lower extremity strength and foot deformities. He has the signs and symptoms of a toenail fungal infection. He has inappropriate footwear and lacks knowledge or follow-through with self-management of his wound and diabetes. His BMI places Mr. Townsend in class 1 obesity. He is limited in ambulation and leisure activities.

Prognosis and Plan of Care

In general, Wagner grade 1 or 2 ulcers have a good prognosis for wound healing. However, Mr. Townsend's ulcer has been present for more than 2 months and is currently infected. Mr. Townsend has the following multiple risk factors for delayed healing: CAD, peripheral vascular disease, uncontrolled diabetes, peripheral neuropathy, foot deformities and abnormal mechanical stress, poor integumentary quality (anhydrous, cracked, callus), inappropriate footwear, poor self-care, and decreased vision. He is at significant risk for an amputation. Therefore, his prognosis for wound healing is fair, at best. A 25% reduction in wound size in 4 weeks would suggest wound healing may occur. If progressing, complete wound closure would not be expected before 14 weeks.

The following functional goals have been discussed and mutually agreed upon:

1. Mr. Townsend will ambulate independently with partial weight bearing on his left lower extremity with a walker and a padded ankle foot orthosis with a custom insert for 150 feet in three visits.
2. Mr. Townsend's integumentary integrity will be fully restored in 16 weeks.

The following wound-related component goals have been discussed and mutually agreed upon:

1. Skin hydration will be restored and callus will be removed within 3 days.

2. Wound bed will contain 90% healthy granulation tissue and <5% slough in 1 week.

3. Wound surface area will be decreased by at least 25% (to ≤4.3 cm^2) over the next 4 weeks.

4. Mr. and Mrs. Townsend will verbalize an understanding of skin care protection techniques and methods to enhance wound healing in three visits.

5. Ankle dorsiflexion +10° B and gastrocnemius length to neutral dorsiflexion B in 2 weeks to decrease plantar foot stress.

Mr. Townsend will be seen twice daily while in the hospital. Physical therapy interventions will include coordination, communication, and documentation; patient/client-related instruction; integumentary repair and protective techniques; electrotherapeutic modalities, physical agents, and mechanical modalities; therapeutic exercises; prescription, application, and fabrication of devices and equipment; functional training; and manual therapy techniques. Upon discharge from the inpatient setting, he will be seen 3–7 days per week pending wound progress and self-care skills.

PHYSICAL THERAPY INTERVENTIONS

As with other types of ulcers, physical therapy interventions for patients with neuropathic ulcers consist of a tripartite approach of coordination, communication, and documentation; patient/client-related instruction; and individualized procedural interventions.

Coordination, Communication, and Documentation

The management of patients with neuropathic foot ulcers can be significantly enhanced by using a holistic approach.[1, 8, 95, 96] In addition to the patient, the patient's significant others, the physician, and the surgeon, team members might include an endocrinologist and a diabetic educator to assist with insulin and/or oral hypoglycemic agent dosages. A podiatrist may be needed to assist with proper footwear, toenail care, callus removal, and wound care. A vascular surgeon may be necessary to remediate impaired macrocirculation to prevent ulceration or to assist with wound healing. An orthotist may assist with the development of temporary footwear to allow wound healing and permanent footwear to prevent ulcer recurrence, or a prosthetist may be called upon after an amputation.

Medical nutrition therapy provided by a registered dietitian is invaluable in providing patients with proper nutritional information regarding a diabetic or weight loss diet, helpful hints regarding variation in meal planning, and keys to eating out while maintaining their diet.[97–99] For patients with type 2 diabetes, the loss of as little as 5–10% of body weight can improve insulin sensitivity, glycemic control, blood pressure, and serum lipid levels.[97] Chaplaincy or psychological counseling may be beneficial to assist patients with the many stresses involved in living with a chronic illness. A medical social worker may be able to provide information about obtaining medical equipment and supplies as well as securing financial assistance through public assistance programs or private insurers.[96] This interdisciplinary patient care must be consistent and highly coordinated to successfully manage such a complex and multifaceted disease process.

Patient/Client-Related Instruction

It is imperative that individuals with diabetes be provided with the knowledge and resources to increase their control over this chronic disease process.[1, 8, 96, 99] Patients must be thoroughly informed of the disease process and medical management of diabetes. They must be made aware of the findings of the Diabetes Control and Complications Trial and the United Kingdom Prospective Diabetes Study regarding the ability to substantially decrease long-term complications, though at the risk of hypoglycemic episodes.[64, 66, 100] They also need to understand the role of exercise and basic safety guidelines when exercising. They must be informed of ways to reduce the risk factors known to contribute to neuropathic ulcers in an attempt to prevent ulceration or reulceration and to improve the potential for wound healing if an ulcer is present.

Because patients with diabetes are at increased risk for ulceration, clinicians should instruct them in proper shoe wear and foot care guidelines (see Box 13–2).[40] Clinicians should teach patients to check for proper shoe fit, to break new shoes in slowly to

---

BOX 13–2   Foot Care Guidelines

1. Inspect feet daily. Use a mirror to see bottoms of feet and check between toes. Have a family member or friend check if you are unable to adequately see all aspects of your feet.

2. Always wear socks with your shoes.

3. If wearing socks with seams, wear them inside out, so the seam does not cause undue pressure on the tips of the toes.

4. Inspect soles and inside of shoes for foreign objects prior to donning.

5. Shoes should be properly fitted, comfortable, and easy to don. There should be a break-in period.

6. In cold weather, wear insulated boots or heavier socks. Be sure shoes allow room for heavy socks.

7. Do not walk barefooted.

8. Do not use hot water bottles or heating pads to warm your feet. Use heavy socks instead.

9. Do not soak your feet.

10. Do not use acids or chemicals on your feet unless directed by your physician.

11. Wash feet daily and dry well between toes. Apply moisturizing lotion liberally, but not between toes.

12. Bath water temperature should be comfortably warm (between 105°F and 110°F). Test water temperature with your elbow or a thermometer or set hot water heater not to exceed this temperature.

13. Trim nails straight across and file gently.

14. Always remove shoes and socks when visiting your doctor.

15. Have regular foot exams by your physician or podiatrist.

16. Have a physician or podiatrist remove corns, calluses, or ingrown toenails.

17. Call your health care provider immediately if you detect a new wound or if your foot becomes swollen, red, or painful. Stay off your foot until you see a clinician.

18. Maintain good diabetes control.

19. If you smoke, quit.

---

avoid blisters, and to ensure that there are no foreign objects in their shoes before donning them.[37, 40] Patients should apply lotion[21] to the feet to prevent callus formation and powder between the toes to prevent excess moisture, which may become a breeding ground for bacteria. Wearing white cotton socks and changing them daily will help absorb perspiration and make it easier for patients to identify drainage from a new wound. Padded socks may be helpful in distributing foot forces.[21] Patients should also perform daily foot checks using a mirror to assess all aspects of the feet for reddened or open areas to identify ulcerations early, thereby decreasing the likelihood of serious infection or amputation.[40, 101] If any skin changes are noted, the patient should contact the physician immediately. Patients with poor eyesight should have a significant other inspect their feet for signs of trauma or infection. Whenever being assessed by a health care provider, patients should remove both of their shoes and socks to allow inspection of their feet. Because the toenails are predisposed to fungal infections causing thickening of the nails, patients should have their toenails cut often and with the aid of a podiatrist if necessary.[28, 87] Lastly, patients should avoid putting heating pads or ice on their feet to prevent serious thermal damage due to insensitivity.[28] Individuals with neuropathic ulcers must also be instructed in ways to

improve the chance of wound closure, such as limiting weight bearing and improving glycemic control. Although there is little information on the effect foot care programs have on the incidence of ulceration, these programs have been proven to significantly decrease the rate of amputation[36, 102] as well as reduce medical costs and diabetes-related complications.[40] A recent clinical trial[89] did find a tenfold decrease in diabetic foot ulcerations in patients who utilized an infrared thermometer to measure foot temperature twice daily at the standard sensation testing locations. Patients were instructed to decrease weight-bearing activity while skin temperature at any location was elevated by 4° F (2.2° C) or more.

Unfortunately, instructing patients in the management of diabetes and its long-term complications does not guarantee adherence to suggested regimens. In fact, adherence with diabetic regimens has been shown to be as low as 10–20%,[103] while adherence to weight-bearing and removable footwear regimens in patients with neuropathic ulcers has been found to be 60%.[104] In one study, patients who missed more than half of their scheduled appointments for diabetes management were 54 times more likely to develop a foot ulcer and 20 times more likely to have an amputation when compared to those who regularly went to scheduled appointments.[105] As mentioned previously, one of the key predisposing factors in the development and progression of diabetic (neuropathic) ulcers is sensory neuropathy. This lack of sensation, and lack of pain, may make it difficult for patients to truly believe the serious nature of their condition. Because these patients do not perceive pain, they may inaccurately assume they are not at risk for injury. Clinicians should use the assessment of sensory integrity as a teaching tool for patients with or without ulcers. If a patient lacks normal sensation on any aspect of the foot, the clinician can then demonstrate just what that amount of pressure should feel like on a sensate area, such as the volar aspect of the forearm, before again testing the foot while the patient visually observes the monofilament as it is applied. In this way, the patient may better comprehend what this lack of sensation "feels" like and the significant impact that sensory neuropathy might have on wound development and progression, leading to increased adherence to the plan of care. Excellent interdisciplinary coordination of services and the involvement of the patient's significant others in the care plan can also help increase adherence by avoiding duplicitous care and improving the often fragmented approach to patient management.[1] Chapter 9 provides strategies for enhancing patient adherence.

Procedural Interventions

Precautions

Clinicians should be aware of three precautions when working with patients with neuropathic ulcers. First, because of the chronicity of some neuropathic ulcerations, decreased inflammatory response, and possible concomitant vascular disease, many of these patients do not demonstrate the cardinal signs of infection when infected.[106] Clinicians should request an order for a wound culture and sensitivity coupled with appropriate antibiotic therapy for ulcers that fail to respond to conservative interventions. In addition, patients with osteomyelitis cannot be managed successfully without surgical intervention. Second, because of the extremely high risk of sensory loss, patients with diabetes should be educated in foot care guidelines and be provided with appropriate footwear.[40] Third, when working with patients with diabetes it is important to monitor for signs of hypoglycemia.[1] Patients should be scheduled for therapy after mealtime to avoid the potential for hypoglycemic episodes. Hypoglycemia is of particular concern in patients with infected ulcers. Blood sugar levels tend to increase due to an infection, leading to delayed wound healing.[1, 83] In response to the infection, the

physician will generally increase the patient's hypoglycemic agent dosage and prescribe appropriate antibiotic therapy. However, once the infection is under control, the patient will likely be overmedicated, increasing the risk of a hypoglycemic episode. Patients should be queried regularly about their blood sugar control, and any adverse changes should be reported to the physician.[1]

Integumentary Repair and Protective Techniques

Request for Further Medical Testing

An order for a bone scan or x-ray should be requested if there is exposed capsule or bone to rule out the presence of osteomyelitis.[72, 73, 83] If osteomyelitis is present, the infected bone must promptly be surgically removed before allowing the wound to close.[81] An order for a wound culture and sensitivity should be requested if the patient presents with the signs and symptoms of infection[72] or if wound progress is slower than expected. If the wound is infected, the physician should initiate appropriate antibiotic therapy.[83, 89]

Local Wound Care

Highlights of local wound care specific to patients with neuropathic ulcers are included here. Refer to Chapters 5–7 for more details. Callus should be pared flush with the epithelial surface[1, 5, 8, 9, 40, 73] to encourage epithelial cell migration across the wound bed.[3] Daily or twice-daily application of a petrolatum-based moisturizer to the feet can minimize dry, cracked skin caused by autonomic neuropathy.[40] Lotions should not be applied between the toes as this may lead to maceration[41] and increase the risk of fungal infections. If enclosing the toes within a bandage, gauze or toe spacers should be placed between the digits to absorb moisture, provide padding, and reduce shearing forces. If using clean technique for toe ulcerations, toe caps may be easier to don and maintain in position than traditional gauze dressings. Modalities, such as negative pressure wound therapy,[107] ultrasound, and electrical stimulation, as well as growth factors (Oasis and becaplermin)[108–110] may be useful adjuncts for wounds that are slow to heal (see Chapters 7 and 8).[5, 7]

Total Contact Casting

Total contact casting is an efficient and effective method of treating grades 1 and 2 neuropathic ulcers.[5, 7, 41, 61, 62, 71, 81, 108, 111–114] **Total contact casts** are essentially modified short leg casts traditionally used in fracture management. Total contact casts use smaller amounts of cast padding to promote a more "total contact" fit. The toes are enclosed within the cast to protect them from external trauma, such as toe stubbing, and from foreign objects entering the casts.

Total contact casts may assist with wound healing in many ways. First, the cast is carefully molded to the patient's foot and lower leg (see the Figure 13–4 series). This allows weight-bearing forces to be dispersed over a larger area, reducing plantar pressures. Second, the rigidity of the cast assists with edema control, thereby improving local circulation. Third, the cast immobilizes the foot and ankle, leading to a reduction in shearing forces. Fourth, the cast completely encloses the patient's insensate foot, protecting it from trauma and microorganisms. Last, the cast may assist with increasing patient adherence as it allows the patient to be active without undue hardship.

Total contact casts are contraindicated in the presence of gangrene or osteomyelitis (grade 3, 4, or 5 ulcers).[73, 112] Other contraindications include fluctuating edema, active infection, and patients who may not properly care for the cast.[73] Patients with ABIs less than 0.45 should not be casted because of decreased arterial supply. Patients with fragile skin may benefit from a **walking splint**—a total contact cast that is bivalved to allow it to be removed for more frequent monitoring of the skin and wound. Patients with bilateral grades 1 and 2 ulcers may have both feet casted simultaneously if their mobility continues to be safe. If not, the more severe ulcer should be casted first and appropriate footwear chosen for the noncasted foot.[114]

Total contact casts require skill to apply correctly. Sensory neuropathy makes patients unable to perceive improperly fitted casts, increasing the risk of trauma from an ill-fitting cast. Originally, the total contact cast was made from plaster, but plaster is inferior to fiberglass casting in three ways. First, the innermost layers of plaster require approximately 24 hours to dry, preventing the patient from early ambulation. Second, this increased drying time may contribute to maceration of the surrounding tissues or wound infection by allowing microbes to penetrate through the wet plaster. In contrast, fiberglass casting is quick to set and dry, allowing the patient to ambulate within 30 minutes. Third, plaster casts are heavier and less durable than fiberglass casts.

Another controversy with total contact casting revolves around the use of a walking heel or a cast shoe. The walking heel is meant to protect the plaster cast from contact with the ground and to allow heel and toe clearance during the stance phase of gait.[71] With the recent advances in footwear, most clinicians favor the use of a cast shoe to a walking heel. The cast shoe may decrease the risk of falls by allowing greater contact with the support surface and by more closely approximating the height of a traditional shoe worn on the uninvolved side. The cast shoe has a rocker-bottom design, which facilitates rollover of the foot during stance phase, while still protecting the cast from ground contact. Patients may prefer the cast shoe over the walking heel for cosmetic reasons. Appendix D contains detailed instructions for constructing a fiberglass total contact cast with a cast shoe and instructions for patients receiving a total contact cast.

☑ *Checkpoint Question #3*
_____

Give two reasons why it is important for patients with diabetes to apply moisturizing lotion to their feet.
_____

Therapeutic Exercise

Gait and Mobility Training

As discussed previously, patients with neuropathic ulcers commonly continue to ambulate on their wounds because they lack any painful feedback from even severely damaged tissues. It is believed that 90% of neuropathic ulcers are caused by abnormal pressure.[5] Ideally, these patients should be taught how to ambulate using a non-weight-bearing pattern to eliminate continued trauma to the affected area.[9, 60] However, for the vast majority of patients with diabetes,

this would be an impossible task because they lack the strength, endurance, and/or balance to safely maintain a non-weight-bearing status.[1] Additionally, this gait pattern would lead to severe functional limitations, making patient adherence unlikely.

There are several ways to safely unload the affected tissues.[5, 22, 37, 73] First, rather than attempting to promote a strict non-weight-bearing pattern, the patient could be instructed in partial weight bearing on the involved extremity. To address the balance deficits commonly found in these patients, a walker may be superior to crutches in assisting patients to maintain a partial

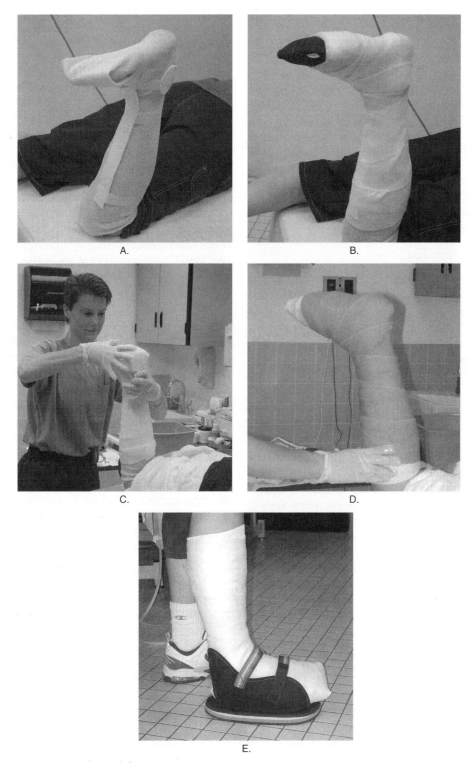

FIGURE 13–4   Construction of a total contact cast. *A.* The wound is covered with a thin primary dressing. The lower extremity is protected with a stockinette and felt pads are applied over bony prominences (malleoli, tibial crest). *B.* The toes are covered with thick foam padding, and a thin layer of cast padding is applied to the lower extremity. *C.* Fiberglass cast tape is applied. *D.* Cast tape is molded to the lower extremity with a moistened elastic bandage. *E.* Completed total contact cast with removable cast shoe.

weight-bearing status because it provides a greater base of support. Wheelchair use should be considered for patients who cannot safely unweight the involved extremity or for patients with an amputated uninvolved lower extremity. Second, patients with ulcers of the great toe or forefoot may benefit from using a step-to pattern to decrease plantar pressures to these areas by up to 53% during ambulation.[115] Alternatively, if patients take slower steps and use a shuffling gait pattern in which there is decreased heel strike and push-off, forefoot plantar pressures can be reduced up to 63%.[116] Third, footwear can be modified to reduce plantar pressures during ambulation (see the following section on devices and equipment).[5]

Range of Motion Exercises

Because limited joint range of motion is believed to play a role in the development and progression of neuropathic ulcers,[1, 40, 43, 44, 117–119] it would be wise to specifically assess great toe extension, talocrural dorsiflexion, and subtalar joint motion.[72, 89] Appropriate stretching exercises should be initiated if any of these motions is significantly limited.[8, 45]

Aerobic Exercise

Attaining and maintaining tight glycemic control will help maximize the body's ability to heal.[1] Clinicians can assist with proper glycemic control by developing an appropriate aerobic exercise program.[99] Aerobic exercise is known to assist in lowering hyperglycemia.[98] Many patients with type 2 diabetes are overweight. Aerobic exercise can help these individuals with weight loss, which, in turn, can lead to improved glycemic control.[98, 120] It is recommended that patients with diabetes participate in a minimum of 150 minutes of moderate-intensity aerobic activity per week.[1]

Prescription, Application, and Fabrication of Devices and Equipment

Temporary Footwear

Temporary footwear must allow safe ambulation while providing adequate pressure relief and room for bandages.[73] Inserts made of felt or foam can be customized to unweight ulcerated areas and better distribute forces over the surface of the foot.[50, 121] These materials "bottom out" fairly quickly and may need to be replaced before the ulcer is closed.

Patients not meeting the criteria for total contact casting may benefit from one of the many varieties of **padded ankle-foot orthoses**[41] or walking shoes available on the market today.[5] Both orthoses and walking shoes can be removed for wound care/inspection and bathing. Because these devices are not total contact, they should allow space for insoles to reduce pressure on the wound or the entire plantar surface of the foot. Orthoses or walking shoes should be made of soft materials, allow room for bandages, and completely enclose the foot.[113] Both should have a rocker-bottom to facilitate a smooth gait pattern and decrease shear forces.[5] The advantage of the padded ankle-foot orthosis is that it further reduces shear forces by immobilizing the ankle and foot. The advantages of the walking shoe are that it is relatively inexpensive, more stable, lighter, less bulky, and cosmetically more appealing to most patients. When comparing a removable padded ankle-foot orthosis with an irremovable orthosis of the same construction and a total contact cast, recent studies found neuropathic ulcer healing to be greatly enhanced with the irremovable devices.[122, 123] This would seem to indicate that pressure and shear relief as well as patient adherence to the prescribed device are fundamental to wound healing success.[104] Clinicians would be wise to repeatedly counsel patients who are prescribed removable footwear of the importance of adherence to wearing instructions or use an irremovable device, such as a total contact cast or irremovable padded ankle-foot orthosis, if adherence is suspect. See Table 13–5 for a summary of the characteristics of total contact casts, padded ankle-foot orthoses, and walking shoes.

Permanent Footwear

Permanent footwear must protect the foot and minimize plantar pressures and shear forces[35] to decrease the risk of ulceration or reulceration.[5, 8, 35, 113, 124, 125] Detailed information on the prescription of appropriate footwear is beyond the scope of this chapter and many excellent resources are available on this topic.[126, 127] However, some general suggestions regarding shoe construction and fit can assist novice clinicians in determining appropriate permanent footwear for their patients with diabetes.

First, shoes should be of the appropriate size. Shoes should be approximately $\frac{1}{2}$ inch longer than the longest toe. This is easily assessed with the patient standing by palpating for the distance between the

TABLE 13–5 Characteristics of Total Contact Casts, Padded Ankle-Foot Orthoses, and Walking Shoes

Characteristics	Total Contact Cast	Padded Ankle-Foot Orthosis	Walking Shoe
Ulcer grade	1, 2	1, 2, 3, 4	1, 2, 3, 4
Removable	No	Yes	Yes
Pressure distribution	Total contact	Insole to distribute pressure	Insole to distribute pressure
Shear forces	Greatly decreased	Decreased	Minimally decreased
Rocker-bottom	Yes	Yes	Yes
Enclosed toes	Yes	Yes	Yes
Weight	Moderate	Heavy	Light
Cosmesis	Fair	Fair	Good

end of the shoe and the end of the patient's longest toe. There should be a snug heel fit. Proper heel fit is assessed by monitoring for pistoning within the heel counter when the patient ambulates. The last, or shape, of the shoe should match the shape of the patient's foot, so that if the patient's foot has a curved shape, the shoe is similarly curved. This can be assessed by placing the sole of the shoe against the plantar aspect of the patient's foot. The width of the shoe at the ball of the foot should be snug enough to prevent the clinician from pinching excess material at the dorsum of the shoe but should not be so snug as to constrict the foot. Many patients require an extra-depth toe box to allow space for pressure-relieving insoles or foot deformities such as clawing of the toes.[37, 40, 113] Without this space, patients risk dorsal toe ulcerations from undetected pressure against the top of the shoe. Patients should try on shoes at the middle of the day when foot size is stabilized.[127] Patients should increase wearing time of new shoes gradually, starting with 2 hours per day, and feet should be carefully inspected upon shoe removal for signs of injury.[40]

Second, shoes should be constructed of soft, moldable materials to decrease pressure on the foot.[37] Patients should be discouraged from wearing shoes with heel heights greater than 1 inch because they decrease stability and increase plantar pressures and shear forces.[37] Patients should be instructed to purchase shoes that tie rather than slip on because this style decreases the shearing forces when donning and

doffing and accommodates for swelling of the foot as the day goes on.[37] Soft inserts can distribute weight-bearing forces across the surface of the foot, reducing contact pressures by as much as 50%.[113] Patients lacking protective sensation but without foot deformities should have unmolded soft inserts, whereas patients with deformities should be fitted with custom-molded inserts.[40, 41]

Patients with severe foot deformities or amputations[128] should be referred to a skilled shoemaker or orthotist.[1] Customized footwear may include rocker-bottom soles to accommodate for decreased flexibility or insoles molded to the exact contour of the foot.[113] Recent advances in technology allow customized footwear to be both therapeutic and cosmetic, thus increasing patient adherence, while still reducing the risk of ulceration.[128]

Manual Therapy Techniques

The potential for limited joint mobility to contribute to plantar ulceration has already been discussed. In addition to stretching exercises, joint mobilizations may assist in improving joint mobility.[129] For example, imagine you are working with a patient who has a neuropathic ulcer at the plantar aspect of the first metatarsophalangeal joint and limited great toe extension. In addition to traditional stretching exercises, you might choose to perform distraction and dorsal glides to this joint to increase extension range of motion.

CASE STUDY: Mr. Richard Townsend

PART 3

Interventions

The following highlights some of the key procedural interventions that will be incorporated into Mr. Townsend's plan of care.

Coordination, Communication, and Documentation: Mr. Townsend's physician has been contacted regarding his ABI findings and a request for a toe brachial index was made. Mr. Townsend was placed on a broad-spectrum antibiotic while the culture result was pending, and the physician ordered a topical bacitracin due to the patient's allergy to sulfa.

A consult with a certified diabetic educator to assist with following an appropriate meal plan for blood sugar control, blood pressure control, and weight loss was also requested. A referral to a pedorthist for a right custom shoe and insert was made, and a left shoe and insert will be fabricated if satisfactory wound healing occurs. A podiatrist consult was requested for toenail care.

Patient/Client-Related Instruction: Mr. and Mrs. Townsend will be instructed in the etiology of neuropathic ulcers and the potential for improvements in diabetes-related complications, including delayed wound healing or amputation, if improved glycemic control is attained and maintained. He will be instructed in the importance of limited weight bearing and shear forces to his wound as well as protection of his right lower extremity. Mrs. Townsend will be instructed in how to perform skin checks. They will be instructed to apply moisturizing lotion to both lower extremities to improve skin hydration.

Procedural Interventions
- Local wound management will consist of pulsed lavage with suction to irrigate the wound, to decrease wound infection, to enhance granulation tissue formation and quality, and to promote epithelialization. Calluses will be removed via sharp debridement. High-voltage pulsed current will be initiated to assist with infection control and wound healing with an initial setting of 100 Hertz, negative polarity, and a submotor intensity of 75–200 volts for 30 minutes twice daily. A moisturizing lotion will be used on intact skin. The wound will be dressed with a skin sealant to the periwound, bacitracin ointment to the wound, a gauze pad, and a roll gauze.
- Therapeutic exercises will include gastrocnemius and soleus stretches and strengthening exercises for his hip abductors and extensors, knee flexors and extensors, and ankle dorsiflexors. Carefully monitored aerobic exercise, such as an upper body ergometer, will be considered in the outpatient setting once his infection is better controlled.
- Prescription, application, and fabrication of devices and equipment: a walking splint with a custom-formed insole to reduce weight bearing and shear forces to the wound and plantar foot will be fabricated.
- Functional training will include gait training with a walker to further unload Mr. Townsend's left foot and improve his stability while ambulating with the walking splint.
- Manual therapy may include talocrural and/or tibiofibular joint mobilizations if therapeutic exercise alone is not enough to regain dorsiflexion.

Reassessment

Mr. Townsend's response to interventions will be monitored at all times. His wound will be formally reassessed every other day and plan of care modified if there are any adverse effects or if no improvements are noted after 2 weeks of treatment.

 Checkpoint Question #4

Your patient has a grade 3 neuropathic foot ulcer. You want to unload the ulcer to enhance healing. State three intervention options.

MEDICAL AND SURGICAL INTERVENTIONS

Because of their multifactorial etiology, neuropathic ulcerations can be frustrating for patients, significant others, and medical professionals. However, many studies have demonstrated that the risk of ulceration can be reduced, and the potential to heal after ulceration can be greatly enhanced, by minimizing the risk factors discussed earlier.[1, 29, 36, 41, 54, 55, 65] Although medical and surgical interventions are clearly beyond the scope of physical therapy, they are included here to provide a better understanding of the valuable roles these disciplines play in the management of neuropathic ulcerations.

Medical Interventions

Physicians play a vital role in the management of patients with neuropathic foot ulcerations by assisting with glycemic control, prescribing appropriate antibiotic therapy, and selecting necessary radiological assessments.

Glycemic Control

The results of the United Kingdom Prospective Diabetes Study and the Diabetes Control and Complications Trial clearly indicate that intensive therapy with the goal of near normal blood sugar control can reduce the development and progression of the long-term complications of diabetes.[33, 56, 64, 65, 100, 130–132] A 1% decrease in hemoglobin A_{1c} is associated with a 25% decrease in microvascular complications and a 36% reduction in amputations.[6, 8] In addition, better blood sugar control can improve the body's ability to resist infection and fight existing infections.[29, 53–55, 83] Interestingly, 25% of all people with diabetes do not develop complications regardless of their glycemic control.[133] This can be particularly disconcerting to patients with diabetes who develop complications despite following their suggested regimens and to clinicians who are attempting to emphasize the importance of maintaining glycemic homeostasis. In addition to dietary management and exercise, hypoglycemic agents are the mainstay of treatment for diabetes.[1] Patients with type 1 diabetes require insulin therapy. Patients with type 2 diabetes are generally started on oral hypoglycemic agents, such as sulfonylureas and biguanides. If adequate glycemic control is not attained, insulin may be used either alone or in combination with oral antidiabetic agents.[1, 134] Because the disease course of type 2 diabetes is characterized by the progressive deterioration of beta-cell function, it is essential that pharmacological interventions are regularly reviewed and modified to attain and maintain euglycemia as the disease progresses.[1]

Management of Neuropathic Paresthesias

Physicians may prescribe medications to control neuropathic pain and paresthesias.[23, 134] Anticonvulsants, such as gabapentin, and tricyclic antidepressants, such as amitriptyline, have been shown to decrease the severity of neuropathic pain.[21, 39] Topically applied capsaicin, chili pepper extract, depletes the area of substance P, thereby reducing pain sensation as well.[21] If pain is not adequately controlled, the physician may prescribe opioids or refer the patient to a pain management center.[39]

Management of Concomitant Arterial Insufficiency

Physicians may prescribe medications such as dalteparin to improve local tissue oxygenation and assist in wound healing in patients with concomitant peripheral arterial occlusive disease.[134, 135]

Antibiotic Therapy

Individuals with neuropathic ulcers have both an increased risk of infection and a decreased immune response.[73, 83, 136] A recent study noted that roughly 9% of neuropathic ulcerations were infected at the time of initial examination.[89] Of these, the vast majority of infections was confined to soft tissue, but 20% presented with osteomyelitis.[89] Without appropriate antibiotic coverage, these wounds are unlikely to heal. As with other open wounds, a wound culture and sensitivity is able to detect wound infection and allows for the identification of the offending organism(s). Cultures of neuropathic ulcers average four to five different microbes, including gram-positive, gram-negative, aerobic, and anaerobic organisms, with the most common being group A *Streptococci* and *Staphylococcus aureus*.[37, 83, 101, 137] The goal of antibiotic therapy is to provide broad-spectrum antimicrobial activity that penetrates into the involved tissue with relatively few side effects.[134] Some physicians discourage the use of antibiotics unless the ulcer extends into bone or the signs of a deep space infection are present.[81] However, the standard of care on initial presentation of infection appears to be to obtain a wound culture and prescribe a broad-spectrum antibiotic.[137] This treatment is later fine-tuned based on the sensitivity of the cultured organisms to the various types of antibiotics.[83, 138] In this way, it is possible to combat the infection immediately, thus avoiding a potential spread of the infective process while minimizing the risk of antibiotic resistance by limiting the exposure to ineffective or inappropriate antibiotics.[73, 139]

Antibiotics can be administered orally, topically, or intravenously.[134] There is some debate as to whether topical antibiotics, such as bacitracin or Neosporin, are effective in combating infection,[73] but the consensus appears to be that topical agents are safe and effective when the appropriate guidelines are followed.[140] Previously, intravenous antibiotics required hospitalization, but it is now possible for patients to receive intravenous antibiotics on an outpatient basis, thus reducing the overall cost of medical care and the disruptions to the patient's lifestyle.

Radiological Assessment

In addition to basic medical testing for wounds in general, radiological assessment is particularly helpful in guiding appropriate interventions for patients with neuropathic ulcers.[22] Neuropathic fractures and osteomyelitis are identified by radiological assessment.[37] Conventional x-rays can assist with the identification of a fracture found in acute Charcot foot as well as the presence of any foreign bodies.[22, 73, 83] Vessel wall calcification in patients with severe vascular disease may also be evident on radiographs. Radiographic evidence of osteomyelitis does not show up until approximately 50% of bone mass has been lost.[141] Therefore, the gold standard for the detection of osteomyelitis is the bone scan.[142, 143] Wounds with exposed joint capsule or bone should be assessed for osteomyelitis.

Surgical Interventions

Sometimes neuropathic ulcers require surgical intervention. Surgeons and podiatrists may perform debridement, incision and drainage, antimicrobial bead implantation, and/or amputation.

Debridement

Necrotic tissue is an excellent medium for organisms to grow. Surgical debridement may be more efficient than debridement in a physical therapy setting if a wound contains large amounts of necrotic tissue. Immediate surgical debridement is required in the presence of osteomyelitis.[7, 37, 101] Surgical debridement for osteomyelitis may range from shaving away the infected portion of bone, to performing an osteotomy, to amputating the entire bone.[5, 83] Surgical treatment for osteomyelitis is followed by appropriate antibiotic therapy.[83]

Incision and Drainage

The cardinal signs of an abscess are redness, swelling, increased local temperature, and, occasionally, tenderness. The classic presentation of a deep space infection is similar to that of an abscess except the patient is likely to have a systemic temperature and there may be purulent drainage from the wound. Because of their aggressive, polymicrobial nature, these infections will spread without prompt surgical exploration, drainage, and debridement (e.g., **incision and drainage**) followed by appropriate antibiotic therapy.[73, 81, 83]

Antimicrobial Bead Implantation

A recent advance in the surgical treatment of neuropathic foot ulcers is the implantation of antimicrobial beads (see color image 12). After surgical debridement, a string of beads impregnated with the appropriate antibiotic agent is implanted within the wound.[107] The antimicrobial beads can be made in a number of sizes to match the size of the wound. The beads serve a twofold purpose. First, since the antibiotic is delivered directly to the affected area without having to pass through the body's circulation, it is theorized to be more effective than oral or intravenous antibiotic therapy. Second, the beads can remain in the foot to serve as a biological spacer. This means that the patient does not need to build as much granular tissue to fill the area of previously devitalized tissue, making wound healing faster. The beads can also be removed at any time.

Surgery to Address Abnormal Foot Function or Limited Tissue Perfusion

Various surgical techniques can be employed to try to improve abnormal foot function in patients with neuropathic ulcerations. For example, limited great toe extension has been successfully managed with joint arthroplasty[123] and restricted ankle gastrocnemius length has been treated with surgical tendon lengthening,[45] resulting in accelerated wound closure and decreased rates of ulcer recurrence. Surgical stabilization of Charcot deformities and reduction of abnormal biomechanics have also been successful.[9] While sensory neuropathy and offloading abnormal plantar pressures and shear forces are of prime importance for all patients with neuropathic ulcers, clinicians must remember that wound healing is limited in the absence of satisfactory tissue perfusion and oxygenation. Patients with diabetes have increased rates of microvasculature and macrovascular disease.[1, 24] Therefore, some patients with neuropathic ulcers may benefit from consultation with a vascular surgeon for revascularization options.[1, 40]

Amputation

Gangrenous wounds, Wagner grades 4 and 5, require amputation. If there is no sign of ascending infection, the treatment of choice for a gangrenous toe is usually amputation of the digit. In the presence of an abscess or metatarsal osteomyelitis, the involved ray is resected and left open. When the infection is resolved, the wound is surgically closed.[144] If there is extensive gangrene or infection, or when the functional structure of the foot or lower extremity has been destroyed, the affected areas are amputated and allowed to close by secondary intention.[139]

CHAPTER SUMMARY

Diabetes mellitus is a disorder of carbohydrate, protein, and fat metabolism related to alterations in the body's ability to produce or use insulin. The resulting hyperglycemia damages a variety of body tissues. Of those diagnosed with diabetes, 10% have type 1 diabetes and 90% have type 2 diabetes. There are many risk factors contributing to neuropathic ulceration and delayed wound healing, including vascular disease, neuropathy, mechanical stress, abnormal foot function, inadequate footwear, impaired healing and immune response, poor vision, ulcer and disease characteristics, inadequate professional care, and inadequate patient education. Independently, each risk factor, other than hyperglycemia, does not pose much of a threat. However, risk factors are interrelated, making their combined impact significant. Neuropathic ulcers may be classified using the Integumentary Preferred Practice Patterns, Wagner's classification system, or both to better coordinate patient care among different disciplines. In addition to basic local wound care techniques, physical therapy interventions for patients with neuropathic ulcers should emphasize patient/client-related instruction and may include direct interventions including total contact casting, therapeutic exercise, footwear modifications, and manual therapy techniques.

REVIEW QUESTIONS

1. Does improved blood sugar control affect wound healing? Why or why not?

2. The physician's history and physical on Patient X state that the patient has signs of autonomic neuropathy. State three structural changes you might expect to find when examining Patient X's feet.

3. You have previously instructed Patient D in how to ambulate non-weight bearing with a walker to try to unload his neuropathic ulcer. However, every time he enters the clinic, he is walking without it. Describe three reasons why Patient D might be nonadherent and three alternative methods of unloading the ulcer.

4. You are working with Patient E's neuropathic foot ulcer on the plantar aspect of his first metatarsophalangeal joint. After debriding the ulcer, you notice regularly arranged fibrous tissue in the wound bed. What is this tissue and what should you do?

5. You are asked to examine Mr. W, who has a diagnosis of neuropathic ulcer. Use the wound in color image 19 to answer the following questions.

   a. What tests and measures would you perform on Mr. W?

   b. Document wound and periwound characteristics as you would in the patient's chart.

   c. Should you debride this wound? Why or why not?

   d. Does the wound appear infected?

   e. Describe how you might bandage this wound.

   f. Describe other interventions you might include in your plan of care.

   g. Are there any consults you would request for this patient? Provide your rationale.

PEARSON
myhealthprofessionskit™

Use this address to access the Companion Website created for this textbook. Simply select "Physical Therapy" from the choice of disciplines. Find this book and log in using your username and password to access images, video clips, and additional learning tools.

REFERENCES

Go to myhealthprofessionskit.com to view this chapter's references.

14

Burns

Chapter Objectives

After reading this chapter, learners will be able to:

1. Differentiate the etiology of burn wound injuries from other types of open wounds.
2. Classify the depth of a burn wound injury.
3. Estimate the size of a burn wound injury as a percent of total body surface area.
4. Classify the severity of a burn wound injury.
5. Describe the adverse effects burn wound injuries can have on various tissues, organs, and physiological processes and the clinical relevance of these effects.
6. Design an interdisciplinary approach for the management of patients with burn wound injuries.
7. Describe precautions clinicians should be aware of when working with patients with burn wound injuries.
8. Integrate the keys to local wound care for patients with burn wound injuries.
9. Select physical therapy procedural interventions for patients with burn wound injuries including integumentary repair and protective techniques, therapeutic exercise, devices and equipment, and physical agents and mechanical modalities.
10. Discuss possible medical and surgical interventions for patients with burn wound injuries.

Key Terms

Burn shock
Conversion
Deep partial-thickness burn
Escharotomy
Fasciotomy
Full-thickness burn

Full-thickness skin grafts
Lund–Browder classification
Rule of nines
Split-thickness skin grafts
Subdermal burn

Superficial burn
Superficial partial-thickness burn
Zone of coagulation
Zone of hyperemia
Zone of stasis

INTRODUCTION

There are greater than 2 million burn injuries per year in the United States,[1] including over 40,000 hospitalizations and 4,000 deaths.[2] Higher surface area involvement and presence of inhalation injuries are associated with greater mortality.[3, 4] One-third of burn victims are children.[3] In fact, fire and burn injuries are the second leading cause of death in children between 1 and 4 years of age, and the third leading cause of death in children under 19 years of age.[5-7] Most burn injuries occur in the home,[3] primarily in the kitchen and bathroom, and an estimated 75% of all burn injuries and deaths are preventable.[6] Child abuse is reportedly responsible for 10–30%[6, 8] of pediatric burn injuries,[5] most often via scalding.[9]

Burn injuries cause destruction to the integument as well as a host of other physiological changes that can affect every body system. This chapter begins with a discussion of the pathophysiology of the three types of burn injuries: thermal, chemical, and electrical. Next, the classification of burn injuries, including depth, size, and severity, is presented. This is followed by a discussion of the pathophysiological effects of burn injuries on key tissues and the clinical consequences of these effects. Finally, the chapter presents a thorough description of physical therapy and medical and surgical interventions for the management of burn wound injuries.

ETIOLOGY OF BURN INJURIES

Burns occur when energy is transferred from a heat source to the body. If heat absorption is greater than heat dissipation, cell temperature rises and may reach a point where cell death occurs. There are three types of burn injuries: thermal, chemical, and electrical (see Table 14–1). Thermal burns are the most common type of burn injury and result from direct or indirect contact with a flame, hot liquid, or steam.[3] The severity of a thermal burn injury is proportional to the contact time, temperature, and type of insult sustained. Brief exposure to temperatures greater than 120°F can cause tissue destruction, while only 5 seconds of exposure to temperatures above 140°F can cause a full-thickness burn.[10]

Thermal energy is produced when strong acids or alkalis react with body tissues.[11] If enough thermal energy is generated, a chemical burn injury may result. Although typically smaller in surface area than thermal burns, chemical burns are more likely to cause full-thickness skin damage and account for 2–7% of all burn unit admissions.[12] The severity of a chemical burn injury is related to the contact time with the skin as well as the type, concentration, and amount of chemical.[10] The burning process continues until the chemical is removed or sufficiently diluted.[13] If acidic chemicals come in contact with the integument, skin proteins neutralize the acid, causing coagulation necrosis and limiting the extent of tissue injury.[12, 13] In contrast, alkaline chemicals denature the proteins within the skin,[13] causing liquefaction necrosis and deeper penetration of tissue damage.[12] Therefore, burns resulting from alkaline chemicals tend to be more severe than burns due to acids.[1] In addition to direct cutaneous damage from chemicals, inhalation of the fumes created by chemical spills can lead to pulmonary dysfunction.[12, 14] Although the thought of a chemical burn may lead one to envision a high school chemistry experiment gone awry, most chemical burns are the result of either assaults or industrial accidents with compounds, such as cement and asphalt.

TABLE 14–1   Types of Burn Injuries

Burn Type	Examples	Factors Influencing Severity
Thermal	• Direct contact with flame, hot liquid, steam • Indirect contact with flame, hot liquid, steam	• Contact time • Temperature • Type of insult
Chemical	• Acids • Bases • Industrial accidents • Assaults	• Alkali burns are more severe • Contact time • Chemical concentration • Amount of chemical
Electrical	• Low voltage • High voltage	• AC burn injuries are more severe • Contact time • Voltage

There are over 4,400 electrical burn injuries per year in the United States, resulting in 800–1,000 deaths.[3] From 4% to 7% of burn unit admissions are due to electrical injuries, and up to 20% of those admitted are children.[12] Recall that resistance is the impedance to the flow of electricity. Dry skin has a high resistance, whereas skin that is wet or moist with sweat has less resistance.[15] Blood vessels and nerves have low resistance and are good conductors of electricity. Bone and muscle have higher resistances. Resistance to electrical flow results in heat production. The skin, because of its large external surface area, is able to dissipate this heat better than deeper tissues.[16] Electrical injuries commonly present with a depressed or charred entrance wound and a larger, explosive-appearing exit wound.[17] Although there may be little or no integumentary damage between these two wounds, the passage of electrical current through deeper, less resistant tissues typically results in healthy-appearing skin covering deeper tissue necrosis.[12, 18] Forty-four percent of electrical burn patients have concomitant musculoskeletal dysfunction including fractures[11] and muscle necrosis.[19] Early and late neurological injuries, such as carpal tunnel syndrome and other mono- and polyneuropathies, are also common.[15] The flow of electricity through the body may also induce cardiac dysrhythmias, cardiac arrest, and pulmonary arrest.[15, 18] Finally, acute single- and multiorgan system dysfunction, such as renal failure, may occur and has a high mortality rate.[19]

The severity of an electrical injury depends on the type of current, duration of contact, and voltage.[1] At a given voltage, alternating current, such as a standard household outlet, penetrates the skin more readily than direct current, such as the third rail of an electric train, and produces three times the amount of tissue damage.[3] Contact with electrical currents produces tetanic muscle contractions, making release of an electrified object more difficult, prolonging contact time, and leading to more extensive injuries.[15] Electrical injuries are described as being either low- or high-voltage injuries. Low-voltage injuries result from currents from 120 to 240 volts and account for 43–66%[12, 20] of all electrical injuries. Low-voltage injuries typically result from household accidents, such as children biting electrical cords or putting metal objects into electrical outlets. In contrast, high-voltage injuries result from currents greater than 1,000 volts. Power lines or lightning strikes are the usual culprits. With voltages this high, tissue resistance is negligible,[12] making extensive deep tissue damage probable. Almost 80% of high-voltage victims will require at least one amputation, and nearly a quarter require fasciotomies or escharotomies to reduce local tissue pressure.[16, 19] High-voltage currents may arc across the patient's skin surfaces, causing additional integumentary damage[11] and the need for extensive surgical debridement.[20]

CASE STUDY: Miss Amy Kim

This case study is referenced throughout the chapter.

PART 1

History

Amy Kim is a 19-year-old Asian female seen this morning in an acute care hospital for physical therapy and wound management. Her primary language is English. She is a sophomore in college and has a work-study job 10 hours per week in the university library reshelving books. She lives in a dormitory on campus with two roommates with a shared bathroom.

Wound History: According to her medical record, Miss Kim's ex-boyfriend poured alcohol over her and then lit her on fire yesterday. She reports significant pain at rest on her anterior trunk and left upper extremity. She reports inability to use her left upper extremity at this time due to pain and bandages.

Past Medical History: Miss Kim had her tonsils removed at age 10 and has no known allergies.

General Health Status: Miss Kim reports she was in excellent health prior to this event and that she enjoys participating in recreational flag football and jogging.

Current Medications: Miss Kim is currently on a Demerol PCA pump and oral hydrocodone.

Other Available Data: Laboratory values available from the patient chart include hematocrit = 48%, white blood cell count = 11,000/mm^3, platelets = 250,000/mm^3, albumin = 4.5 g/dL, blood glucose 145 mg/dL, BUN 30 mg/dL, creatinine 0.9 mg/dL. TcPO$_2$ 97% on room air. Body temperature 100.0°F.

CASE STUDY Continued

Systems Review

Cardiovascular/Pulmonary System: Heart rate: 106 bpm, blood pressure 80/50 mm Hg, respiratory rate 11 bpm. Minimal distal left upper extremity edema.

Musculoskeletal System: Gross assessment reveals range of motion deficits in left shoulder elevation, left elbow, and right cervical sidebend due to pain. Height: 68 inches (1.73 m). Body weight: 125 pounds (56.8 kg). Body mass index (BMI) = 19 kg/m^2.

Neuromuscular System: No gross deficits noted in gross coordinated movement or motor control.

Gastrointestinal System: No problems noted.

Urogenital System: Miss Kim has an indwelling catheter that was placed on admission yesterday.

Integumentary System: Burns noted on Miss Kim's anterior and left lateral thorax, neck, and left upper extremity.

Communication, Cognition, Language, and Learning Style: Miss Kim avoids eye contact and does not volunteer information unless specifically asked. Miss Kim states that she is afraid her boyfriend will try to hurt her again. Miss Kim reports she learns best by demonstration. She verbalizes an understanding of her situation and a willingness to participate in wound management interventions.

CLASSIFICATION AND CHARACTERISTICS OF BURN INJURIES

Burn injuries are classified by the level of tissue involvement and by the amount of surface area affected. Together, burn size and depth are used to determine the overall severity of a burn injury as well as assist with making a wound healing prognosis.

Depth of Burn Injuries

Historically, burn depth was described in terms of degrees (e.g., first-degree burn). However, burn injuries are more accurately categorized by the level of tissue involvement,[10] similar to the Integumentary Preferred Practice Patterns in the *Guide to Physical Therapist Practice* (see Figure 14–1). Because skin depth varies in different anatomical locations and individual burns are not uniform in depth, classification can be difficult. Burns affecting the palms of the hands and the soles of the feet may initially appear to be quite deep, but may actually be less severe because of the thickness of the skin in these locations. Clinicians should be cautious with their assessment of burn depth immediately after chemical exposure because it takes up to 24–72 hours for a chemical burn to fully develop, making the determination of the depth of these injuries particularly problematic.[11] Clinicians should use burn depth and patient and wound characteristics to make their prognosis for wound healing.

Superficial Burns

Superficial burns, also known as first-degree burns, involve only the epidermis.[21] These burns fit into Integumentary Preferred Practice Pattern B: Impaired Integumentary Integrity Associated with Superficial Skin Involvement. Superficial burns, such as a sunburn or minor flash burn,[22] are characterized by dry, bright red, or pink skin that blanches under pressure.[23] The erythema is due to irritation of the underlying dermal vasculature and may be delayed for several hours after exposure.[24] Although a mild edema may be seen around the eyes with facial burns,[24] superficial burns generally do not cause edema because the dermal vessels remain undamaged.[25] No blisters are formed.[13] However, the skin may exfoliate (peel) several days after exposure.[11] The skin maintains its barrier function,[21] including its impermeability to bacteria and ability to regulate the body's fluid content. Superficial burns resolve spontaneously in 3–5 days without scarring.[23, 24]

Superficial Partial-Thickness Burns

Superficial partial-thickness burns, also known as superficial second-degree burns, involve the epidermis and papillary dermis (see color image 20).[21] These burns fit into Integumentary Preferred Practice Pattern C: Impaired Integumentary Integrity Associated with Partial-Thickness Skin Involvement and Scar Formation. Superficial partial-thickness (SPT) burns

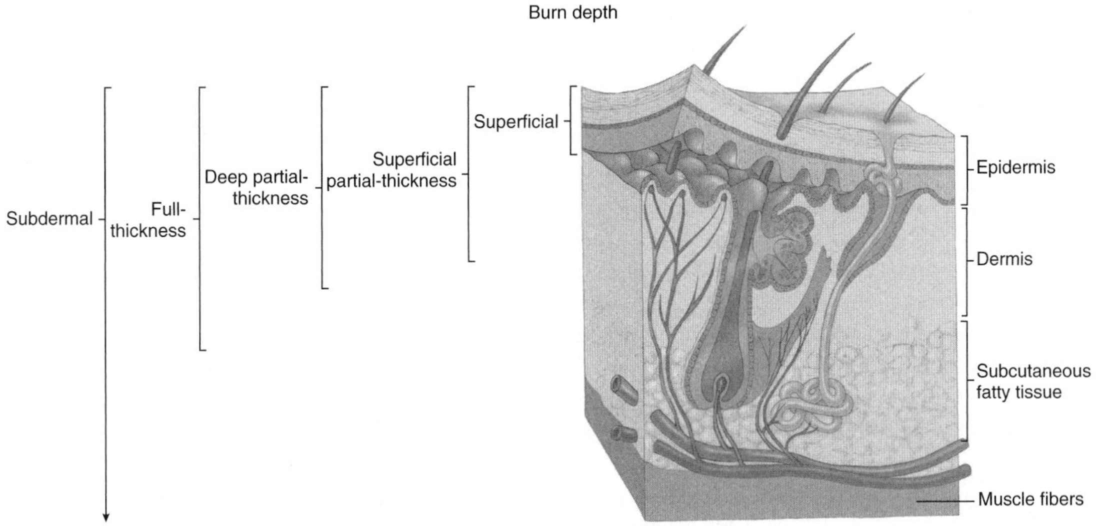

Burn depth

FIGURE 14–1   Depth of tissue involvement in burn wound injuries.
Source: Emergency Care 9/e by Limmer/O'Keefe/Grant/Murray/Bergeron.

may result from severe sunburns, brief contact burns, scalds, flash burns, and brief contact with dilute chemicals.[1, 22] These burns are characterized by moist, weeping, blistered skin.[1, 21] Dermal inflammation causes local erythema and edema. Compromised vascular integrity allows fluid and proteins to leak into the interstitium exacerbating moderate edema.[25, 26] Like superficial burns, SPT burns blanch under pressure. However, immediate capillary refill is the hallmark of SPT burns.[26] SPT burns are usually extremely painful because of exposed nerve endings.[14] The area may be particularly sensitive to pressure and air.[23] A large amount of wound drainage is possible, especially if blisters are removed or broken. SPT burns heal within 10 to 14 days with minimal or no scarring.[5, 10] However, there may be pigment changes due to melanocyte destruction.[24] After wound closure, hypersensitivity and itching are common.

Deep Partial-Thickness Burns

Deep partial-thickness burns, also known as deep second-degree burns, involve the epidermis and dermis (see color image 21).[21] These burns also fit into Integumentary Preferred Practice Pattern C: Impaired Integumentary Integrity Associated with Partial-Thickness Skin Involvement and Scar Formation.[22] Deep partial-thickness (DPT) burns may result from contact with hot liquids or objects, flash burns, or chemical burns. These burns have extensive damage to dermal vessels and are characterized by mottled areas of red with white eschar.[21] Although typically absent,[21] DPT burns may have large or ruptured blisters.[24] Because some pain receptors remain intact, DPT burns may be painful or have areas of insensitivity.[23] DPT burns blanch to pressure; however, unlike SPT burns, capillary refill is sluggish.[1, 26] When assessing sensation, areas of DPT burns have decreased pinprick sensation but intact pressure sensation.[13, 26] DPT burns may convert into full-thickness burns,[27] especially if they become infected or if adequate tissue perfusion is not restored.[21, 28]

Because some of the epidermal appendages, such as hair follicles and sebaceous glands, are spared, DPT wounds are able to reepithelialize both from the periphery and from these islands of epithelial tissue.[1, 13] Healing time for DPT burns varies with wound size. Smaller wounds may heal within 3 weeks, while larger wounds may take several additional weeks to achieve wound closure.[21] Physicians may choose to perform skin grafting procedures on patients with extensive areas of DPT burns.[10, 21] DPT burns result in scarring and pigment changes.[1] Hypertrophic scarring and contracture formation are possible.[1] After wound closure, the new tissue may have fewer sebaceous glands, resulting in pruritus, scaling, and skin that is easily abraded.

Full-Thickness Burns

Full-thickness burns, also known as third-degree burns, result in destruction of the epidermis and dermis to the subcutaneous tissues.[11, 21] Adipose tissue may be exposed.[11, 21, 24] These burns fit into Integumentary Preferred Practice Pattern D: Impaired Integumentary Integrity Associated with Full-Thickness Skin Involvement and Scar Formation.[22] Full-thickness (FT) burns may result from an immersion scald injury, prolonged contact with a flame or steam, contact with electrical currents, or exposure to chemicals.[21, 29] Infection can convert a partial-thickness burn injury into a full-thickness injury.[11, 30] FT burns may initially be red, but quickly become mottled white, gray, or black.[21] The white areas represent ischemia, while the red discoloration is likely due to hemoglobin from the destruction of red blood cells.[24, 25] The necrotic tissue may even appear charred, and thrombosed vessels may be visible.[21] The eschar generally appears leathery, rigid, and dry.[21, 26] The area should be thoroughly examined for exposed deep tissues, such as tendons, muscle, fascia, ligament, joint capsule, and bone. FT burns involve little surface pain because of the destruction of all cutaneous nerve endings[27] and are insensate to pressure and temperature.[21, 26] However, this does not mean FT burns are not painful. Burns are rarely all one depth.[26] Therefore, less severely damaged areas surrounding FT burns are likely to be excruciatingly painful. Because the epidermis has been completely destroyed, FT burns heal by epithelial cell migration from the wound margins and wound contraction.[13, 17] Only small FT wounds will heal on their own.[17] Most FT wounds require surgical debridement and some form of surgical closure, such as skin grafting.[13, 21] Scarring from FT burns is likely.[23] Because hair follicles and sebacious glands do not regenerate, these are absent in scar tissue.[31] FT burns are at increased risk for hypertrophic scarring and contractures.

Subdermal Burns

Subdermal burns, sometimes referred to as fourth-degree burns, result in destruction beyond the dermis and into fat, muscle, tendon, and/or bone.[13, 21] These burns fit into Integumentary Preferred Practice Pattern E: Impaired Integumentary Integrity Associated with Skin Involvement Extending into Fascia, Muscle, or Bone and Scar Formation.[32] Subdermal burns are typically caused by electrical injuries, prolonged thermal contact, or exposure to strong chemicals.[3] Subdermal burns have a charred or mummified appearance.[21] They are dry and typically have minimal edema. These areas should be assessed for exposed tendons, muscle, fascia, cartilage, capsule, and bone. The surface of subdermal burns is insensate. These burns will not heal without extensive surgical intervention, including fasciotomy, escharotomy, and grafting. Amputation is often necessary,[21] and muscle paralysis may occur due to permanent nerve damage. See Table 14–2 for a summary of depth of tissue involvement in burn wound injuries.

Estimation of Burn Size

In addition to the depth of a burn injury, the clinician must also measure burn size. Unlike other types of wounds, burn injuries may be irregular in shape and cover an extensive amount of surface area. Therefore, it may be both impractical and pointless to perform wound tracings or to take traditional length and width measurements. Instead, burn wound size is generally described in terms of percentage of total body surface area (TBSA).[10] There are three generally accepted methods to calculate the percentage of TBSA affected: the rule of nines, the Lund–Browder classification, and the palmar method. Areas of superficial burns are never included in these calculations.[11]

Rule of Nines

The **rule of nines** divides the integument into areas roughly equivalent to 9% of TBSA.[10, 21] Using this method, the head, the front and back of each upper extremity, the front of each lower extremity, and the back of each lower extremity all represent 9% of TBSA. The anterior trunk and the posterior trunk each equal 18% of TBSA. The perineum represents 1% of TBSA. The rule of nines consistently overestimates the size of a burn injury.[33] There is also some variability in the estimates of burn size when using the rule of nines; however, clinician reliability improves with experience.[33] Despite these flaws, the rule of nines is the fastest and easiest method of determining the percent of TBSA involved in a burn wound and is a universally recognized method of assessing burn size.[10]

Lund–Browder Classification

With relatively larger heads and smaller lower extremities, infants and young children have different body proportions than adults.[26] The **Lund–Browder classification** takes into account these variations in the distribution of body surface area when determining the size of a burn injury.[10] For example, the head and face of an infant account for 18% of TBSA, while in the adult this same locale accounts for a mere 9% of

TABLE 14–2   Depth of Burn Injuries

Burn Depth	Involved Tissues	Clinical Presentation	Prognosis
Superficial	• Epidermis	• Dry, red skin without open areas • May exfoliate	• Heal in 5 days without scarring
Superficial partial-thickness	• Epidermis • Papillary dermis	• Weeping, blistered skin • Blanches to pressure with quick capillary refill • Moderate edema • Large amounts of drainage possible • Extremely painful	• Heal in 10–14 days • May have minimal scarring
Deep partial-thickness	• Epidermis • Dermis	• Mottled red and white areas • Painful • Blanches to pressure with slow capillary refill • Decreased pinprick but intact pressure sensation	• Small wounds heal in 3 weeks • Reepithelialize from periphery and spared epidermal appendages • Large wounds may be managed surgically • Result in scarring and pigment changes
Full-thickness	• Epidermis • Dermis • Damage to the subcutaneous tissue	• Mottled appearance • Dry, rigid, leathery eschar • Thrombosed vessels may be visible • Lack pain, pressure, and temperature sensation	• Require >3 weeks to close • Small wounds heal by epithelial cell migration from perimeter and wound contraction • Usually require surgical closure • Result in scarring • May have contractures
Subdermal	• Epidermis • Dermis • Destruction through the subcutaneous tissues	• Charred • Mummified • Dry • Exposed deep tissues	• Require surgical interventions • Amputation and paralysis possible • Result in scarring

TBSA (see Figure 14–2). Therefore, this method of estimating burn size is more appropriate for children under 16 years of age.[5, 34] Despite its complexity, the Lund–Browder classification is preferred by pediatric burn units.[3, 26]

Palmar Method

The palmar method uses the area of the palmar surface of the hand to determine burn size. However, some authors estimate the size of the palm to represent 1% of TBSA,[5, 24] while others estimate it at 0.5%[35] or 0.8%.[26] This inconsistency makes the palmar method highly unreliable. Additionally, the estimation of the "number of palms" that would be required to cover large burns, such as the anterior thigh and trunk, is unlikely to be very accurate. For these reasons, clinicians should not use the palmar method to estimate the size of a burn injury.

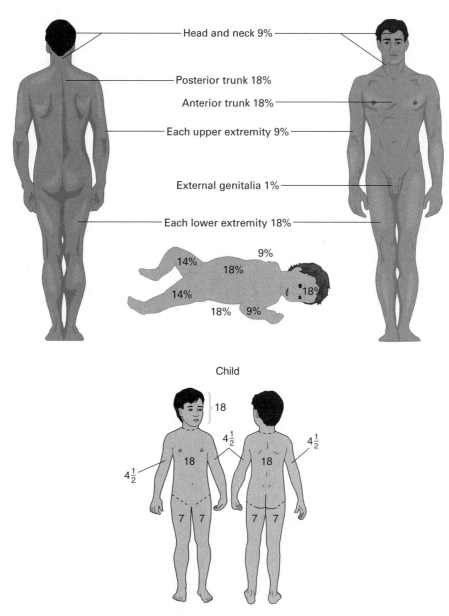

FIGURE 14–2 Determining burn wound size.

Source: Emergency Care 9/e by Limmer/O'Keefe/Grant/Murray/Bergeron..

TABLE 14–3   Burn Severity

Classification	Adult		Child	
	%FT	%PT	%FT	%PT
Minor	<2	<10	<1	<5
Moderate	2–5	10–20	1–5	5–10
Major	>5	>20	>5	>10

%FT, Percentage of total body surface area burn that is a full-thickness burn injury.

%PT, Percentage of total body surface area burn that is a partial-thickness burn injury.

Burn Severity

The depth and size of a burn injury are used to determine severity. The American Burn Association categorizes the extent of burn injuries as minor, moderate, and major (see Table 14–3).[30] These categories can help clinicians to determine the most appropriate setting for patient management. However, clinicians are cautioned that burn size has not been found to correlate with patient pain complaint[14] as a burn wound covering 5% of TBSA may be as painful as one covering 50%. Major burn injuries also include partial- or full-thickness burns involving most of the hands,[16] face, or genitalia; circumferential burns; electrical burn injuries; severe or extensive chemical burn injuries; and burn injuries with concomitant inhalation injuries.[21, 30]

Minor burn injuries are usually treated on an outpatient basis[1, 30] assuming burns do not cover critical areas, pain is adequately controlled by oral medications, and there is no suspicion of abuse.[6, 35] These patients will likely need some form of assistance at home for activities of daily living or for burn wound care. Moderate burn injuries are generally managed on an inpatient basis in a community hospital[30] because of the greater integumentary involvement and potential for concomitant organ system dysfunctions. Patients with major burn injuries are generally managed in specialized burn units.[3] In some cases, the attending physician may choose to manage the patient within the community hospital setting after consultation with a burn unit team. The American Burn Association recommends that patients with major burn injuries, burn injuries associated with major trauma, or burn injuries with significant comorbidities be referred to a burn unit.[3, 10]

 Checkpoint Question #1

You are called to the emergency room to examine a patient who spilled hydrochloric acid on his left hand while conducting an experiment in chemistry class earlier that morning. The wound bed is blistered and draining. The patient is able to detect light touch and pressure within the burned area. When digital pressure is applied to the wound bed, the area blanches and capillary refill is rapid. How would you classify the depth of this burn injury?

PATHOPHYSIOLOGY OF BURN INJURIES

Extensive integumentary trauma results in loss of the barrier function of the skin, leading to massive fluid loss, increased risk of infection, and hypothermia. However, in the case of large or severe burns, the assessment and treatment of the integument are of secondary importance.[35] A major burn causes a massive, sustained physiological stress response. Systemic complications of severe burn injuries, such as dysfunction of the cardiovascular, pulmonary, immune, and other organ systems as well as alterations in metabolism, can be life threatening. The acute and long-term psychological effects of a burn injury must also be considered.

The circumstances surrounding many burn injuries may result in associated injuries, such as fractures or head injuries due to falls or anoxia due to smoke inhalation, which must also be identified and addressed. This section reviews the wide-reaching effects a burn injury can have on body systems. The global clinical consequences of each of these pathophysiological responses are briefly highlighted, but more in-depth clinical information is provided within the section on physical therapy interventions.

Integumentary System

The first step in burn management is to stop the burning process. The patient must be safely removed from contact with heat sources or electrical current, and all nonadherent clothing and jewelry should be removed. If powdered chemicals are present, they should be brushed off the skin.[13] Chemical burn injuries should be thoroughly irrigated with massive quantities of water for at least 20–30 minutes.[18]

Integumentary damage due to burn injuries is divided into three concentric circles known as the zones of coagulation, stasis, and hyperemia (see Figure 14–3). The **zone of coagulation** is the central portion of the burn. This region has suffered irreparable damage and is characterized by coagulation, ischemia, and necrosis.[10, 28] The zone of coagulation may expand for up to 48 hours after the initial burn injury.[7, 36] The **zone of stasis** surrounds this central necrotic region and represents an area of cellular injury and compromised tissue perfusion.[10] Red blood cells and platelets aggregate and may form microemboli, further impeding local circulation. Unless adequate perfusion is restored within 1 to 2 days after injury, these cells will not survive.[5] This process of widening and deepening of the original area of necrosis is known as **conversion.**[5] For example, a DPT burn may be converted into an FT burn injury if improperly managed.[28] The **zone of hyperemia** represents the outer edges of tissue affected by the burn injury.[10] These tissues receive the least thermal energy and sustain only minimal cellular injury. This area is characterized by erythema due to vasodilation and generally recovers within 7 to 10 days of injury.[28]

Consequences for Clinicians

The depth of a burn injury can be affected by physical therapy interventions. Bandages that are too tight, splints that cause excessive pressure, and positioning without sufficient tissue unloading further impede the already precarious circulation in the zone of stasis, ultimately exacerbating the clinical condition. Patients who have lost protective sensation or who are incoherent because of injury or medication will be unable to sense these forms of tissue trauma and must be meticulously monitored. Refer to the section on local wound care for specific details regarding treatment of the integument.

Cardiovascular System

Burn shock is a complex clinical syndrome that develops when perfusion is unable to meet the demands of body tissues.[5] As skin cells die, they release enzymes that increase capillary permeability,[1] allowing intravascular fluid, proteins, and electrolytes to leak out of the vessels.[26] Burn injuries also cause venous dilation and a massive release of histamine and other inflammatory mediators.[10] In combination, these factors cause a massive fluid shift from the vasculature to the interstitium.[26] Additional fluid is lost directly from burned areas through evaporation at a rate five to ten times faster than through intact skin.[5] This hemodynamic

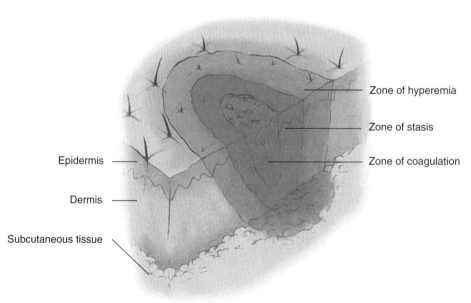

FIGURE 14–3 Zones of injury.

Source: Paramedic Care: Principles & Practice—Trauma Emergencies by Bledsoe/Porter/Cherry.

Zone of hyperemia

Zone of stasis

Zone of coagulation

Epidermis

Dermis

Subcutaneous tissue

instability causes hypovolemia and edema.[28] Cardiac output may be decreased by as much as 50% for the first 2–4 days after a severe burn.[10] The delayed release of bradykinin further compromises tissue perfusion by causing widespread vasoconstriction.[37] All of these factors—hypovolemia, increased capillary permeability, edema, and vasoconstriction—result in a decrease in circulating blood volume. Because the red blood cells remain within the vasculature, the increased hematocrit and blood viscosity slow blood flow, further impairing circulation and increasing the potential for microemboli.[1] These physiological responses deprive tissues of oxygen and nutrients and cause waste products to accumulate. Tissue necrosis, organ dysfunction, and even death may occur as a result.[10]

The administration of large quantities of intravenous fluids is needed to counteract the effects of burn shock.[33, 38, 39] Many times patients with significant burn injuries will have a central line placed because of the difficulties of obtaining and maintaining peripheral access sites in areas of uninjured skin.[10] Although capillary integrity is generally restored to the uninjured areas within 36 hours,[7] the effects of this massive fluid shift take considerably longer to resolve.[40] The larger the burn, the greater the risk of burn shock and the more urgent the need for fluid resuscitation.[26] Patients with burns covering more than 15% TBSA are at high risk for burn shock.[28, 33]

Consequences for Clinicians

Although physical therapists and physical therapist assistants do not manage burn shock and compromised circulation directly, they must understand this physiological process for several reasons. First, clinicians must recognize that fluid resuscitation is of primary importance.[10] Intravenous lines should not be disconnected for ease of skin care or other therapeutic interventions, and increased care must be taken to ensure intravenous lines are not compromised.

Second, clinicians must be aware of the effect these cardiovascular changes can have on the patient's vital signs.[10] Blood pressure generally decreases as a result of hypovolemia. However, an increase in blood pressure may signal anxiety or inadequate pain control and should be further investigated.[6] Within hours of a burn injury, patients develop sinus tachycardia in an attempt to maintain cardiac output at an acceptable level. In response to a burn injury, adult patients will generally have a resting heart rate between 100 and 120 beats per minute, and children will have a heart rate between 120 and 170 beats per minute.[34] This increase in resting heart rate means patients will have lower cardiac reserves for any increase in activity, such as mobility training and range of motion exercise. Therefore, patient response to these activities must be carefully monitored. Cardiac dysrhythmias are common after electrical injuries,[3] and these patients are generally placed in units where cardiac activity can be monitored.

Third, clinicians must monitor and manage edema. Not only can edema limit normal range of motion and function, but it can also limit venous return and increase the risk of progressive arterial occlusion.[3] Peripheral pulses in all extremities should be palpated frequently or identified by Doppler ultrasound if necessary.[10] Because burned tissues are inelastic, extremities with circumferential burn injuries can create a tourniquet-like effect due to the accompanying edema. Vascular occlusion may result in ischemia and distal tissue necrosis.[18] Compartment syndrome, when compartmental pressures rise from a normal range of less than 9 mm Hg to greater than 30 mm Hg,[29] must be rapidly identified and managed surgically, usually by means of escharotomy or fasciotomy, to reduce tissue pressures and prevent permanent tissue loss and/or amputation.[10] Clinicians must watch for and report these signs if observed.

Pulmonary System

Pulmonary dysfunction—including pulmonary edema, acute respiratory distress syndrome, pneumonia, and inflammation—is a major cause of morbidity and mortality after burn injuries.[3] Inhalation injuries are responsible for up to 20% of burn mortalities.[41] Carbon monoxide, produced by the combustion of organic materials, has 200–220 times greater affinity for binding oxygen than hemoglobin.[42] Carbon monoxide poisoning and smoke inhalation account for half of all deaths[42] that occur after the first 12 hours of a burn injury.[43] Lung tissue may be directly traumatized by the inhalation of toxic gases impairing the mucociliary escalator and damaging the cell membranes of the lower airways.[41] Increased pulmonary vascular resistance due to vasoconstriction and decreased lung compliance due to direct trauma to lung tissues can rapidly result in hypoxemia.[11] Severe airway inflammation may lead to occlusion, asphyxia, and even death.[41] Inhalation injury may damage the mucociliary elevator, preventing clearance of debris, exfoliating epithelial cells, and bacteria from the airways.[14, 42] Circumferential or large torso burns[35] may limit chest expansion, impairing ventilation.[44] Pain, fear, and severely limited mobility may also lead to reduced pulmonary inflation, further contributing to hypoxia. Finally, hemodynamic instability and burn shock may lead to pulmonary edema, resulting in impaired gas exchange within the lungs.

Consequences for Clinicians

Pulmonary involvement should be suspected in patients with singed facial hair, carbonaceous sputum (sputum that is black and contains particulate matter including carbon), a history of a closed-space injury, or burns to the face, neck, or torso.[41] In patients who present with these findings, hoarseness, cough, or dyspnea should be closely monitored.[41] Aggressive pulmonary hygiene must be encouraged.[42] Clinicians must monitor for signs of increasing difficulty breathing and report these changes to the physician immediately. It is estimated that 50% of burn unit patients will require intubation at some point.[41]

Metabolism

The basal metabolic rate may double or even triple with severe burn injuries, and this hypermetabolism has far-reaching effects.[5, 45] The stress of a burn injury causes the release of cortisol and catecholamines, resulting in an increase in heat production to counteract the heat loss from burned areas. As a result, core body temperature (100.4–102.2°F) and skin temperature are elevated.[7, 30] There is an increase in resting oxygen consumption and excessive nitrogen loss due to an increase in catabolism.[45] Sustained hyperglycemia, increased fat catabolism, and a decrease in body mass are predictable.[45] This hypermetabolic response peaks 7–17 days after injury and slowly returns to normal as wounds approach closure.[10]

Patients with severe burn injuries have significantly greater nutritional requirements than normal because of the need to repair tissues directly and indirectly affected by burns.[10, 30] Malnutrition is possible without proper nutritional interventions,[34] including a high-protein, high-calorie diet.[27] Increased protein intake is essential for the body to build the collagen necessary for tissue repair and regeneration.

Consequences for Clinicians

Nutrition is a priority for patients with burn injuries. Rehabilitation should be scheduled around patient meals, and clinicians should encourage food and water intake. Air temperature and, for patients undergoing hydrotherapy, water temperature should be set to prevent additional insensible heat loss. Heat lamps and blankets may be beneficial. Wounds should remain bandaged except for local wound care.

Immune System

Sepsis and infection are common and can be significant complications of burn injuries for various reasons.[10] It is estimated that up to 75% of burn deaths may be due to infection.[46] First, the often extensive integumentary surface area involvement impairs the barrier function of the skin.[34, 47] Endogenous bacteria present on the skin's surface,[47] in hair follicles, and in glands, as well as exogenous bacteria from hospital personnel and equipment, may cause infection.[48] However, burn injuries also change the normal skin microflora, which may lead to an increase in the number of pathogenic bacteria. Second, decreased tissue perfusion reduces the ability of immune cells to reach the affected areas.[10] Third, for reasons yet unknown, neutrophils that are able to reach the site of injury are less effective in destroying microbes that are encountered.[30] Fourth, eschar, blister fluid, and residual topical agents provide excellent media for bacterial proliferation. Fifth, burn wounds, especially FT burns, may be open for extensive periods of time. Sixth, malnutrition due to poor enteral intake or inadequate parenteral supplementation is associated with infection and impaired burn wound healing.[45] Last, the body's immune system is compromised by the sustained physiological stress of a severe burn injury. In addition to wound site infections, infections may also arise from intravascular and urinary catheters.[36] Pulmonary involvement increases the risk of respiratory infections, such as pneumonia.[3]

Consequences for Clinicians

To help reduce the risk of wound infection and sepsis, clinicians should perform aggressive debridement and strive to achieve wound closure or skin coverage as soon as possible.[36] Prophylactic use of topical antimicrobials should be standard. The use of a topical antimicrobial for major burn wounds reduces mortality rates by 10% compared to no topical agent.[49] The most common bacteria present early after a burn wound injury is *Staphyloccocus aureus*.[46, 47, 50] However, burn wounds that remain open more than 2–3 weeks are more likely to have significant numbers of *Pseudomonas aeruginosa* and a higher incidence of methicillin-resistant *Staphylococcus aureus* (MRSA).[46, 47, 50] Because of the changing nature of colonizing and infecting bacteria over time, clinicians must carefully monitor for signs and symptoms of infection and contact the physician if they suspect changes in topical agent or pharmacotherapy may be needed. Additionally, to decrease the risk of resistant bacterial strains, prophylactic antibiotic use should be reserved only for patients with the highest risk of infection.[36, 50] Clinicians should consistently follow rigorous infection control techniques for all patients with burn wounds. Sterile technique should be instituted with patients who have large burn injuries or are immunocompromised to reduce the risk of infection. In addition, clinicians should encourage good pulmonary hygiene to decrease the risk of pulmonary compromise.

Other Organ Systems

Hypovolemia, tissue hypoxia, or sepsis may cause multisystem organ dysfunction.[10] Central nervous system dysfunction, including hallucinations, delirium, personality changes, and seizures, may also occur. If untreated, permanent brain damage can result.[34] Decreased kidney perfusion and hypovolemia result in reduced renal blood flow and glomerular filtration rates and may lead to acute kidney failure.[10] Kidney failure may also result from the release of large amounts of myoglobin into the bloodstream due to extensive muscle damage.[10] Gastrointestinal dysfunction,[10] such as decreased peristalsis, ileus, and ulcers, is common, especially in patients with wounds involving greater than 20% TBSA. Pain medications[11] and the psychological stress of a burn injury may also lead to gastrointestinal dysfunction. Last, organic compounds may be absorbed through the skin.[18] Therefore, topical exposure to organic compounds not only results in chemical burns, but may also cause systemic toxicity.

Consequences for Clinicians

Swift correction of hypovolemia and burn shock can limit the severity of organ dysfunction. Because mobility can assist with circulation and edema control, gastrointestinal motility, and psychological well-being, early controlled mobility is encouraged.

Psychological Dysfunction

The side effects of medication,[51] the disruption of normal routines, and the emotional trauma of a burn injury may result in acute psychological dysfunction.[52] It is common for patients with burn injuries to experience sleep disturbances, nightmares, confusion, delirium, or even hallucinations.[53] Posttraumatic stress disorder, depression, disturbed sleep, and anxiety are normal responses to severe burn injuries.[51, 52] For the first few days after a severe burn injury, anxiety[54] and fear of death and pain[54] are common. The patient may appear uncooperative, withdraw from social interaction, or exhibit inappropriate behaviors.[10] As patient recovery continues, the patient will likely become more verbal and have increased complaints or demands. It is estimated that 73% of patients with burn injuries continue to have sleep disturbances after discharge from the hospital and anywhere from 25% to 65% of patients with burn injuries experience depression during the first year after their injury.[51] Patients with burns report feeling more vulnerable and more frail.[55] Later in the rehabilitation process, depression is not uncommon and may result from financial concerns due to the loss of abilities and/or fear of social isolation due to changes in personal appearance.[56] Risk factors for lasting or prolonged psychological dysfunction include pre-morbid psychopathology, burns that involve large surface areas, and burns that result in disfigurement.[51] However, more recent studies seem to suggest no correlation between burn wound size, amount of disfigurement, and psychopathology.[57] When children with burn wound injuries were compared with children with fractures, the children with burns had higher depression scores, were more anxious, were more lonely, avoided social contact and new social situations more, and confided in their parents less.[58, 59]

Consequences for Clinicians

Experimental evidence suggests that pain, anxiety, and depression are interrelated in patients with burn injuries.[51] A coordinated and consistent approach to patient care promotes trust and security.[43] Patient education, in tandem with adequate control of pain and anxiety, may help mitigate psychological dysfunction following burn injuries.[1, 54] Clinicians should explain procedures prior to performance and repeat instructions as necessary, especially early on, as patient recall may be limited.[10] Promoting patient independence, providing limited choices, and increasing patient control in the rehabilitation process can increase patient adherence and minimize potential adverse effects.[60] Involving patients' families and significant others can help them cope with fear and anxiety.[53] Goal setting,[1] counseling,[51] chaplaincy, and job retraining may also be beneficial.[10] Clinicians should notify the physician if psychological dysfunction increases or persists more than 6 months post-injury. In such cases, intensive therapy and/or medications should be considered.[40] See Table 14–4 for a summary of the effects burn injuries can have on body systems.

TABLE 14–4 Summary of the Effects Burn Injuries Can Have on Nonintegumentary Body Systems

Tissue/Body System	Dysfunction	Clinical Relevance
Cardiovascular system	• Increased capillary permeability • Edema • Hypovolemia • Impaired perfusion • Burn shock • Resting tachycardia • Hypotension • Dysrhythmias • Compartment syndrome	• Monitor vital signs • Be aware that patient has limited cardiac reserves • Monitor peripheral pulses • Monitor and manage edema • Make necessary referrals
Pulmonary system	• Smoke inhalation • Carbon monoxide poisoning • Pulmonary edema • Increased pulmonary vascular resistance • Hypoxia • Dyspnea • Pneumonia • Acute respiratory distress syndrome	• Perform and encourage aggressive pulmonary hygiene • Monitor oxygen saturation • Make necessary referrals
Metabolism	• Increased metabolic rate • Insensible heat loss • May be at risk for malnutrition • Sustained hyperglycemia	• Remember that patient hydration and nutrition take priority over all other interventions • Maintain warm environment • Keep wounds covered • Make necessary referrals
Immune system	• Impaired skin barrier function • Impaired neutrophils	• Use sterile technique as needed • Use topical antimicrobials • Achieve wound closure as soon as possible • Make necessary referrals
Other organ systems	• Kidney failure • Decreased gastrointestinal peristalsis • Ulcers • Ileus	• Monitor for signs and symptoms of burn shock • Encourage mobility • Make necessary referrals
Psychological dysfunction	• Disrupted sleep • Confusion/delirium • Inappropriate behavior • Depression • Posttraumatic stress disorder	• Be coordinated and consistent in patient management • Educate patient and caregivers • Control pain and anxiety • Promote patient independence • Involve patient's support system • Make necessary referrals

CASE STUDY: Miss Amy Kim

PART 2

Tests and Measures

Integumentary Integrity: Position: anterior and left lateral thorax, anterior and left lateral cervical region, and part of the left brachium and forearm. Presentation: superficial partial-thickness (SPT) and deep partial-thickness (DPT) burns covering approximately 18% total body surface area. Wound bed contains 90% yellow slough and 10% closed blisters on her lateral trunk. Wound drainage: moderate, thin, serous. No wound odor is present. Periwound: WNL. Temperature: WNL.

Sensory Integrity: Decreased pin prick in areas of DPT, which is primarily on the left upper extremity.

Circulation: Pulses: B radial, ulnar, and brachial pulses 2+. Capillary refill: on intact skin 2 seconds B, in wounds varies based on location from 1 second on superficial partial-thickness wounds to 4 seconds on the left upper extremity.

Gait, Locomotion, Balance: Miss Kim requires minimal assistance with bed mobility and transfers to a wheelchair due to pain and medical devices (IV, catheter, bandages). She ambulates with stand-by assistance while pushing her IV pole.

Pain: Patient reports 6/10 trunk and left upper extremity pain.

Range of Motion: Cervical SB L18°/R10°, left shoulder flexion 120°, left shoulder abduction 95°, left elbow 25°–100°. All motions are limited by complaint of pain. Passive motion is approximately equal to active motion and limited by pain with an empty endfeel.

Evaluation and Diagnosis

Miss Kim has superficial and deep partial-thickness burns consistent with Integumentary Preferred Practice Pattern C: Impaired Integumentary Integrity Associated with Partial-Thickness Skin Involvement and Scar Formation. The size and extent of Miss Kim's burns are considered moderate in severity. Her laboratory data and vital signs are consistent with a hypermetabolic state. Because Miss Kim does not have any areas of full-thickness skin involvement, is a young and otherwise healthy nonsmoking adult, and has <20% total body surface involvement, she can be cared for in the acute care setting. She should be monitored for burn shock, although this is unlikely. Even though Miss Kim's burns are fairly extensive, they are not circumferential, so she is not at risk for compartment syndrome. While Miss Kim does not have an inhalation injury, she is at risk for pulmonary dysfunction due to the combined effects of pain medication–induced respiratory depression, decreased activity/mobility, and thoracic burns that may cause her to take more shallow breaths to decrease chest expansion. She has limited left upper extremity and cervical motion and is at risk for contracture formation. Because Asians are more likely to have problems with excessive scar formation, Miss Kim has a risk of hypertrophic scarring in the areas of DPT burns. She is limited in activities of daily living and functional activities. Because Miss Kim's injuries occurred as the result of domestic violence, she is at risk for posttraumatic stress disorder or depression. Her physical safety must be addressed by the appropriate personnel.

Prognosis and Plan of Care

Superficial partial-thickness burn wounds typically heal in 10–14 days with minimal to no scarring. Deep partial-thickness burns of this size typically heal in about 3 weeks and there is a possibility of hypertrophic scarring during maturation and remodeling. Because of her good general health and young age, Miss Kim's prognosis is very good.

The following functional goals have been discussed and mutually agreed upon:

1. Miss Kim will be able to dress and reach into her closet with her left upper extremity without deviation in 7 days.
2. Miss Kim will be independent in all functional mobility in 3 days.
3. Miss Kim and her roommates will be independent with wound and scar management to allow full wound closure, including the ability to verbalize the signs and symptoms of a decline in wound status, infection, and abnormal scar formation, and an action plan for same in 2 weeks.

CASE STUDY   Continued

The following component goals have been discussed and mutually agreed upon:

1. Miss Kim and her roommates will be independent in bandaging her wounds in 3 days.
2. Miss Kim will be independent with a home exercise program for ROM, positioning, and deep breathing in 3 days.
3. Wound surface area will be decreased to <5% TBSA in 2 weeks.
4. Wound beds will be 95% granular in 2 days.
5. L elbow and cervical AROM will be restored in 4 days.
6. L shoulder self-assisted or active elevation ≥165° in 4 days.

Miss Kim will be seen two times per day while she is an inpatient. Physical therapy interventions will include coordination, communication, and documentation; patient/client-related instruction; integumentary repair and protective techniques; physical agents and mechanical modalities; and therapeutic exercises. Upon discharge from the hospital, physical therapy will continue daily for a total of 2 weeks of interventions.

 Checkpoint Question #2

Your 28-year-old patient sustained circumferential full-thickness burns to the right upper and lower extremities after being trapped in his bedroom when his house caught on fire. Describe how the patient's injuries might affect the following areas and the rehabilitation consequences of these dysfunctions.

a. The cardiovascular system
b. The pulmonary system

PHYSICAL THERAPY INTERVENTIONS

As with other types of wounds, physical therapy interventions for patients with burn wound injuries consist of a tripartite approach of coordination, communication, and documentation; patient/client-related instruction; and individualized procedural interventions.

Coordination, Communication, and Documentation

Physical therapy services for patients with burn injuries must be coordinated with the patient, caregivers, and other disciplines to maximize outcomes.[10, 40, 60] Because patients with severe burn injuries commonly have multiple, significant, concomitant medical conditions, coordination of care can be quite challenging. In addition to working toward achievement of disciplinary-specific patient goals, each team member should take advantage of every opportunity to reinforce the goals set by other disciplines.[40] For example, consider Mr. G, a patient with extensive trunk and right upper extremity burns. While performing wound care in the Hubbard tank, the physical therapist may have the patient try to assist with the removal of residual topical agents. By having Mr. G use his right hand to hold the gauze sponge to perform this procedure, the goals of the occupational therapy plan of care, functional use of the right hand, can be reinforced. Extensive communication, initially and at regular intervals, may be required to ensure that all necessary aspects of patient management are addressed without duplication of services. For example, the overlapping expertise of physical and occupational therapists is often an area of confusion. A survey of burn units found that physical therapists perform the majority of functional training and wound management, while occupational therapists are primarily responsible for activities of daily living training.[61] Regardless of the specific means used to delegate services, a consistent approach to patient management will promote patient trust and a sense of security.[43] Weekly, or even daily, patient rounds may facilitate communication among team members.

Pain is a pervasive feature of burn wound injuries that must be successfully addressed by the wound care team. Although prescribing and distributing pain medications is a standard intervention, the burn care team should also assist with pain modulation by using nonpharmacological approaches. Educating patients on what to expect from a procedure before it is performed can allay fear and anxiety.[54] Explaining that a whirlpool may cause a stinging sensation in the burned area, and that this is normal, may better prepare the patient for the experience. Distracting patients through conversation, with music,[54] or, in the case of children, with toys may reduce anxiety and pain perception.[5] Describing specific time- or outcome-based end points for each treatment session or functional activity may enhance patient cooperation. Rest periods during interventions may also be beneficial. Some patients respond favorably to mental imagery, breathing exercises, or relaxation techniques to help manage pain and anxiety. Whenever possible, patients should be given some control over their rehabilitation. By having patients assist with removing bandages or old topical agents or choose the order of interventions, patient compliance may be enhanced and anxiety lessened.

In addition to the attending physician and physical and occupational therapy professionals, holistic management of patients with burn wound injuries may include a number of other disciplines. A surgeon's role within the interdisciplinary team may consist of surgical debridement, escharotomy/fasciotomy, grafting procedures, or even amputation. Depending on the patient's status, other physicians, such as specialists in infectious disease and internal medicine, may need to be called upon to manage multisystem dysfunction. Nursing staff are vital to acute patient care to assist with patient positioning, patient/caregiver education, adequate pain control, and dressing changes.[10] Patients with inhalation injuries or other pulmonary compromise will likely benefit from the expertise of a respiratory therapist. Burn wound injuries, especially if severe, can have both acute and long-lasting psychological effects on patients. Therefore, a psychologist, psychiatrist, and/or chaplaincy may help patients to work through these issues.[51] A medical social worker can assist with discharge planning and obtaining any equipment or devices necessary to promote patient independence. If abuse is suspected, both the physician and the medical social worker should be informed immediately to investigate the patient's social situation. Vocational rehabilitation is a vital component to community reintegration of a severely injured adult burn patient. Recreational therapy may be more appropriate for young patients. A registered dietitian can ensure the patient is receiving the appropriate high-calorie, high-protein diet to maximize healing and lessen the adverse effects of the hypermetabolic response to a burn injury. Refer to Chapter 9 for more details regarding nutrition and wound healing.

Patient/Client-Related Instruction

Patients with burn wounds must be provided with the knowledge and resources to recover from their injury.[40] Because interventions for burn wound injuries are frequently painful and anxiety provoking, patients must be instructed in ways to help control their pain. Clinicians should also prepare patients as much as possible for each intervention prior to performance, including rationale and expected sensations, to reduce patient anxiety.[40] Before a patient is discharged to an outpatient setting, the clinician must instruct the patient/caregiver in how to care for the wound, including irrigation, bandaging, and positioning. A home exercise program should be initiated to remediate any impairments in range of motion, strength, endurance, or mobility.[62] Prior to discharge from an outpatient setting, patients and caregivers must be informed of the importance of proper skin care and scar management. Newly closed wounds and scar tissue are at increased risk for future skin breakdown and contractures. Therefore, patients should be instructed to liberally apply moisturizers to scar tissue, minimize friction, protect scar tissue from sun exposure, and perform at least daily skin checks of any insensate areas. The importance of long-term (up to 2 years post–wound closure) compression over deep burn and donor scars cannot be overemphasized (see the following section on scar management).[10] Clinicians must inform patients of the benefits of compliance with suggested interventions as well as the risks of noncompliance.

Procedural Interventions

Precautions

Clinicians should be aware of special precautions for patients with burn wound injuries (see Box 14–1). Although patients should be universally screened for the possibility of domestic violence, this screening is paramount when working with patients with burn injuries. In one study, nearly 30% (93 out of 321 consecutive) of patients admitted to a pediatric burn unit had been abused or neglected. Children found to be at greatest risk were under 2 years of age, were members of single-parent or low-income families, or sustained a scald injury.[8, 9] The most likely perpetrator is the child's mother's boyfriend.[9] Burn injuries that may be consistent with abuse include injuries that are shaped like familiar objects, such as cigarette butts, curling irons, or fireplace tools, and submersion pattern injuries, such as burns to the palmar aspect of the hands, burns to the plantar aspect of the feet, and circumferential distal extremity burns.[7] Patients presenting with these qualities or with inconsistent reports of the mechanism of injury should be carefully assessed.[5] If abuse or neglect is suspected, the clinician is obligated to inform the attending physician and social services immediately.

Clinicians working with this patient population must anticipate and try to prevent complications based on patient presentation.[10, 38] Given the same burn depth and percent of TBSA, children with burn injuries are more likely to have a contracture than adults.[7] The number of contractures is proportional to wound size, with the majority of contractures being of the hand, face, neck, and axilla.[63] Early, aggressive infection control and pulmonary hygiene, early range of motion, early mobility training, early reconditioning, and positioning to prevent contracture formation and pressure ulcers should be standard practice[10, 15] Patients with sensory deficits or alterations in mental status should be monitored for signs of excessive or adverse pressure. Unstabilized fractures, recent skin grafts, and recent applications of biological or synthetic dressings are contraindications for range of motion exercises.[15] Splinting may be necessary to improve static positioning or to protect grafts.[15] Exposed tendons must be prevented from dehydration by using moist dressings.

Integumentary Repair and Protective Techniques

Local Wound Care

This section contains highlights of local wound care specific to patients with burn injuries, including debridement, infection control, dressings, and scar management. Refer to Section II of the text for further details. Because burn wound management procedures are associated with increases in pain levels,[64] clinicians should ensure adequate pain control prior to local wound care. Patients taking oral medication may benefit from taking their pain medication about 20–30 minutes prior to wound care procedures or other therapeutic interventions.[5] Likewise, patients using patient-controlled analgesia (PCA) pumps may benefit from a bolus dose about 10 minutes prior to these procedures and should be allowed to self-medicate during treatment when necessary.[10, 13]

Debridement

Most burn wound injuries require repeated bouts of mechanical, sharp, and/or enzymatic debridement.[10, 13] Debridement will decrease the inflammatory response, help control or reduce the risk of infection, and enhance wound healing. Some topical agents, especially creams, will form a thin film, or pseudoeschar, over the wound bed. This film may be mistaken for eschar or may be difficult to remove. Debridement may be more tolerable when performed during peak medication time or underwater during hydrotherapy.[7]

With each treatment session, the clinician should ensure that all previously applied topical agents and exudate are removed to prevent the risk of bacterial colonization.[35] Clinicians should shave any facial hair remaining in or around facial burns to prevent bacterial colonization of hair follicles.[1] As with all other types of wounds, eschar and necrotic tissue should be debrided as expediently as possible. Any foreign debris within the wound bed should also be removed. However, tar and asphalt should not be debrided.[37] These substances adhere and bond to the skin, and any attempts to remove them will severely traumatize the skin underneath.

Open blisters should be removed[5, 21, 26] using sharp debridement to reduce the risk of infection and to avoid increasing the size of the wound by tearing or pulling at the skin adhered to the edge of the blister. The debridement of closed blisters is an area of intense controversy.[13] Most clinicians agree that large or thin-walled blisters likely to open spontaneously, blisters that cross a joint, and blisters that restrict joint motion should be debrided. In the past it was recommended that closed, intact blisters should be left as "nature's Band-Aid" and the risk of infection would be less by not opening the overlying skin. However, more recent literature suggests that blister fluid contains substances that suppress white blood cells, inhibit fibrinolysis, and increase the inflammatory response.[16, 25, 48, 65] Additionally, blister fluid provides an ideal environment for bacterial proliferation.[11] For these reasons, it is suggested that all blisters, both open and closed, be debrided.[1, 5, 16, 26]

Enzymatic debriding agents, particularly collagenase, have been used to assist with burn wound debridement.[13] Typically, enzymatic ointments are used in combination with a topical antimicrobial and concomitant sharp debridement. One study found that partial-thickness burns treated with Santyl and Polysporin powder debrided eschar 24% faster and healed wounds 16% faster than standard burn care.[66] However, since the improvements with enzymatic debridement found in this study were only a matter of 2–3 days, the clinical significance of this intervention is minimal. Enzymatic debridement is generally reserved for smaller burns, and its effectiveness appears to be highly variable.[67] For further information regarding all forms of debridement, refer to Chapter 5.

Infection Control

Preventing infection is of primary importance in treating patients with burn injuries. Sterile technique should be used for patients with extensive surface area burn injuries or patients who are immunocompromised. Clean technique is sufficient for those with smaller, more superficial burn injuries or those being seen on an outpatient basis.[5, 35] In addition to using proper infection control procedures,[40] antimicrobial therapy is standard. Systemic antibiotics are generally not prescribed prophylactically[5, 30] because concomitant hypovolemia and reduced tissue perfusion would likely compromise their effectiveness. Therefore, topical antimicrobials are the mainstay of infection control in this patient population.[10]

Silver sulfadiazine 1.0% cream (Silvadene, Thermazene) is the most commonly used antimicrobial for burn wound injuries.[10, 49] Silver sulfadiazine is effective against gram-positive and gram-negative bacteria, including *Staphylococcus aureus* and *Pseudomonas aeruginosa*. Its broad spectrum of action, ability to penetrate burn eschar, and soothing feeling upon application make it ideal for most patients.[68] Silver sulfadiazine

should be applied in a thin layer about 1/16-inch thick either directly to the wound or indirectly to a nonadherent impregnated gauze before being covered with a gauze dressing.[10] The moistness of the wound bed may make direct application difficult, and hypersensitivity may make this method painful. While there is some debate as to the ability of silver sulfadiazine to penetrate burn eschar and potential for inhibition of epithelialization,[5] silver sulfadiazine remains the standard of care for initial burn management.[49, 64] Mafenide acetate cream (Sulfamylon) is better able to penetrate eschar[1, 68] and is especially beneficial in the treatment of ear burns to prevent chondritis (red, swollen, painful, infected ear cartilage).[29] Mafenide acetate may be applied in the same manner as silver sulfadiazine or left open to the air. Mafenide acetate may cause mild burning[5] or stinging for up to 30 minutes after application.[13] Both topical agents must be thoroughly removed and reapplied two times per day for maximum effectiveness.[10] Because silver sulfadiazine and mafenide acetate both contain sulfa, they should not be used to treat patients with allergies to sulfa.[5] In such cases, bacitracin is the antimicrobial of choice.[10] Although some sources advocate the use of silver nitrate solution (0.5%)[13] or sticks (95%) as a topical antimicrobial agent for burn care,[1, 17] these are unable to penetrate eschar and do not have as broad a spectrum of activity as the previously mentioned topical agents. Therefore, clinicians would be wise to reserve silver nitrate (sticks) for cauterizing hypergranular tissue and not for the management of bacterial load in burn injuries.[68]

The signs and symptoms of a burn wound infection are similar to the classic signs and symptoms of infection discussed in Chapter 6. Increasing erythema, increasing pain, edema, and a foul wound odor may develop.[35] There is an increase in purulent drainage, requiring more absorptive dressings.[7] Previously red granulation tissue may become pale.[69] There may be an increase in necrotic tissue within the wound bed and conversion to a deeper wound.[69] Systemic signs of a burn wound infection include fever,[21] temperature fluctuation, increasing tachycardia, and altered levels of consciousness.[69] The most common offending agent is *Staphylococcus aureus*,[46, 47, 50] followed by *Pseudomonas aeruginosa*, *Streptococcus pyogenes*, *Escherichia coli*, *Proteus* infections, and methicillin-resistant *Staphylococcus aureus* (MRSA).[35, 48] If these signs and symptoms are present, the clinician should suspect an infection and report these findings to the physician immediately. The clinician should request an order for a culture and sensitivity and inquire about the use of a broad-spectrum antibiotic while the offending microorganism is being identified. Treatment for burn wound infections includes aggressive debridement, systemic antibiotics, and continuation (with modifications as needed based on the culture results) of topical antimicrobial therapy.[21, 35] Whirlpool treatments may also be beneficial in decreasing bacterial load.

Dressings

The most commonly used dressing for burn wound injuries is a topical antimicrobial agent covered with a nonadherent impregnated gauze and a bulky gauze dressing.[5, 21] This dressing combination provides a means of controlling infection, protecting the granulating wound bed from trauma, distributing pressure, and absorbing wound exudate.[13] Whenever possible, dressing bulk should be limited to allow for improved range of motion, well-fitting splints, and enhanced function.[13] Heavily draining wounds may benefit from the addition of an alginate dressing.[13, 68] Burn wound surfaces should not be allowed to touch each other. For example, if a patient has a burn injury involving the entire hand, each digit should be wrapped individually.[13] A spiral technique should be used to prevent a tourniquet-like effect. Small, uninfected burn wounds may be covered with moisture-retentive dressings such as sheet hydrogels or hydrocolloids.[10] Small, superficial, uninfected burns may be covered with a semipermeable film.[10] Short-stretch compression bandages or self-adherent elastic wraps should be used for edema control[13] and to decrease scarring.[40, 70, 71] Skin grafts, skin substitutes, and biological/synthetic dressings may also be used to cover burn wound injuries.[10, 15] These interventions are discussed in the following section on surgical interventions.

Scar Management

Burn scars may require 6 months to 2 years to mature.[37] The scar tissue is fragile and prone to breakdown from friction, shear, and trauma.[72] During the remodeling phase, scar tissue should be gently cleaned daily using a mild, nonperfumed soap and water. A moisturizer should be applied several times per day to prevent dryness, cracking, and skin breakdown. Gently massaging the moisturizer into closed burn scars may result in even better relief of itching, pain, and anxiety.[73] The use of moisturizers is particularly important after FT burns as these areas have lost the ability to sweat and self-lubricate. Blisters may occur if scars are exposed to friction or shear forces. For example, a patient with an FT burn injury to the thigh may experience blistering

from the rubbing of his pant leg against the scar tissue. If blistering occurs, the blisters should be opened with a sterile needle and covered with a light, nonadherent gauze dressing.[72] It is important to identify and resolve the cause of the blister whenever possible. In this case, the patient should be instructed to wear loose-fitting pants made of a soft material (such as light sweatpants), rather than stiff and abrasive jeans.

Hypertrophic scarring and keloids are possible complications of the remodeling phase of burn wound healing.[15] Abnormal scarring may occur in 30–70% of patients with burn wounds.[74, 75] Individuals with darker skin tones, particularly those of Asian or Afro-Carribean descent,[31, 76] have a two to three times higher incidence of hypertrophic scarring than those with lighter skin.[75, 77] Warning signs of potential scar problems include limited range of motion, new onset of joint restriction, banding of scar tissue (see Figure 14–4) with range of motion, or blanching with stretching of scar tissue.[78] The Vancouver Scar Scale, also known as the Burn Scar Index, is a reliable method used to describe the quality of scar tissue after a burn injury.[17, 74, 79–81] This scale rates four scar qualities: vascularity, pliability, pigmentation, and height. Scores range from 0 to 14, with higher scores representing more severe scarring (see Table 14–5). More severe scars may benefit from aggressive interventions to modify scar tissue quality and appearance. Clinicians may also use the Vancouver Scar Scale to

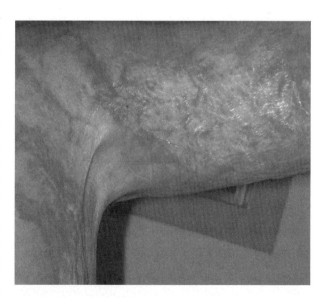

FIGURE 14–4 Banding of scar tissue after deep partial-thickness and full-thickness burns to the trunk and left upper extremity closed with skin grafts.

TABLE 14–5   Vancouver Scar Scale*

Subscale	Score	Description
Vascularity	0	Normal
	1	Pink, slight increase in local blood supply
	2	Red, significant increase in local blood supply
	3	Purple, excessive vascularity
Pliability	0	Normal
	1	Supple
	2	Yielding
	3	Firm
	4	Banding, ropes that blanch with range of motion but do not limit motion
	5	Contracture
Pigmentation	0	Normal
	1	Hypopigmentation
	2	Mixed pigmentation
	3	Hyperpigmentation
Height	0	Flat
	1	<2 mm
	2	2–5 mm
	3	>5 mm

*Adapted from Baryza MJ, Baryza GA. The Vancouver Scar Scale: An administration tool and its interrater reliability. *J Burn Care Rehabil.* 1994;15:181–188.

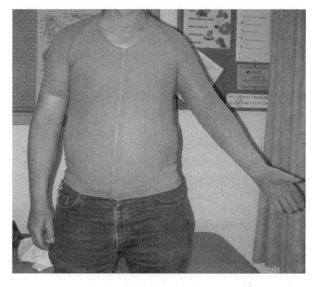

FIGURE 14–5   Compression garment worn to help control hypertrophic scarring on a patient with scarring after deep partial-thickness and full-thickness burns to the trunk and left upper extremity.

monitor the success (or lack of success) of such interventions.

Scar mobilization may help remodel scar tissue quality and appearance.[81] Compression wraps and garments are used prophylactically to prevent excessive scarring and to modify scar tissue if problems do arise.[51, 81] Self-adherent compression wraps, short-stretch bandages, and tubular bandages are used to manage scar formation while wounds are closing.[15, 17] Patients with extensive burns, DPT burns, or FT burns are generally fit for compression garments[37] for the affected areas as the wounds approach closure (see Figure 14–5). Because it is more efficient to prevent abnormal scarring than to treat hypertrophic or keloid scars,[81] a good rule of thumb is that burn wounds requiring 2–3 weeks to heal should be treated with compression, but compression is *mandatory* for those requiring more than 3 weeks to heal. The use of zippered garments may help reduce friction during donning and doffing. Garments should be worn at all times except when bathing until remodeling is complete, approximately 12–24 months after wound closure.[15, 82] Unfortunately, the adherence with these suggestions has been reported to be as low as 41%. Nonadherent patients reported the garments caused discomfort, were too hot, or restricted their activities.[83] Therefore, in addition to ensuring proper fit, clinicians should thoroughly educate patients with burn wound injuries on the purpose and importance of the use of compression garments, including potential complications of nonadherence.[40]

Silicone gel sheets or pads may help to reduce or prevent scarring of healed, intact, burned skin[31, 77, 84, 85] and are particularly helpful in small areas, such as the fingers or hands, and in body creases, such as the cubital fossa. The greatest gains in scar tissue modification, including increased pliability, decreased scar thickness, improved vascularity, decreased pain, and decreased itching, occur over the first 2 months of use, but significant improvements continue for at least 6 months.[77] In addition, silicone gel sheeting can assist with hypertrophic scar modification even if initiated as late as 4 years after a burn wound injury.[31, 77] Silicone gel sheets and pads may be secured with a light gauze wrap or used in combination with compression therapy.[37] Silicone sheets and pads are more expensive than traditional dressings but may be washed and reused multiple times,[84] making them a cost-effective treatment option. Patients with facial burns are commonly fitted for a form-fitting face moulage, or mask, to provide therapeutic compression while maximizing cosmesis.[7, 56] Gentle scar mobilization using a moisturizing agent, ultrasound, and paraffin (using either the dipping or paintbrush method pending the area to be treated) may also be used to help remodel scar tissue.[17] These interventions may be initiated as soon as the wound is closed. Refer to Chapter 8 for further details on the use of ultrasound as an adjunct to modify scar tissue. See Box 14–2 for the highlights of local wound care for patients with burn injuries.

Therapeutic Exercise

Positioning, range of motion exercises, mobility training, breathing exercises, and aerobic exercise are the five essential components of a therapeutic exercise/activity program for the rehabilitation of a patient with burn injuries.[10] Supervised exercise programs are associated with a significant reduction in contracture formation.[62] Interventions must address both the burned areas as well as the areas not directly involved in the original injury. The use of functional goals can increase patient adherence and satisfaction and improve reimbursement for services.[40, 86] Some sample goals (without time frames) for patients with burn injuries are provided in Box 14–3.

Positioning

Proper positioning can enhance wound and scar healing, reduce edema, prevent and reduce contractures, prevent pressure sores, and improve pulmonary hygiene.[10, 15] Burn wounds should be bandaged so that no two burned surfaces touch each other. Pressure ulcers develop in 5% of hospitalized burn patients.[29] Therefore, clinicians should monitor for signs of pathological pressure and assist patients with frequent position changes. Patients should be positioned to limit friction and shear forces to enhance wound healing and limit scar breakdown. For example, patients with burn injuries to the posterior trunk and buttock should not lay supine with the head of the bed elevated, as this would increase shear forces to the affected areas. Positioning programs should also assist with edema reduction.[16] Edematous limbs should be elevated above the level of the heart when feasible.

> **BOX 14–2   Keys to Local Wound Care for Patients with Burn Wound Injuries**
>
> **Debridement**
> - Mechanical
> - Sharp
> - Enzymatic
>
> **Infection control**
> - Sterile technique for patients with extensive burns or patients who are immunocompromised
> - Standard use of topical antimicrobials
>
> **Dressings**
> - Absorb drainage
> - Protect from trauma
> - Allow range of motion/function
> - Do not allow burn surfaces to touch one another
> - Control edema
>
> **Scar management**
> - Apply moisturizer
> - Protect from friction and shear forces
> - Perform scar mobilization
> - Use compression garments
> - Consider silicone gel sheets or pads for smaller areas
> - Consider ultrasound or paraffin to help scar remodel
>
> **Educate patient/caregivers**
> - Local wound care
> - Skin/scar management
> - Positioning

Controlling edema can increase range of motion and improve overall patient function. Patients with respiratory impairments should be positioned to maximize lung segment ventilation and oxygen saturation.[1]

Proper patient positioning helps prevent contracture formation and loss of function.[5, 10, 15, 16, 40, 62] In general, the position of comfort (i.e., the position that places the least tension across the burn wound) will be the predicted position of contracture. It is easier to prevent contractures than to resolve these impairments once they have occurred. The astute clinician must be

---

> **BOX 14–3   Sample Functional Goals for Patients with Burn Injuries**
>
> The following chart includes some examples of objective and measurable goals that might be helpful when working with patients with burn wounds. *Note:* Time frames have not been included.
>
> - Improve respiratory abilities to allow patient to clear secretions independently.
> - Patient will be independent in bed mobility to prevent pressure sore formation.
> - Increase range of motion in affected areas to allow patient to feed him- or herself independently.
> - Increase lower extremity strength and range of motion to allow patient to transfer independently.
> - Improve mobility to allow patient to independently ambulate 100 feet indoors in 2 minutes.
> - Increase aerobic capacity to allow patient to ambulate through the grocery store without resting.
> - Patient and caregiver will be independent with scar management to limit future complications.

able to anticipate potential contractures based on burn location, burn depth, burn size, and patient status. Table 14–6 provides a guideline for patient positioning based on burn location. Patients should be encouraged to sleep and rest in positions that prevent contracture formation.[56] However, although static positioning can be beneficial in preventing contractures, range of motion exercises, active movement, and early return to function are more efficient and should be encouraged as soon as patient status allows.

Range of Motion Exercises

Range of motion exercises[5, 17, 40, 56] should be performed twice daily.[7] Every joint should be moved through its full range to maintain or restore full motion as soon as possible. If patients are able to participate, active or active-assisted range of motion is preferred to passive exercise because alternate, repeated muscle contraction can assist with edema reduction[25] and the restoration of functional movement. In patients with major burns, thermally injured and noninjured extremities should be exercised both to assist with edema control and to minimize the effects of deconditioning. Bandages may restrict full motion, and the friction between the bandages and wound during movement may traumatize the wound bed and increase patient discomfort.

Therefore, range of motion exercises are most effective when performed during dressing changes. Range of motion exercises may be better tolerated when combined with immersion hydrotherapy and well-timed pain and/or anxiety medications. In addition to straight-plane range of motion exercises, functional movement patterns and purposeful activities may increase patient adherence, increase the frequency of movement, and enhance overall patient function. Clinicians should specifically target ranges that discourage contracture formation.[72] For example, if an inpatient presents with a volar upper extremity burn injury, the clinician might choose to place the patient's telephone and food tray slightly farther away from the patient to encourage active elbow extension. Patients should be provided with a home exercise program to increase or maintain motion during the remodeling phase of wound healing when skin contraction forces will increase the tendency to lose tissue extensibility.[87] Loss of motion should be managed aggressively through range of motion exercises, stretching, positioning, and splinting when necessary.[10] Shoulder pulleys may be beneficial for patients with shoulder or axillary burn injuries and loss of motion.

Contraindications to range of motion exercises include nonstabilized fractures, cardiovascular instability, extubation within 8 hours of treatment, and exposed tendons.[87] Most surgeons will allow gentle range of motion exercises to begin 4–5 days after graft placement.[10, 16]

Mobility Training

Mobility training to increase functional independence should be initiated as soon as the patient is medically able.[15] Patients should wear loose-fitting nonconstrictive clothing to avoid impeding circulation or mobility. Patients with lower extremity burns or grafts should have a compression wrap on before getting out of bed. In addition to limiting edema, compression will prevent venous pooling, enhance venous return, and reduce the risk of a deep vein thrombosis.[78]

Breathing Exercises

Patients who have respiratory involvement, extensive torso burns, or who will require more than a few days of limited mobility should be instructed in some form of breathing exercise.[1, 40] Deep breathing and incentive spirometry exercises may work well for adults. The use of straws, singing games, and bubble blowing may be more appropriate for young children.[7]

TABLE 14–6   Predicting and Preventing Contractures Based on Burn Wound Location

Burn Location	Predicted Position of Contracture	Contracture Prevention Position
Anterior neck	Cervical flexion	Supine without a pillow, small towel roll to support cervical lordosis
Axilla/shoulders	Adducted, restricted elevation	Abducted at least 90 degrees and externally rotated
Cubital fossa	Elbow flexion	Elbow extension
Volar wrist/hand	Wrist flexion/digit flexion	Wrist extension, digit extension
Dorsal wrist/hand	Wrist extension/MCP extension	Neutral wrist with metacarpophalangeal joints 90 degrees flexed, interphalangeal joints extended
Anterior thigh/hip	Hip flexion	Flat supine, hips extended
Posterior knee	Knee flexion	Knee extension
Ankle	Plantar flexion	Neutral or slight dorsiflexion

Aerobic Exercise

Aerobic exercise may be initiated early in the rehabilitation process. Some patients may be so deconditioned that mere active range of motion exercises and mobility training will be aerobic activities. Acute burn injuries create tremendous physiological stress and resting tachycardia, limiting cardiac reserves. Therefore, although aerobic exercise is a vital component of the rehabilitation program, patient response to increases in activity should be carefully monitored. For example, during the acute stage of rehabilitation, clinicians should modulate activity to prevent heart rate from exceeding 20 beats per minute above the patient's resting heart rate. As healing occurs and burn shock resolves, clinicians should strive to attain and maintain the patient's target heart rate between 50% and 70% of maximum predicted heart rate.

Prescription, Application, and Fabrication of Devices and Equipment

At times, passive positioning and range of motion exercises are not enough to maintain or increase motion, and the use of splints or braces should be considered.[16, 40] Splints and braces may also be used to immobilize and protect graft sites,[16] exposed tendons, fractures, or peripheral nerve injuries.[10] Splints may be particularly effective with young children, patients who are nonadherent with positioning programs, and patients with altered mental status. Superficial burns rarely require splinting. The hand is the most commonly splinted area.[88] In fact, some clinicians may choose to splint a thermally injured hand prophylactically upon admission. However, because splints limit active movement and may inhibit function, clinicians may defer the use of splints unless range of motion is decreasing or not improving as expected.[16] In addition to static splints, dynamic splints may be beneficial by allowing motion while still providing a low-load, long-duration stretch to the affected area. Dynamic splints are used more often during the maturation and remodeling phase of burn wound healing and can be particularly effective in the management of elbow and knee flexion contractures by allowing patients to use their arms for activities of daily living and to ambulate but still receive a low-intensity stretch while at rest. When using splints, it is important to perform frequent skin checks to detect the early warning signs of excessive pressure. If redness lasts more than 20 minutes after splint removal, the splint should be modified to prevent pressure necrosis.[87] Other devices and equipment that may prove valuable for patients with lower extremity burn injuries include assistive devices, such as walkers and crutches, to enable early mobility.

Physical Agents and Mechanical Modalities

Immersion of the affected area in a whirlpool,[68] with or without agitation, can assist with burn wound care by removing old topical agents, decreasing the pain of exposure of burned areas to the air, and allowing increased ease of motion.[7] Hydrotherapy may help to soften burn eschar, assist with the removal of necrotic tissue, and decrease the pain of debridement.[10, 13] The use of whirlpool additives is contraindicated for patients with chemical burn injuries to prevent possible adverse chemical interactions. Some clinicians prefer to use the showering method in which patients are suspended over a whirlpool tub and rinsed off.[13] The showering method may reduce treatment time, lower treatment cost, and prevent autocontamination from an infected area to a noninfected open area, which can occur during immersion hydrotherapy.[72] Both methods must be used in combination with wiping or washing to effectively reduce bacterial load. Ninety-two percent of burn units surveyed used immersion or shower-method hydrotherapy.[89] Ideally, hydrotherapy sessions should be relatively short, less than 30 minutes,[89] and whirlpool temperature should be between 90 and 100°F. To avoid an increase in peripheral edema, water temperature should be lower and treatment time shorter for patients who are treated in extremity tanks.[25] Patients who are being treated while in the hospital or burn unit generally receive hydrotherapy once or twice per day.[89, 90] Pulsed lavage with suction or irrigation with normal saline[72] may be preferred for smaller or less severe burn wound injuries or patients who are hydrophobic. Facial burns are best managed with irrigation. This method is commonly used in the home care setting.

During the maturation and remodeling phase of wound healing, ultrasound, paraffin baths, silicone gel sheeting,[84] compression, and low-level laser therapy[91, 92] may help modify scar tissue and, thereby, increase range of motion and improve cosmesis. Refer to Chapter 8 for specific details regarding the use of physical agents and modalities.

CASE STUDY: Miss Amy Kim

PART 3

Interventions

The following highlights some of the key procedural interventions that will be incorporated into Miss Kim's plan of care.

Coordination, Communication, and Documentation: A consult with a medical social worker was requested to assist with coordination of patient safety issues including contacting local law enforcement and resources Miss Kim may find helpful, such as counseling and community resources for individuals affected by domestic violence. Physical therapy sessions will be coordinated with nursing staff around patient mealtimes and her pain medication schedule. If needed, a bolus of pain medication will be requested prior to wound management sessions.

Patient/Client-Related Instruction: Miss Kim will be instructed in the normal course of burn wound healing and she will be informed of potential adverse effects of her injuries, such as scarring, contractures, and respiratory compromise. She will be instructed in methods to minimize the risks of these adverse outcomes. She will be instructed in positioning and an exercise program to reduce edema, improve motion, and enhance respiratory function. To reduce anxiety and pain perception, the method and purpose of all procedures will be thoroughly explained to Miss Kim prior to performance.

Procedural Interventions
- Local wound management will consist of whirlpool in a Hubbard tank twice daily. Range of motion exercises and sharp debridement of slough, exudate, and blisters will be performed while in the whirlpool. A time limit will be placed on wound care sessions to minimize Miss Kim's pain and anxiety. When out of the whirlpool heat lamps and warming blankets will be used to keep Miss Kim warm and comfortable during bandaging. A moisturizer will be used on intact skin. The burns will be dressed with a

CASE STUDY Continued

petrolatum-impregnated nonadherent gauze coated with a 1/16-inch layer of silver sulfadiazine cream and covered with a thick gauze pad to absorb drainage. A roll gauze will be used to secure the left upper extremity bandage. A self-adherent elastic wrap, such as Coban, will be used to control edema and decrease the risk of abnormal scarring. A piece of elastic netting will be used to secure the gauze pads to her trunk. For convenience, the cervical wounds will be dressed with bacitracin two to three times per day and left open to the air.

- Therapeutic exercises will include active and active-assisted left elbow and shoulder range of motion exercises as well as cervical active range of motion exercises. Miss Kim will be instructed in deep breathing exercises, such as inspiratory spirometry. Functional activities, including walking in the halls and encouraging Miss Kim to use her left upper extremity for reaching, bed mobility, and dressing will be encouraged.

Reassessment

Miss Kim's response to interventions will be monitored during each session. In addition, she will be monitored for signs and symptoms of depression or posttraumatic stress disorder, such as inappropriate or uncooperative behavior or sleep disturbances. If these problems are noted, the physician and social worker will be notified.

 Checkpoint Question #3

Your patient is a 3-month-old infant who presents with superficial partial-thickness burns of bilateral lower extremities. The burns extend circumferentially from 5 cm above the ankle distally to the plantar aspect of his feet. The patient's parent reports the burns were sustained while bathing.

   a. Does the parent's explanation of the wound etiology warrant further investigation?

   b. In addition to the physician, should you report your findings to any other team members? Why?

MEDICAL AND SURGICAL INTERVENTIONS

Although medical and surgical interventions are clearly beyond the scope of physical therapy, they are presented here to provide a better understanding of the valuable roles these disciplines play in the management of patients with burn wound injuries.

Medical Interventions

Physicians are essential in the acute management of patients with severe or extensive burn injuries. Three key areas require rapid physician identification and response.[44] First, physicians must successfully manage burn shock to prevent severe, and potentially life-threatening, complications. Rapid fluid resuscitation with intravenous fluids is essential, the achievement of which is measured by urinary output.[10] Second, physicians must monitor and manage cardiac dysfunction including dysrhythmia and arrhythmia that may be a direct or indirect result of the burn wound injury in order to maintain perfusion to vital organs. Third, physicians must identify and manage inhalation injuries and pulmonary dysfunction,[44] such as pulmonary edema, carbon monoxide poisoning, and acute respiratory distress syndrome (ARDS), to ensure adequate tissue oxygenation.[14]

Pharmacological Management

In addition to prescribing medications to prevent and manage infection, physicians must also address patient pain complaint, both in the acute phase and throughout the healing process. Patient pain complaint[64] and anxiety increase for the first 4–7 days after a severe burn injury.[93] Because patient pain complaint and anxiety are correlated, clinicians must ensure adequate control of both pain and anxiety.[38] Anxiety may stem from psychological trauma from the injury, loss of independence, fear of death, and the ongoing need for painful interventions.[51] Anxiety typically increases during dressing changes and decreases within a half hour after the conclusion of the session.[93] The patient commonly experiences three types of pain: background, procedural, or breakthrough.[53] Background pain is constant pain directly associated with the burn injury and may be due to damaged nerve endings and/or the inflammatory response to the injury. Procedural pain is related to local wound care techniques and other therapeutic interventions. Typically, pain is increased for up to 30 minutes after local wound care procedures.[93] Breakthrough pain is more intense, episodic pain that is not relieved by regularly scheduled medication.

Ideally, patient pain should be maintained at less than 4 on a 0–10 pain scale (0 = no pain, 10 = most intense pain imaginable).[93] Patients with minor burn injuries may only require nonsteroidal anti-inflammatories.[14] In contrast, patients with more severe burn injuries may initially require intravenous medications[14] such as morphine or meperidine. PCAs are beneficial in controlling background pain, while bolus doses of a short-acting narcotic may help reduce procedural pain.[94] Anxiolytics, such as benzodiazepines, may be beneficial and decrease the need for pain medication since pain perception is affected by anxiety.[14, 38, 51] Antidepressant medications may also help with pain modulation.[51] However, because it may take 2–4 weeks for these drugs to reach a therapeutic level,[95] antidepressant medication is typically prescribed only for patients with burn injuries that are likely to require more than a few weeks of intensive therapy.[94]

Undermedication is thought to be a major problem in the care of patients with burn injuries.[14] Clinicians should not withhold or limit pain medication for fear of patient addiction or dependence. Rather, clinicians should monitor the efficacy of the patient's pain management on an ongoing basis and report any problems to the physician.[10] Flexible dosing schedules that allow for hourly changes in patient pain perception and rescue doses for breakthrough pain, if needed, should be a standard of care for patients with burn injuries.[14] Patients should be transferred to oral medication as soon as possible to facilitate transfer to an outpatient setting. Whenever possible, patient treatment should occur after the medication has had time to take effect.

Sixty percent of patients with burn wound injuries complain of itching,[96] with an average severity of 7.6 on a 0–10 scale, in the affected areas. Itching appears to be more common for lower extremity burns (100%) than upper extremity burns (70%), while facial burns do not appear to cause pruritus.[97] Although nonperfumed moisturizers, including lanolin-based creams, cocoa butter,[73] vitamin E, and aloe,[23] are routinely used to try to lessen this complaint,[5] frequently these topical interventions are insufficient. Most patients benefit from the use of antihistamines, such as Benadryl, to control pruritus; however, this rarely results in complete relief.[73, 97]

Surgical Interventions

Surgical interventions, such as debridement, escharotomy/fasciotomy, grafting, or the placement of skin substitutes, are commonly required for moderate and major burn injuries and may be necessary for some minor burn injuries.

Surgical Debridement

Early surgical debridement is commonly performed on patients with medium and large full-thickness and subdermal burns.[10, 13, 21] Surgical debridement may occur as early as the day of or the day after a burn injury, with the majority of surgeons waiting until after the first week.[56] The advantages of this early debridement include a shortened inflammatory process, reduced risk of infection, decreased pain, earlier wound closure, and shorter hospitalization.[36, 98, 99] However, surgical debridement is not without risks, including physiological and psychological stress as well as the potential to excise some areas of healthy tissue. Many times, especially with patients who have extensive burns, multiple surgical debridements may be required because of the stress of surgery, blood loss, and lack of skin coverage/donor sites.[5, 10]

Escharotomy/Fasciotomy

An **escharotomy** is a surgical incision through burn wound eschar and into the subcutaneous tissues to release tissues that may be constricting circulation.[10] The massive edema that may accompany a burn injury and the inelastic nature of eschar may cause progressive vascular occlusion.[7] By making carefully planned midmedial and midlateral surface incisions, the surgeon can allow the tissues to expand, improving tissue perfusion.[26] An escharotomy may be indicated in the following circumstances: unidentifiable distal pulses with

Doppler ultrasound, cyanosis distal to a burn wound injury, increasing delay in capillary refill, new or increasing paresthesias, or increasing deep tissue pain complaint.[11] Clinicians should monitor for these overt signs of impaired perfusion and, if observed, notify the physician immediately. In contrast, a **fasciotomy** involves making a surgical incision through the fascia to release pressure and improve distal circulation.[10] Fasciotomies are most commonly performed after electrical burn injuries that result in severe muscle trauma.[16]

Skin Graft

Skin grafting is the mainstay of significant burn wound closure[98] and should be considered for FT or DPT burns[13] if the wound is not expected to close within 3 weeks.[37] Wounds must be free of necrotic tissue and infection prior to grafting. Often, one or more surgical debridements are performed prior to grafting to clean the wound bed. Planning for skin grafts should begin within the first 3–5 days postinjury. Xenografts and cadaveric allografts may be used to provide temporary skin coverage.[98] However, because these grafts are composed of foreign tissues, the host body may reject the graft.[27] Therefore,

autografts harvested from uninvolved areas are the preferred method of skin coverage.[98] The harvest site is determined by the size and extent of skin coverage needed. When possible, skin is harvested from less noticeable areas such as the buttocks, thigh, or trunk. However, choices may be limited in patients with extensive burn injuries. Once a site is chosen, the area is shaved and thoroughly cleansed. Next, a dermatome, a cutting instrument used to remove a thin layer of skin, is used to shave away the desired thickness of healthy skin to be used for the grafting procedure.

There are two types of skin grafts: split-thickness and full-thickness. **Split-thickness skin grafts** involve removing the epidermis and a portion of the dermis.[10] Split-thickness grafts are either meshed or sheet grafts. Meshing involves making regularly placed incisions throughout the graft, allowing it to be stretched to cover a larger area (see Figure 14–6).[10] The wider the ratio of the meshing (the larger the spaces that are made within the graft), the greater the expansion, and the larger area the graft will be able to cover.[5] The spaces created by meshing also allow the wound to drain.[17] The new skin graft is stapled or sutured in place or a fibrin glue may be used.[16] A nonadherent dressing, such

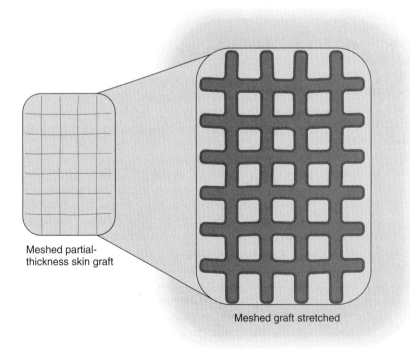

Meshed partial-
thickness skin graft

Meshed graft stretched

FIGURE 14–6 Stretching a meshed graft allows the graft to cover a larger wound bed by increasing the size of the interstices.

as Xeroform and a gauze wrap, is applied in surgery and left in place for several days.[13, 100] Alternatively, the graft may be covered with a coarse mesh gauze soaked with normal saline, and the outer dressing is changed every 1–5 days.[66] A self-adherent elastic wrap and elevation are used to limit edema,[71] if feasible, and the area is immobilized for 5–10 days.[1, 5] A fibrin clot forms between the grafted skin and the burn wound bed, and, within 24 hours, angiogenesis begins. Collagen is then deposited by the body to secure the graft tissue to the recipient area. The new graft is very fragile and must be protected from shear forces, excessive pressure, and movement until the graft takes (adheres to and obtains vascular continuity with the wound bed) in about 5 days.[10] Until the new vessels are fully formed, they lack normal vasomotor tone. Therefore, grafted areas should be bandaged with a light compression dressing whenever they will be placed in a dependent position.[68] The grafted area then heals by epithelializing the interstices from the meshed graft and wound contraction. Because grafts with high ratios of meshing and large interstices must build more new tissue, these grafts will require greater time to heal. In addition, grafts with wider ratios are more prone to hypertrophic scarring than grafts with smaller ratios.[5] Meshed split-thickness skin grafts heal with a scar that has a telltale mesh-like pattern.

In contrast, sheet split-thickness grafts are placed directly on the recipient site without meshing. Sheet grafts contract less because of the higher dermal content and do not leave this mesh-like pattern, making them more functional and more cosmetically appealing than meshed grafts.[17, 101] However, because sheet grafts are not expanded by way of the meshing process, they are generally reserved for use on smaller burn wounds or on patients with minimal TBSA involvement with large areas for potential donor sites.[10] Split-thickness sheet grafts may also be used in areas where cosmesis is more critical, such as the face or dorsal hands, if a full-thickness graft is not possible. The donor site of a split-thickness skin graft becomes a new partial-thickness wound. In general, the donor site is more painful and drains more than the recipient site.[43] The donor site may be covered with a nonadherent gauze dressing or, more commonly, with a moisture-retentive dressing, such as a semipermeable film or hydrocolloid.[10]

Full-thickness skin grafts involve removing the epidermis and dermis. The donor site then undergoes primary closure or, if large, is covered with a split-thickness skin graft.[68] Full-thickness skin grafts contain larger amounts of dermal tissue, making them the most durable and most cosmetic type of autograft.[17, 98] However, full-thickness skin grafts also require greater vascular support from the recipient area and greater initial protection in order to take.[43] With the exception of a longer immobilization period, full-thickness skin graft recipient sites are bandaged the same as partial-thickness skin graft sites. Full-thickness skin grafts are generally reserved for use on the face, feet, and hands.[16]

Regardless of the type of graft, failure may occur for several reasons: infection, the presence of eschar, insufficient immobilization after graft placement, or collection of fluid underneath the graft.[10] Clinicians must ensure a clean, uninfected wound bed prior to grafting and protect the graft from excessive movement, pressure, and shear forces acutely. Graft take may be improved with the use of negative pressure wound therapy.[16, 21, 98] A healthy skin graft should be pink in color. Split-thickness grafts may have a pebbled appearance, while full-thickness grafts should be similar in appearance to the donor site.[102] A graft that appears white is probably ischemic, while a red wound may be inflamed or infected. If graft discoloration occurs or if there is increased drainage, loosening of the graft edges, or blistering, the surgeon should be contacted.[10]

Skin Substitutes

Patients with extensive burn injuries have a limited number of donor sites. In addition, skin grafting creates a new wound at the donor site. Therefore, recent advances in medical technology have led to the creation of skin substitutes, which can provide early skin coverage for patients with extensive burn injuries.[10] Skin substitutes may be used on DPT and FT wounds as well as donor sites.[21, 103–105] Ideally, skin substitutes would be readily available, have a low risk of infection, have few adverse effects, provide permanent wound closure, provide good cosmesis, and be an affordable price.[106] Unfortunately, this is not the case. While several products are available on the market, including AlloDerm, Biobrane, Epicel®, and Transcyte™, all provide only temporary skin coverage at a steep price.

The most successful skin substitutes are bilayered dressings consisting of an epidermal analog, which provides a barrier function, and a dermal analog, which provides a scaffolding for fibrovascular ingrowth.[98, 107] To date, no one product has proven superior,[38, 106, 108] however, the two most commonly used skin substitutes are Biobrane and Integra. These are both collagen-based, bilayered dressings that can be applied directly to the clean, granular wound bed. After placement, these dressings are covered with a light compression dressing for 1–2 days to increase adherence to the wound bed.[109] A bulky dressing[110] may be placed over the skin substitute for protection or it may be left open to the air.[111, 112] In contrast to skin grafts, the involved area does not need to be immobilized,[109] although some surgeons prefer to briefly immobilize if crossing a joint.[110] While in place, skin substitutes decrease wound contraction,[109, 111] resulting in a more cosmetically appealing scar[109] and lowering the risk of contractures.[106] As Biobrane-covered wounds heal, the edges of the dressing will become opaque and peel away from the patient's skin as epithelialization progresses. These areas should be trimmed as needed.[16, 112] After 2–3 weeks, the dermal component of the dressing has been incorporated into the patient.[109] The outer silicone layer is then removed and a thin skin graft is required to achieve permanent wound closure.[13, 98, 112]

Alternatively, cultured epithelial autografts can be used to achieve early wound closure.[5, 98, 104] Using this procedure, keratinocytes from the patient are sent to a laboratory and grown for 20–30 days. The newly grown graft is sutured or stapled over the clean wound bed.[1] Because cultured epithelial autografts lack a dermis, they are very fragile and less durable than the previously mentioned bilayered skin substitutes. Typically, the area is immobilized for about 2 weeks after graft placement and excessive pressure must be meticulously avoided.[27]

Because skin substitutes are extremely costly (Biobrane supply cost of $359 U.S. versus approximately $11 U.S. if using a nonadherent gauze dressing),[109] and there is little research demonstrating the superiority of skin substitutes with standard burn care or skin grafting on minor burn wounds. Skin grafting remains the mainstay of surgical wound closure[38] and the use of skin substitutes is currently reserved for patients with significant or major burns.[105] Box 14–4 presents the benefits of skin substitutes for patients with burn injuries.

CHAPTER SUMMARY

There are three types of burn injuries: thermal, chemical, and electrical. Burn severity is dependent upon contact time, intensity (temperature, concentration, or voltage), and type of insult. Burn wound injuries are classified based on the level of tissue involvement, ranging from superficial to subdermal.

> **BOX 14–4   Benefits of Skin Substitutes**
>
> - Decrease evaporative water loss
> - Maintain warm, moist wound environment
> - Provide physical barrier to reduce risk of infection
> - Provide thermal insulation
> - Protect deeper tissues
> - Promote granulation tissue formation
> - Decrease pain
> - Allow coverage of larger areas than would be possible with skin grafting alone
> - Cannot be rejected by host tissues
> - Require less frequent dressing changes
> - Allow some visualization of wound bed
> - Allow movement due to elasticity
> - Decrease wound contraction
> - Enhance wound healing
> - Result in more cosmetically appealing scar formation

Because burn wounds may be quite large, burn size is generally estimated as a percentage of total body surface area using either the rule of nines or the Lund–Browder classification. In addition to causing extensive integumentary damage, burn injuries can directly or indirectly affect almost every body system, including the cardiovascular, pulmonary, and immune systems. One of the most significant sequelae of a burn injury is burn shock, a complex clinical syndrome that develops when perfusion is unable to meet the metabolic demands of body tissues. Burn injuries may also result in short- or long-term psychological dysfunction. Clinicians must understand how these sequelae can affect the patient and the rehabilitation process. Because burn injuries can be very painful, the clinician should ensure adequate pain control is achieved both in and out of therapy. Key wound management procedures for patients with burn injuries include debridement, infection control, dressings, and scar management. In addition to these wound management techniques, physical therapy interventions for patients with burn wound injuries should emphasize patient/client-related instruction and may include direct interventions such as therapeutic exercise, hydrotherapy, and assistive devices and equipment to improve positioning and mobility. Patients with significant burn injuries may require multiple surgical interventions including surgical debridement, escharotomy, fasciotomy, and skin grafting. Some patients with large burns may benefit from the use of skin substitutes to facilitate early wound coverage.

REVIEW QUESTIONS

You are examining a 6-year-old inpatient with a burn wound injury covering the anterior surface of both lower legs from the knee to the toes. She sustained the burn injury when a leaf fire got out of control, igniting her shoes and part of her pants. The accident occurred about 15 hours ago. You notice two large ruptured blisters. The wound bed has a mottled appearance and blanches to pressure, but capillary refill is sluggish. The patient has decreased pinprick sensation but is able to detect pressure in the affected area.

1. How would you classify the depth of this burn injury?
2. Give two estimates of burn size.
3. What is your prognosis for wound healing?
4. Describe the local wound care procedures you would initiate.
5. What range of motion limitations do you anticipate may occur?
6. How might you prevent or limit these impairments?
7. What mobility problems do you anticipate this patient might incur? How might you address these issues?

PEARSON
myhealthprofessionskit

Use this address to access the Companion Website created for this textbook. Simply select "Physical Therapy" from the choice of disciplines. Find this book and log in using your username and password to access images, video clips, and additional learning tools.

REFERENCES

Go to myhealthprofessionskit.com to view this chapter's references.

Lymphedema

Chapter Objectives

After reading this chapter, learners will be able to:

1. Describe the etiology of lymphedema.
2. Explain the risk factors contributing to lymphedema.
3. Describe and choose key physical therapy tests and measures to assess patients with lymphedema.
4. Define and describe the staging system for classifying lymphedema.
5. State the typical characteristics of lymphedema
6. Design an interdisciplinary approach in the management of patients with lymphedema.
7. Describe precautions clinicians should be aware of when working with patients with lymphedema.
8. Integrate the keys to local wound care for patients with lymphedema.
9. Select physical therapy procedural interventions for patients with lymphedema, including integumentary repair and protective techniques, therapeutic exercise, manual therapy techniques, and physical agents and mechanical modalities.
10. Discuss possible medical and surgical interventions for patients with lymphedema.

Key Terms

Anastomosis
Dynamic insufficiency
Elephantiasis
Filiariasis
Lipedema
Lipolymphedema
Lymph
Lymph capillaries
Lymph collectors

Lymphangiomotoricity
Lymphangions
Lymphatic load
Lymphatic territories
Lymphedema
Lymphorrhea
Mechanical insufficiency
Papilloma
Papillomatosis

Primary lymphedema
Secondary lymphedema
Sentinel lymph node
Seroma
Stemmer's sign
Thoracic duct
Transport capacity
Watershed

INTRODUCTION

The lymphatic system serves two key functions: regulation of fluid balance and assistance with infection control as part of the immune system. Normally, 18 liters of fluid are removed from the interstitial space per day, 80–90% via the veins and 10–20%, or about two to four liters, via the superficial and deep lymphatic vessels.[1–3] Lymphedema occurs when there is an imbalance between the amount of fluid needing to be removed from the interstitium and the lymphatic system's capacity to transport this fluid.[4] In North America and Europe, lymphedema most often occurs secondary to treatment, surgery, and/or radiation, for various forms of cancer. It is estimated that there are 3–5 million people in the United States living with lymphedema.[5] The National Cancer Institute estimates that 26% of women with breast cancer will develop lymphedema, while the National Institutes of Health estimates that 23% of breast cancer survivors will develop lymphedema within 2 years of treatment and up to 45% within 15 years of treatment.[6] In the United Kingdom, 25–30% of patients with breast cancer develop lymphedema.[4] Similarly, lymphedema developed in 21% of patients with ovarian cancer, 30% of patients with cervical cancer, and 28% of patients with endometrial cancer.[7] As many as 70% of men after prostate cancer will develop lymphedema.[3] The increase in limb size and volume can lead to patient complaints of limb heaviness, paresthesia, achiness, skin tightness, poor-fitting clothing, altered cosmesis, decreases in range of motion, limitations in activities of daily living, and is associated with adverse skin changes.[6, 8–10] Impaired lymphatic flow also causes an increased risk of local infection.[6, 8, 9]

This chapter provides a brief overview of the lymphatic system, followed by a review of the etiology of lymphedema and lymphedema-related tissue damage. Next, the classification of lymphedema is outlined along with physical therapy tests and measures commonly used assess lymphedema. Finally, the chapter presents a thorough description of physical therapy, medical, and surgical interventions. To assist with comprehension and learning proper techniques, extensive images and videos are available on the website accompanying this textbook. However, learners are urged to examine more detailed resources, attend an advanced continuing education course with laboratory sessions covering lymphatic drainage techniques, or attend a lymphedema certification course for improved results.[11–14]

LYMPHATIC SYSTEM OVERVIEW

Lymphatic Anatomy

The lymphatic system is composed of two interconnected drainage systems (see Figure 15–1). The superficial lymphatic system is located in and drains the skin and subcutaneous tissues, roughly paralleling the venous system.[15] The deep lymphatic system drains muscles, tendons, nerves, periosteum, joints, and internal organs.[2] The two systems are connected by perforating vessels. The interstitial space contains fibers, collagen, white blood cells, and proteins, which bind to water and serves as a reservoir for cells within the extracellular matrix.[16]

The initial lymphatics, or **lymph capillaries,** are a two-dimensional network of millions of open-ended vessels in the papillary dermis connected vertically to vessels in the reticular dermis to form a more three-dimensional drainage system.[15, 16] With a diameter of roughly 100 μm,[15] lymph capillaries are wider than blood capillaries and have an incomplete basement membrane, which makes them highly permeable. Anchoring filaments connect the lymph capillaries with collagen and elastin fibers within the extracellular matrix.[15] Increased pressure within the interstitium pulls on these filaments, opening lymphatic channels, allowing fluid and other material to move from areas of high pressure into the lower pressure lymphatic system.[5] Because lymph capillaries are larger and more permeable than blood capillaries, they can absorb larger particles, such as proteins and bacteria, from within the interstitium.[5] Once absorbed into the lymphatic system, this fluid is called lymph. **Lymph** is a fluid made up of water, protein, dead or dying cells and cellular components, fatty acids, foreign material, and debris.[3, 17, 18]

The initial lymphatics lead to larger vessels called precollectors, which are approximately 150 μm in diameter.[15] Precollectors have tight endothelial junctions, a few unidirectional valves to direct lymphatic flow,[19] and three underdeveloped layers of muscle.[5] Precollectors flow to larger **lymph collectors.** Lymph collectors have diameters of 100–600 μm with well-developed muscular walls similar to veins consisting of a tunica intima, tunica media, and tunica adventitia. Valves divide the lymph system into functional units called **lymphangions.** In a typical arm collector, there are 60–80 lymphagnions while there are 80–100 lymphagnions in a typical leg collector.[15] See Figure 15–2.

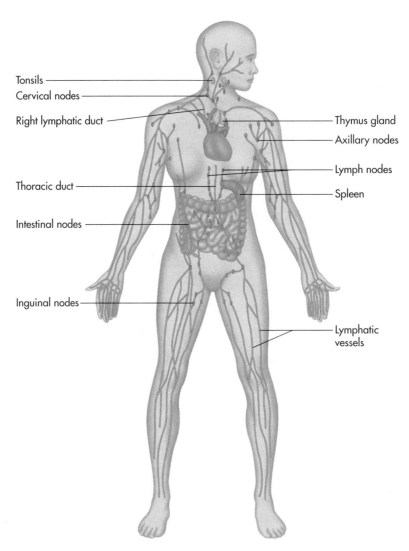

Tonsils

Cervical nodes

Right lymphatic duct

Thymus gland

Axillary nodes

Lymph nodes

Spleen

Thoracic duct

Intestinal nodes

Inguinal nodes

Lymphatic vessels

FIGURE 15–1   Components of the lymphatic system.

Lymph flows into progressively larger vessels toward clusters of regional lymph nodes.[17] Lymph nodes can be round, oval, kidney-shaped, or spindle-shaped and range in size from 0.2 cm to 3 cm. [15, 16] The total number of lymph nodes ranges from 600 to 700, with 100–200 nodes located within the mesentery.[15] The greater the lymph node size, the fewer the number of regional lymph nodes that will be present.[15] The lymph nodes are arranged in a string-like fashion and serve as filter stations[1] in which specialized white blood cells known as lymphocytes identify and destroy foreign material and assist with normal immune function. Surgical removal of regional lymph nodes or lymph node fibrosis reduces this filtration ability,

potentially impeding lymph transport and increasing the risk of local infection.[3] Some collateral lymph collectors exist that skip over regional lymph nodes.[15] These vessels can be a valuable drainage mechanism if lymph nodes are damaged or have been surgically removed. The average person has 10–24 axillary lymph nodes[15] and 8–15 inguinal lymph nodes. Efferent lymph vessels leaving lymph nodes enter into still larger lymphatic trunks that eventually join the venous system at the neck.

Figure 15–3 demonstrates the direction of normal lymph drainage. Lymph from the lower extremities and the genitals passes through the inguinal lymph nodes into the left and right lumbar trunks before

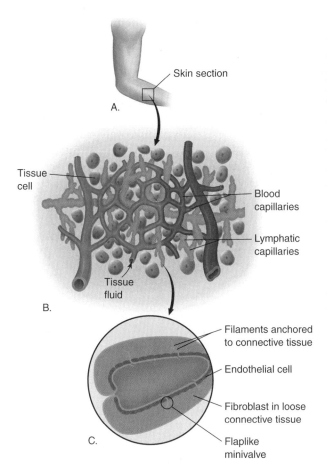

FIGURE 15–2 The superficial lymphatic system. *A.* Skin section. *B.* Relationship between a capillary bed of blood vascular system and lymphatic capillaries. *C.* Lymphatic capillaries are blind-ended tubes in which adjacent endothelial cells overlap each other, forming flaplike minivalves.

emptying into the centrally located **thoracic duct,** the largest lymphatic trunk. Lymph from the gastrointestinal system also drains into the thoracic duct, which parallels the vena cava and aorta before finally re-entering the general circulation at the left venous angle[3, 17]: the internal jugular vein and the subclavian vein.[15] Lymph from the left upper extremity filters through the axillary lymph nodes before emptying into the left subclavian vein, while the right upper extremity empties into the right subclavian vein,[17] aka the right venous angle.[3] The left side of the head and neck drains directly into the left subclavian vein while the right side of the head and neck drains into the right subclavian vein.[3, 17, 20]

Lymphatic territories are areas of skin made up of several adjacent lymph collectors that drain to the same regional lymph nodes. Lymphatic territories are separated by natural boundaries called **watersheds.**[3] In general, lymph fluid flows from the periphery of a watershed toward the regional lymph nodes. The sagittal watershed divides the body into left and right sides, while the horizontal watershed near the umbilicus divides the body into superior and inferior halves. For example, the right axillary lymph nodes receive lymph drainage from the right upper extremity as well as from the right anterior and posterior thorax above the umbilicus and below the clavicles.

There are two collateral pathways that allow lymph to flow between lymphatic territories. First, because the initial lymphatics have no valves, lymph within these vessels can flow in any direction. Lymph will naturally flow from areas of higher lymphatic pressure to areas of lower pressure.[5] Manual techniques, discussed later in the intervention section, can be used to take advantage of this anatomical connection to try to reroute fluid from congested or damaged areas to healthy regions. Because lymph capillaries are very small, only a very small amount of lymph can move across a watershed via lymph capillaries. Also, this is a very local phenomenon. The area of skin that can be drained from one lymph territory to another via the initial lymphatics is necessarily right on the border between lymphatic territories and is believed to occur over only about a 2–3 cm overlap.[15] Second, interterritorial **anastomoses** exist.[5] Anastomoses of peripheral collectors allow regional lymph nodes from one area to use regional lymph nodes from another area as a supplemental or alternative drainage system.[15] These connections are generally located at the shortest distance between regional lymph nodes, such as the anterior axilloaxillary pathway. In addition to these two collateral pathways, two final routes clinicians can take advantage of for rerouting lymph from clogged areas include perforating vessels and the vasa vasorum.[3] Lymphatic perforating precollectors provide connections between the superficial and deep lymphatic system at the parasternal nodes, the paravertebral nodes, and within the intercostal spaces. The vasa vasorum, a network of vessels found in larger vessels, provides another pathway to connect the lymphatic system with the venous system at the cephalic vein within the deltopectoral groove and at the femoral vein just medial to the sartorius muscle.

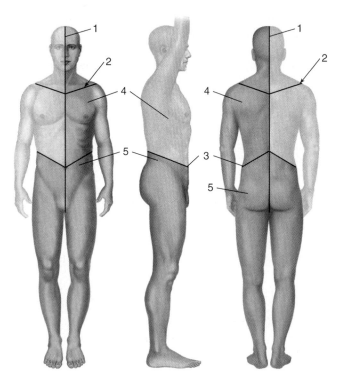

FIGURE 15–3   Normal lymph drainage pattern. The thoracic duct empties roughly 3 liters of lymph per day from the lower extremities, genitals, left trunk, left upper extremity, and left side of the head and neck into the left subclavian area (shaded regions). The right lymphatic duct empties another liter of lymph per day from the right upper extremity and the right side of the head and neck (unshaded regions). 1. Anterior and posterior sagittal watersheds. 2. Anterior and posterior superior horizontal water sheds. 3. Anterior and posterior horizontal water sheds. 4. Upper quadrants. 5. Lower quadrants.

Lymphatic Physiology

The movement of fluid between the blood capillaries, the interstitium, and the lymphatic system is governed by hydrostatic and osmotic pressure,[21] according to Starling's Law.[22] An overly simplistic way of thinking of this is that hydrostatic forces within capillaries and the interstitium push water away from these areas (see Figure 15–4). At the arterial end of the capillary, blood pressure is greater than interstitial pressure, effectively pushing water into the intersitium (ultrafiltration) while at the venous end interstitial pressure is greater than intracapillary pressure and 80–90% of this fluid is reabsorbed back into the capillary (reabsorption). In contrast, the hydrophilic nature of plasma and interstitial proteins pulls water toward them. The capillary basement membrane is semi-permeable, allowing approximately 50% of the circulating plasma proteins to enter the interstitium per day.[3] These proteins are too large to be reabsorbed at the venous end of the capillary. When interstitial pressure is greater than intralymphatic pressure, water and proteins flow into the lymphatic system and

lymph is produced.[15] Table 15–1 identifies some of the factors that influence ultrafiltration and reabsorption. As noted previously, the lymph system also absorbs dead or dying cells and cellular components, fatty acids, foreign material, and debris. All of these substances are collectively referred to as the **lymphatic load.**

In a healthy lymphatic system, lymph moves centrally through a variety of ways. First, skeletal muscle contractions alternately compress and decompress the lymph vessels, which help push lymph centrally through the unidirectional valves.[19] Second, the respiratory pump, as described in Chapter 11, helps move fluid through alternating pressures within the chest.[1, 3, 23] Third, the pulsations of the aorta can assist with movement of lymph within the thoracic duct.[15] Fourth, the smooth muscle within lymphangions spontaneously contracts 3–12 times per minute to propel lymph centrally.[5, 24] This inherent **lymphangiomotoricity,** the frequency and strength of lymphagnion contraction, is key in decreasing edema overnight while patients are recumbent because the lower extremity lymphatics are in a gravity-lessened position, as well as in patients who are immobile or have motor neuron damage.[24] Lymph

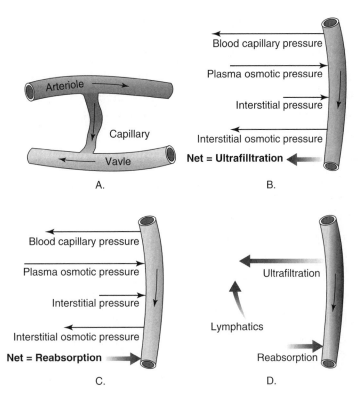

FIGURE 15–4   *A–D*. Lymphatic physiology. *A*. Arrows depict the direction of blood flow. *B*. At the arterial end of the capillary, the net of hydrostatic and osmotic forces favors ultrafiltration. *C*. At the venous end of the capillary, the net of hydrostatic and osmotic forces favors reabsorption. *D*. During homeostasis, the excess fluid and proteins deposited in the interstitium is picked up by the lymphatic system. As a result, edema is not present.

angiomotoricity can transiently increase to 20 times per minute with exercise.[25] An increase in lymph volume, or preload within the lymphangion, increases the force of lymphangion contraction, leading to greater lymph fluid proplusion.[2, 5] Last, sympathetic stimulation can increase lymphangiomotoricity.[2]

ETIOLOGY OF LYMPHEDEMA AND LYMPHEDEMA-RELATED TISSUE DAMAGE

Lymphatic Insufficiency

In general terms, **lymphedema** occurs when the lymphatics are unable to accommodate for and remove this protein-rich fluid from the interstitium resulting in fluid stagnation and edema. Lymphedema may result

from **dynamic insufficiency** in which the lymphatic system is unable to accommodate for and transport an increase in lymphatic load. Conversely, the lymphatic load may be normal but the lymphatic system is unable to transport this load due to some sort of **mechanical insufficiency.** A combination of dynamic and mechanical insufficiency is also possible.[24, 26] Figure 15–5 demonstrates examples of dynamic, mechanical, and combined insufficiency. It is important to remember that edema is a temporary inability of the body to remove excess fluid. Traumatic edema is mostly water.[27] In contrast, lymphedema is an abnormal accumulation of protein-rich fluid,[2, 3, 28] meaning there is more than 1 gram of protein per 100 mL of fluid.[5] With lymphedema, fibrinogen in the interstitium cannot be absorbed by the lymphatic system and accumulates in the interstitial space. Macrophages migrate to this area of high protein and activate fibroblasts. Over time, connective tissue proliferates and there is an

TABLE 15–1 Factors That Influence Ultrafiltration and Reabsorption

Increase in Ultrafiltration	Increase in Reabsorption
Increase in capillary pressure	Decrease capillary pressure
• Vasodilation	• Diuretics
• Heat	• Dehydration
• Inflammation/trauma	
• Infection	
• Venous insufficiency	
• Venous thrombosus	
• Dependent positioning	
• Pregnancy	
• Congestive heart failure	
Decrease in tissue pressure	Increase in tissue pressure
• High elevation	• Muscle pump
• Airplane travel	• Compression bandage
• Adipose tissue	• Compression garment
Increase in interstitial proteins	Decrease in interstitial proteins
• Relative increase with diuretics	• Manual techniques to promote lymph drainage
• Wound	
Decrease in plasma proteins	
• Protein malnutrition	
• Liver disease	
• Kidney disease	

increase in collagen formation, leading to fibrosis.[15] This fibrotic tissue hardens, leading to sclerosis and induration.[15]

While lymphedema itself is rarely painful, it is problematic for several reasons. Patients with lymphedema generally complain of a feeling of heaviness or weakness in the involved extremity. Paresthesias may be present. In addition, edema may result in decreased function due to the inability to easily move the fluid-laden limb.[10] The resulting edema can also be quite disfiguring. Lymphedema causes an increased risk of infection, delayed wound healing, and local tissue hypoxia.[18, 29] The increased limb size requires a greater diffusion distance for oxygen and nutrients to reach body cells[27] and increased tissue pressure caused by this swelling can collapse the lymphatic capillaries, further inhibiting lymph transport. This has been confirmed with dye tests near open wounds.[27] The high protein content of lymphedema is especially problematic. Protein molecules within the interstitium cause tissue fibrosis, further impairing fluid removal and placing the skin at risk for secondary changes and ulceration.[30] Because protein molecules are hydrophilic, lymphedema self-perpetuates[10] by drawing more water from within the vasculature into the interstitial space.[30] Last, this protein serves as a ready food source for bacteria should a break in the skin occur.[18, 31]

More specifically, lymphedema may be primary or secondary.[1, 27] **Primary lymphedema,** accounting for approximately 10% of all cases, occurs without any obvious cause and is the result of congenital malformation or impairment of the lymphatics.[18] Primary lymphedemas are usually described by the type of lymphatic vessel abnormality or the age of onset (see Box 15–1). [5, 15, 16, 32] It is important to remember that individuals may be born with anatomical variations in

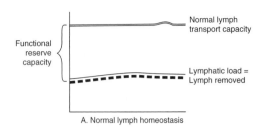

FIGURE 15–5A   Normal lymph system homeostasis. As with heart rate, the lymph system normally operates below maximum transport capacity and can increase the amount of lymph to be transported to match the lymphatic load.

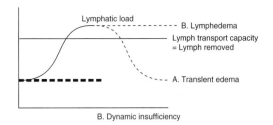

FIGURE 15–5B   Dynamic insufficiency. If the lymphatic load exceeds the transport capacity of the lymphatic system, edema will occur. A. The edema will be transient if the functional reserve capacity of the lymphatic system can compensate for the increased lymphatic load over time. This is commonly seen after an injury such as a sprained ankle, causes a transient increase in lymphatic load. B. A prolonged increase in lymphatic load, as may occur with chronic venous insufficiency, can lead to chronic edema or lymphedema.

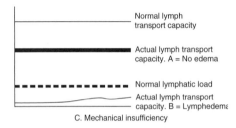

FIGURE 15–5C   Mechanical insufficiency. If there is a decrease in the maximal transport capacity of the lymphatic system, mechanical insufficiency can result. A. If the remaining transport capacity continues to exceed the lymphatic load, no overt signs of lymphedema occur. B. If the remaining transport capacity is less than the lymphatic load, lymphedema will occur. This may be seen in patients who have had a large number of axillary lymph nodes removed due to breast cancer.

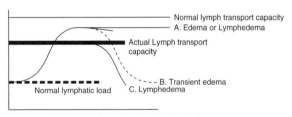

FIGURE 15–5D   Combined dynamic and mechanical insufficiency. A. If there is an increase in lymphatic load in an individual with a previously compromised lymphatic transport capacity, lymphedema will occur. This may be seen in a patient who has had axillary lymph node irradiation and then has an infection in the affected upper extremity. The increased lymphatic load now overwhelms the lymphatic system and the limb swells. B. If the infection is controlled quickly and the lymphatic load decreased, this lymphedema may be temporary if the lymphatic system is able to compensate over time for the transient increased load. C. Over time the prolonged increased workload of the already damaged lymphatic system may further compromise the lymphatic system, lowering its transport capacity even further, causing lymphedema.

their lymphatic systems without overt signs of lymphedema. The onset of lymphedema may occur after a minor trauma,[33] such as a sprained ankle. Hormonal changes that occur with puberty may be the triggering factor. Alternatively, the lymphatic system may simply fatigue and no longer have the functional reserve capacity to compensate for the decreased lymphatic **transport capacity** caused by the structural abnormalities. Primary lymphedemas may affect any body region but most often affect the lower extremities.[32, 34] Lymphedema is rare in children and should be suspected in a child who has more than one attack of erysipelas (localized redness and inflammation of the skin usually caused by *Streptococcus pyogenes*).[32]

Some of the more common forms of primary lymphedema are listed in Box 15–2.[32, 35–38]

Secondary, or acquired, **lymphedema** may result from a disruption in, or damage to, the lymphatic system.[1, 3] The most common cause of secondary lymphedema, affecting 129 million people worldwide, is

BOX 15–1	Primary Lymphedema Classifications
Types of Primary Lymphedema Based on Vessel Abnormality	
Aplasia	• Lack of lymphatic vessels in a body region therefore no lymphatic drainage in this area
Hypoplasia	• Lymphatic vessels are narrower than normal leading to significantly less lymphatic drainage • Comparable to arterial stenosis
Hyperplasia	• Lymphatic vessels are wider than normal • Comparable to varicose veins • Accounts for roughly 15% of all cases of primary lymphedema
Lymph node fibrosis	• Most commonly seen in inguinal lymph nodes
Types of Primary Lymphedema Based on Age at Onset	
Congenital lymphedema	• Present at birth or within the first year of life • Accounts for 6–12% of all primary lymphedemas
Lymphedema praecox	• Onset between one and 35 years of age • Accounts for 77–94% of all primary lymphedemas
Lymphedema tarda	• Onset after 35 years of age • Accounts for 11% of all primary lymphedemas

filiariasis.[27, 37] Filariasis is caused by the bite of a mosquito that is infected with a parasitic worm. The worm is transferred to its human host and lives in the lymphatics of infected individuals. Parasitic offspring circulate within the patient's blood. The parasites' waste products are toxic to the patient's lymphatic system: lymphangions are first weakened then paralyzed; lymph endothelium and valves are damaged, causing vessel dilation and incompetence; and inflammation increases the lymphatic load. Host immune response leads to fever, lymph adenitis, and lymph node fibrosis.[37] While not endemic to the Western world, it is images of this severe, disfiguring lymphedema, also known as **elephantiasis,** that patients may conjure up unless educated by health care professionals.

In the United States, however, secondary lymphedema is most often seen following medical or surgical procedures that disrupt lymph flow, such as a mastectomy, lymph node dissection, lymph node biopsy, or radiation therapy.[30, 39] After the lymph transport capacity is reduced, the body attempts to reach homeostasis by responding to edema and lymph stagnation in several ways.[16] Lymphangiomotoricity can increase. Collateral pathways and unblocked collectors can be utilized to decongest the affected region. Lymph capillaries can be used to move fluid across watersheds to less congested territories. Lymph angiogenesis and lymph–vein or lymph–lymph anastamoses can develop in response to pathology, such as chronic inflammation, tissue injury, or lymphedema.[28] Macrophages may engulf excess interstitial proteins.[15]

While secondary lymphedema after cancer treatment can be evident the day of surgery, there is typically a latency period while the lymph system is able to compensate for its reduced transport capacity. Degenerative changes of the lymphatic system include lymph endothelium hyperplasia or sclerosis, thickening of the collagen fibers in the subendothelial layer, decreases in lymphangion muscle fiber density, lymph lumen occlusion, and/or valve dysfunction.[24] Secondary lymphedema can develop at any time after cancer treatment[18] and has been diagnosed as late as 30 years

BOX 15–2	Inherited Forms of Lymphedema
Klinefelter	• XXY chromosome disorder • Common features: gynecomastia, lack of body/facial/ sexual hair, mitral valve prolapse
Klippel–Trenaunay syndrome	• Common features: multiple vascular malformations—capillary, veins, lymphatics. • May also have polydactyly, syndactyly, hyperhydrosis
Lymphedema–distichiasis syndrome	• Lymph node and lymph vessel hyperplasia leads to retrograde flow
Milroy's disease	• Autosomal dominant condition • Mutation of vascular endothelial growth factor (VEGF) receptor 3 • Only affects lower extremity lymphatics • Generally present at birth, evident within first year of life • Common features: deep toe creases, upturned nails, prominent veins, papillomatosis, cellulitis, hydroceles
Meige's syndrome	• Autosomal dominant condition • Affects lower extremities • Onset near puberty
Noonan syndrome	• Three gene mutations • Common features: facial abnormalities, webbed neck, dysphagia, cardiac defects, generally have lymphedema but may not
Prader–Wili syndrome	• Genetic disorder • Higher incidence in males • Common features: hypotonia, hypogonadism, hyperphagia, obesity, decreased mentation
Turner syndrome	• XO chromosome disorder • Present at birth • Common features: infertility, absent menstruation, small testes, gynecomastia, tall stature

after cancer treatment.[6] However, it is now believed that 80% of breast cancer patients who develop lymphedema will do so within the first 3 years of treatment.[6]

Another leading cause of secondary lymphedema is chronic venous insufficiency. Patients with chronic venous insufficiency may develop secondary lower extremity lymphedema for two reasons.[1, 30] First, venous hypertension pushes higher than normal amounts of fluid and proteins into the interstitium, which then increases the lymphatic load.[27] Eventually, the overloaded lymphatic system may be unable to compensate for this increased volume.[27] Second, the edema created by venous insufficiency increases the distance that fluid must travel to reach the lymphatics, and the pressure created may obstruct the lymphatic channels. Similarly, patients who have undergone vein stripping procedures are at risk for lymphedema. Lymphedema may also masquerade as venous insufficiency. Patients with paralysis may develop lymphedema due to loss of muscle pump.[1] Patients who are obese are at increased risk of developing lymphedema,[1] especially after surgery.[20]

Lipedema and Lipolymphedema

Lipedema is a bilateral symmetrical increase in adipose tissue deposition in the abdomen, buttocks, and lower extremities with sparing of the feet.[37, 40] Lipedema is thought to be due to an imbalance in pituitary, thyroid, and sex hormones and occurs almost exclusively in females. The onset of fatty deposition occurs around puberty while the onset of swelling may occur at this time, after a minor trauma, or at menopause.[3] Patients with lipedema are tender to palpation, have palpable subcutaneous nodules, tend to bleed or bruise easily, have deep skin folds, and may have a familial history of "big legs."[37] Lipedema is sometimes called diet-resistant because the increased thickness of the subcutaneous adipose tissue[37] is unaffected by diet and patients may develop eating disorders in an attempt to control the disfiguring increase in lower extremity size.[40] Many of these patients may be improperly diagnosed as being morbidly obese.

The superficial lymphatics in patients with lipedema are dysfunctional: they may have a wider lumen and decreased angiomotoricity.[15, 40] The increased tissue compliance of adipose tissue along with these anatomical changes are thought to allow more fluid to accumulate in the affected regions, leading to **lipolymphedema**.[15] Lipolymphedema differs from lymphedema in several key ways. First, as noted previously, the pathophysiology and anatomical areas affected are different. Second, pitting and fibrosis are rare with lipolymphedema while tenderness and pain are the norm. Third, edema tends to be symmetrical and elevation has no effect on swelling. While initially spared, foot edema may occur with lipolymphedema due to lymphatic overload and retrograde flow. Infections are uncommon with lipedema but may be frequent with lipolymphedema.[40] Last, and most unfortunately, due to these differences, patients with lipolymphedema will experience only small improvements from the common intervention strategies for lymphedema.[15, 37, 40]

BOX 15–3 Risk Factors Contributing to Lymphedema

- Lymph node status
- Radiation therapy
- Surgical complications
- Time since surgery
- Increased body mass index
- Air travel without compression
- Inflammation/increased lymphatic load
- Decreased lymphatic return
- Individuals prone to scar tissue formation

RISK FACTORS CONTRIBUTING TO LYMPHEDEMA AND LYMPHATIC INSUFFICIENCY

The subsequent list of risk factors for lymphedema are roughly divided into the following categories (see Box 15–3): lymph node status, radiation therapy, surgical complications, time since surgery, increased body mass index, air travel without compression, inflammation/increased lymphatic load, decreased lymphatic return, and individuals prone to scar tissue formation. Some of these risk factors are modifiable, while others are not. However, the potential for successful outcomes for patients with lymphedema is enhanced if risk factors are identified and corrected or controlled for as much as possible.

Lymph Node Status

Surgical removal of lymph nodes increases the risk of lymphedema. In general, patients who have had more lymph nodes removed are at greater risk of developing lymphedema.[41] In a typical axillary lymph node dissection, more than 10 lymph nodes are removed.[42] In contrast, a **sentinel lymph node** biopsy removes only the first lymph node receiving lymph from the tumor. Because patients who have a mastectomy have more extensive lymph node dissection, these patients are at greater risk for lymphedema than those who undergo a sentinel lymph node biopsy and lumpectomy (20–25% for patients undergoing mastectomy vs. 8% for those undergoing a lumpectomy).[6, 41, 43–45] Patients with more advanced disease and those with more positive lymph nodes are more likely to develop lymphedema.[5, 41, 43, 44, 46, 47]

However, the first crucial decision for these patients is *not* how best to decrease their risk of lymphedema, but how best to treat their primary disease process (e.g., their cancer).

There does not appear to be any association between the onset of lymphedema and breast reconstruction surgery, regardless of type of reconstruction procedure performed.[44] This is likely because no further lymph node trauma occurs during reconstruction and no additional radiation therapy is performed.

Radiation Therapy

Recent advances in breast-conserving therapy for the treatment of breast cancer has led to the erroneous assumption that the side effects of this treatment are also less frequent and/or less severe. The myth that patients who can be treated with a lumpectomy do not get lymphedema is clearly dispelled by the abundant research linking radiation therapy, which is the standard of care after a lumpectomy, to lymphedema. One study of patients who underwent lumpectomies and axillary radiation cites 26% of patients developed arm lymphedema, 21% developed breast lymphedema, and 38% reported arm tightness.[42] Radiation therapy after ovarian and uterine cancer is also associated with an increased risk of lymphedema, regardless of the type of surgery performed or number of lymph nodes removed.[7] The greater the dosage of radiation, the greater the risk of lymphedema.[2] Likewise, wider radiation fields and radiation specficially to the axilla increased the risk of lymphedema.[2, 43, 48] The increased risk for developing lymphedema in women who have tumors in the upper outer breast quadrant[5] is likely due to the higher levels of radiation to the axillary lymph nodes.

Radiation therapy increases the risk for lymphedema in several ways.[15] Radiation causes perilymphatic and lymph node fibrosis. It damages regenerating and traumatized lymph vessels. Radiation also decreases the immune response. In addition, the skin damage caused by radiation therapy, such as erythema, connective tissue sclerosis, dermal atrophy, anhydrous skin due to decreased sweat gland density, and vascular fibrosis, decrease the effectiveness of the skin barrier by making the skin more vulnerable to friction, shear, pressure, and UV rays. Again, the key decision here is *not* how to decrease the risk of lymphedema, but how to best treat the patient's primary disease process. That being said, radiation oncologists are now more aware of the risks of treatment and have been able to take advantage of many technological advances in radiation therapy, such as fractionated radiation doses, blocking devices, and more focused radiation beams, to try to minimize the risk of lymphedema.

Surgical Complications

A **seroma** is a localized accumulation of serum within the tissue. If a seroma develops after breast cancer surgery, it is generally noted as a pocket-like collection of fluid within the fascial planes of the thorax. Seromas may be along the anterior chest wall in the region of the surgical incision, lateral chest wall, or posteriorly. To decrease the risk of seroma formation, a drain is placed in the area of tissue excision. The drain is left in place until the amount of new drainage into the drain is less than a few milliliters per day, about 1–2 weeks after surgery. A seroma feels full and may be slightly warm to palpation. The patient may complain of fullness or tightness in the involved area. Seromas that occur after breast cancer may limit shoulder range of motion. Small seromas, just like small joint effusions, may be resorbed by the body without medical intervention. However, large seromas or seromas in combination with wound dehiscence should be drained by a physician either with a needle or surgically, via incision and drainage with repeat drain placement. Seromas typically occur in the absence of infection but the two may occur simultaneously. In the case of a post-operative infection, the classic signs of infection are generally present (see Chapter 6). Seroma formation or post-operative infections increase the risk of lymphedema in patients with breast cancer.[5, 42, 44, 49] Unfortunately, early post-operative lymphedema is sometimes disregarded by both medical professionals and patients as simple post-operative inflammation.[50] Therefore, lymphedema education is paramount.

Time Since Surgery

The risk of developing lymphedema increases over time for patients who have had surgical lymph node removal or lymph node radiation.[26] This may be the result of mechanical lymphatic insufficiency over time (lymph system fatigue) or the combined effect of an additional lymphatic load from a trauma or infection on an already mechanically impaired lymphatic system.

Increased Body Mass Index

Increased body mass index is an independent risk factor for the development of lymphedema.[43–46, 49, 51, 52] In the United States, 75% of morbidly obese patients have lower extremity lymphedema.[53] Excess adipose tissue can alter lymph flow by compressing lymphatic vessels[54] and by decreasing tissue pressure. Other complications related to obesity that adversely affect lymphedema include hemosideran deposition, hyperkeratosis, cellulitis, deepening of skin folds, fibrosis, lymphorrhea, and papillomatosis.[53]

Without significant weight loss, long-term improvement in lymphedema is unlikely to occur in patients with lymphedema.[53] This can be particularly problematic for several reasons. First, individuals with some forms of cancer, particularly some types of breast cancer, are treated with drugs that lead to weight gain while simultaneously decreasing their energy and ability for physical activity. Second, patients who are obese and develop secondary lower extremity lymphedema may have a difficult time losing weight due to the combination of a sedentary lifestyle, deconditioning, and the extra burden of moving an edematous limb (or limbs). Third, morbidly obese patients are more likely to be homebound with little social interaction and their compliance with weight loss and exercise tends to be limited.[53] Fourth, patients who are obese are also more likely to have difficulty breathing when recumbent, leading them to sleep upright with their extremities in more dependent positions, further limiting lymphatic return.[54] While one study found nearly a threefold increase in risk for lymphedema in women with breast cancer who had larger breasts,[5] this is more likely due to the effect obesity has on breast size rather than being an independent risk factor. Obesity is also a risk factor for the development of lymphedema in children.[32]

Air Travel Without Compression

Air travel without the concomitant use of a compression garment or bandaging is linked to the onset of lymphedema.[42, 50, 55] This is likely due to the decrease in atmospheric pressure on a body while in flight. The cabin of an airplane is pressurized to the equivalent of 5,000–8,000 feet above sea level.[3] Therefore, while in flight there is a significant decrease in atmospheric pressure against the body, allowing it to swell. An at-risk extremity may not be able to reabsorb this increase in lymphatic load over time. It is therefore recommended that individuals at risk for lymphedema wear compression (>20 mm

Hg for an upper extremity and >30 mm Hg for a lower extremity) to off-set this decrease in atmospheric pressure, thus decreasing the tendency for increased ultrafiltration into the interstitium during flight.[6, 56] At-risk individuals should also perform range of motion exercises, breathing exercises, move about the cabin when able, and remain well hydrated to improve lymphatic return, particularly during longer flights.[50] By extension, it is also recommended that when at-risk individuals travel to or through areas of higher elevation, such as someone from New Orleans (approximately at sea level) going to Denver (approximately 1 mile above sea level), should use some form of compression to offset the decrease in atmospheric pressure.

Inflammation/Increased Lymphatic Load

In the past, health care providers erred on the side of caution by severely limiting the use of an at-risk limb. Blanket statements such as "never lift more than 5 pounds" were routinely made without regard for other risk factors and individual patient characteristics. The argument for limiting upper extremity use after breast cancer treatment is upheld by a study involving 52 patients in which greater levels of reported use of the affected extremity was associated with an increased chance of having lymphedema.[49] However, several more studies document that regular exercise, strength training, and unrestricted use of an at-risk extremity either has no effect or may actually decrease the risk for developing lymphedema.[8, 43, 44, 51, 57–60]

Perhaps a more useful way of looking at this issue is to consider inflammation as a risk factor for individuals with a compromised lymphatic system. Inflammation is a risk factor for lymphedema because it causes an increase in lymphatic load. From this viewpoint, it is easy to see how muscle overuse can lead to microtrauma and inflammation, which may upset the delicate balance between an at-risk individual's lymph transport capacity and lymphatic load. In fact, at least one study supports that avoiding strenuous use of an affected extremity decreases the risk of an individual developing lymphedema.[61] However, it is *not* necessarily the *amount* of lifting one performs, but a combination of factors, including repetitions, frequency with which the load is imposed, as well as a muscle's current conditioning to handle these interrelated factors.

☑ *Checkpoint Question #1*

Describe whether you think the following individuals are at low or high risk for developing lymphedema. Provide your rationale.

  a. A competitive female tennis player who had a single axillary lymph node removed from her dominant arm with no radiation therapy painting an entire room.

  b. A sedentary, overweight male who had a complete inguinal lymph node dissection followed by radiation therapy hiking the Inca trail.

In addition to muscle overuse, the risk for lymphedema is increased by other things that can cause inflammation in an at-risk area,[26, 42] such as thermal trauma from a sunburn, chemical trauma from an allergic reaction, or mechanical trauma from a sprained ankle. Therefore, anything that has the potential to increase lymphatic load in the affected area should be controlled as much as possible. Because aggressive massage therapy techniques, such as deep tissue work or rolfing, are likely to cause muscle inflammation, these techniques should be avoided in at-risk areas.[50] Because sitting in a hot tub causes vasodilation, which increases the lymphatic load, patients at risk for lymphedema should be educated to avoid prolonged exposure and to decrease the water temperature, if not avoid this activity altogether.[56]

Local infection increases the risk of lymphedema,[42] likely due to the associated inflammation that occurs with infection. Anything that has the potential to breach the skin in an affected area should be limited due to the local decrease in immune response as well as the accompanying inflammatory process to heal the wound. This is why breast cancer patients have been told "no needle sticks" in the affected extremity.[42] For the same reasons, patients are recommended to wear gardening gloves if at risk for upper extremity lymphedema and proper footwear if at risk for lower extremity lymphedema.[56] While one study found no increased risk of lymphedema in patients at-risk for lymphedema who had needle sticks in the affected extremity,[26] the sample of only 14 patients and a limited follow-up time make generalization difficult. In contrast, larger trials over longer periods of time have found that patients who practice risk-reducing behaviors, such as this, have fewer symptoms of lymphedema than those who do not adhere to such precautions.[42]

Decreased Lymphatic Return

Clothing, jewelry, or anything that has the potential to restrict lymphatic or venous return should be avoided.[56] Likewise, tourniquets and blood pressure cuffs should be avoided on at-risk limbs because they decrease lymphatic return. A small sample of 25 patients who had elective hand surgery after breast cancer treatment found no new cases of lymphedema during the study period but 50% of those with lymphedema had a "temporary" (several months) worsening of their lymphedema despite the use of a local anesthetic and extremely limited tourniquet time during surgery.[62] The study does not describe what interventions were required to stabilize lymphedema in these patients. Therefore, patients should be counseled on the risks of elective surgery on an extremity with, or at risk for, lymphedema.

Individuals Prone to Scar Tissue Formation

Some patients, such as those at risk for keloids (see Chapter 3), are more prone to scar tissue formation and fibrosis than others. For these individuals, the trauma of surgical lymph node removal can be exacerbated by an abnormal increase in collagen deposition post-surgery. This excess collagen is problematic for two reasons. First, it poses a physical barrier to lymph flow. Second, the hydrophilic nature of the protein collagen will draw more water into the interstitium.

CASE STUDY: Mrs. Julia Prentice

This case study is referenced throughout the chapter.

PART 1

History

Mrs. Prentice is a 64-year-old female seen this afternoon in out-patient physical therapy for lymphedema management. Her primary language is English. She lives with her retired husband in a two-story house. Mrs. Prentice works in a real estate office where her job involves sitting at a computer and frequent phone calls. She enjoys working in her flower garden and going to visit her grandchildren in Hawaii.

Lymphedema History: Mrs. Prentice reports her left hand began swelling intermittently about 2 months ago and she sometimes cannot put on her wedding ring due to swelling.

Past Medical History: Mrs. Prentice has a history of osteoarthritis and osteopenia. She was diagnosed with left breast cancer 15 years ago and underwent a lumpectomy with removal of five axillary lymph nodes. She had three rounds of chemotherapy followed by 28 treatments of axillary radiation. She was diagnosed with diabetes mellitus 3 months ago at her annual physical when her fasting blood sugars were found to be 140 mg/dL. She has no allergies and is not sensitive to adhesives.

General Health Status: Mrs. Prentice reports she is in excellent health. She has lost 10 pounds with her dietary changes after being diagnosed with diabetes. She notes she has been checking her blood sugar two to three times per day, alternating between her left and right hands for reach test as she was taught in her diabetes education class.

Current Medications: Multivitamin with calcium and iron. She occasionally takes acetaminophen or ibuprofen for headaches or joint pain.

Other Available Data: Mrs. Prentice reports her fasting blood glucose is now 95 mg/dL when she wakes and her only measurement above 120 mg/dL was 1 week ago after splurging at a wedding reception. She does not recall her hemoglobin A1c laboratory values from her physical or recent physician follow-up last week but recalls the physician was pleased that her level had decreased.

Systems Review

Cardiovascular/Pulmonary System: Heart rate: 76 bpm, blood pressure 124/80 mm Hg, respiratory rate 14 bpm, slight left upper extremity edema noted above the elbow with slight pitting.

Musculoskeletal System: No deficits noted in gross assessment of range of motion and strength. Height: 5 feet 7 inches (1.70 m). Body weight: 175 pounds (79.4 kg). Body mass index (BMI) = 27.4 kg/m^2.

Neuromuscular System: No gross deficits noted in gross coordinated movement or motor control.

Gastrointestinal System: No problems noted.

Urogenital System: No problems noted.

Integumentary System: No open wounds are present. Mrs. Prentice's medial left brachium feels full and slightly warm to palpation. Mrs. Prentice's distal left second and third intermetacarpal region appear full compared to the right.

Communication, Cognition, Language, and Learning Style: No deficits noted. Mrs. Prentice reports she learns best by demonstration followed by repetition. She demonstrates an understanding of her situation and a willingness to participate in lymphedema management interventions.

PHYSICAL THERAPY TESTS AND MEASURES FOR LYMPHEDEMA

Clinicians should perform various tests and measures to assess lymphedema and identify changes in patient status. This section highlights some of the key tests and measures presented in Chapter 4 that are critical to perform on patients with, or at risk for, lymphedema: anthropometrics, circulation, and sensory integrity.

Anthropometrics

Circumferential Measurements

Circumferential measurements have high intra- and interrated reliability.[63] In addition, there is a high correlation between volumetric displacement and circumferential measurements,[64] although this is somewhat lower in patients who are obese.[65] Volumetric displacement, once considered the gold standard, is rarely used to evaluate patients with lymphedema due to the increased time, instrumentation, potential for wound contamination, and substantial limb size of many patients. No significant differences in limb volume calculations were found when measuring limb segments every 3, 4, 8, or 12 cm. For greater efficiency of measurement, clinicians should include landmarks required for garment fitting as well as any additional landmarks to include areas of deformity, lobules, or significant edema. While it may be tempting to measure just the affected limb in cases of unilateral lymphedema, clinicians should be cautious in comparing new measurements of the affected limb with initial measurements of the unaffected limb as the control limb has also been found to decrease slightly in volume over the course of treatment.[63] The decrease in control limb volume may be due to total body weight loss, may represent a subclinical lymphedema in the contralateral side, or may be the result of improved lymphatic efficiency in the unaffected limb due to lymphedema interventions.[63]

After taking circumferential measurements, a programmable calculator can be used to calculate limb volume using a mathematical formula based on a truncated cone.[64] Alternatively, several computer software programs are available and can also be used to track volume changes over time. Most programs can be used to compare initial measurements to current measurements as well as compare the affected to the unaffected side to determine the percent difference in limb volume.

Body Mass Index (BMI)

Body mass indices should be calculated on all patients with, or at risk for, lymphedema (Figure 15–6).[66, 67] Patients who are obese should be counseled on the effect obesity has on lymphedema and referred to a nutritionist as needed.[66] Clinicians may use changes in body weight as a measure of change in patients with lymphedema. Body weight changes are particularly useful in patients with severe lymphedema, unilateral or bilateral lower extremity lymphedema, and patients with irregular limb shapes including lobules, which make the calculation of limb volume via the truncated cone method less accurate.

Circulation

Clinicians must perform a vascular assessment prior to initiating treatment. While arterial insufficiency and deep vein thromboses (DVT) can occur in the upper extremity, these problems occur much more frequently in the lower extremity. Therefore, a vascular assessment is absolutely critical in patients with lower extremity lymphedema. Pulse assessment, using a Doppler ultrasound as needed, must be performed on all patients. An ankle-brachial index (ABI) or toe-brachial index (TBI) should be performed on all patients with lower extremity lymphedema (refer to Chapter 10).[68, 69] Recall that an ABI may not be accurate on patients with diabetes. Patients with signs and symptoms of severe arterial insufficiency, including intermittent claudication, pain with elevation, distal toe wounds, and/or wounds with a dry, pale, or necrotic wound base, should be referred to a vascular surgeon for further examination. Refer to Chapter 11 on how to screen the lower extremity for DVTs.

FIGURE 15–6   Body mass index calculation.

$$\text{BMI (metric calculation)} = \frac{\text{Patient weight in kg}}{\text{height in meters}^2}$$

$$\text{BMI (U.S. calculation)} = \frac{\text{Patient weight in pounds} \times 703}{\text{height in inches}^2}$$

Body Mass Index (kg/m^2)	Interpretation
<18.5	Underweight
18.5–24.9	Normal Weight
25.0–29.9	Overweight
30.0–34.9	Obese—Class 1
35.0–39.9	Obese—Class 2
≥40.0	Obese—Class 3

Sensory Integrity

Clinicians must assess sensory integrity in all patients with lymphedema. Patients with lymphedema often report a feeling of heaviness, fullness, and tightness. Patients with lower extremity lymphedema are also likely to report pruritus.[6] Nerve entrapments, such as carpal tunnel syndrome and tarsal tunnel syndrome, can be caused by tissue distention, edema, and inflammation in this population. Neuropathy may be caused by diabetes or chemotherapy, particularly breast cancer treatment using taxanes.[68] These types of nerve dysfunctions can impede the patient's ability to detect skin trauma or ischemia that can be caused by poor bandaging technique, poor garment fit, or too much compression to an arterial insufficient limb. Patients with nerve dysfunction must be particularly meticulous with skin care and skin inspection to prevent undue harm.[6] Last, clinicians must be aware that some pain complaints may not be due to edema[67] and alternative sources, such as metastases, arterial insufficiency, compartment syndrome, or musculoskeletal causes, must be considered.

CLASSIFICATION AND CHARACTERISTICS OF LYMPHEDEMA

Classification

The *Guide to Physical Therapist Practice* provides physical therapists with valuable patient management for lymphedema as well as general wound care. The

TABLE 15–2   Classification of Lymphedema

Classification	Descriptor	Characteristics
Stage 0	**Latent**	• No edema present • Reduced transport capacity of the lymphatic system • Most commonly due to surgery or radiation
Stage 1	**Reversible**	• Edema that pits when digital pressure is applied • Greatly or completely reduces with elevation • No secondary skin changes
Stage 2	**Spontaneously Irreversible**	• Does not pit when digital pressure is applied • Does not reduce substantially with elevation • Skin becomes fibrotic or brawny • May have frequent skin infections
Stage 3	**Lymphostatic Elephantiasis**	• Extreme increase in limb volume • Deep skin folds and papillomas present • Frequent skin infections

Unilateral lymphedema is further classified based on a side-to-side comparison of circumferential measurements or limb volume.

Severity	Circumferential Measurement Difference	Volumetric Difference
Mild	• <3 cm difference	<20% increase in limb volume
Moderate	• 3–5 cm difference	20–40% increase in limb volume
Severe	• >5 cm difference	>40% increase in limb volume

Integeumentary Preferred Practice Patterns may be used as an adjunct to describe wound status in this patient population, however, the preferred practice pattern for patients with lymphedema is Cardiovascular/Pulmonary Pattern 6H: Impaired Circulation and Anthropometric Dimensions Associated with Lymphatic System Disorders.[70] This practice pattern describes the components of the examination, evaluation, diagnosis, prognosis, and interventions for patients with lymphedema. Most other disciplines utilize the staging system to classify lymphedema (see Table 15–2).[3, 25] Both methods attempt to guide intervention strategies but the narrower scope of the staging system allows the classification of lymphedema to more precisely describe the severity of the pathology and direct appropriate interventions. Physical therapists working with this patient population would be wise to use both systems to better coordinate patient care among different disciplines. Unilateral lymphedema may be further classified based on a side-to-side comparison of circumferential measurements[70] or percent increase in limb volume.[5, 18] Clinicians should be cautious with their assumptions of lymphedema severity based solely by comparing side-to-side differences in circumferential measurements as this may misrepresent overall volume changes.[6] Side-to-side comparisons are not relevant for patients with truncal, facial, genital, or bilateral involvement.

It is believed that lymphedema increases over time and that stage 1 lymphedema will progress to stage 2 if left untreated.[1, 3, 20, 30] The early signs of lymphedema include pitting edema that improves with elevation and compression. Edema may be exacerbated at the end of the day secondary to dependency and resolve in the morning after sleeping. As severity increases, edema may no longer be resolved with changes in elevation due to the hydrophilic qualities of high-protein lymphedema fibrosis.[25] The distinguishing characteristic of stage 3 lymphedema are extreme increases in limb volume and **papillomas,** or cauliflower-like projections of the epithelium caused by distended and dilated superficial lymphatics.[18, 28]

Characteristics

To facilitate identification of ulcer and integument integrity similarities and differences, typical characteristics of various types of ulcers are described using the "5PT" method: pain, position, presentation, periwound, pulses, and temperature.

Pain

A poll[9] about pain perception conducted on patients with lymphedema revealed that patients reported several different types of pain in the involved area. Forty-four percent reported a deep ache or pressure sensation, 26% stretch pain due to the increased weight of the limb, 21% neuropathic pain, and 9% had pain from infection or inflammation. These findings are consistent with other studies in patients with primary and secondary lymphedema. If a patient truly complains of pain, rather than discomfort, heaviness, or the above sensations, further evaluation or referral is indicated.[2]

Position

Secondary lymphedema occurs distal to the area of lymphatic obstruction or damage. The clinician must know the type and extent of treatment a patient has undergone. Sometimes this is obvious, such as a patient who had a right breast lumpectomy, sentinel node biopsy, and axillary radiation. Other times, such as treatment for prostate cancer, the clinician must seek out what portions of the lymphatics have been disrupted. For example, were both left and right inguinal lymph nodes excised? All areas that drain to the affected area should be carefully examined.[67, 71] The clinician must also know what tissues were included within the radiation field and thoroughly examine these areas for signs of radiation damage.

Wound Presentation

Lymphorrhea, or weeping, is not unusual.[18] This occurs when there is no overt, measurable open wound but beads of fluid form on the skin surface and trickle down the limb because the skin is stretched beyond its ability to maintain a barrier.[72] Drainage is typically serous, but may be purulent if infected, and can be significant, quickly soiling patient clothing, bedding, and striking through bandages. *Streptococcus* is the most common cause of skin infections[73] but *Pseudomonas aeruginosa* infections are not uncommon and result in blue-green drainage and a characteristic smell. Lymphorrhea can occur in any lymphedematous area but is most common in the lower extremity followed by the inguinal region.[72] Ulcerations may occur in the affected region spontaneously or after minimal trauma. Copious wound drainage is the norm and wound beds are commonly covered with slough.

Periwound and Structural Changes

The integument should be thoroughly examined to determine the extent of skin and lymphatic involvement. Secondary cellulitis may be present.[74] In addition to open wounds and lymphorrhea, clinicians must be alert for more subtle tissue changes such alterations in texture. Areas of soft pitting edema may become fibrotic over time or with increased disease severity. Hair loss or loss of sweating response in affected areas is likely. Intact skin may become dry, flakey, and scaling. The skin may be thickened and hyperkeratotic, particularly if the lower extremity is affected.[75] Skin may have an orange peel–like presentation, known as peau d'orange.[68] Skin folds may deepen,[74] especially at the wrists and ankles. Thickening of the dorsal aspect of the digits may result in a positive **Stemmer's sign,** or the inability to pinch a skin fold on the dorsal aspect of an edematous digit.[1] When positive, this test confirms the presence of lymphedema.[1, 3] However, because false-negative test results are possible, a negative test does not exclude the diagnosis.[20] Lipodermatosclerosis is commonly seen in patients with combined venous and lymphatic insufficiency.[68] **Papillomatosis,** or a cobblestone-like appearance of the epithelium, is seen in stage 3 lymphedema. Scaling intact skin or thickened nails may indicate a fungal infection (see Chapter 17). Box 15–4 describes common integumentary changes due to lymphedema.[1, 2, 5, 6, 18, 20, 28, 31, 67–69, 73, 74, 76]

BOX 15–4   Integumentary Changes Commonly Seen in Patients with Lymphedema

- Xerosis
- Hyperkeratosis
- Fibrosis
- Hair loss
- Deep skin folds
- Lichenification
- Lipodermatosclerosis
- Papillomas
- Lymphorrhea
- Vesicle or blister formation
- Papillomatosis
- Dermatitis
- Ulceration
- Infections
- Bacterial: cellulitis, *Streptococcus, Pseudomonas*
- Fungal: tinea pedis, *Candida*

At times it may be difficult to differentiate between lymphedema and chronic venous insufficiency (CVI). Indeed, as previously discussed, CVI may lead to lymphedema. However, patients with CVI without lymphatic insufficiency generally present with varicosities, pitting edema that reduces overnight and increases at the end of the day, lipodermatosclerosis, and a negative Stemmer's sign.[20] The distinction between patients with CVI with and without lymphatic involvement is critical as dual-system involvement requires more intensive interventions and generally takes longer to reach expected goals.

Pulses

Pulses are generally present and normal in patients with lymphedema. However, if there is significant edema, palpating pulses can be difficult and a Doppler ultrasound may be required.[67, 77]

Temperature

The skin in an edematous area may be warm due to increased volume without being clinically infected.[67] Skin reactions in areas treated with radiation may be erythematous, inflamed, and warm to the touch.

PROGNOSIS FOR LYMPHEDEMA AND LYMPHEDEMA-RELATED SKIN DAMAGE

All studies have shown some degree of improvement with integrated physical therapy interventions for patients with all types of lymphedema.[3, 15, 38, 78] However, the amount of improvement with treatment varies widely, due to differences in measuring change over time as well as differences in treatment frequency, duration, clinician skill level, and clinician technique. Patient-related variables such as time since onset, type of lymphedema (primary vs. secondary), stage and severity of lymphedema, and risk factors present must also be considered.[5, 50] According to the Preferred Practice Pattern 6H: Impaired Circulation and Anthropometric Dimensions Associated with Lymphatic System Disorders, patients with mild lymphedema will require 5–10 visits, those with moderate lymphedema 8–16 visits, and those with severe lymphedema 14–24 visits per episode of care.[70]

In general, earlier diagnosis and early interventions (education, compression, exercise, with or without manual therapy) results in more successful outcomes.[5, 60, 79] Greater clinician skill level and higher levels of patient adherence also result in better outcomes. Some amazing results have been reported, such as a 90% decrease in lower extremity edema after 15 visits over an 8-week time frame,[80] and 26% decrease in upper extremity volume after 4 weeks of treatment.[81] Average volume reductions of 59% for patients with upper extremity lymphedema and 68% for lower extremity lymphedema over 16 days of treatment have

been reported. Sixty-two percent of patients with genital lymphedema had completed resolution with treatment.[82] Overall, variations in volume reduction can be expected to range from 22% to 73% over 6–36 visits.[5] Patients with lipolymphedema and lymphedema associated with widely spread stage IV cancers will have the smallest improvements. Lifetime use of compression and weight management is almost always required to prevent recurrence or exacerbation.[83]

CASE STUDY: Mrs. Julia Prentice

PART 2

Tests and Measures

Landmark	Distance from tip of third digit	Left upper extremity	Right upper extremity
Palm at MCP	8.0	19.5	19.6
Smallest wrist	0	16.5	16.4
Mid-forearm	14.5	22.0	21.0
Elbow	24.5	26.0	25.2
Mid-brachium	35	30.0	27.7
Proximal brachium	44	31.9	30.2

All measurements in cm.

Circumferential Measurements Circumferential measurements of her hands and digits are symmetrical despite the fullness noted in her second and third intermetacarpal regions. She has a negative Stemmer sign.

Integumentary Integrity: Position: Left upper quadrant. Presentation: L anterior chest wall and LUE appears slightly anhydrous, thin skinned, and has a slightly darkened color compared to the right side. There is 1+ pitting of the distal third of Mrs. Prentice's medial brachium. Periwound; NA. Temperature: slight increase in right medial brachium skin temperature.

Sensory Integrity: Patient is able to identify 4.17 monofilament BUE and 2.83 monofilament in each hand.

Circulation: Pulses: radial, ulnar, and brachial 2+. Capillary refill: 3 seconds B.

Gait, Locomotion, Balance: Without assistive device, deviation, or difficulty.

Pain: None.

Evaluation and Diagnosis

Mrs. Prentice has stage 1 left upper extremity lymphedema consistent with Cardiovascular/Pulmonary Pattern 6H: Impaired Circulation and Anthropometric Dimensions Associated with Lymphatic System Disorders. Mrs. Prentice has several risk factors for lymphedema including being 15 years post-removal of five axillary lymph nodes, post–radiation therapy, and increased body mass index (although her body mass index has recently improved from being class 1 obese to overweight). She has less than a 3 cm interlimb circumferential measurement difference, which would be further classified as mild lymphedema.

CASE STUDY Continued

Prognosis and Plan of Care

Mrs. Prentice is a relatively healthy individual who has made significant positive changes in her eating and lifestyle after being recently diagnosed with diabetes. Unfortunately, her frequent blood sugar testing on her left (as well as her right) upper extremity may have upset the delicate balance between her lymphatic load and lymphatic return. Her prognosis to reach the stated goals is good.

The following functional goals have been discussed and mutually agreed upon:

1. Mrs. Prentice will be able to consistently don and doff her wedding ring in 2–3 weeks.
2. Mrs. Prentice will be independent with wear and care of her compression garments in 2–3 weeks.
3. Mrs. Prentice will verbalize understanding of proper skin care and methods to decrease her risk of lymphedema exacerbation or recurrence.

The following lymphedema-related component goals have been discussed and mutually agreed upon:

1. Mrs. Prentice will be independent with a home exercise program to assist with left upper extremity lymph drainage within three treatment sessions.
2. Mrs. Prentice and her husband will be independent with multilayer compression bandaging of her left upper extremity within five treatment sessions.
3. Mrs. Prentice and her husband will be independent with manual lymph drainage techniques within 2 weeks.
4. No pitting in the right medial brachium within 1 to 2 weeks.
5. Mrs. Prentice's maximal interlimb circumferential difference will be less than 1.5 cm in 3 weeks.

Mrs. Prentice will be seen four to five times per week for 2 weeks, then weekly for a total of 3 weeks. Physical therapy interventions will include coordination, communication, and documentation; patient/client-related instruction; therapeutic exercises, physical agents and mechanical modalities, manual therapy techniques, and prescription and application of compression garments.

PHYSICAL THERAPY INTERVENTIONS

Coordination, Communication, and Documentation

Unfortunately, patient education on lymphedema precautions is clearly lacking, as the highest reported percentage of at-risk patients receiving education is thought to be only 57%.[42] There are several barriers to lymphedema education. The first is lack of health care provider education in the area of lymphedema.[79] The second is linking at-risk patients with qualified health care professionals. Part of the difficulty comes from the current health care system, which divides patient care by discipline rather than considering the holistic needs of the patient. In the current system, surgeons rarely see lymphedema during the short post-operative course that they follow cancer patients. This short duration of patient contact can lead to the mistaken perception that lymphedema occurs to "other surgeons' patients" rather than the understanding that the risk for lymphedema increases over time as well as with the various other risk factors discussed previously. In addition, the rare cases of immediate post-operative lymphedema are frequently dismissed as post-operative edema rather than being correctly identified as lymphedema. Likewise, surgeons may not fully appreciate that post-operative infections or seromas are harbingers of future lymphedema.

In the current system, opportunities exist to have standing post-operative orders for physical therapy for all patients who will have lymph node biopsies or dissections. Another opportunity to enter these patients into an appropriate prophylactic education program could be to have radiation oncologists and oncologists screen patients to see if education has been provided and, if not, generate an order for physical therapy at that time. These proactive lymphedema education programs, which educate all at-risk patients rather than only generating referrals after lymphedema has developed, result in decreased incidences of lymphedema, improved quality of life, and have reduced medical expenses by as much as 58%.[60, 79]

In addition to nurses, physicians, and rehabilitation specialists, coordination of care for patients at risk for, or with, lymphedema should include several key disciplines. Patients with a new or repeat cancer diagnosis may benefit from the expertise of counselors, clinical psychologists, social workers, or local support groups. Certified nutritionists can assist with weight management, both for patients who are overweight and need a weight loss program as well as those who may be struggling to maintain their body weight during cancer treatment.[18]

Patient/Client-Related Instruction

Because of the latency period prior to the development of most cases of secondary lymphedema, education is critical to lymphedema prevention, early lymphedema identification, and positive outcomes.[5] Patient/caregiver education reduces the risk for lymphedema, but does not guarantee that lymphedema will not occur nor that this information will be incorporated into patient practice. Patients who perceived themselves as being more vulnerable, who perceived that lymphedema posed a sufficient health risk to them, or who perceived that preventive behavior would decrease the potential for lymphedema development, were more likely to be adherent to lymphedema precautions.[61] Therefore, the challenge to clinicians is to help make these links for at-risk patients. In addition, clinicians must instill upon patients that risk factor reduction is a lifelong commitment that demands adaptive behaviors[55] and not just temporary activity avoidance or transient changes in routines. Box 15–5 provides guidelines for patients with, or at risk for, lymphedema.[3, 4, 6, 15, 42, 55, 56, 84] Education guidelines have several key components. Patients must be taught risk factors for lymphedema development and lymphedema exacerbation, as well as methods to control and treat lymphedema. Patients must be taught methods to avoid breaks in the skin of an affected area, which could introduce bacteria into the body, and what to do if an open wound occurs. Patients must be taught to avoid activities that decrease lymphatic return or increase cutaneous blood flow to the affected area.

Procedural Interventions

Precautions

When patients with a history of cancer present with a new onset of swelling, the first action should be to rule out cancer recurrence as a cause.[15, 18] Patients who have not been previously screened by a physician should be quickly referred for reassessment and clearance prior to initiating physical therapy. Physical therapy interventions can occur concurrently with cancer treatment. However, performing only physical therapy for lymphedema that is caused by a tumor obstructing the lymphatic system is not only unlikely to succeed, it also delays cancer diagnosis and possible treatment options.[85] Patients without a history of lymph node trauma (surgery or radiation) who have a new onset of lymphedema should be referred to a physician to rule out cancer.

As with venous insufficiency, compression is one of the key interventions for lymphedema and lymphedema-related tissue damage. Compression must be modified for patients with arterial insufficiency and is not appropriate for those with severe arterial insufficiency.[68, 69] Significant patient limb size, deep skin folds, and equipment limitations may limit the ability to perform an ankle-brachial index. Figure 15–7 provides an algorithm for screening patients with lymphedema for arterial insufficiency. This patient population has the propensity for skin sensitization, so proper skin care should be emphasized. Whirlpool therapy should be avoided in patients with lymphedema because, similar to venous insufficiency, this intervention will exacerbate the causative pathology.

Lower extremity lymphedema is a risk factor for developing a deep vein thrombosis (DVT).[86] Additional risk factors for DVT include cancer surgery, radiation therapy, and tamoxifen use.[86] DVT screening should therefore be performed in this patient population. Currently there is considerable debate as to when compression therapy can be initiated in oncology patients with DVTs. In ambulatory patients on appropriate anticoagulation therapy, graduated compression therapy (garments or bandages) has resulted in faster edema resolution and decreased pain without increasing the risk of a pulmonary embolism.[86] In contrast, in nonambulatory oncology patients with DVTs compression should be used with caution.[86]

BOX 15–5   Guidelines for Patients With or At Risk for Lymphedema

Do

- Perform daily skin checks.
- Bathe daily using a mild, nonperfumed soap and pat your skin dry.
- Treat any open areas.
  - Wash the area with soap and water.
  - Cover with an antimicrobial ointment and a bandage.
  - Check the wound daily.
  - Report any signs of infection or wound deterioration to your health care provider.
- Drink plenty of noncaffeinated, nonalcoholic fluids.
- Use moisturizing lotion.
- Protect your extremity from injury.
  - Wear gloves for yard work and washing dishes.
  - Trim nails carefully.
  - Use sunscreen and insect repellent when appropriate.
  - Use an electric razor if shaving the affected limb.
- Attain or maintain an ideal body weight.
- Exercise regularly and in moderation.
- Do wear a compression garment for strenuous activity of the involved area.
- Follow your health care provider's instructions regarding bandaging and compression garments.

Do Not

- DO NOT allow any injections, piercings, or tattoos in your affected extremity
- DO NOT allow your blood pressure to be taken in your affected extremity
- DO NOT wear constrictive clothing or jewelry
- DO NOT scratch skin in an affected area even if it itches.
- DO NOT use hot tubs or saunas or take long hot showers.
- DO NOT apply heating pads to affected areas.
- DO NOT walk barefoot if you have lower extremity lymphedema.
- DO NOT perform heavy lifting or extreme exertion with your affected extremity.

Integumentary Repair and Protective Techniques

Request for Further Medical Testing

Patients with lymphedema are at increased risk for infection[2] due to decreased local immunity, increased diffusion distances for white blood cells, and more proteins within the interstitium providing a ready source of food for bacteria to grow and multiply. Clinicians should request an order for a wound culture and sensitivity in patients with a new onset or worsening of edema concurrent with the signs and symptoms of an infection.[42, 85] Patients with the signs and symptoms of an infection, with a new onset of edema, or an increase in prior lymphedema who do not have an open wound should also be referred to a physician for assessment of cellulitis

and prompt antibiotic prescription.[4] Physical therapy interventions in this case delays the appropriate use of antibiotics, increases the risk of septicemia, and by not addressing the trigger for lymphedema may result in less optimal outcomes. Once appropriate antibiotic therapy has been initiated therapy can be initiated or resumed.[87]

Skin Care

Proper skin care is critical to decreasing the risk of open wounds, infection, and wound recurrence. The skin must be kept clean and dry with particular attention paid to areas with secondary skin changes.[31] Because of the increased risk of skin sensitivity,[79] highly alkaline soaps should be avoided as they remove the skin's normal acidic protective coating.[15] Low pH moisturizers, lotions, and ointments may be used to

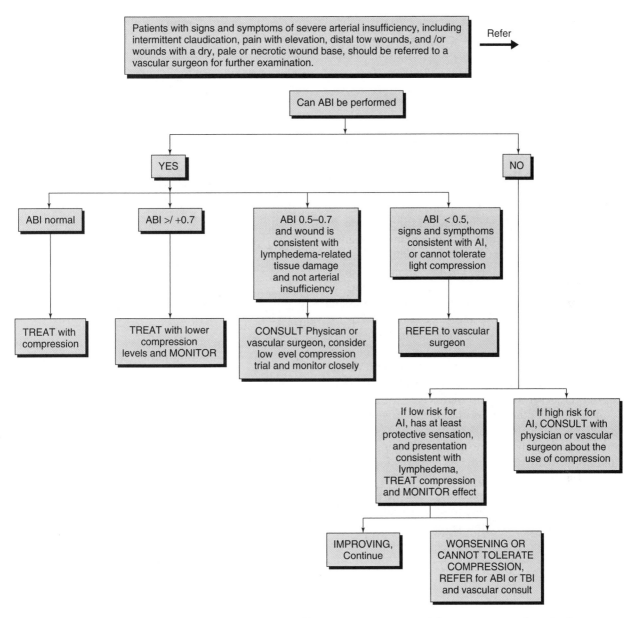

FIGURE 15–7   Screening algorithm for arterial insufficiency in patients with lower extremity lymphedema.

improve skin texture.[4, 76] To decrease the risk of folliculitis, use caution with thick emollients, apply in the same direction as hair growth, and ensure full removal with each skin cleansing.[75] Moisturizers also help with softening scaling hyperkeratotic skin that commonly develops in patients with lower extremity lymphedema,[69] making it easier to remove. Patients with skin sensitivity may do well with moisturizers that contain lanolin alcohol rather than the less purified lanolin.[15] Care should be taken to thoroughly dry

between skin folds and between digits to prevent fungal infections. Topical antifungals may be used prophylactically in these high-risk areas as well as to treat topical fungal infections.[75] To prevent recurrence, antifungals should be continued for at least 1 week after lesions have resolved.[75] Topical steroids, such as cortisone, may be used short term to decrease skin inflammation.

Any breaks in the skin of a limb with, or at risk for, lymphedema should be washed with soap and water followed by application of a prophylactic topical antimicrobial and primary dressing, such as a gauze wrap.[3, 31] Papillomas must be protected from shearing forces from bandages or patient clothing.

Local Wound Care

Box 15–6 describes the keys to local wound care for patients with lymphedema. A skin sealant or moisture barrier should be used to protect periwound skin from maceration and prevent new ulceration. Absorptive, nonadherent dressings, such as a thick gauze pad, semipermeable foam, or alginate, are good options.[31, 72, 88] Adhesive dressing should be avoided to prevent further integumentary trauma upon removal. As with other wounds, dressing absorption and dressing change frequency must match wound drainage.[79] If infection is present, the dressing must be changed at least daily. Dressing changes may need to be more frequent during the day when the limb is more dependent.[72] Given the cost of wound dressings and the potential for large quantities of drainage with patients with lower extremity lymphorrhea,[72] sanitary pads may be an appropriate cost-saving alternative.

The physical therapy management of wounds due to lymphedema must address both the wound and wound etiology to be successful. Edema should be minimized with some form of compression therapy similar to those used to manage venous insufficiency. Compression bandaging, devices, and garments are discussed in Chapter 11 and in more specific detail in the following section. After compression is initiated, wound drainage and lymphorrhea generally decrease significantly due to decreased ultrafiltration and improved lymphatic return. Enhanced venous return in patients with lower extremity lymphedema or with combined lymphovenous insufficiency also reduces drainage. Compression therapy also reduces limb volume, assists with reshaping limb deformities caused by swelling, and decreases tissue fibrosis.

As with other wounds, debridement of slough and necrotic tissue should be performed as needed.[31] Papillomas, dried exudate, and thick layers of hyperkeratotic skin may make debridement exceptionally challenging in patients with lymphedema. Pulsatile lavage with suction and specialized debridement tools, such as curettes, are particularly useful.[31, 89, 90]

Fungating wounds are more common in primary cancers such as breast and penile cancers. These wounds appear as deep necrotic ulcers with hypertrophic granulation tissue.[85] These wounds tend to have copious, foul-smelling drainage even though they may not be infected. As tumor cells invade local blood vessels, excessive wound site bleeding may occur.[85] Treatment of these wounds includes protecting the surrounding tissue from maceration and excoriation using moisture barriers and absorptive dressings. Charcoal dressings provide odor and moisture control. Alginates are helpful by providing significant absorption as well as acting as a hemostatic agent. Absorptive silver dressings may decrease bacterial load, thereby assisting with odor control. For patients in palliative care, it is also important to consider bandage wear time and ease of dressing changes when choosing skin and wound care products.[85] Other factors to consider in palliative care include alleviating symptoms, improving function, and improving quality of life.[71] In some cases, this may mean using compression bandaging to ease the aching of an edematous limb while in other cases compression bandaging may unnecessarily inhibit patient mobility.

BOX 15–6   Keys to Local Wound Care for Patients with Lymphedema

• Protect the surrounding skin
  ◦ Skin sealant/moisture barrier
  ◦ Lotion to intact skin
  ◦ Antifungal as needed
• Beware of skin sensitization
• Absorptive dressings
• Compression
• Educate patient/caregivers

Therapeutic Exercise
Patient Positioning

Gravity has a strong effect on venous drainage and ultrafiltration. There is no change in intralymphatic pressures when patients with normal lymphatics move from a recumbent to an upright position. However, in patients with lymphatic obstructions, intralymphatic pressures increase with this positioning change.[24] Therefore, patients should be counseled on the importance of elevating affected areas above the level of the heart for brief periods during the day as well as during sleep.[68] Positioning is particularly important and most likely to have the greatest effect for patients with stage 1 lymphedema because there is more pitting and less fibrosis present.[18] Due to the greater fibrosis, positioning limbs to allow gravity-assisted lymphatic and venous drainage is less likely to improve edema in patients with stage 2 or 3 lymphedema[18] but may slow edema progression by decreasing ultrafiltration forces. Patients who are obese are at increased risk for sleep apnea, making them more likely to choose to sleep in a chair with their legs in a dependent position exacerbating lower extremity lymphedema.[18] To maximize outcomes, these patients should be counseled to sleep in bed on a small wedge if needed, elevate their legs at or above the level of their heart, and may need to be referred for a sleep study for CPAP (continuous passive airway pressure) assessment.

Active Range of Motion Exercises

Active range of motion exercises allow muscle pumps to move fluid proximally within the veins and lymphatic system.[15, 68, 73] When there is damage to either of these systems, active range of motion exercises become even more pivotal to avoiding fluid and protein stagnation and propelling fluid forward.[24] An increase in lymph angiomotoricity was found in patients with lymphedema who performed simple active range of motion exercises.[24] Compression concomitant with exercise further enhanced lymphatic return.[24]

Flexibility Exercises

As noted in Chapter 11, suboptimal ankle dorsiflexion impairs calf muscle pump efficiency.[91] Therefore, patients with lower extremity lymphedema with restricted range of motion should be instructed in gastrocnemius and soleus stretching exercises. Patients with flexibility restrictions in other affected areas are likely to benefit from stretching exercises as well because they create a greater range of joint excursion that will improve muscle pump effectiveness.[15]

Anaerobic Exercise

Contrary to prior assumptions, strength training is not a factor in the development or progression of lymphedema.[8, 57–59, 92] Strength training is actually negatively correlated with the development of lymph-edema.[44, 59, 60, 93] Again, the key to strength training exercises for patients with or at risk for lymphedema is a gradual increase in duration and intensity of exercise[56] to avoid muscle overload.[50] While strength training programs for patients at risk for lymphedema have noted a very slight (5 ml), transient (resolving in less than 24 hours), nonclinically, and nonstatistically significant increase in limb volume when *not* wearing a compression garment,[94] patients should monitor their affected limb after activity to ensure no adverse changes in limb volume have occurred.[56] In addition, most clinicians suggest their patients wear compression when exercising and during more strenuous activities to increase the effectiveness of the muscle pump and to decrease ultrafiltration in case of overuse.[50]

Aerobic Exercise

Because aerobic exercise assists with lymphatic return as well as attaining and maintaining an ideal body weight, it is a valuable component of lymphedema management. Patients who are obese or deconditioned may be tempted to find excuses for not being able to exercise.[79] The successful lymphedema therapist is able to develop an individualized exercise program[50] that is appropriate for each patient and provides methods to increase adherence, such as the use of an exercise log, group exercise classes, linking the patient with available community resources, or finding appropriate activities the patient finds enjoyable.

Breathing Exercises

Breathing exercises can be incorporated into the therapeutic exercise program of patients with lymphedema to improve the respiratory pump and lymphatic return.[15] This low level of exercise can be successfully incorporated into a program for all patients.

Manual Therapy Techniques

Manual therapy techniques for lymphedema management, alternately called manual lymphatic drainage, simple lymph drainage, or lymphatic massage, are key to the management of more advanced lymphedema.[73, 95] Four leaders in the field of manual techniques for lymphatic drainage are Casley-Smith, Foldi, Leduc, and Vodder.[3, 15, 20, 96] There are no studies that clearly demonstrate an advantage of one technique over any other. However, patients treated by massage therapists received less complete information and education regarding proper self-care than those treated by clinical professionals.[97] In addition, these technically trained

---

BOX 15–7   Benefits to Manual Therapy Techniques for Patients with Lymphedema

- Increases lymph formation
- Propels lymph proximally
- Increases lymph angiomotoricity
- Reroutes stagnated lymph fluid via:
  - Lymph capillaries
  - Interterritorial anastomoses
  - Perforating pre-collectors connecting the superficial with the deep lymphatic system
  - Connections between the lymphatic system and the vaso vasorum
- Encourages development of collateral circulation
- Reduces sympathetic nervous system stimulation while promoting parasympathetic response
- Decreases pain and promotes relaxation
- Fibrotic techniques can decrease firmness within tissues caused by interstitial proteins
- Edema techniques can be used to remove excess fluid from small areas of the extremities

---

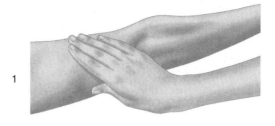

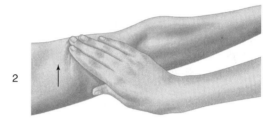

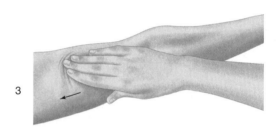

FIGURE 15–8   "J"-shaped stroke.

individuals are not educated in differential diagnosis, medical contraindications, or other key components for the successful management of patients with lymphedema. Therefore, licensed health care providers, particularly those with advanced training in lymphedema, are the practitioners of choice. This section describes the benefits of manual therapy and basic manual techniques. Including manual therapy techniques appears to consistently result in improved volume reduction and an increased likelihood of maintaining this reduction over time with self-treatment.[50, 55, 81] Box 15–7 lists the benefits of manual therapy for patients with lymphedema.[2, 3, 15, 73, 96]

As with all manual therapy techniques, there is room for variation and individual differences, both based on clinician and patient-related factors. However, a few key principles must be adhered to. First, because the superficial lymphatics are within the skin, all strokes consist of gentle pressure. Aggressive "massage" will compress and obstruct the superficial lymphatics. Rather, manual contact points should have just enough force to maintain contact with the patient's skin. Lymph flow can be maximized by using large surface contact points and by molding to the body's contours. Strokes generally consist of two phases. The

working, or pressure, phase is basically a skin stretch in the shape of a right angle or a "J" (Figure 15–8). First the skin is stretched perpendicular to the lymph collector, theoretically pulling on the anchoring filaments within the interstitium to open lymph capillaries. Then the skin is stretched parallel to the lymph collector, theoretically pushing fluid forward in the desired direction. The greater the skin stretch, the more lymph is created and propelled forward. During the relaxation phase, manual contact is maintained with the patient's skin but it is allowed to recoil to its original position. The stroke is then repeated.

Manual techniques may be used to soften tissue fibrosis.[73] In this case, more aggressive manual contacts are used. Manually picking up the skin, separating it from the subcutaneous tissue underneath, then kneading or bending the thickened skin in a "U" shape can be used to help break up adhesions and fibrosis (Figure 15–9). Limb encircling techniques can be used on areas of pitting edema within

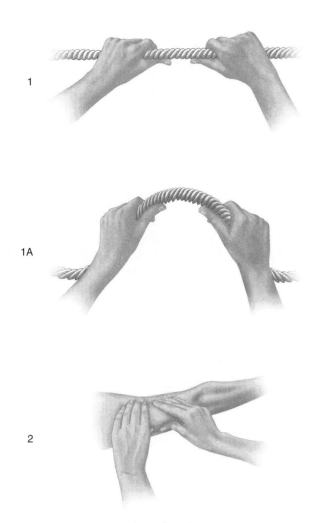

FIGURE 15–9   "U"-shaped stroke.

an extremity. This technique involves the clinician completely encircling the affected area with his or her hands. The clinician then squeezes the extremity, compressing his or her hands together, then gently pushing the skin proximally about a centimeter,

effectively milking the fluid away from the congested area. The stroke can be repeated several times in the same location or the manual contacts can be advanced proximally about a half of a centimeter at a time. Fibrotic and edema techniques are more aggressive and generally lack the soothing/analgesic effect found in the skin stretching techniques described previously.

All manual therapy techniques begin with the concept of clearing the proximal lymph system before moving distally.[2, 3, 15, 96] Since the lymph system joins the venous circulation at the venous angles of the neck, treatment begins here before progressing to the next distal segment. Figure 15–10 describes a basic pattern for performing manual techniques for a patient with right upper extremity lymphedema due to breast cancer after a lumpectomy, sentinel lymph node biopsy, and radiation therapy. Sample clinician and patient handouts as well as videos of manual techniques to promote lymph drainage are available on the accompanying Website. Learners are urged to examine more detailed resources, attend advanced continuing education courses in lymphatic drainage techniques, or attend a lymphedema certification course for improved results.[11, 12 13, 14]

Table 15–3 lists contraindications and precautions for manual therapy techniques and their rationale.[3, 15] One frequently encountered precaution is treating irradiated skin. Manual therapy techniques can be performed to irradiated skin, provided it is intact. Techniques should be less vigorous by applying less tension and less friction to irradiated skin.[15] It is also helpful to work from the central-most damaged skin outward toward peripheral healthy tissue[15] before trying to follow traditional lymph drainage flow patterns. These modifications can also be followed over intact skin near an open wound in a patient with lymphedema.[15]

Checkpoint Question #2

List the anastomoses that can be used to move fluid from a congested left lower extremity in a patient who had an inguinal node dissection and radiation.

Physical Agents and Mechanical Modalities

Compression therapy reduces ultrafiltration, enhances venous return, improves the effectiveness of muscle

pumps, and increases lymph angiomotoricity.[24] Compression may also decrease fibroblast proliferation and collagen production, reducing tissue fibrosis.[21] Without compression, lymphedema is unlikely to resolve. If any edema reduction occurs with the other

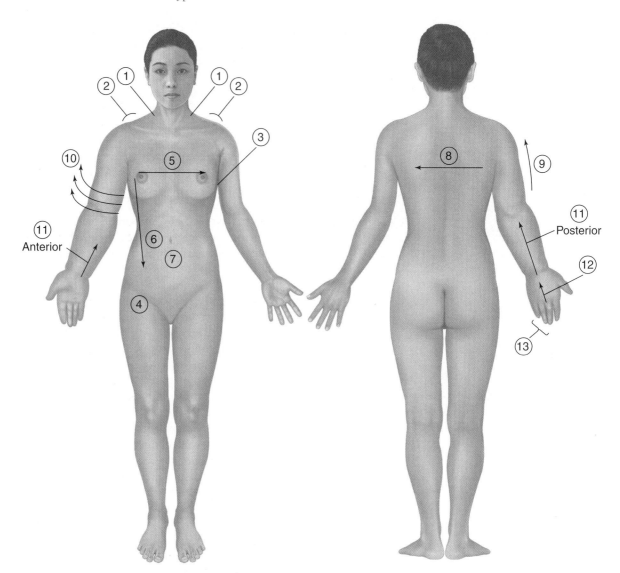

FIGURE 15–10   Manual therapy for a patient with right upper extremity lymphedema due to breast cancer after a lumpectomy, sentinel lymph node biopsy, and radiation therapy: (1)Venous angles at the neck; (2) Shoulder collectors; (3) Left axillary lymph nodes; (4) Right inguinal lymph nodes; (5) Anterior axillo-axillary pathway; (6) Right axillo-inguinal pathway; (7) Deep breathing; (8) Posterior axillo-axillary pathway; (9) Lateral brachium; (10) Re-routing from medial to lateral brachium; (11) Anterior and posterior forearm; (12) Back of hand; (13) Fingers.

components of treatment, it is unlikely to be maintained without the concomitant use of compression because of the loss of tissue elasticity.[15] Chapter 11 provides detailed information on the basics of compression therapy and its use for patients with venous insufficiency ulcers. Much of this information is relevant to the treatment of patients with lymphedema. This section reviews some of the key concepts and provides insights into more specific techniques and information based on research with patients with lymphedema, including multilayer compression bandaging, compression garments, and compression bandage alternatives. Last, this section reviews the most recent information on the use of compression pumps for patients with lymphedema.

TABLE 15–3   Precautions and Contraindications for Manual Therapy Techniques for Patients with Lymphedema

Precaution / Contraindication	Rationale	Modification
Deep vein thrombosis	Do not treat in the area of an acute deep vein thrombosis. The fear is that manual techniques may dislodge the clot, causing a potentially life-threatening pulmonary embolism.	Treat adjacent areas. Await medical clearance prior to treating affected region.
Active infection	Do not treat patients with an active infection. Fear of spreading infection.	Wait until appropriate antibiotic therapy has been initiated and infection shows signs of resolving.
Open wound	Do not treat areas with breaks in the skin.	Treat adjacent intact skin.
Metastatic disease	Fear of spreading cancer via the lymphatics, although there are no documented cases of this.	Manual therapy can be used as part of a palliative care program. Manual therapy may be initiated after discussion with the patient, care giver, and health care team.
Congestive heart failure	Fear of systemic fluid overload.	Condition must be controlled prior to lymphedema treatment. Treatment should begin gradually and in segments with careful monitoring of patient response.
Asthma	Fear that parasympathetic stimulation will provoke an asthma attack.	Asthma must be controlled prior to initiating treatment. Treatment should begin gradually and in segments with careful monitoring or patient response.
Patients with arterial disease	Treatment of the neck may dislodge an atherosclerotic plaque, leading to an ischemic cerebrovascular event.	Avoid treatment of the neck.
Patients with AAA, diverticulitis, diverticulosis, irritable bowel syndrome, Crohn's disease, ulcerative colitis, or who have had recent abdominal surgery	Deep abdominal techniques may aggravate or worsen these conditions.	Do not perform deep abdominal techniques.
Patients who are currently pregnant	Fear deep abdominal techniques may harm the fetus or uterus.	Do not perform deep abdominal techniques.

AAA, abdominal aortic aneurysm

Multilayer Compression Bandaging

 Compression bandaging is performed short term during intensive treatment to reduce edema.[98] Compression bandaging may also be required during periods of exacerbation when limb volume changes preclude proper garment fit or during air travel when more precise compression of an edematous limb is required.[3, 15] Multilayer compression bandaging with short stretch compression bandages is one of the most important methods of reducing edema in patients with lymphedema. These bandages have a low resting pressure, making them comfortable for the patient at rest and a high working pressure in which the sub-bandage pressure increases significantly with muscle contraction.[27, 73] Similar to multilayer compression bandage systems used for patients with chronic venous insufficiency ulcers, multilayer compression bandaging uses the principles of Laplace's law to provide graduated compression from the distal to the proximal extremity. While not ideal, tubular compression bandages such as those used for venous insufficiency can also be used to assist with edema control for patients with lymphedema.[55] Table 15–4 provides key information on multilayer compression bandaging.[3, 15, 27, 69, 73, 79, 99] Some key differences between compression bandaging for CVI and lymphedema are discussed below.[98]

☑ *Checkpoint Question #3*

Describe LaPlace's law.

TABLE 15–4   Multilayer Compression Bandaging for Lymphedema Management

Type of Bandage	Purpose
Cotton liner	• Decreases risk of skin sensitization • Absorbs sweat
Digit bandaging	• Uses elastic gauze rolls • Reduces digit edema if present • Prevents edema due to more proximal compression • Assists with decreasing distortion caused by swelling
Cotton padding	• Distributes compression more evenly, making bandage more comfortable • Creates a conical shape to the limb • Fills skin folds • May decrease bandage slippage
Foam padding	• Can be washed if contaminated by wound drainage or exudate • Provides more cushioning than cotton padding • May further decrease bandage slippage • Cut into strips can facilitate drainage by creating high and low areas of pressure • Chip bags and foam mats assist with decreasing tissue fibrosis
Custom-made compression pads	• Ideal for breast, inguinal region, and localized trunk edema • Generally held in place with clothing
Short-stretch compression wraps	• Smaller widths applied distally • Larger widths applied proximally • Avoid circular turns • Increase layers to increase compression

Lymphedema treatment includes bandaging of the digits. Compression of the foot/ankle or palm/wrist will increase venous and lymphatic pressure within the toes and fingers and also blocks drainage from these areas,[100] thus increasing the risk of edema if these areas are unaffected or worsening any edema that is already present. Because of the small circumference of digits, high compression levels created by short-stretch compression wraps are not required for digits. Therefore, two to four layers of a specialized form of elastic gauze bandage is used to safely compress the digits. There is no compelling evidence that toe bandaging must be performed in patients with lower extremity lymphedema without toe involvement. Patients with arterial insufficiency, especially those with small vessel disease, may best be treated without toe bandaging as at least one study noted a decrease in toe perfusion with compression bandaging from the metatarsophalangeal joints to the knee in patients.[100] Toe bandaging may need to be a point of compromise for patients without toe edema, particularly those with limited dexterity or ability to reach their own toes. If toe bandaging is not used, patients must be carefully monitored for the development of toe edema and bandage modifications, such as toe caps or toe bandaging, must then be reconsidered. Isotoner gloves may be used as an inexpensive alternative to finger/hand bandaging for patients with limited dexterity and minimal or no hand edema.[28]

Padding assists with distributing compression more evenly and absorbing drainage. Rolled foam, while more expensive than cotton padding, provides more cushioning, can be washed if it becomes contaminated by wound drainage or exudate, and may assist with softening tissue fibrosis.[3, 20, 101] Foam can also be cut to fill tissue folds and skin creases that can occur, particularly at the wrist and ankle. Foam strips can be used to create higher compression locally, such as between the metacarpals and metatarsals in cases of dorsal hand or foot edema. Chip bags and foam mats can be made from cut pieces of different densities of foam. When placed over fibrotic tissue, active movement of the limb and the different foam densities act as a form of massage to soften these areas. Custom-made compression pads can be applied to edematous areas such as the lateral trunk, breast, or inguinal region for treatment of local edema in these locations.[28]

Short-stretch compression bandages are applied in the same manner and with the same precautions as with patients with CVI (see Chapter 11). To prevent skin trauma, bandages should be taped in place rather than using metal clips provided with the bandages by the manufacturer. Clinicians should strive to apply compression bandages with even tension and rely on the other variables of Laplace's law to create a more comfortable and consistent compression gradient. To increase efficiency and enhance patient comfort, check compression after each bandage is applied. If uncomfortable to the patient consider consistently decreasing tension with all bandages, reducing the number of layers short-stretch compression bandages applied, increasing the amount of cotton padding, applying foam padding to localized areas of discomfort, or using foam for all padding if global discomfort is reported. Old bandages should be washed to restore their elasticity and replaced if they are no longer effective.

Three major problems with multilayer compression bandaging are bandage bulk, bandage slippage, and decreased functional mobility. Patients should be instructed to have loose-fitting clothing to accommodate for the increase in limb circumference. Bandage bulk is particularly problematic for patients with lower extremity lymphedema and temporary footwear will likely be needed to accommodate.[102] Walking shoes with velcro closures,[102] a lace-up shoe that is one size larger, or a slipper-type shoe with a nonslip bottom are good alternatives. Backless footwear should be avoided as this may increase the risk of falls.[102] Patients may require an assistive device for safe ambulation due to footwear changes and bandage bulk.

Several strategies can be employed to limit bandage slippage. A significant decrease in sub-bandage compression occurs over time due to limb volume reduction. In one study, sub-bandage compression at the ankle was reduced by half just 2 hours after bandage application, resulting in a 48% limb volume reduction.[78] Decreases in sub-bandage compression were less significant with subsequent applications, indicating an initial rapid decrease in limb volume followed by slower rates of volume reductions. To maintain effective compression and combat bandage slippage, initial bandage application should feel snug and be applied at higher tensions.[78]

Foam padding generally leads to less slippage than cotton padding. Applying masking tape over the front and back of bandages in the shape of an "X," particularly at elbows, knees, and areas of deformity, can decrease bandage slippage. Placing a larger cotton liner over the completed bandage will decrease friction between the bandage and clothing or the environment without additional compression. In contrast, applying an outer layer of flexible cohesive bandage will decrease bandage slippage but will also increase overall bandage compression. For patients with lower extremity lymphedema, compression shorts, biking shorts, panty hose, or applying a hip spica bandage can decrease bandage slippage.

Functional mobility can be improved by trying to limit compression bandage bulk as much as possible. Function can be improved somewhat by proper patient positioning when applying compression bandages. Patients should fully spread their fingers while wrapping the hand and make a fist when wrapping the forearm. Patients should stand if at all possible when wrapping from the knee to the hip. Last, patients should perform active range of motion exercises immediately after bandage application to assist with loosening bandages slightly, allowing for a greater functional range of motion.

Although cumbersome and time consuming, compression bandaging provides better volume reduction than compression garments[55] and is more effective than any other individual treatment component.[15] While the basic principles of compression must be followed, individual variations are required to accommodate for differences in limb size, limb shape, limb deformity, and patient mobility. Decreasing bandage complexity will not only decrease patient/caregiver stress levels when applying, but will also improve safe application and increase treatment adherence. Patients without the dexterity to apply their own bandages should engage the help of others. If this is not possible, use of a tubular bandage, more frequent treatment sessions, or increased bandage wearing time should be considered.

Many lymphedema "experts" will staunchly adhere to the notion that compression must be applied the length of the extremity. However, the astute clinician must consider individual patient preferences and patient differences, and accommodate for compression modifications to increase adherence. For example, after patient discussion, compression may be limited to below the knee[103] without toe bandaging for a patient who has limited edema above the knee, no current digit edema, lives alone, has difficulty reaching his foot, and has a job requiring significant mobility. As with manual therapy techniques, there is no one best method for performing compression bandaging for lymphedema management. The accompanying website provides videos of multilayer compression bandaging for a patient with lower extremity and upper extremity lymphedema. Box 15–8 lists contraindications and precautions for compression bandaging.[3, 15, 79, 87, 99, 103]

Compression Garments

While it may be tempting to prescribe compression garments to combat lymphedema and avoid the much

BOX 15–8	Precautions and Contraindications for Compression Bandaging for Patients with Lymphedema
Arterial insufficiency	• Reduce compression • May need to avoid toe compression • Educate patient on signs and symptoms of too much compression such as paresthesias, color change, or pain, and action plan for same
Radiation damage with intact skin	• Take steps to avoid bandage slippage • Consider applying topical amorphous hydrogel or hydrogel pad to the involved skin
Congestive heart failure	• Obtain physician clearance, particularly if poorly controlled • Initiate compression at lower levels • Initiate compression in segments, first below knee/elbow, and monitor systemic effects
Deep vein thrombosis	• Await medical clearance
Open wound	• Follow proper infection control procedures • Adjust dressing, padding, and bandage change frequency based on wound drainage
Infection	• Wait until appropriate antibiotic therapy has been initiated and infection shows signs of resolving
Weak, immobile, or insensate patient	• Decrease compression • Monitor skin

more time-intensive and cumbersome compression bandaging described above, there is no evidence that compression garments alone are effective in reducing lymphedema.[50] Therefore, once limb volume has stabilized with compression bandaging and other treatment methods,[10, 104, 105] compression garments are used for the long-term management of lymphedema. Prophylactic compression garments for use during high-risk activities may be obtained at any time. Compression garments successfully maintain edema reduction and decrease fluid accumulation in at-risk individuals.[3, 15, 83, 103] Garments are available in a wide variety of sizes, styles, colors, and compressions. Given the variety of manufacturers and sizes, the majority of patients will be able to fit in off-the-shelf garments. Patients who are obese, who have disproportionate limb sizes, who have deformities, or who require a more individualized style (such as toe caps) will require custom garments. There is no universal terminology for garment sizing or measurement landmarks.[106] Therefore, clinicians should carefully check

manufacturers' instructions regarding proper patient positioning, measurement, sizing, and compression. Tables 15–5 and 15–6 provide a sample measurement form and Figure 15–11 provides examples of various garment styles that are available. Male patients with genital edema may benefit from the compression of regular athletic compression shorts, a garment with a Whitaker pouch for compression, or ongoing compression bandaging.[107] A jock strap may be used to support swollen genitalia. Female patients with genital edema may benefit from regular athletic compression shorts, with or without the extra compression provided by a sanitary napkin or gauze pad, or specially made compression pads.

Compression garments can be made from a variety of materials. Patients with skin sensitivities would benefit from garments with higher cotton content rather than more synthetic components.[15] Compression garments are made in one of two ways. Round, or circular, knit garments are made in a continuous, circular manner such that garment size and shape are

TABLE 15–5   Upper Extremity Compression Garment Measurement

Patient Name:

Date:

Landmark	Distance from tip of third digit	Left upper extremity	Right upper extremity
A₁. Palm at MCP			
A. Smallest wrist			
B. Mid-forearm			
C. Elbow			
D. Mid-brachium			
E. Proximal brachium			

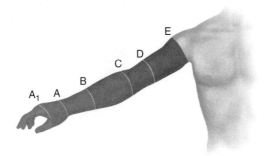

All measurements in cm.

TABLE 15–6   Lower Extremity Compression Garment Measurement

Patient Name:
Date:

Landmark	Distance*	Left Lower Extremity	Right Lower Extremity
Z. MTP			
Y. Base of fifth metatarsal			
X. Diagonal from posterior heel across anterior ankle joint	XXXXXXXXX		
A. Smallest ankle			
B. Achilles tendon–gastrocnemius junction			
C. Widest calf			
D. Knee joint line			
E. Distal third of thigh			
F. Proximal third of thigh			
G. Proximal thigh			

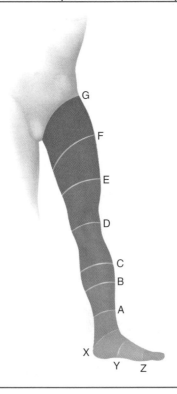

All measurements in cm.
*Distance from the tip of the distal posterior calcaneus

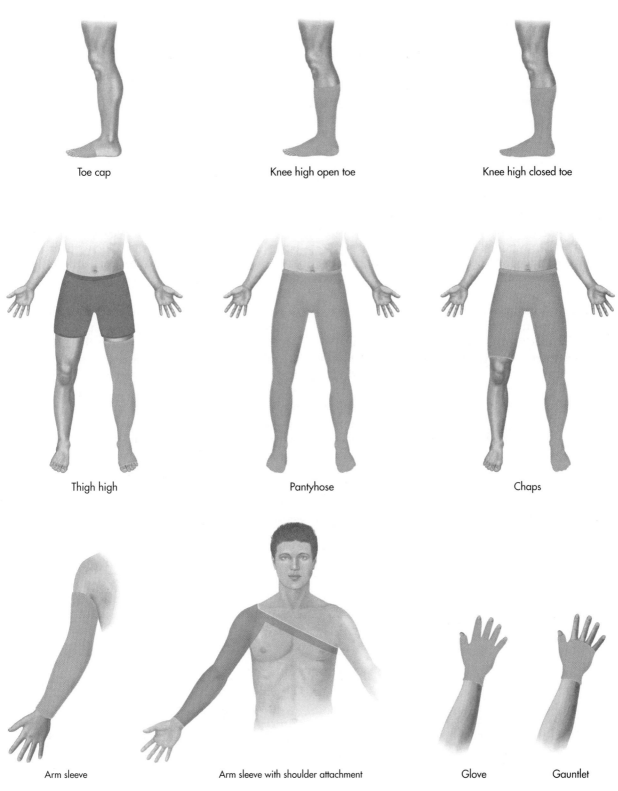

FIGURE 15–11   Compression garment styles.

adjusted by altering the number of stitches used. Circular knit garments are generally thinner, making them more cosmetically appealing. In addition, they are best for milder edema and "normally" shaped limbs.[106] In contrast, flat knit garments, sometimes referred to as made-to-measure,[83] are knitted flat and then the ends are stitched together. Flat knit garments, therefore, have a seam and this method allows the manufacturer to adapt the garment shape and size. Flat knit garments are thicker and more robust than circular knit garments. Flat knit garments, therefore, are best for patients with more severe edema who require higher levels of compression and for those with limbs that do not fit in standard-size garments due to excessive size or deformity.[106] While all patients should be counseled to maintain an ideal body weight and continue self-treatment of lymphedema to maintain limb volume, this is particularly important with the more precise fit of flat knit and custom garments.[15, 106]

In addition to determining the size and style of garment, clinicians must determine the amount of compression desired. As noted in Chapter 11, just as there is no universal standard for compression nomenclature, terminology varies by limb (upper extremity vs. lower extremity) and by manufacturer (German, British, or French standard compression values). For the greatest clarity, clinicians would be wise to state the desired numeric value of compression level in mm Hg (which is the highest compression at the ankle or wrist) in addition to noting the manufacturer's specific "compression class" designation. While there is little compelling research, the information in Table 15–7 can be used as a general guide for clinicians.[3, 15, 18, 99] Note that, as with patients with CVI, patient adherence to garment use is paramount to successful long-term management. Some of the barriers to garment adherence include physical difficulties donning or removing garments, cost, and cosmesis.[83, 108] Clinicians must include patients and caregivers throughout the decision-making process.[108] Current research supports that to increase patient adherence, whenever feasible, clinicians should prescribe the lowest compression possible. Patients who require higher levels of compression can sometimes be managed with a combination of garments.[18] For example, a patient with BLE lymphedema that is severe in the lower legs and feet may do well wearing a panty hose–style garment with 30–40 mm Hg compression and then a second knee-high compression garment that is 20–30 mm Hg compression to better control the lower leg edema. This combination approach will allow easier garment donning and avoid undue compression proximally that would make toileting cumbersome. The negative to this approach is that the patient must pay for three garments versus one. However, the overall cost may not be that much different if a custom garment is avoided. Note that the total compression on the patient is not strictly additive and patient response must be monitored. Other methods known to increase patient adherence is to consider whether a knee-high rather than thigh-high or panty hose–style garment will be sufficient and to prescribe gauntlets rather than gloves whenever feasible. Patients who have not had hand involvement need not be fitted for a compression glove or gauntlet.

TABLE 15–7   Compression Garment Standards

Compression Level	Description	Indications
10–21 mm Hg	Light compression	• Mild lymphedema • Lipedema • Palliative care compression garments • Prophylactic upper extremity compression garments • Lower extremity edema control in pregnant women
15–32 mm Hg	Medium compression	• Moderate to severe lymphedema, upper extremity lymphedema • Mild lower extremity lymphedema
30–40 mm Hg	Strong compression	• Moderate to severe lower extremity lymphedema
>40 mm Hg	Very strong compression	• Stage 3 lower extremity lymphedema

Several accessories are available to assist patients and caregivers with donning and doffing garments safely, easily, and properly (see Figure 15–12).[18, 108] Garments should be donned shortly after waking. Lotions should not be put on immediately prior to attempts to don garments as this will make donning more difficult and may damage the garment.[18] Garments should be laundered daily following manufacturer's guidelines. Some garments must be hand-washed, while others can be machine-washed on delicate cycle. Detergents should be nonperfumed, such as Dreft or Ivory, while petroleum-based detergents, such as Woolite, can damage garments. Washing garments after each use also helps restore garment elasticity.[5, 15] Garments should lie flat to dry or put on fluff cycle in dryer without fabric softeners.[28] Once an appropriate garment has been determined, the patient should obtain a second set,[18] allowing one pair to be worn while the other is being laundered. When worn and cared for properly, garments can be expected to last 6 months.[83]

Alternative Compression Devices

Patients with tissue changes, such as fibrosis, or with open wounds require continuous compression to control their edema (with the exception of time required for wound care, skin care, and manual techniques to the affected areas). Unfortunately, compression garments cannot be used during sleep because of their imprecise fit and the potential for skin trauma. Patients may choose to continue multilayer compression bandaging at night. Alternately, patients can choose from several varieties of easily donned, nonelastic, orthotic compression devices.

In addition to CircAid, described in Chapter 11, other manufacturers including FarrowWrap™, Jovi, Peninsula Medical, and Solaris have created similar devices specifically designed for the treatment of upper or lower extremity lymphedema.[55, 109] Nonelastic canvas/Velcro systems are appropriate for more severe edema,[55] while devices that contain foam fillers enhance patient comfort and integumentary protection and are appropriate for mild to moderate lymphedema. Some manufacturers utilize convoluted foam to provide alternate areas of high and low pressure, while others stitch foam channels in an attempt to redirect lymph flow to complement manual therapy techniques. Velcro straps or closures available on some of these devices accommodate for a small amount of variation in limb size. Compression is typically low, 15–20 mm Hg, as the patient is typically recumbent when wearing these devices. However, additional compression can be provided by an outer lycra compression sleeve (Figure 15–13) or velcro straps combined with a pressure gauge. Typically, these

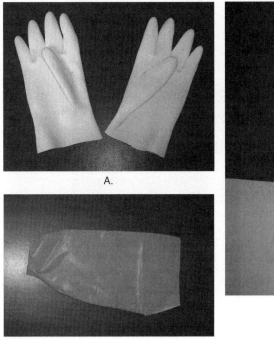

A.

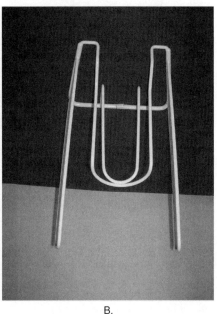

B.

C.

FIGURE 15–12 Donning aides for compression garments. *A.* Donning gloves. *B.* Donning frame. *C.* Donning slide

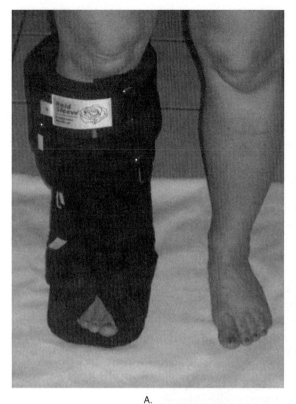

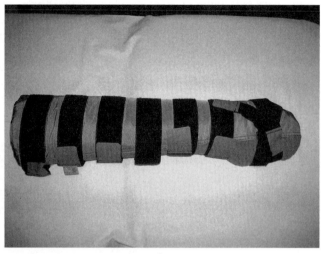

A.   B.

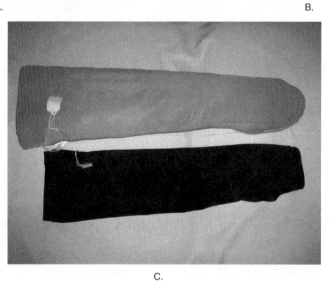

C.

FIGURE 15–13   Alternative compression devices for *A.* below knee lymphedema, *B.* moderate to severe arm lymphedema, and *C.* mild to moderate arm lymphedema.

have a 1-year warrantee and last several years with proper wear and care. The cost of these devices varies based on manufacturer, sizing, style, and compression but typically will range from $500 to $1,000 for a ready-made device and up to $2,400 for a custom device. Alternative compression devices may not be covered by insurance.

Device bulk leads to a significant decrease in patient mobility or inhibition of upper extremity function during wear time and severely restrict their use as a daytime compression option. However, the benefits of these alternative compression devices include ease of donning (most patients can do independently), quick donning (seconds vs. 5–15 minutes for bandaging), and low long-term cost (compared to replacing worn bandages) may make the high one-time cost worthwhile for some patients. Patients may also use these devices in the case of an active infection when garments are contraindicated and may fit poorly due to a slight increase in limb volume.

Compression Pumps

Compression pumps are standard procedure for immobilized and post-surgical patients to decrease the risk of deep vein thrombosis.[110] In the past, pumps were thought to be key to lymphedema reduction: simply apply compression for a period of time and physically squeeze excess fluid out of a congested extremity. Compression pumps were initially made from a single-chamber, air-filled sleeve that was pulled onto an edematous extremity. With advances in technology, multichamber sequential compression pumps[110] were made to try to recreate a pumping or milking effect in an attempt to more successfully remove fluid from the affected extremity. Before and immediate post-pump circumferential measurements consistently note a reduction in limb size. However, compression pumps are not compatible with current knowledge of the anatomy, physiology, or pathology of lymphedema[15] and are actually thought to exacerbate lymphedema.[2, 111] First, compression levels set on the pump can vary drastically from the actual tissue compression created by the device.[112] Second, while compression may decrease ultrafiltration and venous hypertension, compression pumps collapse or further damage lymphatic vessels,[110] obstructing lymph flow rather than promoting lymphatic drainage.[2, 15] Third, volume reductions noted post–compression pump application are solely the result of decreases in local interstitial fluid content without a parallel decrease in interstitial protein levels. While distal limb circumference may decrease, there is no overall volume reduction as there is no place for the fluid to go without treating the affected proximal quadrants or rerouting the lymphatic fluid. By leaving behind high levels of interstitial proteins, once compression is stopped, tissue oncotic pressure will pull more water from the vasculature back into the interstitium and tissue fibrosis will increase due to higher protein levels. Anecdotally, many clinicians have reported an increase in tissue fibrosis at the proximal end of the compression sleeve, proximal or truncal edema, or genital swelling with the use of compression pumps. Poor patient adherence, high cost of equipment, and significant treatment time should also be considered. In fact, one study found 47% of patients who were issued a compression pump used the device less than one time a week or not at all.[113] For these reasons, compression pumps are not recommended for lymphedema management.

There are rare instances in which a compression pump may be considered. Candidates must be free of comorbidities including arterial insufficiency, deep vein thrombosis, infection, complex regional pain syndrome, congestive heart failure, and proximal edema.[50] Patients must not have tissue fibrosis and must be unable to perform compression bandaging. In addition, patients must either be able to perform or have caregiver assistance for manual techniques[110] to assist with protein removal from the affected area and drain the affected and neighboring quadrants. Pumps that are multi-chambered and sequential are more likely to be effective.[113, 114] Ideally, compression will also be applied to the affected trunk quadrant. To be effective, compression pumps must be used for at least an hour a day. They must also be used in combination with daytime compression garments, exercise, and proper skin care to prevent fluid reaccumulation.[50] Compression must not be so high as to cause, or increase, pain. Research in this area is extremely sparse and the majority is sponsored by pump manufacturers. However, reasonable pump settings might include intermittent compression with a longer relief time,[114] such as a cycle time of 20 seconds on and 40 seconds off, at a compression of up to 40 mm Hg for an upper extremity and 50–60 mm Hg for a lower extremity.[110]

Low-Level Laser

There is limited evidence that low-level laser therapy may be effective as an adjunct in reducing lymphedema. It is thought that laser treatment may promote lymphangiogenesis, increase lymphangiomotoricity, stimulate macrophages, and decrease tissue fibrosis.[6, 109] To date, insufficient data exists to support this intervention as a standard of care.[50]

Integrating Treatment and Promoting Self-Management

The gold standard of treatment for patients with lymphedema is an integrated approach to patient care presented in Box 15–9, sometimes referred to as complete decongestive therapy, complex decongestive therapy, complex physical therapy, or CDT.[3, 5, 15, 26, 50] The best results seem to come from a stepped approach divided into an early, intense decongestion phase followed by a

BOX 15–9   **Keys to Successful Management for Patients with Lymphedema**

- Patient/caregiver education
- Skin care
- Compression therapy
  - Multilayer compression bandaging short term
  - Compression garments long term
- Therapeutic exercise
  - Active range of motion
  - Breathing exercise
  - Aerobic exercise
- Manual techniques to promote lymph drainage

self-management phase.[2, 3, 15, 55, 80, 81, 96, 115] During the first phase, patients are treated frequently, up to daily in an out-patient setting or twice daily in an in-patient setting. While no two patients are alike, sample treatment goals and time frames for the first phase of integrated treatment are listed in Table 15–8. The key result of phase one is to make patients and caregivers independent with managing this lifelong disease process[28] and knowing when to seek out medical assistance in the future.

Phase two is an ongoing phase of self-management in which the patient/caregiver continue with the minimal interventions required to maintain edema reduction. If there has been a plateau in edema reduction and some differences in limb volume persist, patients may need to continue all portions of treatment. Other patients may be able to reduce to basic skin care and the use of a compression garment solely for high-risk activities. The key to this phase is the ability of the patient and/or caregiver to monitor their condition and act swiftly and appropriately if negative changes occur. In patients with more severe lymphedema, intensive phase one treatments may need to be repeated in 3–6 months' time. This rest time allows the body to have a chance to stabilize and the lymphatic system may be able to continue to decongest.[3, 15]

The clinician must ensure proper patient/caregiver performance of each treatment component before moving onto the next. While it may be tempting to teach a wide variety of manual techniques or highly complex bandaging, keeping techniques simple[96] will result in better patient adherence and quicker skill development without sacrificing outcomes. Three tests of mastering compression bandaging can include (1) visual observation of practice bandaging in the clinic; (2) pre- and post-weekend circumferential measurements with patient/caregiver bandaging over the weekend; and (3) visual inspection of bandaging on return to the clinic.

MEDICAL AND SURGICAL INTERVENTIONS

Medical Interventions

Although medical and surgical interventions are clearly beyond the scope of physical therapy, they are presented here to proved a better understanding of the valuable roles these interventions play in the management of patients with lymphedema.

TABLE 15–8   Sample Phase One Treatment Goals

Treatment Goal	Time Frame
1. Patient/caregiver will verbalize understanding of skin and wound care, risk factor reduction, and treatment rationales.	1 week
2. Patient/caregiver independent with home exercise program.	1 week
3. Patient/caregiver independent with multilayer compression bandaging.	1–2 weeks
4. Patient/caregiver independent with manual techniques to promote lymph drainage.	2–3 weeks
5. Patient limb volume will be reduced by ___ %.	2–4 weeks
6. Tissue fibrosis will be resolved.	2–4 weeks
7. Restore skin integrity so there are no open wounds or lymphorrhea.	2–4 weeks

Medical Testing

Medical testing may be required to rule out serious disease, complications, and pathologies. The following patients should be assessed and cleared by a physician prior to initiating physical therapy: those with a history of cancer, congestive heart failure, chronic obstructive pulmonary disease, kidney disease, liver disease, bleeding disorders, or protein deficiencies.[68] Patients with high pain levels should also be assessed by a physician given that this is atypical of uncomplicated lymphedema. Some typical characteristics suspicious for malignant lymphedema include a rapid onset and progression of painful edema in combination with weight loss or decreased appetite.[15] Collateral veins, ulceration, and supraclavicular fossa edema also warrant referral to rule out metastatic disease.[15] Stewart–Treves syndrome, or lympangiosarcoma,[2] is a rare complication of severe, untreated lymphedema.[3] This very aggressive form of cancer has a 5-year survival rate of only 5–29%.[32]

There are medical tests that can demonstrate lymphatic anatomy and lymph flow. However, clinical examination and a thorough history,[18] in combination with the screening tests noted above, are normally sufficient to diagnose lymphedema. A diagnostic ultrasound can be used to assess axillary and inguinal lymph nodes.[15] Direct lymphography is no longer used due to complications with the dye used.[3] Indirect lymphography with a water-soluble contrast medium is injected subcutaneously into the dorsal hand or foot to visualize the lymphatic system in 40–60 cm segments.[15] Lymphscintigraphy is a nuclear medicine test that uses a radioactive tracer to identify the sentinel lymph node or lymphatic obstruction.[15] In patients who have had medical interventions to the lymph system, such as node excision or radiation therapy, it is reasonable to assume that the lymph transport capacity has decreased, making lymphscintigraphy irrelevant.[22] In addition, when lymphscintigraphy was used to assess lymph flow in patients after breast cancer surgery, it did not satisfactorily differentiate lymphedema severity,[22] limiting the significance of the test.

CASE STUDY: Mrs. Julia Prentice

PART 3

Interventions

The following highlights some of the key procedural interventions that will be incorporated into Mrs. Prentice's plan of care.

Coordination, Communication, and Documentation: Mrs. Prentice's diabetic educator was contacted to educate her on the risks of checking blood sugars, performing any laboratory testing, or blood pressure measurements on a limb that is at risk for lymphedema.

Patient/Client-Related Instruction: Mrs. Prentice will be instructed in the importance of skin protection techniques, minimizing lymphatic load and maximizing lymphatic return. Specifically, Mrs. Prentice will be instructed to only check her blood sugar in the fingers of her right hand. She will be instructed to request her blood pressures be taken only in her right upper extremity. She will be instructed to apply a hypoallergenic moisturizer daily to her left upper extremity and twice daily to her left anterior chest wall. She will be instructed to wear gardening gloves and wash them frequently to prevent skin trauma or infection while gardening. She will be instructed to wash any open skin areas within her left upper quadrant with soap and water then cover with a topical antimicrobial and an adhesive bandage until the skin is closed. She will be instructed in the use of daily compression as well as the use of compression when traveling by plane to visit her grandchildren. She will be instructed in how to self-measure her upper extremities on a monthly basis to ensure her lymphedema is controlled and an action plan if her swelling starts to return.

Procedural Interventions

- Local lymphedema management will consist of washing, patting dry, and applying a moisturizer to Mrs. Prentice's left upper extremity and anterior chest wall, multilayer compression bandaging of Mrs. Prentice's left upper extremity, manual lymphatic drainage using the anterior and posterior axilloaxillary as well as the left axilloinguinal pathway.

- Therapeutic exercises will include active range of motion exercises of her neck, trunk, and left

(Continued)

upper extremity to promote muscle pumping and proximal fluid return. She will also be instructed in a walking or biking program of her choice to assist with continued weight loss as well as promote lymphatic drainage.

- Mrs. Prentice will be prescribed both a short fingered glove as well as a left upper extremity compression sleeve with 20–30 mm Hg compression. A glove should be included because of her history of intermittent left hand swelling. While she *may* be able to wean off the glove with careful monitoring of her hand swelling, compression from her wrist proximally without distal compression is likely to allow a return of her hand lymphedema.

Reassessment

After $2\frac{1}{2}$ weeks of physical therapy, Mrs. Prentice's left upper extremity circumferential measurements are within 1 cm of her right, her left hand looks normal compared to her right, and there is no pitting edema. She is also able to easily get her wedding ring on and off. She and her husband verbalize and demonstrate understanding of self-management strategies for her stage 0 left upper extremity lymphedema. She is able to independently don and doff a short-fingered glove and arm sleeve. While wearing her garments, she has no difficulty with computer or phone use.

Medical Interventions

Medical interventions should be directed toward any heart, liver, lung, or kidney pathologies present. If consistent with the patient's overall plan of care, oncological interventions should be initiated as indicated.

Management of Risk Factors

Obesity is a leading risk factor in all types of lymphedema and weight gain after breast cancer surgery may be the number one risk factor for developing lymphedema.[45] Therefore, physicians can help reinforce the need for patients to attain and maintain an ideal body weight[6, 18] through proper diet and exercise.[54] Weight management is particularly important in children with primary lymphedema.[68]

Pharmacological Interventions

The infection rate of breast cancer patients with lymphedema may be as high as 42%, while up to 31% of patients with primary lymphedema may be expected to have an infection at some time.[32] Patients with cellulitis should be given a standard 2-week course of antibiotics.[9, 75] Oral amoxicillin, clindamycin, penicillin, or erythromycin are usually prescribed and if there are no signs of improvements, the patient is changed to intravenous antibiotics.[9] Physicians may prescribe topical antimicrobials and/or oral antibiotics to manage wound infection.[31] Topical corticosteroids may be prescribed to decrease inflammation, erythema, and puritus.[104] In addition to interventions directed toward treating lymphedema, physicians may prescribe analgesics, gabapentin, or amitriptyline for the pain and discomfort associated with lymphedema.[9] Nonsteroidal anti-inflammatories (NSAID) should be used with caution as one side effect of this class of medication is fluid retention.[9]

While it may seem tempting for physicians to prescribe a diuretic to decrease edema, these drugs are likely to worsen lymphedema in the long run as they increase the concentration of proteins within the interstitium, exacerbating tissue fibrosis while simultaneously risking hyponatremia, hypotension, and dehydration.[2, 27, 73, 111] That said, patients with severe lymphedema, peripheral edema, and heart failure may be given diuretics short term to decrease life-threatening fluid overload.[9, 27, 29] In addition, patients who require a diuretic to control hypertension should continue to take their medication as prescribed.[9] In contrast, calcium channel blockers should not be used to manage hypertension in patients with, or at risk for, lymphedema.[2, 26] Calcium is required for smooth muscle contraction and this medication may decrease lymphangiomotoricity.

Theoretically, benzopyrenes, coumarin, and flavonoids may help control lymphedema by reducing capillary permeability, stimulating macrophages, and inhibiting the production of inflammatory mediators.[2, 9] However, these medications are hepatotoxic and, therefore, are not currently used in the treatment of lymphedema.[2, 9, 50]

Surgical Interventions
Debridement

Patients with lymphedema who have large, necrotic wounds that are slow to respond to autolytic, enzymatic, or sharp debridement may benefit from surgical debridement.

Microsurgical Procedures

Lymph nodes that have been removed do not spontaneously regenerate.[15] However, animal studies have documented partial lymph node regeneration with the ability to transport a smaller volume of fluid than prior to node excision.[15] In adulthood, lymphangiogenesis occurs along with blood vessel angiogenesis, albeit at a slower pace.[28] Inflammatory cytokines, tumor necrosis factor alpha (TNFα), fibroblast growth factor (FGF), and vascular endothelial growth factor (VEGF) all appear to be able to trigger lymphangiogenesis to some extent.[28] However, adult lymphangiogenesis is primarily associated with pathology, such as cancer or chronic inflammation.[28]

Recent advances in medical technology have made it possible to perform microsurgery on the lymphatic system. Lymphatic-venous anastomoses, lymph vessel bypass surgery, and lymph vessel transplantation, while in no way standard treatment options, are currently being performed on animal models and experimentally on humans.[2, 9, 15, 116] Even if these connections are made, the long-term patency of the repaired vessel is unknown. Lymph node transplantation surgery has been tried in combination with growth factors such as VEGF in the hope that lymphatic vessels will spontaneously regrow.[28, 116, 117] However, even if successful, researchers fear there may be a fine line between stimulating lymphatic growth and stimulating cancer recurrence or metastatic spread through the repaired lymphatic system.[116] To date, the few studies with successful lymph vessel surgery demonstrated only minimal limb volume reduction.[15, 32]

Debulking Surgeries

Debulking surgeries are used in extreme cases of lymphedema that have failed standard interventions and in which patients have severe functional impairment due to limb volume or repeated infections. These procedures are not curative and have significant risks of infection, nonhealing, and poor cosmesis. Debulking surgeries include radical excision of subcutaneous tissues[15] with primary closure or staged skin grafting.[2] These procedures also remove the superficial lymphatic system. Therefore, there is a risk of a return or worsening of edema. Additionally, manual techniques cannot be used in the region because there is no longer a superficial lymphatic system with which to work.[3]

Elective Surgery to an Extremity with Lymphatic Insufficiency

As mentioned previously, patients with or at risk for lymphedema should avoid activities that risk puncturing the skin or causing inflammation to decrease the chance of worsening or creating lymphedema. Patients with lower extremity lymphedema should be particularly wary of having vein surgery as the surgery would likely worsen their edema.[15] Patients with upper extremity lymphedema and their physicians should carefully consider all nonsurgical options prior to operating on an at-risk or lymphedematous arm due to the very real potential the condition will worsen.[62] Suggested modifications in surgical technique include using the shortest possible tourniquet time, applying the tourniquet at the least effective compression, and prophylactic antibiotics. Pre- and post-operative circumferential measurements should be taken to track changes in limb volume. Post-operatively, patients should be instructed to wear compression garments or bandages until their follow-up visit when repeat measurements can be taken. Patients who had previously performed manual techniques or exercise should restart these interventions unless contraindicated by the type of surgical procedure performed (e.g., shoulder active range of motion exercises should not be performed immediately after a rotator cuff repair).

CHAPTER SUMMARY

Lymphedema is an abnormal accumulation of protein-rich fluid that may be caused by anatomic abnormalities in the lymphatic system or by trauma to a normal lymphatic system. Clinicians must stress lifelong prophylactic behaviors for patients at risk for the lymphedema. If untreated, lymphedema is a progressive disorder that causes patient discomfort, alters cosmesis, causes skin changes, and increases the risk of open wounds and infection. To better coordinate care among disciplines, lymphedema should be classified using the staging system in addition to the Integumentary and Cardiovascular Prefered Practice Patterns. Local wound care for patients with lymphedema-related wounds includes protecting the surrounding tissue, absorptive dressings, compression, and patient/caregiver education. An integrated approach to lymphedema management should also include therapeutic exercise and manual techniques to promote lymph drainage to unaffected areas.

REVIEW QUESTIONS

1. You have been working with a patient with severe trigger finger in her right upper extremity. She had a mastectomy and axillary lymph node dissection 3 years ago and has transient swelling in her right arm unless she wears her compression garment daily. Her trigger finger is not responding to conservative treatment, is painful nearly all of the time, and limits the use of her dominant hand. She is to have hand surgery next week. What recommendations do you have for the patient and the surgeon to decrease the risk of exacerbating her lymphedema?

2. Your patient has a history of left upper extremity lymphedema after a lumpectomy with 10 lymph nodes removed followed by radiation to her affected axilla and breast. After treatment, her limb volume has returned to the same size as her unaffected limb. Answer her questions about self-care and provide your rationale.

   a. Do I still need to wear my compression garment during the day?

   b. Do I still need to wear my compression garment when I fly?

   c. Do I still need to worry about blood pressures being taken in my left arm?

   d. Can I get in the jacuzzi now, as long as I keep my left arm out?

   e. Do I still need to self-measure my arm?

3. You are working in an out-patient clinic and are evaluating Mr. Gerard. Mr. Gerard had a right total knee replacement 4 weeks ago and just completed home health. His past medical history is positive for osteoarthritis, hypertension, and diabetes. When you examine him, you find his right knee circumference is 6 cm greater than his left, he has 2+ pitting edema in his right calf, 1+ in his dorsal right foot, and a positive right big toe Stemmer's sign. He has hemosideran deposition bilaterally. His pedal pulses are normal and his feet are warm (not hot) to touch. His right knee passive range of motion is 15–80 degrees and limited by swelling rather than pain. You believe the patient has venous insufficiency.

   a. What additional tests and measures might you want to perform to rule in or out your assessment?

   b. You discuss your findings with the referring physician and are given additional orders to treat Mr. Gerard for venous insufficiency with secondary lymphedema due to post-operative edema. Mr. Gerard and his wife consent as well. Discuss why you would choose or not choose to perform the following interventions over the next three visits.

      i. Ice with compression and elevation.

      ii. Have Mr. Gerard perform active and active assisted range of motion exercises with his right leg while lying or standing.

      iii. Have Mr. Gerard perform rocking or full revolutions on a stationary bicycle.

      iv. Measure for a below-knee compression garment.

      v. Measure for a thigh-high compression garment.

      vi. Perform multilayer compression bandaging.

      vii. Perform manual lymph drainage.

myhealthprofessionskit

Use this address to access the Companion Website created for this textbook. Simply select "Physical Therapy" from the choice of disciplines. Find this book and log in using your username and password to access images, video clips, and additional learning tools.

REFERENCES

Go to myhealthprofessionskit.com to view this chapter's references.

Miscellaneous Wounds

Chapter Objectives

After reading this chapter, learners will be able to:

1. Describe the presentation and appropriate interventions for abrasions.
2. Describe the presentation and appropriate interventions for skin tears.
3. Describe the presentation and appropriate interventions for surgical wounds.
4. Describe the presentation and appropriate interventions for traumatic wounds.
5. Describe the presentation and appropriate interventions for bite wounds.
6. State the etiology of radiation burns.
7. Describe the presentation and appropriate interventions for radiation burns.
8. Instruct patients and caregivers in precautions for the management of radiation burns.
9. Describe the presentation and appropriate interventions for pyoderma gangrenosum.

Key Terms

Fistula   Pyoderma gangrenosum   Radiation fibrosis

INTRODUCTION

Section II of this text provides the clinician with the basic framework to successfully manage patients with open wounds. Chapters 10–15 provide information about specific types of wounds commonly seen by physical therapists and procedural interventions that may be required based on wound etiology. The same approach to wound examination and management is required, regardless of wound etiology, patient population, or clinical setting. The clinician must obtain a detailed patient history including general demographic information, lifestyle and functional status, past and current general medical history, and past and current wound history. This will provide the clinician with a wealth of information including allergies, sensitivities, and factors that may adversely affect wound healing as well as insights into wound etiology, interventions, and healing potential. The clinician then performs a screening examination of the cardiovascular/pulmonary, musculoskeletal, neuromuscular, gastrointestinal, urogenital, and integumentary systems to identify risk factors or impairments that may require physical therapy interventions or referral to, or consultation with, other disciplines. Finally, the clinician performs a comprehensive integumentary examination. The clinician must objectively document wound characteristics, including location, wound size, tunneling or undermining, wound bed, wound edges, wound drainage, and wound odor. The clinician should note the characteristics of the periwound and associated skin including structure and quality, color, epithelial appendages, edema, and temperature. Circulation and sensory integrity should also be assessed.

After gathering this information, the clinician must classify the wound into the appropriate Integumentary Preferred Practice Pattern based on the depth of tissue involvement and determine a wound healing prognosis. The clinician's interventions then must consist of a tripartite approach of coordination, communication, and documentation; patient/client-related instruction; and procedural interventions. In addition to any procedural interventions required to remediate contributing factors, the clinician must determine appropriate local wound management procedures, including debridement, infection control, dressing and bandage selection, and the use of modalities or physical agents as adjuncts to facilitate wound healing. Interventions should be directed toward achieving objective, measurable goals and functional outcomes. Ideally, the desired outcome of wound management is wound healing: the wound bed is completely resurfaced with epithelium, and the tissue is remodeled so that its strength approaches normal. However, regardless of wound type, a short-term goal is to obtain a clean, moist, warm, granular wound bed while protecting the wound, periwound, and intact skin. Keeping this basic framework in mind, this chapter highlights additional insights into the management of miscellaneous types of wounds that health care providers are likely to see during their career, including abrasions, skin tears, surgical wounds, other traumatic wounds, bite wounds, wounds due to radiation fibrosis, and pyoderma gangrenosum.

ABRASIONS

An abrasion is a wound caused by friction to the skin's surface and may result in a superficial or partial-thickness wound. Abrasions may result from "skinning one's knee" in a fall, "road rash" from falling off a bicycle, a "raspberry" from sliding into home plate, or a "floor burn" from sliding across a gym floor.

Presentation

Some abrasions, such as floor burns, may be free from gross contamination. Others, such as road rash, may be grossly contaminated. Superficial abrasions may bleed slightly, whereas deeper abrasions will have a moderate amount of bleeding due to the involvement of dermal vessels. Abrasions are generally accompanied by a mild stinging sensation, which increases during irrigation or bathing. Unlike other types of wounds, abrasions rarely go on to become chronic wounds and are rarely the primary reason for referral to physical therapy services. However, contaminated abrasions are at risk for infection without proper wound management. Abrasions that occur in older adults, the immunocompromised, or individuals with multiple medical conditions can also lead to serious complications, including infection and sepsis, if not managed properly. Therefore, clinicians should monitor all patients for signs of integumentary trauma and initiate appropriate interventions before adverse effects can occur.

Interventions

Abrasions should be thoroughly irrigated with water or normal saline to remove foreign debris and bacteria.[1] Extensive abrasions that are grossly contaminated may benefit from whirlpool therapy to help debride loosely adhered devitalized tissue and debris. Selective or nonselective debridement may be required. This may be particularly challenging because of the potential for large areas of deeply imbedded debris. Although generally contraindicated, short-term mechanical debridement, such as scrubbing or wound cleansing, may be appropriate in this situation. Clean wounds can be covered with a moisture-retentive dressing (refer to Chapter 7). Contaminated wounds may be treated with a broad-spectrum topical antimicrobial, such as silver sulfadiazine, and a gauze dressing.

 Checkpoint Question #1

What tissues are involved in an abrasion?

Skin Tears

Skin tears are traumatic wounds resulting from shear or friction forces that separate the epidermis from the underlying dermis resulting in a partial-thickness wound (see Figure 16–1). Occasionally, both the epidermis and dermis may be separated from the underlying subcutaneous tissues resulting in a full-thickness wound.[2] Skin tears may occur from improper turning and lifting procedures, sliding down in bed when the head of the bed is raised, or bumping into objects, such as a wheelchair leg rest. It is estimated that 80% of skin tears occur on the arms and hands.[2] Older adults are particularly at risk for skin tears due to age-related skin changes such as decreased dermal thickness, decreased skin elasticity, decreased sweat gland production, and flatter rete pegs.[3, 4]

Presentation

The Payne–Martin Classification System for Skin Tears is commonly used to describe skin tears (Table 16–1).[4] Skin tears may occur without tissue loss and present in a linear fashion, similar to an incision, or may present as a

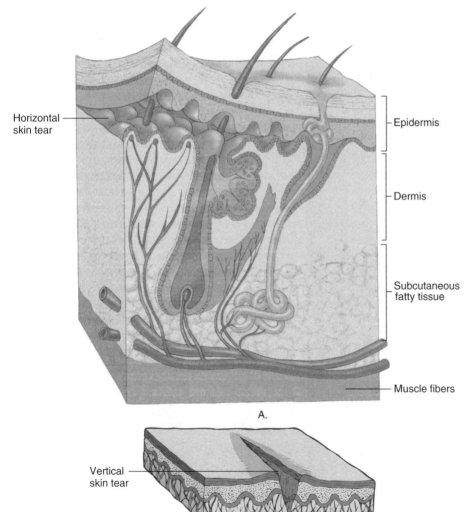

Horizontal skin tear

Epidermis

Dermis

Subcutaneous fatty tissue

Muscle fibers

A.

Vertical skin tear

B.

FIGURE 16–1   Skin tears occur when the epidermis is separated from the underlying dermis either A. horizontally or B. vertically. Although at times the wound edges can easily be approximated, sometimes they are jagged or avulsed, making approximation impossible.

Source: A. Emergency Care 9/e by Limmer/O'Keefe/Grant/Murry/Bergeron. B. Medical Terminology: An Anatomy and Physiology Systems Approach, 2/e by Fremgen/Frucht.

TABLE 16–1 Payne–Martin Classification System for Skin Tears

Type	Presentation
Category I	No tissue loss
• IA: Linear	• Epidermis and dermis pulled apart
• IB: Flap	• Epidermal flap covers dermis
Category II	Partial tissue loss
• IIA: Scant tissue loss	• </= 25% epidermal loss
• IIB: Moderate to large tissue loss	• >25% epidermal flap loss
Category III Skin tear with complete tissue loss	No epidermal flap

flap of epidermal tissue covering the underlying dermis. Wound edges can readily be approximated. Alternatively, shear and friction forces may result in partial tissue loss, resulting in jagged wound edges, or the epidermis may be completely sheared off.[2] Skin tears may have slight serous drainage. If there is damage to the dermis, the wound may bleed. Bleeding may be significant in patients taking anticoagulants. Pain is generally minimal, and there is no functional impairment.

Interventions

The wound should be gently irrigated with saline and patted dry. The wound edges should be approximated if possible. Skin tears that can be completely approximated may be best treated with a skin sealant.[5] Detached or nonviable pieces of epithelium should be carefully debrided. A moisture-retentive dressing should be applied, such as an amorphous hydrogel, nonadherent gauze, and gauze square secured with a roll gauze or self-adhesive wrap.[4] Adhesives should be avoided[4] unless the patient's skin is able to handle removal without further skin trauma. In such a situation, a skin sealant and a semipermeable film may be beneficial. A film dressing has several advantages. It allows visualization of the wound bed; it can be left on for up to 1 week; it is flexible; it is water impermeable, allowing the patient to wash or bathe; and it has a high moisture-vapor transmission rate, preventing fluid accumulation beneath the dressing.

SURGICAL WOUNDS

There are three types of surgical wounds that may be encountered in a physical therapy setting: muscle flaps and skin grafts, wound dehiscence, and wounds that have been surgically debrided and left to close by secondary intention. Refer to Chapters 11, 12, and 14 for information on the management of muscle flaps and skin grafts.

Surgical Wounds Treated with Primary Closure

Many surgical wounds are closed with sutures, staples, or tissue adhesives (also known as skin glue; see Chapter 7). With normal wound healing, these wounds need little direct treatment. For the first 24–48 hours, the area should be kept clean and dry. A small amount of bleeding, seeping, or wound drainage can be expected over the first day or so. The area should be observed for signs of infection, such as excessive redness or induration. Some physicians recommend the use of a topical antimicrobial, such as triple antibiotic, be applied with a clean swab to decrease the risk of infection. It should be protected from friction and tension. Generally, this requires the use of a gauze dressing or adhesive strips across the incision site. Patients should be cautioned not to immerse the body part in a tub or pool until the incision is fully closed. A physician, nurse, or physical or occupational therapist may remove the stitches or staples after the incision is fully re-epithelialized, in about 7–10 days.

Clinicians should be aware of two precautions when working with patients with primarily closed wounds. First, the risk of superficial skin infection appears to be four times greater with the use of staples than with stitches.[6] Therefore, wounds closed with staples require extra vigilance, and the clinician may be wise to use a topical antimicrobial and gauze dressing. Second, some patients may have a delayed sensitivity or allergy to one or more of the chemical agents within a tissue adhesive. While rarely severe, this can require the use of oral steroids to control the ensuing inflammatory reaction and pruritus.

Dehisced Surgical Wounds

Several patient factors are related to wound dehiscence. First, malnutrition, particularly deficiencies of vitamins A, C, and B complex, may decrease wound tensile strength,[7,8] increasing the potential for dehiscence. By correcting for these deficiencies, wound healing may be enhanced. Second, patients with diabetes are at increased risk of wound dehiscence.[9] Optimizing blood sugar control prior to planned surgeries may improve surgical wound healing.[10] Third, recall from Chapter 3, steroids have a deleterious effect on all phases of wound healing. Therefore, patients on steroids long term are at risk for wound dehiscence and delayed wound healing.[9, 11–13] Because smoking causes vasoconstriction, smokers are also at risk for wound dehiscence.[9, 14] Preoperative smoking cessation programs should be considered for patients who smoke, especially if they have other risk factors for delayed wound healing.[14] For these patients, vigilant monitoring of the surgical incision for dehiscence and optimizing the wound healing environment are vital. For example, by keeping the patient warm and providing adequate pain relief, vasoconstriction can be minimized. In addition, immediately postoperatively, patient oxygen saturation should be measured. Patients with inadequate tissue perfusion may require supplemental oxygen short term.

Surgical wound dehiscence may result from too much tension across the wound edges.[9] By controlling for these mechanical forces, the clinician can facilitate wound closure. For example, consider an obese patient who had an exploratory laparotomy. The incision dehisced 3 days after surgery and the patient is referred to physical therapy for wound management. The wound is unlikely to close in a timely manner if interventions are solely directed toward attaining or maintaining a clean, moist, granular wound bed because the wound etiology, excessive tensile forces due to patient movement, and soft tissue folds were not addressed. An abdominal binder or Montgomery straps (see Chapter 7) should be used to help approximate the wound edges and reduce tensile forces across the wound bed.

Surgical wound dehiscence may also occur due to underlying infection and abscess formation.[9] Copious surgical irrigation and sometimes surgical drains are used to minimize the risk of dehiscence[15] due to infection. Any bacteria present within a closed surgical wound will flourish within these warm, moist confines. Eventually, a sinus tract may form, allowing purulent material to escape and alerting the patient and health care provider to the infection. In this scenario the wound is likely to present with the classic signs of infection along with a necrotic or slough-covered base. Sinus tracts that connect two epithelial surfaces, such as the gastrointestinal tract and the skin, are called **fistulas.** Fistula formation may be intentional (as with an iliostomy), a complication after gastrointestinal surgery, or occur spontaneously.[16] Many times surgical wounds are closed using multiple layers of sutures, and it is possible for an infection to be confined to the superficial layers. However, it is also possible that the infection was able to spread to tissue layers beyond the level of the surgical procedure before becoming clinically evident. A wound culture and sensitivity should be performed. In general, the surgeon will initially prescribe a broad-spectrum antibiotic, changing to a more specific antibiotic after obtaining the results of the wound culture. Local wound management in this case would consist of wound irrigation, debridement, and obtaining and maintaining a moist wound environment. Because infection is present, or at least suspected, moisture-retentive dressings should not be used unless they are changed daily until all clinical signs of infection have resolved. The use of modalities such as pulsed lavage with suction, electrical stimulation, and ultrasound is contraindicated in surgical wounds involving body cavities. However, these modalities may be appropriate to facilitate wound healing in other locations.

Surgically Debrided Wounds

Wounds that have been surgically debrided and allowed to close by secondary intention have been discussed in various places throughout the text. These wounds should be almost 100% granular after surgery. Hence, local wound management interventions should be directed toward enhancing granulation tissue formation, wound contraction, and epithelialization.[17] Debridement and whirlpool therapy are not indicated. If there is no sign of infection, a moisture-retentive dressing may facilitate wound closure. It is important to fill any dead space within cavity wounds and deep wounds.[15] Adjunctive interventions, such as electrical stimulation and negative pressure wound therapy, may be beneficial. Additional interventions may be needed to address wound etiology or to assess for nutritional deficiencies that may contribute to delayed wound healing.

OTHER TYPES OF TRAUMATIC WOUNDS

Presentation

Traumatic wounds may result from a wide variety of situations including gunshots, motor vehicle accidents, falls, and industrial accidents. As such, wound presentation, including size, depth, and degree of contamination, is highly variable. The clinician should be aware of concomitant injuries, including fractures, spinal cord injuries, and head injuries, that may affect the course of rehabilitation.

Interventions

The clinician should follow standard wound healing principles when working with traumatic wounds. Contaminated or infected wounds should be irrigated and debrided as needed. The clinician should strive to attain and maintain a warm, moist wound environment by covering the wound and either adding moisture or absorbing wound drainage as needed. The area should be protected from further trauma, if necessary, by a bulky dressing. The cause of wound trauma must be identified and addressed, if necessary. For example, if a patient sustained a partial-thickness wound in a fall, it is important to find out why the patient fell. Was the patient careless? Is the patient's balance impaired? Does the patient have orthostatic hypotension? Is the patient in need of an eye examination? Is the patient at risk for future falls? Failure to identify and address the cause of a traumatic wound may place the patient at risk for future injury. Clinicians should ensure that patients with puncture wounds have current tetanus vaccinations.

 Checkpoint Question #2

Your patient presents with a crush injury to the right forearm after being partially trapped in a printing press. There are several open wounds, all with various amounts of foreign material within the wound beds.

a. Should you suggest the use of a topical antimicrobial? Defend your answer.

b. Should you cover the wounds with a moisture-retentive dressing such as a semipermeable foam? Defend your answer.

BITE WOUNDS

Every year in the United States 4–5 million people will experience a bite wound.[18] Approximately one-half of all Americans will have sustained a bite wound at some point during their lifetimes.[19] While the majority of bite wounds does not require substantial medical interventions,[18] these wounds may become infected, cause disfigurement, and, rarely, lead to death.[18, 20–22] This section addresses dog, cat, human, and spider bite wounds. Because poisonous snake bites and scorpion stings create a serious systemic problem rather than a local wound healing problem, these bites are not addressed in this text. These patients must be treated with appropriate antivenom and be closely monitored for cardiac arrhythmias.

Animal and Human Bite Wounds

Dog bite wounds account for 80–90% of all bite wounds.[23] Dog bites can cause lacerations, puncture wounds, and crush injuries. Dog bite wounds typically have jagged edges and at least minimal tissue loss. Cat bite wounds account for 5–15% of all bite wounds and are primarily puncture wounds.[23] Human bite wounds represent only 2–3% of all bite wounds.[23] Human bite wounds are described as an actual bite wound or a closed fist injury, as may occur when a person hits someone in the mouth.

In addition to the standard history and examination for all patients with open wounds, the examination of a patient with a bite wound must include a few additional key pieces of information for appropriate treatment (see Box 16–1).[18, 20, 23] Patients who have not had a tetanus shot in the last 5 years should receive a booster shot.[22] Patient risk factors for infection should be assessed. The exact date and time of the wound should be noted. The patient should describe how the bite wound occurred. For example, animals that are unprovoked or are behaving erratically may have rabies.[20] All animal bite wounds must be reported to the local health department.[18] Physicians should prescribe hyperimmune serum and active immunization[20] for patients at risk for rabies.

Bite wounds vary considerably in size and depth, ranging from superficial skin involvement to damage extending into the subcutaneous tissue, fascia, muscle, tendon, and even bone. The wound beds must be thoroughly examined and probed to assess for involvement of deeper tissues. The clinician must assess the function

---

BOX 16–1   Key History and Examination Points for Animal and Human Bite Wounds

Patient History

Day and Time of Bite

Tetanus vaccine/booster in the last 5 years?

At risk for infection due to any of the following:

    <2 or >50 years of age

    History of corticosteroid use

    Diabetes

    Cancer

    HIV+/AIDS

    SLE

    Prosthetic joints or valves

    Asplenic

    Vascular disorder affecting area of bite wound

    Wrist or hand bite wound

Wound Examination

    Depth of tissue involvement

    Local nerve, muscle, tendon, and vasculature function

    Signs of local infection

If Animal Bite:

Is the animal a household pet known to the patient?

Does the animal have a current rabies vaccination?

Was the animal provoked?

Was the animal exhibiting abnormal behavior prior to the bite?

Is the animal available for observation and examination?

If Human Bite:

Name of biter

Is the biter known to have any communicable diseases, such as:

    Hepatitis

    HIV/AIDS

    Syphilis

Is the biter available for a blood test if this information is unknown?

---

of local nerves, tendons, muscles, and vasculature in the area to determine the extent of tissue damage. Patients with exposed joints or ruptured tendons must be treated surgically.[20] In closed fist bite wounds, if deep tissues are exposed, an x-ray should be requested.[20]

All wounds should be thoroughly irrigated with copious amounts of water or saline.[20, 22–24] Cleansers or antibiotic solutions should not be used, as these are likely to irritate the patient's tissues.[22] However, some physicians advocate the short-term (1–3 days) use of antiseptics, such as adding chlorazene to the whirlpool or povidone–iodine soaks, for bite wounds in patients at risk for infection. In such cases, the risk for infection must clearly outweigh the delayed wound healing these substances are known to cause. The wounds should be inspected for the cardinal signs of infection, including erythema, excessive edema, and purulent or excessive drainage. All devitalized tissue and foreign material should be debrided.[23, 24]

Most bite wounds are polymicrobial, with an average of four different microbes per bite.[20] These microbes arise from the normal bacterial flora within the biter's mouth as well as the normal surface bacteria on the victim's skin.[20] It is estimated that 2–20% of dog bite wounds and 5–50% of cat bite wounds[18, 22, 23] will become infected, while 10–50% of human bite wounds will become infected.[23] Human bite wounds tend to be more serious for two reasons. First, the human mouth has more varied microflora.[22] More importantly, however, is the etiology of the closed fist bite wound.[25] When a person strikes someone in the mouth with a clenched fist, the victim's teeth are likely to lacerate the thin skin on the dorsum of the hand and can penetrate into the patient's tendons, joint capsule, or even into bone, implanting bacteria into these deeper tissues. Next, as the patient opens his or her clenched fist, the tendons will glide proximally, bringing these bacteria under the intact proximal skin. Therefore, a relatively benign-looking human bite wound may lead to a delay in proper management and serious infection. Box 16–2 lists the most common infections resulting from bite wounds.[18, 20–22, 25]

It is important to note that at the time of a bite wound, it is not possible to predict if a patient will develop an infection, nor which of the pathogens present will be the cause of an infection.[21] Therefore, prophylactic antibiotics are indicated only in certain instances: patients who are at risk for infection due to a compromised immune system and patients with full-thickness closed fist injuries.[20, 26, 27] Patients presenting with signs of infection should have both aerobic and anaerobic wound cultures.[20] Because most infection-causing bacteria in bite wounds are resistant to penicillin, the physician should initially prescribe a broad-spectrum antibiotic empirically based on bite pathology, such as a combination of amoxicillin and fluoroquinolones.[20, 28] Once the culture results are available, this regimen is modified if needed.[23] Pulsed lavage with suction or whirlpool may be warranted to

---

BOX 16–2   Most Common Infectious Agents in Bite Wounds

Dog and Cat Bite Wounds

- Aerobes:
  - Pasteurella multocida
  - *Staphylococcus*
  - *Alpha-hemolytic Streptococci*
  - *Eikenella corrodens*
  - *Afipia febis* (cat)
  - *Bartonella henselae* (cat)
  - *Francisella tularensis* (cat)
- Anaerobes:
  - *Actinomyces*
  - *Fusobacterium*
  - *Prevotella*
  - *Porphyromonas*

Human Bite Wounds

- *Viridans Streptococcus*
- *Strepococcus pyogenes*
- *Staphylococcus aureus*
- *Eikenella corrodens*
- *Haemophilus influenza*

---

reduce wound bioburden and promote tissue proliferation. Unsutured wounds should be covered with a gauze dressing. If muscle, tendons, or nerves are exposed, a moist wound environment is imperative and an impregnated gauze or an amorphous hydrogel may help reduce trauma to the wound bed during dressing changes. The use of splints or assistive devices may be required in cases of peripheral nerve damage, lower extremity bite wounds, or wounds that extend beyond the subcutaneous tissue. Bite wounds involving the wrist or hand should be immobilized in the position of function and elevated when possible.[23, 29] Electrical stimulation may be beneficial for slow-healing wounds because of its ability to combat infection and promote granulation tissue formation.

Suturing acute bite wounds remains somewhat controversial. Most sources agree that nonpuncture, noncrush wounds seen within 24 hours of the bite, without clinical signs of infection, that do not involve the wrist, hand, or deep tissues may be safely sutured.[22, 29, 30] However, some physicians choose only to suture bite wounds in which concerns for cosmesis clearly outweigh the risk of infection, such as facial bite wounds.[23] Patients with acute bite wounds should have a follow-up appointment with the clinician within 24 to 48 hours to assess for signs of infection.[22] Patients treated with antibiotics should be reassessed in 1–5 days to ensure appropriate coverage.[22] If a sutured wound shows signs of infection on follow-up, a culture should be taken and empiric antibiotic coverage initiated by a physician. Some or all of the sutures should be removed and the wound should be thoroughly irrigated before bandaging.[21]

Spider Bite Wounds

Every year in the United States, approximately 10,000 spider bites are reported to poison control centers.[31] However, spider bites are very difficult to diagnose, as less than 20% of patients with documented spider bites actually felt the bite occur[31] and the spider is seldom seen. In Brazil, the wolf spider has been blamed for necrotic ulcers for decades. These suspected spider bite wounds were treated with antivenom, an expensive and potentially dangerous intervention. A recent study found that only half of the suspected bite wounds were caused by the wolf spider,[32] placing patients at undue risk of the serious side effects of the antivenom (serum sickness) and increasing treatment cost. In the United States, only 45% of suspected spider bites were actually caused by spiders.[33] Impetigo, varicella zoster, toxic epidermal necrolysis, pyoderma gangrenosum, cellulitis, and community-acquired MRSA are frequently misdiagnosed as spider bites.[33–35] There is no test to conclusively diagnose a spider bite.[36, 37] Luckily, only two types of spider bites endemic to the United States will require medical intervention: the black widow and the brown recluse.[34]

The black widow is the most venomous spider in the United States and is 15 times more poisonous than a rattlesnake.[36] From the genus *Latrodectus*, the black widow is a large black spider with an hour glass–shaped red mark on its abdomen and is indigenous to every state except Alaska. Patients who sustain a black widow spider bite are acutely, systemically ill within 1 to 3 hours of the bite. The bite itself may go unnoticed or the patient may feel a stinging sensation. The bite wound is small, without necrosis,[38] and is surrounded by erythema that develops into an urticarial rash (see Chapter 17). Black widow venom contains a neurotoxin that depletes motor nerve endings of acetylcholine, causing muscle depolarization and weakness. In addition, patients experience headaches, pain disproportionate to the size of the bite wound that quickly spreads to the abdomen and back, nausea, vomiting, hyperreflexia, dyspnea, diaphoresis, tachycardia, hypertension, and restlessness.[36] Medical interventions, including antivenom, if tolerated, tetanus booster, muscle relaxers, and nonsteroidal anti-inflammatory medications are key. Ice can be applied to the bite wound to decrease local pain.[36] The bite wound itself rarely requires medical attention.

In contrast, the wound caused by a brown recluse spider bite may require medical treatment. The brown recluse spider, *Loxosceles reclusa*, is also known as the fiddle-back spider because of the characteristic fiddle-shaped brown marking on its dorsum. The brown recluse is about 10 mm long and lives in quiet, enclosed spaces such as attics, basements, boxes, and under rocks.[32] They hibernate in the fall and winter and are more active in the spring.[38] However, identification is not that simple as there are several types of brown spiders; some brown recluse are black, tan, or yellow in color; and the markings on some brown recluse spiders may be distorted or faded.[34] The brown recluse is only endemic to a swath of the United States west to Nebraska and Texas, east to Georgia, south to the Gulf of Mexico, and north to Indiana, Illinois, and Missouri.[32, 35] Alternative wound etiologies must be sought for patients outside of this geographic region.

Brown recluse spiders will bite only defensively,[32] and the majority of these bites is thought to heal without complications in 3–5 days.[34, 38] Brown recluse bites are diagnosed by clinical presentation alone[39] because the bite itself may go unnoticed[33] and fewer than one-quarter of patients experience pruritus or fever.[31] Envenomation causes local edema, vasodilation, blood vessel degeneration, and hemorrhage. Reddish blisters or bullae (see Chapter 17) may erupt.[37] Within 24 hours, the bite wound has a characteristic presentation of red inflammation, blue thrombosis, and white ischemia. In about 20% of bite wounds, this leads to a centrally necrotic area within 3–4 days, progressing to eschar in 5–7 days.[40, 41] Spider venom interacts with the patient's basement membrane and extracellular matrix,[42, 43] liquefying local fat stores and extending the size of the wound to a maximum of 1.7×2.3 cm in half of all cases,[31] but may extend up to 30 cm in diameter.[38] The mean wound healing time ranges from 5 to 17 weeks.[31, 38] Systemic reactions may occur, including fever up to 105°, nausea, malaise, joint pain, seizures, hemolysis, thrombocytopenia, and rarely renal failure and death.[31, 33, 38, 40, 42, 43] Patients with these more severe systemic reactions tend to have less significant skin involvement.[38] Differential diagnosis should include tick bite, Lyme disease, and necrotizing fasciitis.[33, 44]

Treatment remains controversial,[40] partly due to the difficulty in properly diagnosing a brown recluse bite wound. Physician supervision is required due to the potential systemic complications and for pharmacological management. Following basic wound management principles presented within the text, including aggressive debridement of necrotic tissue and moist wound healing with dressings based on wound presentation, are the norm.[38] Superficial heat should be avoided as it may increase necrosis.[31] Topical nitroglycerine patches to improve local ischemia have had mixed results.[34, 40] Early surgical excision is contraindicated as it may spread the spider's venom and prolong the inflammatory response.[37] However, this may be beneficial in large, stable bite wounds that are not healing after 6–8 weeks of appropriate local wound care.[34] Up to 3% of patients may require skin grafts.[34] Antibiotics are generally not indicated unless the clinical signs of infection are present.[38] Antihistamines may be prescribed to decrease pain and pruritus.[34] Local and systemic steroids are frequently prescribed, however, there is little evidence as to their effectiveness.[31] Topical dapsone is sometimes prescribed to inhibit the patient's immune response and limit the size of the lesion. However, the results are highly variable and adverse reactions to dapsone can be lethal.[31, 37, 38, 40]

RADIATION FIBROSIS AND RADIATION BURNS

Radiation therapy, along with chemotherapy and surgery, is a standard treatment for cancer. Up to 50% of patients with cancer will receive radiation therapy[4] and of these, half will be long-term survivors.[45] Patients treated with a combination of radiation and chemotherapy are at greater risk for skin reactions than those receiving monotherapy.[46] Unfortunately, the rapidly dividing cells of the skin are highly sensitive to the damaging effects of radiation.[4, 47] The acute effects of radiation result from both direct tissue destruction and indirect damage from free radical production.[47] Radiation delays normal healing by inhibiting the inflammatory response, connective tissue proliferation, granulation tissue formation, angiogenesis, collagen deposition, and fibroblast replication.[48, 49] Radiation tissue injury is dose-dependent.[49] Skin reactions to ionizing radiation also vary based on type of radiation, location, and surface area treated.[4, 50] Other variables affecting the severity of radiation therapy damage include patient age, preexisting diseases, medications, nutrition status, hydration, immune function, and smoking or alcohol use.[50, 51]

Presentation

Mild skin reactions due to vascular congestion and increased capillary permeability[50, 52] are characterized by mild inflammation, slight erythema, and local edema. Dryness may occur due to epidermal and sebaceous gland damage. Low-dose radiation, less than 30 gray, leads to dry desquamation characterized by scaling and hyperpigmentation within the first 2–3 weeks of treatment.[46] The patient may report the skin feels tight, itchy, tender to the touch, and sensitive to the movement of overlying clothing.[50, 51] If radiation exposure is continued over 4 weeks, moist desquamation is likely to occur in the treated area.[46] This is characterized by increased pain, bulla formation, and a fibrinous exudate.[46] Because an open wound with exposed dermal nerve endings now exists, the area becomes more painful and the patient is at risk for infection.[50, 53] Ulcer formation may occur from minor trauma if the demands of wound healing exceed tissue perfusion. In contrast, radiation necrosis occurs if tissue oxygenation is insufficient to even maintain skin integrity.[52] Skin reactions due to radiation therapy are graded on a 4-point scale (see Box 16–3).[51]

Late tissue injury causes **radiation fibrosis** due to the overproduction and decreased degradation of collagen as well as hypovascularity in the treated area.[45, 52, 54] Tissue samples have shown an increased rate of Types I and II collagen synthesis up to 3 years after radiation exposure.[54] The irradiated skin appears discolored, dry, hairless, atrophied, fibrotic, and inelastic.[4, 50] The skin may appear semitransluscent with superficial blood vessels readily visible.[46, 50] Ulceration due to late tissue injury may occur at any time,[50] but on average occurs 9 years after radiation therapy.[53]

Interventions

There is a paucity of research regarding effective treatment for irradiated skin. However, there is consensus that irradiated skin requires protection from mechanical forces, including pressure, friction, and shear forces. Clothing covering the affected area should be loose-fitting and made from nonabrasive fabrics. Adhesives should be strictly forbidden. The patient should be instructed to pat the skin dry after bathing and to avoid scratching the affected area. Because bathing can have a drying effect on the skin, bathing frequency may need to be decreased.[4, 46] Thermal trauma should be minimized by avoiding the use of superficial heat and ice on the affected area. Chemical trauma from harsh detergents or heavy perfumes should also be avoided.[4] An amorphous hydrogel may be gently applied to anhydrous irradiated skin with the area left open to the air, or the area may be covered with a sheet hydrogel.[4, 46, 53] Patients generally report that these dressings are soothing to the skin. Some radiation oncologists prescribe a mild, nonperfumed moisturizing ointment, such as Aquaphor, to be applied to the affected area to help rehydrate the skin.[50] Colloidal oatmeal baths[46] or topical steroids may be prescribed by the physician to help reduce pruritus. These should be used with caution as steroids will cause local vasoconstriction, potentially compromising skin perfusion.[53] If a break in skin integrity does occur, a sheet hydrogel held in place by the patient's clothing or a light roll gauze is the dressing of choice to prevent infection and decrease patient discomfort. The physician may prescribe a broad-spectrum topical antimicrobial, such as silver sulfadiazine, for infected wounds.[46] See Box 16–4 for instructions for patients with irradiated skin. Hyperbaric oxygen[45, 53] and skin grafting[46] have been used to improve healing in problem wounds. Recent studies have shown that pretreatment of the skin to be irradiated with topical ascorbic acid, aloe vera,[50] or curcumin (the active ingredient in the spice turmeric) may delay the onset, decrease the severity, and improve the healing time of radiation skin reactions.[47–49]

BOX 16–3   Skin Reactions Due to Radiation Therapy

Grade 1

- Faint erythema
- Epilation
- Dry desquamation
- Decreased sweating response

Grade 2

- Bright erythema
- Tenderness to palpation
- Moderate edema
- Moist desquamation

Grade 3

- Moist desquamation with pitting edema

Grade 4

- Ulceration or necrosis

BOX 16–4   Precautions for Patients with Irradiated Skin

Do

- Perform daily skin checks.
- Bathe daily or less often using a mild, nonperfumed soap and pat your skin dry.
- Protect your skin from injury.
- Follow your health care provider's instructions regarding the use of topical ointments and moisturizers.
- Treat any open areas.
  - Wash the area with soap and water.
  - Cover as directed by your health care provider.
  - Check the wound daily.
  - Report any signs of infection or wound deterioration to your health care provider.
- Drink plenty of noncaffeinated, nonalcoholic fluids.
- Do apply sunscreen to areas with radiation fibrosis if direct sun exposure is expected.

Do Not

- DO NOT wear constrictive clothing or jewelry.
- DO NOT scratch your skin even if it itches.
- DO NOT use hot tubs or saunas, or take long hot showers.
- DO NOT use adhesive bandages.

 Checkpoint Question #3

You are working with a patient with the diagnosis of right adhesive capsulitis. The patient had a right lumpectomy with three lymph nodes removed 8 months ago after undergoing 3 months of preoperative chemotherapy. She completed 5 weeks of radiation therapy postoperatively. You notice the skin of your patient's right anterior upper quadrant is mildly dark in color and dry in contrast to her left side. Describe why the following interventions would be contraindicated.

a. Myofascial release and soft tissue mobilization to the right pectoralis minor and major to increase range of motion.

b. Ultrasound to the right anterior and inferior glenohumeral joint.

PYODERMA GANGRENOSUM

Pyoderma gangrenosum is a noninfectious, progressive necrotizing skin condition.[55, 56] The etiology of pyoderma is unclear. Half of patients have a systemic inflammatory condition such as ulcerative colitis, Crohn's disease, irritable bowel syndrome, lupus, or rheumatoid arthritis,[57–59] but only 5% of patients with ulcerative colitis have pyoderma.[56] About one quarter of cases of pyoderma begin after some sort of trauma or surgery[56, 60] but another quarter have an insidious onset. Pyoderma most frequently affects patients who are middle-aged.[58] While some studies have found pyoderma to be twice as common among women than men, other studies have shown no gender preference.[61] The pathology of pyoderma gangrenosum is also poorly understood but is believed to be due to neutrophil dysfunction.[62]

Presentation

The classic presentation of pyoderma gangrenosum begins as a small, very painful papule, vesicle, or pustule[58, 63, 64] on the lower extremities and/or trunk.[59] While a single lesion is possible, generally there is a cluster of ulcerations that rapidly expands.[65, 66] Pyoderma rapidly progresses to full-thickness ulcerations[67] with irregular, violaceous borders, which have purulent and hemorrhagic exudates. Because the inflammatory process spreads within the dermis, undermining is the norm. Undermining and lack of dermal support lead to epidermal necrosis.[66] The wound bed is eschar- or slough-covered and the wound edges may be rolled.[55, 59] The periwound is indurated[56] or boggy.[59] The patient may also have fever, malaise, or myalgia.[66] Pyoderma lesions are erythematous due to inflammation but may also have a blue hue from epidermal necrosis.[56]

Despite this typical presentation, pyoderma is misdiagnosed up to 10% of the time, possibly because there is no specific laboratory or histological test to identify the condition.[62] Differential diagnosis includes cancer, vasculitis, primary infection, drug-induced skin reaction, spider bite,[60] and chronic venous insufficiency.[56, 62] Wound cultures and laboratory testing can be used to exclude infection, however, secondary *Staphylococcus* or *Streptococcus* infections are not uncommon.[56] Therefore, pyoderma should be suspected if patients with positive wound cultures do not respond to antibiotics.[56, 62] Pyoderma should also be considered in wounds that are not responding to standard interventions for the presumed etiology, for example, a venous insufficiency ulcer that is not responding to compression and moist wound healing principles. The physician should perform a tissue biopsy in suspected cases of pyoderma to rule out other diagnoses, including malignancy.[63, 64, 68] Microscopic analysis of pyoderma is nonspecific,[55] but typically shows massive dermal neutrophil infiltration, hemorrhage, and epithelial necrosis.[66, 68]

Interventions

Patients with pyoderma gangrenosum require ongoing medical management. While specific intervention strategies remain controversial, the mainstay of treatment includes medication and local wound care. Immunosuppressive agents,[57, 59, 62, 63] such as cyclosporine, and anti-infective agents, such as dapsone, are used to decrease neutrophil overexpression of interleukin. Systemic, topical, and locally injected corticosteroids,[4, 57–59, 62, 63, 66, 68] such as prednisone and triamcinolone, are used to control inflammation.

Local wound care includes gentle and limited debridement of slough and necrotic tissue.[59] Extensive sharp or surgical debridement is contraindicated because it increases the inflammatory response, leading to severe exacerbations.[56, 59, 68] Recently, the use of maggots for biological debridement has shown some promise.[63] Topical antimicrobials, such as silver sulfadiazine, are indicated for sensitive bacterial infections.[69]

Gauze or moisture-retentive dressings should absorb wound exudate and protect the surrounding tissue. Extremity wounds may benefit from elevation and gradient compression.[66] Negative pressure therapy[67] and hyperbaric oxygen[64] have been used with some success. Wounds that have stabilized with medication have been treated successfully with skin grafting.[56, 57, 59, 66]

Differential diagnosis is key. For example, malignancy must be expediently surgically removed while surgical debridement of pyoderma is contraindicated. Even with proper diagnosis, wound healing is extremely slow,[57, 64] with only 69% of wounds resolved after 1 year and 95% after 3 years.[61] Because recurrence is common,[64, 68] physicians generally continue pharmacological management for 6–12 months after wound closure.[56]

CHAPTER SUMMARY

The ideal outcome of wound management is a wound bed completely resurfaced with epithelium and normal tensile strength. To achieve this final product, clinicians should first strive to obtain a clean, moist, warm, granular wound bed. The same basic principles can be applied regardless of wound etiology. Wounds that are at risk for infection, such as grossly contaminated abrasions or traumatic wounds, bite wounds, and dehisced surgical wounds, require thorough irrigation, debridement, and careful monitoring. Clean wounds, such as skin tears and surgically debrided wounds left to heal by secondary intention, require protection. Slow to heal surgically debrided wounds may benefit from adjunctive interventions to stimulate tissue proliferation, such as electrical stimulation or negative pressure wound therapy. Radiation burns require protection. An amorphous hydrogel or nonperfumed moisturizing agent may decrease local discomfort and enhance resolution of mild radiation skin reactions, while sheet hydrogel dressings are the dressing of choice for more severe radiation burns. Patients with pyoderma gangrenosum require prolonged medical management, limited debridement, and appropriate wound dressings.

REVIEW QUESTIONS

1. You are a physical therapist working at a youth outdoor basketball tournament when a player seeks treatment for a large abrasion on his lateral calf sustained while diving for a loose ball on the asphalt basketball court. There is visible debris

covering approximately 75% of the wound bed and the wound has minimal sanguinous drainage.

   a. How would you treat this patient's wound?

   b. What instructions would you give to this patient?

2. While transferring from bed into a wheelchair, your 76-year-old patient bumps her leg on the leg rest, sustaining a skin tear on her posterior calf. Although it is bleeding, the patient does not appear to notice the injury. How should you treat this wound?

3. You are working with a patient with a right forearm ulcer that began 4 weeks ago after a suspected spider bite. The wound initially measured $2.0 \times 4.5\,cm$, had a necrotic base with moderate exudate, and the perimeter was erythematous with minimal induration. After 2 weeks of debridement and dressing changes, the wound measured $3.2 \times 5.3\,cm$. The wound increased in size despite debridement and dressing changes. Describe two potential reasons for this adverse response and how your treatment would be modified for each.

4. You are working with a patient with a nonhealing lower extremity ulcer. The wound has a moderate amount of serous drainage requiring daily dressing changes with a moisture barrier, alginate, gauze pad, and six-ply roll gauze. Although granular, the wound has failed to decrease in size over the past 2 weeks despite patient adherence with your instructions and biweekly physical therapy. During today's visit you notice the patient has mild pitting edema of the foot and ankle, which you had not previously noticed. On questioning the patient, he reports that at the end of the day his leg is usually swollen. He also notes that his therapy appointments have regularly been scheduled in the morning, but that today he came after working all day.

   a. Based on this information, name two potential causes for the patient's edema.

   b. Describe how you will change your interventions based on these hypotheses.

5. A 46-year-old darkly pigmented man has been referred to physical therapy for wound management and therapeutic exercise for venous insufficiency. The patient reports he has a venous ulcer on his right lower extremity that has not responded to topical medication and compression therapy. During the physical examination of the wound, you note the wound margins appear irregular, raised, and undermined with a deep blue halo surrounding the lesion. The patient reports the area is painful and that it has been draining "pus." The patient has a history of ulcerative colitis and asthma.

   a. Given the patient's history and wound presentation, name an alternative etiology for this patient's wound.

   b. How would you communicate your hypothesis to the referring physician?

   c. Given the dark pigmentation of the patient's skin, what other cutaneous signs should you look for when evaluating dark skin?

PEARSON
myhealthprofessionskit

Use this address to access the Companion Website created for this textbook. Simply select "Physical Therapy" from the choice of disciplines. Find this book and log in using your username and password to access images, video clips, and additional learning tools.

REFERENCES

Go to myhealthprofessionskit.com to view this chapter's references.

17

Basic Dermatology

HEATHER HETTRICK, PT, PhD, CWS, MLT, FACCWS

Chapter Objectives

After reading this chapter, learners will be able to:

1. Identify threats to skin integrity.
2. Describe the intrinsic and extrinsic factors associated with aging skin.
3. Recognize primary and secondary lesions associated with dermatological conditions.
4. Describe the diagnostic details of dermatological lesions.
5. Identify common dermatological conditions that may be encountered within a physical therapy setting.
6. Understand the physical therapist's role in the management of selected dermatological conditions.
7. Recognize dermatological conditions that warrant referral to other health care practitioners.
8. Understand common dermatological variants in non-Caucasian skin.

INTRODUCTION

Dermatology is a vast field within the medical profession. This chapter provides an overview of common dermatological conditions that may be encountered in a physical therapy setting. Diseases of the skin manifest differently between individuals and are influenced by extraneous factors. However, most skin disorders present with unique characteristics that contribute to accurate diagnosis and treatment. Understanding basic dermatology will enhance physical therapists'

knowledge of the skin and related pathologies. As health care practitioners, it is important to recognize changes in the skin, such as blemishes or lesions, that may indicate skin-specific or systemic-related problems. With the rise of direct access legislation for physical therapy and the increasing potential for physical therapists to serve as primary care providers, it is paramount that clinicians recognize integumentary pathologies that warrant further consultation or referral. Physical therapists must be familiar with basic dermatology in order to achieve two goals: (1) to identify and recognize threats to skin integrity, common diseases of the skin, and integumentary changes associated with aging; and (2) to facilitate communication with other health care providers to provide optimal care for patients. This chapter introduces the clinician to the basics of dermatology and provides an overview of the most common dermatological conditions encountered in the clinical setting. A glossary at the end of the book provides key terms and definitions related to dermatology. Because dermatology requires visual examination of the skin, the Website accompanying this text provides images of a wide variety of the pathologies discussed within this chapter.

THREATS TO SKIN INTEGRITY AND THE AGING PROCESS

The largest organ of the body, the skin provides a vital role in maintaining homeostasis. In an average adult, the skin covers about 25 square feet and makes up 15% of the body weight. The epidermis and dermis of the skin are equivalent to the thickness of a credit card, yet contain a plethora of vital structures. In fact, one square inch of skin contains 65 hairs, 100 sebaceous glands, 78 yards of nerves, 78 sensory apparatuses for heat, 160 pressure apparatuses for the perception of tactile stimuli, 13 sensory apparatuses for cold, 650 sweat glands, 19 yards of blood vessels and a similar number of lymph vessels, 9.5 million cells, 1,300 nerve endings, 20,000 sensory cells, and 32 million bacteria.[1] The primary functions of the skin include protection, sensation, metabolism, thermoregulation, and communication.[2] Homeostasis is maintained by the stratum corneum. When intact, the stratum corneum protects against excessive electrolyte and fluid loss. The layers of the skin and its elastic qualities also serve as protection against mechanical forces and trauma while melanin protects the skin from ultraviolet radiation. Furthermore, several features of the epidermis work in unison to protect the skin from pathogens: the skin immune system (Langerhans' cells, macrophages, and mast cells), normal skin flora (primarily aerobic gram-positive cocci, diphtheroids, and yeast), acid pH, sebum production, and an intact stratum corneum.[2]

Skin aging occurs from the natural passage of time combined with the cumulative effects of sun exposure. Therefore, skin problems are common in the elderly population. The changes associated with aging skin predispose individuals to skin problems, diseases, and injury. A detailed summary of skin changes associated with aging can be found in Box 17–1.[2, 4] It is particularly

---

BOX 17–1   Skin Changes with Aging

- Decreased amount of ground substance, elastin, and collagen in dermis
- Reduced epidermal turnover
- Flattened epidermal rete pegs and dermal papillae
- Decreased thickness of dermis and hypodermis
- Decreased vascularity, particularly in the capillary loops of dermal papillae
- Changed sebum composition
- Reduced number of sweat glands
- Reduced skin elasticity
- Compacted collagen tissue
- Increased visibility and prevalence of wrinkles
- Decreased vitamin D production
- Reduced barrier function
- Decreased inflammatory response
- Diminished thermoregulation
- Diminished sensory perception
- Thickened nails
- Reduced moisture content of skin
- Reduced immune function due to decreased number of mast cells, Langerhans' cells, and active melanocytes

Source: Bryant R, Rolstad B. Examining threats to skin integrity. *Ostomy/Wound Management.* 2001;47(6):18–27; and Resnick B. Dermatologic problems in the elderly. *Lippincott's Primary Care Practice.* 1997;1(1):14–30.

---

important for clinicians to identify and understand the normal and abnormal skin changes that can occur with aging given the current estimates that 20% of the U.S. population will be over the age of 65 by the year 2025.[3]

In a study of nursing home patients, the two most common skin problems were found to be xerosis and pruritus.[5] Xerosis, or dry skin, affects older adults because they have decreased sweat and sebaceous gland activity. Furthermore, elderly patients are more prone to xerosis due to preexisting disease states, therapies, and medications such as end-stage renal disease, thyroid disease, nutritional deficiency, neurological disorders, malignancy, radiation, anti-androgen medications, and diuretic therapy.[6–8] Xerosis can lead to the development of flaking, fissuring, inflammation, dermatitis, and infection—a vicious cycle that must be controlled to prevent complications. Managing xerosis and understanding the skin changes associated with aging is important for health care providers. In general, people over the age of

65 should reduce the frequency of bathing and only use lukewarm water. Mild, nonirritating soaps and skin cleansers should be used followed by the application of a good moisturizer directly to damp skin. Avoiding abrasives and friction and adding air humidification in dry environments is recommended.[5] Regardless of the age of the patient, proper skin care and management is integral for optimal health. However, extra caution in handling older patients during transfers and positioning will help to reduce the effects of mechanical and physical forces their skin must sustain.

BASIC DERMATOLOGY

The clinician must be able to perform a thorough history and examination and clearly document the clinical presentation of a skin disorder to make an assessment and establish the basis for referral to another health care provider, such as a primary care physician or dermatologist. Because of the repeated and intensive nature of physical therapy encounters, physical therapists may be the first health care professionals to encounter a dermatological condition worthy of further investigation. Therefore, the importance of a thorough systems review during all physical therapy examinations, including patients with chief complaints that are unrelated to integumentary dysfunction, cannot be overstated. Clinicians must be able to recognize skin impairments and succinctly describe and document the clinical presentation in order to discuss the pertinent information with the appropriate health care provider. When suspicious lesions are encountered, referrals should be made either to the patient's primary care physician or directly to a dermatologist to ensure appropriate diagnosis and intervention.

The skin reflects the overall health of an individual. The fundamentals of integument screening, examination, and patient considerations covered in Chapter 4 provide a thorough overview of the considerations relevant to conducting a complete dermatological screening. In dermatology, diagnosis is most frequently made on the objective physical characteristics and location or distribution of one or more lesions that can be seen or felt. Combined with a thorough history, careful physical examination of the skin is paramount in identifying dermatological conditions.[9]

Disorders of the skin are often referred to as rashes or lesions. Rashes are temporary eruptions of the skin such as those associated with heat, childhood diseases, diapers, and drug-induced reactions. A lesion is a pathological or traumatic loss of normal tissue continuity, structure, or function.[10]

Dermatological diseases usually initially present with distinct lesions and have a limited number of clinical manifestations. Many skin diseases and disorders occur in characteristic shapes, arrangements, distributions, and reaction patterns that serve as diagnostic clues.[11] Lesions that are first to appear are called primary lesions, and their identification is the most important aspect of the dermatological physical examination.[9] Macules, patches, papules, plaques, nodules, tumors, wheals, vesicles, bullae, and pustules are all considered primary lesions. Primary lesions may continue to develop or they may be modified by trauma, regression, or other extraneous factors producing secondary lesions. Table 17–1 and Figure 17–1 describe primary lesions

TABLE 17–1   Primary Lesions

Nonpalpable, Flat, Changes in Skin Color	Palpable, Elevated Solid Masses	Superficial Elevations Formed by Fluid Residing in a Cavity between Tissue Layers
Macule—small, up to 1 cm	*Papule*—up to 0.5 cm	*Vesicle*—up to 0.5 cm, filled with serous fluid
Patch—macule larger than 1 cm	*Plaque*—papule with elevated surface larger than 0.5 cm, often formed by coalescence of papules	*Bulla*—vesicle greater than 0.5 cm, filled with serous fluid
	Nodule—range from 0.5 cm to 2 cm, deeper and firmer than papule	*Pustule*—filled with purulent material, variable size
	Tumor—nodule larger than 2 cm	
	Wheal—localized skin edema, irregular, transient, superficial, variable size	

Source: Fitzpatrick TB, Johnson RA, Wolff K. *Color Atlas & Synopsis of Clinical Dermatology.* 4th ed. New York: McGraw-Hill; 2001.

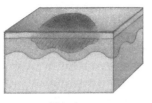

Macule

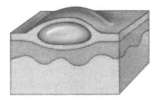

Wheal

FIGURE 17–1   Primary lesions.
Source: Human Diseases: A Systematic Approach, 6/e by Mulvihill/Zelman/ Holdaway/Tomprary/Raymond.

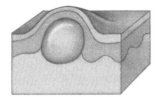

Papule

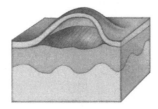

Vesicle or Bulla

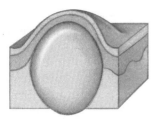

Nodule or Tumor

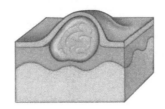

Pustule

according to their clinical presentation and distinctive characteristics. Some primary lesions can be called specialized lesions as they are limited to a few skin diseases. These include burrows, comedones or blackheads, cutaneous horn, follicular plugs, malperforans ulcer, milia, striae cutis distensae, and telangiectasias.[12] Please refer to the glossary for their respective definitions under "Dermatology Terminology."

Primary lesions may progress to secondary lesions. In general, secondary lesions are depressed and manifest below the plane of the skin. Scales, crusts, excoriations/abrasions, fissures, erosions, ulcers, and scars are all considered secondary lesions. Table 17–2 and Figure 17–2 provide the diagnostic characteristics of secondary lesions. Using reaction patterns to describe eruptions, rashes, or skin lesions can assist in formulating a

TABLE 17–2   Secondary Lesions

Lesion	Characteristics
Scales	• Dry or greasy laminated masses of keratin • Pathological exfoliation involving the epidermis • Vary in size and color
Crusts	• Dried blood, serum, or pus mixed with epithelial and bacterial debris • Vary in size, shape, thickness, color, and composition • Commonly referred to as scabs
Excoriations/ abrasions	• Linear or punctate abrasion produced by mechanical trauma, often associated with pruritus and scratching

(continued)

TABLE 17–2   Continued

Lesion	Characteristics
Fissures	• Linear crack or cleft through the epidermis and often into the dermis • Vary in shape, size, and moisture content • Commonly occur in thickened and inelastic skin due to dryness and inflammation
Erosions	• Loss of portions or all of the epidermis only • Heal without scar tissue • Sometimes areas of erosion are referred to as denuded
Ulcers	• Vary in size, shape, and etiology • Excavation involving complete loss of the epidermis and a portion of the dermis • Usually heal with scar formation
Scars	• Collagen and connective tissue that replace lost dermis • Size and shape are dependent upon etiology and level of tissue destruction • Hypertrophic and keloid scars are pathological

Source: Odom RB, James WD, Berger TG. *Andrew's Diseases of the Skin Clinical Dermatology.* 9th ed. Philadelphia: W. B. Saunders; 2000.

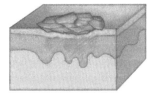

Scale

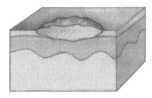

Crust

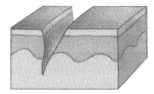

Fissure

FIGURE 17–2   Secondary lesions.

Source: Human Diseases: A Systematic Approach, 6/e by Mulvihill/Zelman/Holdaway/Tomprary/Raymond.

working clinical diagnosis. There are six basic reaction patterns and these are outlined in Table 17–3.

When learning about dermatology, it is important to note seasonal skin diseases, military dermatoses, and dermatoses of non-Caucasian skin, particularly African Americans.[12] See Table 17–4. These are unique conditions affecting the skin that warrant consideration. Certain dermatological conditions have an increased incidence during the seasons of the year and should be considered during skin assessment.

For countries ravaged by war and natural disasters, complications such as lack of personal hygiene, lack of adequate food, overcrowding, injuries and epidemic diseases exacerbate stress and can aggrevate existing skin dermatoses, increasing the incidence of the following dermatological conditions:

- Bacterial dermatoses
- Leishmaniasis
- Miliaria
- Pediculosis
- Pyoderma
- Scabies
- Sexually transmitted diseases
- Tinea (feet, groin)

Certain skin diseases are more prevalent among non-Caucasian people and should be considered during evaluation. Additional information on dermatological considerations in non-Caucasian skin can be found at the end of this chapter.

- Acne keloidalis nuchae
- Acral lentiginous melanomas
- Annular form of secondary syphilis
- Dermatosis papulosa nigra
- Granuloma inguinale
- Keloids
- Mongolian spots
- Pigmentary disturbances
- Pseudofolliculitis barbae
- Pyodermas of lower extremities in children

- Seborrheic dermatitis of scalp (related to greasy hair products)
- Tinea capitas
- Traumatic marginal alopecia

The advantage of dealing with the integumentary system, as opposed to other body systems, is that the disorders associated with the skin can be seen and palpated. Recognizing the basic characteristics of lesions is the first step toward formulating a working clinical diagnosis. Other factors must also be taken under consideration such as the shape and configuration of the lesion(s); the arrangement, distribution, and grouping of lesions; the

TABLE 17–3   Reaction Patterns

Reaction Pattern	Description
Papulosquamous	Eruptions in which the primary lesions consist of macules, papules, or plaques with scales. Examples: psoriasis, tinea corporis and versicolor lichen planus, mycosis fungoides, pityriasis rosea.
Eczematous	Various presentations; often difficult to distinguish from papulosquamous. Examples: Acute, subacute, and chronic eczema (poison ivy, atopic dermatitis, lichen simplex chronicus).
Vesicobullous	Consist of fluid-filled blisters. Examples: shingles, herpes simplex, partial-thickness burns.
Dermal	Confined to the dermis. Examples: cutaneous sarcoidosis, granuloma annulare.
Subcutaneous	Confined to subcutaneous tissue. Examples: lipomas, erythema nodosum.
Vascular	Erythema or edema due to changes in vasculature. Examples: superficial burns, urticarial, vasculitis, drug reaction rashes, erythema multiforme.

Source: Goodheart H. *Photoguide to Common Skin Disorders.* 3rd ed. Philadelphia: Lippincott, Williams & Wilkins; 2009.

TABLE 17–4   Common Dermatoses by Season

Winter	Spring	Summer	Fall
Atopic dermatitis	Acne	Candida intertrigo	Acne
Contact dermatitis	Erythema multiforme	Darier's disease	Atopic eczema
Ichthyosis	Pityriasis rosea	Epidermolysis bullosa	Contact dermatitis
Psoriasis	Viral exanthems	Impetigo	Pityriasis rosea
Seborrheic dermatitis		Insect bites	Senile pruritus
Nummular eczema		Miliaria	Tinea of scalp
Xerosis		Poison ivy contact dermatitis	Winter itch
		Polymorphous light eruption	Viral exanthems
		Tinea (feet, groin)	
		Tinea versicolor	

involution and evolution, which deals with the lesions' state of development; and the color, texture, and consistency of the involved tissue. Good technique, including diligent hand washing and standard precautions, warrants that clinicians wear gloves anytime there is potential exposure to blood or body fluids. Skin lesions that disrupt the integrity of the skin or lesions that bleed or drain fluid should be assessed with gloved hands. This will protect the clinician from direct contact with blood and body fluids, and it will protect the patient from potential cross-contamination. Clinicians are not at risk of contracting systemic disorders that affect the skin, skin cancer, pigmentary disorders, or other noninfectious cutaneous disorders. For more accurate palpation and assessment, snug fitting, latex-free gloves should be utilized during an integumentary examination.

A thorough review of the integumentary system is just as important as a comprehensive cardiopulmonary, musculoskeletal, or neuromuscular systems review. Skin assessment differs from a wound assessment, as the patient's entire body should be examined—not just the wound or lesion(s). Visual and physical inspection should not only include the skin, but the hair and nails as well. To assist the clinician in performing a thorough integumentary examination, the following mnemonic can be utilized: ***DERMATOLOGICAL.*** For a complete description of the mnemonic, please refer to Figure 17–3.

D: Describe integrity

  ➤ Skin is intact or presents with injury

   ▪ Classify type of skin injury and location

   ▪ Describe type, shape, arrangement, distribution of injury/lesions

E: Edema

  ➤ Location

  ➤ Pitting verses non-pitting (non-pitting may indicate lymphatic involvement and/or compromise and warrant further investigation)

   ▪ 1+ = barely perceptible depression, <2 mm

   ▪ 2+ = easily identifiable depression, rebounds in <15 seconds, 2–4 mm

   ▪ 3+ = depression rebounds in 15–30 seconds, 5–7 mm

   ▪ 4+ = depression lasts >30 seconds, >7 mm

R: Review sensory status

  ➤ Intact or altered

   ▪ Location

   ▪ Loss of protective sensation, two-point discrimination, heat/cold, deep pressure, pin prick

M: Moisture

  ➤ Dry or moist to touch

   ▪ Dry—flaking, scales, fissures, cracks (hyperkeratosis, xerosis, eczema, dermatitis, psoriasis, rashes)

   ▪ Moist—sweat, incontinence, weeping edema, wound exudate, effluent from stoma, exogenous in nature (i.e., spilled drink in lap)

A: Atrophic changes

  ➤ Shiny, hairless extremities

  ➤ Warrants a vascular consult/examination

T: Turgor/texture

  ➤ Normal

   ▪ Quickly returns to original state

➤ Slow

■ Diminished return to original state (dehydration, effect of aging)

O: Observe nail composition and hair quality

➤ Nails (can reflect the patient's overall health)

■ Color, shape, contour, clubbing, texture, thickness

➤ Hair

■ Hirsutism: excessive body hair

■ Alopecia: hair loss

L: Look and feel for color and temperature variations

➤ Normally smooth, slightly moist, and relatively same tone throughout

■ Tone depends on patient's melanocytes (skin pigmentation continuum: light ivory, deep brown, black, yellow to olive, light pink to dark ruddy pink, or red)

■ Pigmentation

➤ Pallor—mucosa, conjunctiva, distal extremities

➤ Cyanosis—oral mucosa, conjunctiva, nail beds

➤ Jaundice—sclerae, palates, palms

➤ Hyper- or hypopigmentation—may reflect variations in melanin deposits or blood flow

O: Observe skin folds and between the toes

➤ Look for breakdown (denudement or pressure from pannus), yeast/fungal infections, intertrigo, foreign objects

G: Gerontodermatological changes

➤ Normal skin changes with aging

➤ Risks: skin tears, bruising, senile purpura

I: Inquire about allergies and PMH

➤ Are findings exogenous or endogenous in nature?

C: Callus

➤ Indicates area(s) of high pressure or repetitive stress/trauma

➤ Hemorrhagic callus is indicative of ulceration beneath the callus tissue

A: Assess vascular status

➤ Look, listen, feel

■ Color changes

■ Doppler

■ Palpate pulses, capillary refill

L: Lesions (rashes, scars, bruising, hemosiderin, nevi, etc.)

➤ Document location(s), describe presentation, formulate working clinical diagnosis

FIGURE 17–3   Dermatological: Skin assessment mnemonic.

COMMON DERMATOLOGICAL CONDITIONS ENCOUNTERED BY PHYSICAL THERAPISTS

This section focuses on specific dermatological conditions commonly seen in the physical therapy setting, including eczema and dermatitis, urticaria, psoriasis, benign neoplasms and hyperplasias, cutaneous carcinomas, and cutaneous pigmentary disorders. Additional information is provided on systemic disorders affecting the skin, allergies and adverse cutaneous drug reactions, integumentary infections, and common nail disorders. The chapter concludes with a discussion of normal and abnormal variations in non-Caucasian skin that warrant careful consideration by health care practitioners.

Eczema and Dermatitis

Eczema is an inflammatory skin response to any injurious agent.[10] The terms *eczema* and *dermatitis* are often used interchangeably. However, eczema is more commonly used to denote endogenous disease, and dermatitis is more commonly used for exogenous disorders such as irritant or allergic contact dermatitis.[13] In either case, the pathology involves an inflammatory reaction of the epidermis and dermis. Eczematous diseases can often be differentiated from one another by their clinical symptoms and the course of the disease.[14] Table 17–5 describes the type of dermatitis by location.[15]

Patients generally present with xerosis (dry skin). A common saying is "eczema is the itch that rashes."

The constant scratching leads to a vicious cycle of itch → scratch → rash → itch.[16] The acute presentation is often denoted by poorly defined red patches, papules, and plaques with or without scales. The skin also appears edematous with excoriations from frequent scratching. In contrast, chronic cases present with a thickening of the skin known as lichenification. Chronic cases are more commonly found on the neck, flexor surfaces, eyelids, forehead and face, and dorsa of the hands and feet.[16]

Physical therapists and physical therapist assistants may encounter these conditions frequently, particularly dermatitis. Treatment measures are aimed at identifying and removing the causative agent(s). Clinicians should scrutinize the location of the lesions and identify potential allergens by conducting a thorough history with special consideration to the patient's home and work environment. Oftentimes, simple modifications can be made to prevent and/or reduce the potential for recurrence, such as changing soaps or detergents or having a person wear gloves when handling items that irritate the skin.

If a patient presents to the clinic with a suspected dermatitis, it is best to call the patient's physician to discuss treatment options. Treatment often employs the use of topical corticosteroids, which require a physician's prescription. More severe cases may be managed with moist dressings, systemic medications, and, possibly, oral antihistamines. Dermatitis that begins to weep or drain or presents with bullae is more severe and should be managed with dressings. This will protect the areas involved, manage the exudate, and provide an obstacle to prevent other contaminants

TABLE 17–5   Types of Dermatitis

Type	Description	Treatment Considerations
Allergic	• Erythema commonly found on the eyelids	• Determine irritant and avoid exposure.
		• Consider makeup as a possible irritant.
Contact	• Localized erythema common on the hands.	• Determine irritant and avoid exposure.
Hand	• Persistent erythema with scaling on the digits/palms.	• Topical steroids.
Seborrheic	• Erythematous, scaly eruptions on the face, scalp, and body.	• Topical hydrocortisones and tar-containing shampoos.
Stasis	• Erythema, pigment changes, thickening of the skin, and dependent edema.	• Leg elevation, support stockings, exercise, topical and/or systemic management.

Source: Resnick B. Dermatologic problems in the elderly. *Lippincott's Primary Care Practice.* 1997;1(1):14–30.

from entering the tissues. Saline-moistened gauze is usually sufficient unless the physician orders an antimicrobial solution to be used.

Urticaria

Urticaria, commonly known as hives, presents with pruritic edematous wheals that may be pink or red. The most common mediator of urticaria is histamine. A variety of immunological, nonimmunological, chemical, and physical stimuli can cause the release of histamine into the surrounding tissues and circulation, leading to the formation of urticaria.[10] Urticaria may be acute or chronic. Acute urticaria is most commonly associated with foods, medications, or exposure to allergens or chemicals. If daily, or almost daily, episodes of urticaria persist for longer than 6 weeks, then the condition is considered chronic.[10] It is important for physical therapists to recognize the clinical features of physical urticaria, because some patients may develop a reaction after the application of a modality or manual intervention. For example, a patient may develop a reaction with the use of a cold pack or ice massage due to cold-induced urticaria. Other patients may develop reactions to adhesives used to secure electrodes. Therefore, it is important not only to ask the patient about any known reactions, but also to test a small area prior to the use or application of a new modality. Table 17–6 describes the types of physical urticarias and their associated clinical features.

Physicians typically prescribe the use of antihistamines to treat urticaria, although severe urticaria is treated with epinephrine. Colloid or starch baths may also be used to reduce the associated pruritus.[10, 16] Most of the time, urticaria will spontaneously resolve after the offending agent is removed. Patients with chronic urticaria should be examined and treated by a physician.

Psoriasis

Psoriasis is a chronic, recurrent, inflammatory disease of the skin that affects up to 2% of the population in Western countries.[9, 16] The cause of the disease is unknown, although the tendency to develop psoriasis is inherited. The disease is characterized by round, circumscribed, erythematous, dry, scaling plaques of various sizes that are covered by silvery white scales. The disease has a predilection to develop plaques on the scalp, nails, extensor surfaces of the extremities, elbows, knees, umbilical region, and sacral region.[9] The pathogenesis of psoriasis involves an alteration of the cell kinetics of keratinocytes. The cell cycle is

TABLE 17–6   Clinical Features of Physical Urticaria

Type	Clinical Features
Cholinergic	• Presents as small wheals surrounded by bright red flares and intense pruritus • Develops in response to a rise in core temperature, as with external heat, exercise, emotion, or eating spicy foods • Duration, 1–2 hours
Cold	• Appears red or pale, swollen and pruritic • Presents at site of contact with cold water, air, or surfaces • Duration, 30–60 minutes
Dermographism	• Presents as pruritic linear wheals with a bright red flare • Results from stroking or scratching the skin • Duration, 15–30 minutes
Pressure	• Presents as large, painful, or pruritic swelling at a site of pressure • Appears 1–4 hours after pressure application and may last >24 hours
Solar	• Presents as pale or red swelling that is pruritic • Results from exposure to ultraviolet light

Source: Porth C. *Pathophysiology: Concepts of Altered Health States.* 7th ed. Philadelphia: Lippincott, Williams & Wilkins; 2005.

reduced from 311 hours to 36 hours, which results in 28 times the normal production of epidermal cells.[16]

Psoriasis can be classified as either nonpustular or pustular. Pustular psoriasis involves the development of pustules, typically on the palms and soles. However, it may involve the entire surface of the skin, which can be a severe, life-threatening course. Patients may also present with psoriatic arthritis, a chronic, destructive arthritis that mainly involves the interphalangeal joints, the spine, and large joints. Over time, severe deformities can ensue, leading to functional limitations.[16]

Currently, there is no cure for psoriasis; however, with treatment the disease can be converted from an active to a latent state. Treatment may involve systemic or topical interventions prescribed by a physician. Systemic therapy is limited to patients with severe disease whose symptoms require more aggressive measures. Retinoids, topical corticosteroid applications, systemic corticosteroids, and immunosuppressive agents, such as cyclosporin A and methotrexate, are often employed for severe psoriatic episodes.[14] Less severe forms of psoriasis are often managed by a combination of therapeutic interventions. Salicylic Vaseline and colloidal baths help to reduce the thick scales. Physicians typically prescribe topical medications (e.g., anthralin, triamcinolone) to manage the lesions. Oftentimes, dermatologists are the best health care professionals to manage a patient with psoriasis, for they have extensive experience with topical therapies. Because many of these topical agents can have deleterious side effects with long-term use, patients must be closely monitored by a physician.

Coal tar products and ultraviolet (UV) therapy have antiproliferative effects on keratinocytes. Coal tar products, although effective, can be malodorous and stain the skin and clothing. Physical therapists or dermatologists may use UV therapy. This can be implemented as selective ultraviolet (SUV) therapy with long-wave UV-B light or as photochemotherapy, with a combination of a photosensitizing drug and UV-A light (PUVA).[14] Dermatologists generally carry out the photochemotherapy treatments because of drug administration.

The interventions selected to manage psoriasis are dependent upon the site(s), severity, and duration of the lesions; previous treatments; and the age of the patient. It is important for clinicians to recognize the lesions associated with psoriasis and, if necessary, to direct the patient with an exacerbation to a dermatologist for management.

Benign Neoplasms and Hyperplasias

Benign neoplasms and hyperplasias is a broad classification of a variety of skin conditions. It is important for clinicians to be aware of these benign cutaneous presentations and to be able to differentiate these from malignancies or other cutaneous diseases that require immediate medical management. All skin lesions and pigmentation changes should be monitored and assessed regularly. The American Academy of Dermatology and the Skin Cancer Foundation recommend using the ABCDE method to help detect melanoma: A (most early melanomas are *asymmetrical*); B (*borders* of melanomas are uneven); C (*color;* shades of brown, tan, or black are often the first sign of melanoma); D (*diameter;* melanomas tend to grow larger than common moles, 6 mm or greater); and E (*elevation or evolving;* raised above the skin and has an uneven surface and/or any change in size, shape, color, or another trait, or any new symptom such as bleeding, crusting or itching). This simple mnemonic can assist patients and clinicians in identifying lesions that warrant further examination by a physician. For additional information and photographs depicting these changes, please visit www.skincancer.org.

This section reviews the clinical presentation of melanocytic nevi and mongolian spots; capillary hemangiomas, port-wine stains, and cherry angiomas; seborrheic keratosis and skin tags; and lipomas and dermatofibromas, as these are the most common benign neoplasms and hyperplasias that may present in the clinical environment. In most cases, treatment of these benign lesions is not indicated; however, these lesions should be identified and monitored over the course of the patient's life for changes that may be indicative of serious pathology that requires medical attention. More often than not, treatment for cosmetic reasons results in a scar that is less cosmetically acceptable than the initial lesion. Patients should discuss treatment options with their primary care physician or seek a referral to a dermatologist.

Nevi and Mongolian Spots

Melanocytic nevi and mongolian spots are disorders of melanocytes. Nevi, commonly referred to as moles, appear in early childhood and peak in young adulthood. By the third and fourth decade of life, most Caucasian adults present with approximately 30–50 nevi.[14, 16] Typically, nevomelanocytic nevi develop slowly and present as light to dark brown, flat or round tumors, with or without hair, 1–2 mm in size.[14]

It is important to distinguish these nevi from malignant melanomas. Nevi that develop rapidly, change in size or color, weep, bleed, or present with pruritus should be referred to a dermatologist or the patient's primary care physician to determine if the nevi are a form of malignant melanoma.[14, 16]

Mongolian spots are congenital blue-gray macular lesions typically found on the lumbosacral area. These lesions are almost always found (99–100%) in infants of Native American and Asian origin.[16] Mongolian spots disappear in early childhood. It is important for the clinician to recognize mongolian spots so as not to confuse these lesions with bruising or concerns of potential child abuse. For a color photograph of a Mongolian spot, please refer to the accompanying Website.

Capillary Hemangiomas, Port-Wine Stains, and Cherry Angiomas

Capillary hemangiomas, port-wine stains, and cherry angiomas are disorders of blood vessels. Capillary hemangiomas occur almost exclusively in children at or soon after birth, and they disappear spontaneously by the fifth year of life. Capillary hemangiomas are soft, bright red to deep purple, vascular nodules or plaques.[14, 16] These common benign lesions often distress parents because of their cosmetic appearance.

Port-wine stains (clinically termed *nevus flammeus*) are irregularly shaped, red, macular, vascular malformations of dermal blood vessels that present at birth. These lesions do not spontaneously resolve except for the type called median nevus flammeus or "stork bite."[14, 16] Typically, port-wine stains present on the neck, middle of the forehead, glabella, or eyelids.[16] Lateral nevus flammeus may progressively worsen in appearance over the course of the patient's life; however, in most cases, treatment is unnecessary. Like mongolian spots, port-wine stains should not be mistaken for burns or signs of abuse.

Cherry angiomas are very common, asymptomatic, bright red, domed vascular lesions that are typically found on the trunk. These tiny to small benign tumors are commonly seen in older patients; however, they are not of clinical significance other than cosmesis.[16]

Seborrheic Keratosis and Skin Tags

Seborrheic keratosis is the most common of the benign epithelial tumors, particularly in elderly patients.[16] Initially flat, these are well-demarcated, small, brown-pigmented areas. Over time, they can become raised and darker in color with a soft, crumbly surface.[14] In most cases, seborrheic keratoses are harmless consequences of aging, and treatment is not indicated unless a malignant tumor cannot be excluded.[14] If a patient presents with a suspicious lesion, the clinician should refer the patient for examination by a physician for definitive diagnosis. Similarly, skin tags, also known as cutaneous papillomas or fibromas, are commonly seen in older patients, as well as patients who are obese. These are soft, round, skin-color or tan or brown benign tumors that can range in size from less than 1 mm to as large as 10 mm.[14] Other than cosmetic implications, these tumors do not pose a threat to the patient or warrant medical treatment. Clinicians should exercise caution when treating areas with skin tags, particularly when using modalities or manual techniques, to avoid torsion to or rupture of the tumor.

Lipomas and Dermatofibromas

Lipomas and dermatofibromas are also important for clinicians to recognize, as they can be misdiagnosed for other more serious lesions. Lipomas are benign tumors of fatty tissue that can present as single or multiple lesions.[14, 16] Lipomas develop slowly and they are soft, rounded, and movable beneath overlying skin. The cause is unknown; however, in certain regions the fat herniates through the tissue layers. Lipomas should not be mistaken for metastatic tumors or malignant cysts, which can be definitively determined by biopsy. In contrast to lipomas, metastatic tumors and malignant cysts often have associated pain, develop rapidly, and may present with ulcerations.

Dermatofibromas are button-like dermal nodules commonly found on the extremities.[16] They may be domed or depressed below the plane of surrounding skin. When pigmented, these lesions can be mistaken for malignant melanoma. A classic finding is the "dimple sign" where lateral compression with the thumb and index finger produces a dimpling effect with the lesion. In contrast, melanomas will not have a positive dimple sign. Treatment for dermatofibromas is not indicated other than for cosmesis.

Skin Cancers

The American Cancer Society has reported an alarming increase of skin cancers over the past several decades. Exposure to UV radiation, harsh weather conditions, leisure-time activities in the sun, and the decrease in the ozone layer all contribute to this rise.[17] The incidence of skin cancer in individuals with black skin is relatively low, 3.4 per 100,000, compared with 232.6 per 100,000 whites.[17] There are many types of skin cancer, including basal cell carcinoma, squamous cell carcinoma, malignant melanoma, and Kaposi's sarcoma, all of which have further subcategories. It is imperative that clinicians are able to recognize and differentiate skin cancers from other cutaneous lesions so patients can be appropriately referred and treated. Box 17–2 outlines the criteria of suspicious lesions/tumors. A patient presenting with a suspicious lesion should be referred to his or her primary care physician for a biopsy of the lesion. A biopsy will determine whether the lesion is benign or malignant and help to direct the course of care.

Basal Cell Carcinoma

The most common form of skin cancer is basal cell carcinoma (BCC). Basal cell carcinoma has a limited capacity to metastasize. However, these malignant tumors must be treated aggressively, as they can extend widely and deeply, destroying skin, cartilage, and bone.[10, 14] The majority of these tumors (80%) presents on the head, neck, and face, where sun exposure is common.

Nodular ulcerative BCC is the most common type of BCC. It begins as a small, pink or flesh-colored, smooth, translucent nodule that enlarges over time, causing the center of the lesion to become depressed.[10] Oftentimes, the central depression progresses to an ulcer. The lesions can also become keratotic. This can make them difficult to distinguish from normal aged skin because keratosis is a typical finding on aged skin. The next most common form is superficial BCC. Often seen on the back or chest, superficial BCC is difficult to diagnose because it mimics other dermatological conditions. These lesions begin as flat, nonpalpable, erythematous plaques, which slowly enlarge, producing nodular margins and telangiectatic bases.[10]

Squamous Cell Carcinoma

Squamous cell carcinoma (SCC) is the second most common form of skin cancer and represents about 20% of cutaneous malignancies. Most patients who develop one SCC have a 40% risk of developing additional tumors within the next 2 years; therefore, patients with a history of SCC should be evaluated with a complete skin examination every 6–12 months. The risk of nodal or distant metastasis for SCC primary tumors is reported to be 2–6%.[18] Squamous cell carcinoma is a malignant tumor involving the outer epidermis. These tumors metastasize more readily than BCC. Two types of SCC exist: intraepidermal and invasive. Intraepidermal SCC remains confined to the epidermis. At some point in time, it may penetrate into the dermis and metastasize to the regional lymph nodes.[10] At such time, the lesion is considered invasive SCC. Squamous cell carcinomas are keratotic, scaly, elevated lesions with irregular borders and shallow central ulcers. The lesions often appear "meaty" as with hypergranulation tissue. As with BCC, treatment is aimed at the removal of all the cancerous tissue.

All suspicious lesions are biopsied to confirm a diagnosis. Treatment is aimed at complete elimination of the lesion but is contingent on the site and extent of the lesion. Treatment is generally surgical or with cryotherapy performed by physicians. Optimally, function and cosmesis are maintained. It is imperative that patients are checked at regular intervals to assess for recurrence of either BCC or SCC.

Malignant Melanoma

Malignant melanoma is a rapidly progressing, metastatic form of cancer involving the melanocytes.[10] The incidence of malignant melanoma has increased tenfold over the last 40 years.[14] Early recognition of the tumor is essential because the patient's chance of survival is increased with early treatment. The prognosis of melanoma is dependent upon the thickness of the tumor and the level of invasion into the surrounding tissues.

Malignant melanomas differ in shape and size and they can appear anywhere on the body. They present with irregular borders, uneven surfaces, and black or brown discoloration. At times, these lesions bleed and/or ulcerate. The surrounding area is typically red, inflamed, and tender. Dark melanomas are often mottled with white, blue, and red hues representing three concurrent processes: scar tissue formation (white), melanoma growth (blue), and inflammation (red) as the body attempts to localize and destroy the tumor.[10]

Four different morphological types of melanoma have been identified: superficial spreading, lentigo maligna, nodular, and acral-lentiginous.[9, 10, 14] Superficial spreading melanoma accounts for approximately 70% of all melanomas. Typically, it is a flat tumor with a tendency for multicoloration. These tumors are mainly found on the trunk and extremities, and they grow at moderate speed. In addition, these tumors bleed and ulcerate with growth.[9, 10, 14] Lentigo maligna melanoma accounts for 5% of all melanomas, and these tumors occur almost exclusively on the face of older individuals who have had excessive exposure to sunlight. These tumors are slow-growing with irregular borders. They begin as tan macules that gradually darken and spread.[10, 14] Nodular melanoma, which accounts for 16% of all melanomas, is a black to dark brown tumor that grows vertically and horizontally in a nodular fashion.[14] These tumors have a poor prognosis, as they metastasize rapidly. The last type of melanoma is acral-lentiginous melanoma, which accounts for 5–10% of all melanomas. These tumors typically present on the hands and feet, but also appear in nail beds and mucous membranes. Typically, these lesions present as brown patches that spread horizontally.

All tumors that are suspicious of melanoma are surgically excised along with at least a 3-mm margin of healthy tissue to ensure no metastases are present.[14] Treatment measures are dependent upon the severity of the tumor, the location, and its clinical presentation. Skin grafts may be required to repair the deep and wide excisions used to remove the cancer. Immunotherapy, chemotherapy, or radiation therapy may be initiated if the disease metastasizes.[10]

Kaposi's Sarcoma

Kaposi's sarcoma (KS) is a malignancy of the endothelial cells that line small blood vessels.[10] Seroepidemiological evidence exists that may link KS with human herpes virus 8.[16] KS has many clinical variants including classic or European KS, African-endemic KS, immunosuppression-associated KS, and HIV-associated KS. Table 17–7 describes the clinical variants of KS.

TABLE 17–7 Clinical Variants of Kaposi's Sarcoma

Type	Description
Classic or European	• Seen in elderly males of eastern European heritage • Predominantly on the lower extremities, but also lymph nodes and abdominal viscera • Progresses slowly
African-endemic	• Non-HIV-associated • Four clinical patterns: (1) nodular, (2) florid or vegetating, (3) infiltrative, (4) lymphadenopathic
Immunosuppression-associated	• Seen in patients with cancer treated with cytotoxic chemotherapy or recipients of renal transplants • Resolves with cessation of immunosuppression
HIV-associated	• Associated with HIV infection • Extensive systemic involvement • Rapid progression

Source: Fitzpatrick TB, Johnson RA, Wolff K. *Color Atlas and Synopsis of Clinical Dermatology.* 4th ed. New York: McGraw-Hill; 2001.

Regardless of the type, KS generally begins as an ecchymotic-like macule that evolves into papules, plaques, nodules, and tumors. They appear red, pink, or tan and become purple-brown with a green hemosiderin halo over time.[16] Most KS lesions are palpable and they may be local or widespread. Widespread distribution on the lower extremities is often accompanied by lymphedema due to the deep involvement of the lymphatics and lymph nodes.[16]

The lesions associated with KS are not open or ulcerated, and treatment of the lesions themselves usually involves keeping the area dry and clean. No direct interventions are employed, as treatment is aimed at controlling the symptoms of the disease. Furthermore, the lesions are not contagious and HIV cannot be transmitted by contact with KS. It is also important to confirm the diagnosis of KS, as many cutaneous manifestations can mimic the appearance of KS, such as dermatofibromas, hemangiomas, melanocytic nevi, and even stasis dermatitis.[16] As with all suspicious cutaneous lesions, appropriate referral should be made for diagnosis and subsequent management.

Cutaneous Pigmentary Disorders

Normal skin color is composed of four biochromes: (1) melanin (brown), (2) carotenoids (yellow; exogenous from diet), (3) oxyhemoglobin (red), and (4) reduced hemoglobin (blue).[16] Skin color results from a combination of these biochromes. However, the total amount of melanin is the principal determinant. Pigmentary skin disorders are worthy of discussion because of the emotional distress and social stigma these disorders can cause. All pigmentary disorders are the result of altered melanin production. The most common pigmentary disorders are albinism, vitiligo, melasma, ephilides, and letigines.

Albinism

Albinism is a congenital disorder affecting the skin, hair, and eyes. Individuals with albinism have a normal number of melanocytes, but they lack the enzyme, tyrosinase, needed for the synthesis of melanin. Individuals present with pale or pink skin, yellow or white hair, and light-colored eyes. Many also have a variety of ocular problems and are extremely sensitive to light. Because people with albinism are highly susceptible to sunburn and cutaneous damage from UV exposure, measures must be taken to protect the skin from the sun.[10, 16]

Vitiligo

Vitiligo is a pigmentary problem that appears in all races and affects up to 1% of the general population.[16] The lesion is a macular depigmentation (loss of melanocytes) with distinct borders on the face, neck, axillae, and extremities.[16] The etiology is unknown, although it appears to be inherited. It has also been found to be more prevalent in people with thyroid disease, pernicious anemia, and diabetes mellitus.[10, 16] Vitiligo is a chronic disease with a highly variable course. Up to 30% of patients may experience some spontaneous repigmentation, particularly in areas that are exposed to the sun.[16] Spontaneous repigmentation is not completely understood, and it is suspected that a few melanocytes may be dormant in the area to enable repigmentation to occur. Tattooing, makeup, controlled UV exposure, and, at times, surgery are employed as treatment interventions. Patients should be referred to dermatologists for consultation if they are concerned about cosmesis and want to consider cosmetic interventions.

Melasma

Melasma is an acquired light or brown hyperpigmentation that presents most frequently on the face. It is commonly associated with exposure to sunlight, pregnancy, or ingestion of oral contraceptive hormones. However, many cases are idiopathic.[16] Melasma may disappear spontaneously after the cessation of oral contraceptives or childbirth, but it may return with subsequent pregnancies. Because sun exposure can exacerbate the condition, patients should use sunblocks or sunscreens.

Ephilides

Commonly known as freckles, ephilides indicate skin damage from sun exposure. The sun damage causes the melanocytes to become hyperreactive to sunlight.[19] The excess melanin produces results in the formation of a freckle. Although benign, all freckles should be monitored for subtle changes that could indicate a more serious pathology such as skin cancer.

Lentigines

Lentigines, or liver spots, are small brown lesions that occur anywhere on the body that is frequently exposed to the sun.[19] The most common locations for lentigines include the back of the hands, neck, and face. Lentigines are the result of excessive sun exposure and not due to aging as commonly believed.

Systemic Disorders

Certain systemic disorders can involve the integumentary system. Lupus erythematosus and scleroderma are of particular importance for rehabilitation professionals, as patients with these diseases often require physical therapy for nonintegumentary complications. Adverse drug reactions may also cause cutaneous dysfunction. It is important for clinicians to recognize the associated cutaneous complications that can arise from both systemic diseases and adverse drug reactions to hasten referral to physicians and specialists.

Lupus Erythematosus

Systemic lupus erythematosus (SLE) is a serious progressive disease mainly involving the internal organs. SLE primarily affects young women, manifesting in a wide range of signs and symptoms. Cutaneous involvement is present in 80% of the cases of SLE and it is helpful in distinguishing SLE from other disease states.[14, 16] The cutaneous symptoms associated with SLE include the characteristic facial "butterfly rash" and erythematous changes involving the nail folds. The trunk may have macular eruptions, and lesions may be present on the oral mucosa. Patients with SLE may be referred to physical therapy because of the associated symptoms of this generalized disease. Polyarthritis, polymyositis, nephritis, myo- and pericarditis, and central nervous system dysfunction are common symptoms, and patients report varying levels of malaise and fatigue.[14]

In contrast, discoid lupus erythematosus (DLE) is a chronic dermatological disease, without organ involvement, that may last for months or years. DLE primarily involves the neck and face; however, the trunk, upper extremities, and hands may be involved following sun exposure. The skin lesions appear as psoriasiform or annular. The psoriasiform lesions are well demarcated with slight scaling. They evolve into bright red plaques. Annular lesions are bright red with minimal scaling and have a slight depression centrally.[16] The skin lesions are transient and the eruptions may last a day to several weeks, and resolve without scarring.[9]

Sunscreens, sunblocks, and protective clothing are essential for all cutaneous involvement related to lupus, as the sun can cause cutaneous exacerbations. Topical therapies, such as corticosteroids, may be prescribed for skin lesions pending the severity. Generally, the disease dictates the appropriate course of care prescribed by the physician.

Scleroderma

Scleroderma is a slow, progressive, incurable, multisystem disorder that involves the skin and internal organs, primarily the lungs, heart, and gastrointestinal tract. The skin and internal organs undergo inflammatory, vascular, and sclerotic changes.[14, 16] The skin appears hard and smooth and often presents with hypopigmented areas that are immobile or feel "bound down." Sixty percent of patients with scleroderma have limited systemic scleroderma (lSSc), while 40% present with diffuse systemic scleroderma (dSSc). Limited systemic scleroderma presents with a long history of Raynaud's phenomenon and skin involvement limited to the feet, hands, forearms, and face.[16] It also includes the CREST syndrome, which involves the following clinical variants: *c*alcinosis cutis + *R*aynaud's phenomenon + *e*sophageal dysfunction + *s*clerodactyly + *t*elangiectasia.[14, 16] In contrast, patients with dSSc have a rapid onset of symptoms and diffuse involvement of the hands, feet, trunk, and face and present with synovitis, tenosynovitis, and an early onset of internal involvement.[16]

Patients with scleroderma benefit from daily general exercise and physical therapy that emphasize range of motion, therapeutic massage, and gentle warming modalities. Therapeutic massage and warming modalities facilitate tissue extensibility and help manage the fibrotic changes associated with scleroderma. Cold exposure and smoking (vasoconstriction) should be avoided.[9] The majority of patients with scleroderma requires medical management involving systemic medications.

Adverse Cutaneous Drug Reactions

Cutaneous drug reactions are nontherapeutic deleterious effects of a prescribed or over-the-counter medication.[11] Generally, the symptoms are transient and mild, accompanied by pruritus, and resolve promptly after the offending drug is discontinued.[16] Cutaneous drug reactions can mimic nearly all the morphological expressions in dermatology and must be first considered in the differential diagnosis of a rapidly appearing symmetrical skin eruption.[11, 16] At times, however, cutaneous drug reactions can develop into life-threatening diseases, such as toxic epidermal necrolysis (TENS), Stevens–Johnson syndrome (SJS), erythema multiforme minor, or anaphylactic reactions. Drug reactions may be allergic (immunological) or nonallergic (toxic). Allergic-type drug reactions are not dose dependent and are classified as four types of immunological reactions:

- Type I: classic immediate hypersensitivity
- Type II: cytotoxic
- Type III: immune complex
- Type IV: delayed hypersensitivity

Nonallergic drug reactions are the most common type of drug-related eruptions and they may be idiosyncratic or dose related.[11] Although physical therapists do not prescribe medications, early identification of adverse reactions and communication with the referring physician can hasten recovery and prevent serious complications.

Drug-induced cutaneous side effects can vary and cause any type of skin lesion. Ninety-five percent of all drug-induced reactions involve maculopapular rashes, urticarial and angio-edema, and the spectrum of rashes such as erythema multiforme, Stevens–Johnson syndrome, toxic epidermal necrolysis, and fixed drug eruptions.[19] Whenever drugs are suspected to be the causative agent, a thorough and accurate history must ensue. Of particular importance is the type of drug, the time in which the drug was first given, and the point when the symptoms initially began. For example, sulfa-based drugs (sulfonamides) and penicillin are often used in wound management. One of the main problems with these medications is the potential for allergic reactions. Skin rashes, hives, itching, and, at times, difficulty breathing may be induced in patients who are hypersensitive to penicillin.[20] If allowed to progress, anaphylactic reactions may occur. Similarly, the most common reactions to sulfonamide drugs are allergic reactions, gastrointestinal distress, and photosensitivity.[20] More life-threatening reactions may ensue if the medication is not discontinued. A clinician should suspect an adverse cutaneous drug reaction if a patient presents with rapidly appearing skin lesions and/or reports that the lesions began shortly after the initiation of a new topical or systemic medication. Table 17–8 provides an overview of the most common cutaneous rashes caused by drugs.

Rehabilitation professionals may be the first health care providers to notice the reaction or be informed of the reaction by the patient. Objective, subjective, and historical findings should be immediately communicated to the patient's primary care physician. The physician will determine whether to discontinue the drug and/or consider less reactive, alternative medications to manage the patient's condition.

TABLE 17–8   Cutaneous Rashes Caused by Drugs

Cutaneous Eruption	Description	Medications Commonly Associated with Cutaneous Eruption
Acneiform	• Acne-like on any part of the body • Lesions appear suddenly	Anticonvulsant medications, lithium, oral contraceptives, prednisone
Exfoliative dermatitis	• Large areas of skin become scaly and erythematous; slough off • Associated with systemic infections and reactions • May follow other drug eruptions	Gold compounds, penicillin, sulfa drugs, vitamin A
Epidermal necrolysis	• Painful erythema that may blister • Epidermis peels in sheets • Skin appears scalded • Most serious skin eruption, 30% of cases result in death due to secondary infection or from fluid loss	Ibuprofen, penicillin, sulfa drugs
Fixed drug eruption	• Red lesions with well-demarcated borders • Propensity to reappear at same site each time causative drug is reintroduced	Acetaminophen, aspirin, codeine, morphine, penicillin, sulfa drugs, tetracycline

TABLE 17–8 Continued

Urticaria	• Hives with intense pruritus • Edematous, flat lesions • Sudden onset, resolves within 24 hours after offending drug has been discontinued	Aspirin, codeine, ibuprofen, morphine, penicillin, sulfa drugs
Maculopapular	• Flat, erythematous lesions with extensive involvement • Appear within 1 week after initiation of causative drug • Resolve 1–2 weeks after offending drug has been discontinued • Pruritus may or may not be present	Allopurinol, amoxicillin, ampicillin, sulfa drugs
Photosensitive	• Fluid-filled lesions and superficial sunburn • Require the presence of sunlight combined with the offending drug to occur	Anticonvulsants, antipsychotics, ibuprofen, naproxen, sulfa drugs, tetracycline
Purpura	• Small purplish hemorrhages under the skin	Coumadin, diuretics, penicillin, sulfa drugs
Stevens-Johnson	• Small blisters primarily affecting the mucous membranes • May be accompanied by fatigue and fever • Most common type of severe drug eruption • Mortality estimated between 5% and 18%	Barbiturates, lithium, penicillin, sulfa drugs

Source: Zelman M, Tompary E, Raymond J, Holdaway P,Mulvihill M. *Human Diseases: A Systemic Approach.* 7th ed. Upper Saddle River, NJ: Pearson Prentice Hall; 2010.

 Checkpoint Question #1

You are preparing your patient, Ms. G, for an ultrasound treatment to the right lumbar paraspinals when you notice red patches on her skin. On further inspection, you notice that her entire trunk is affected and that there are several excoriated areas.

a. What dermatological condition may these findings represent?
b. What questions would you ask this patient about these findings?
c. What actions should you suggest to the patient?
d. Should you continue with your ultrasound treatment? Defend your answer.

Common Integumentary Infections

The skin is the first line of defense against the environment and sources of infection. Infections are caused by bacteria, viruses, fungi, or parasites and generally occur from a disruption in the skin's integrity. Infections may also spread hematogenously from distant sources within the body.[21] Bacterial, viral, and fungal infections are as numerous as they are diverse.

This section focuses on common bacterial, viral, and fungal skin infections, their clinical presentations, and treatment options.

Bacterial Infections

The most common bacterial skin infections encountered in the clinical setting are impetigo, ecthyma, abscesses, furuncles, carbuncles, and cellulitis.

Impetigo and Ecthyma

The bacteria *Staphylococcus aureus* and *Streptococcus pyogenes* can cause superficial infections of the epidermis (impetigo) or extend into the dermis (ecthyma). The lesions associated with these infections present as crusted erosions or ulcers.[16] Impetigo is one of the most common skin infections in children and infants. It often occurs after injury to the skin or subsequent to existing skin conditions such as atopic dermatitis, eczema, or scabies, where the skin's integrity and ability to protect are compromised. Other epidemiological factors such as warm weather, humidity, young age, prior antibiotic use, poor hygiene, neglect, and crowded living conditions have been implicated in the development of impetigo.[16, 21] Impetigo can manifest as bullous or nonbullous. Bullous impetigo is the most common form and presents with blistering. After several days, the blisters rupture and leave crusted erosions that may last several days to weeks. Impetigo occurs most frequently on the exposed parts of the body such as the face, neck, extremities, and hands. Impetigo is diagnosed by a culture and gram stain, and treated with systemic and topical antibiotics prescribed by a physician. Dressings can be used to protect the areas from scratching, trauma, and other exogenous threats. Standard precautions should be taken to protect both the patient and clinician from cross-contamination.

Ecthyma is a deeper ulcer with a yellow-green crust that extends into the dermis. Lesions begin as a pustule or vesicle on an erythematous base and develop into ulcers with crusting and a violaceous halo. These lesions are painful and are frequently found on the lower extremities of debilitated individuals.[21] The lesions may persist for weeks or months and often result in a scar due to dermal involvement. Diagnosis is confirmed with a culture and gram stain. Treatment involves the use of penicillinase-resistant antibiotics specific against the pathogens *S. aureus* and *S. pyogenes*.[21]

Abscess, Furuncle, Carbuncle

These lesions generally arise from an *S. aureus* infection and represent a continuum of severity. An abscess may arise in any structure or organ of the body. Those present on the skin may originate in the dermis, subcutaneous adipose, muscle, or deeper structures.[16] An abscess usually starts as a tender red nodule. Over time, purulent material develops centrally and is characterized by fluctuance (boggy feel with palpation).

Furuncles (boils) are firm tender nodules in the dermis or subcutaneous tissue near hair follicles. The lesions present with a central necrotic plug filled with purulent material.[16, 21] Furuncles are generally located in hair-bearing regions such as the scalp and posterior neck, beard area, axillae, and buttocks. They range in size from 1 to 2 cm in diameter and may present as a single lesion or in clusters.

Carbuncles are deep extensions of two or more coalescing furuncles.[18] They have interconnecting sinuses and are red, tender, and indurated. They drain purulent material. Patients with these lesions may also experience malaise, fever, chills, and pain. Carbuncles tend to recur despite treatment and often warrant surgical excision to reduce the chance of recurrence.[18]

With all these lesions, moist heat is often applied to promote consolidation and hasten drainage. If the use of heat does not promote consolidation and drainage, an incision and drainage combined with the use of systemic antibiotics should be considered. Topical ointments and basic dressings such as gauze or foams may also be employed to protect the lesion from further trauma and exogenous threats.

Cellulitis

Cellulitis is an acute infection of the dermis and subcutaneous tissues. Cellulitis presents with localized tenderness, induration, fever, malaise, chills, and regional adenopathy.[18] Necrosis and bulla formation may occur, which could result in extensive epidermal sloughing and erosion. Abscess formation and necrotizing fasciitis may also ensue. Cellulitis can be severe, and it often warrants hospitalization and the use of systemic antibiotics prescribed by a physician. Superficial debridement, application of topical medications, and bandages may be administered by physical therapists under the order of the treating physician. Whirlpool is generally discouraged because of the dependency and the potential to exacerbate the existing infection.

Viral Infections: Varicella-Zoster

The varicella-zoster virus (VZV) is a human herpes virus that is responsible for both chickenpox and shingles.[16, 22] Chickenpox is the primary infection and is most common in children less than 10 years old. These lesions are pruritic macules or papules that become vesicles on an erythematous base. Chickenpox is spread through airborne particles or by contact. After the primary infection, the virus lies dormant in the dorsal root ganglia.[22] The virus can become "reactivated" through illness or stress, and it travels along the sensory nerve to the skin and mucosal surfaces it innervates. This is known as zoster or shingles. These lesions present in crops with erythematous papules and vesicles along a dermatome that corresponds to the dorsal root ganglion containing the latent virus.[22] Patients may be left with severe residual pain known as postherpetic neuralgia, even after the lesions have healed.

Treatment for varicella involves the use of antiviral agents. Shingles also responds well to systemic corticosteroids. Pain interventions may be indicated to manage the discomfort associated with postherpetic neuralgia. In both chickenpox and shingles, the course of the virus is self-limiting. Although these lesions do not require direct interventions, physical therapists and physical therapist assistants may use modalities such as TENS to assist patients with postherpetic neuralgia.

Fungal Infections

Superficial fungal infections are the most common of all mucocutaneous infections. These infections are often caused by an overgrowth of resident or transient flora and changes in the microenvironment of the skin.[16] Dermatophytes are fungal organisms that have an affinity for epidermal keratin, including the stratum corneum, nails, and hair.[16, 22] Dermatophytic genera that lead to fungal infections include *Trichophyton, Microsporum,* and *Epidermophyton.*[16, 22]

Tinea Pedis

Tinea pedis, or athlete's foot, is the most common dermatophyte infection. This infection involves the interdigital spaces and plantar surface of the feet. It is characterized by erythema, pruritus, scaling, maceration, and/or bulla formation.[16] The infection can present on other parts of the body, and it is named accordingly: inguinal area (tinea cruris), trunk (tinea corporis), face (tinea faciale), scalp (tinea capitis), and hands (tinea mannum).

Tinea pedis can be contracted by walking barefoot or by wearing occlusive footwear that harbors a warm, moist environment conducive for fungal growth. The arthrospores can survive in skin scales for up to 1 year.[16, 22] Wearing clean, dry socks and shoes, and

cleansing and drying between the toes are the most effective means to prevent tinea pedis. If treatment is indicated, it involves the use of topical and, at times, systemic antifungals prescribed by a physician. When examining a patient's foot, assess the interdigital spaces for signs of tinea pedis and educate the patient regarding appropriate foot care to prevent fungal infections.

Candidiasis

Candidiasis is a fungal infection most frequently caused by the yeast *Candida albicans. C. albicans* is part of the normal flora found in the mouth, gastrointestinal tract, and vagina. Uncontrolled proliferation results in a candidal infection, the presentation of which is dependent upon the anatomical area involved.[22] Keratinized surfaces present as red, pustular, well-defined, scaling eruptions. Mucous membranes present as white, cheesy, adherent masses on red surfaces.[22]

People with decreased immunity, diabetes mellitus, infection, obesity, chronic corticosteroid use, and hyperhidrosis, and those in professions with frequent exposure to water (e.g., bartending, cooking, health care, and floristry) have a propensity to develop a *Candida* infection.[16, 22] Cutaneous *Candida* infections commonly present in moist occluded skin such as the axillae, groin, and redundant tissues such as the breasts and abdominal folds. Treatment employs the use of topical agents and may also include oral antifungals prescribed by a physician. Prevention is key to reduce the risk of infection, including proper hygiene, keeping susceptible areas dry, and using talc powders to absorb perspiration. In wound care, patients may be prone to developing *Candida* infections under occlusive dressings, when exudate is not managed appropriately, and/ or if they have had a long course of antibiotics rendering them susceptible to a fungal infection versus colonization.

All cutaneous infections require careful diagnosis to determine the etiology so proper therapy can be initiated. The earlier treatment is initiated, the less chance the patient has of developing additional deleterious consequences due to the infectious process.

 Checkpoint Question #2

While performing sensory testing on a patient who complains of low back pain, you notice areas of erythema and scaling on the plantar aspect of the patient's right foot.

a. What dermatological condition may these findings represent?

b. What actions should you suggest to the patient?

c. Should you cover the scaling areas with a hydrocolloid? Defend your answer.

Nail Disorders

Cutaneous nail disorders can arise from trauma, infection, and/or systemic disease. A thorough examination of the fingernails and toenails should be a routine part of the integument examination. The normal nail apparatus is comprised of the nail plate and surrounding soft tissue structures. Nails aid in function and protect the terminal digits. Normal nails should appear smooth and translucent, revealing pink tissue beneath. The lunula, white half-moon-shaped structures, should be present at the proximal end of the nail near the cuticle. Changes in nail integrity, texture, color, thickness, and/or clubbing should be noted. For example, thick dystrophic nails can be indicative of circulatory compromise or a fungal infection. Yellow nail syndrome is characterized by thickening and yellow to yellowish-green discoloration of the nails, often associated with lymphedema and compromised respiration. Clubbing of the nails can be idiopathic or acquired, with acquired clubbing usually a consequence of cardiac, pulmonary, hepatic, or gastrointestinal disease.[9] A referral to a dermatologist or podiatrist should be made to determine the etiology of a nail dysfunction and to initiate medical treatment if indicated. Like the skin, the nail and its associated structures can provide insight into the overall health of the individual, providing clues about underlying systemic disease. Depending on the etiology of a nail dysfunction, treatment may involve topical medications for fungal infections or, if the condition is recalcitrant or severe, surgical removal of all or part of the nail apparatus. For systemic conditions, treatment should address the underlying pathology or disease.

Other Considerations for Physical Therapists

In all practice settings, physical therapists need to be cognizant of other cutaneous manifestations that may affect themselves or their patients. Occupational irritants and dermatoses, rare skin conditions, and the use of modalities on patients with alterations in their integumentary system are important considerations in today's clinical environment.

The ubiquitous use of latex gloves and other latex products in virtually all health care settings has resulted in a parallel increase in latex-associated adverse reactions since the adoption of universal precautions (aka standard precautions) by the Centers for Disease Control in 1987.[23] Additional occupational irritants that a physical therapist may encounter include, but are not limited to: fiberglass, silicone, adhesives, and cleansing agents. Long-term use or frequent exposure can predispose the clinician or patient to developing a sensitivity or reaction to such products. Recognizing associated signs and symptoms and initiating appropriate preventative and therapeutic strategies can assist the clinician in maintaining a healthy and safe work environment for both health care providers and patients alike.

Irritant dermatitis and allergic contact dermatitis are two types of dermatitis caused by substances coming in contact with the skin. Irritant dermatitis is an inflammatory reaction resulting from exposure to a substance that causes an eruption in most people who come in contact with it.[9] Allergic contact dermatitis is an acquired sensitivity to various substances that produce reactions in some individuals who have been previously exposed to the allergen.[9] Adverse reactions to latex, fiberglass, silicone, adhesives, cleansing agents, or other allergy-inducing agents can be categorized as irritant dermatitis, allergic contact dermatitis, or immediate hypersensitivity reactions (anaphylaxis, asthma, allergic rhinitis, angioedema, or urticaria).[23] The most common reaction is irritant dermatitis, which is a nonimmunologically mediated dermatitis characterized by dry, pruritic, irritated areas of the skin. The reaction can be a result of prolonged glove wearing, repeated hand washing and drying, incomplete hand drying, the frequent use of sanitizers and cleansers, exposure to powders added to gloves, and exposure to other workplace products or chemicals.[23] The most effective prevention is the avoidance of the irritant and proper hand hygiene. Physical therapists should also be cognizant of other potential irritants for both themselves and their patients. Dressings, gauze wraps, resistive exercise bands and tubing, and linens used in the clinic can all be sources of irritants. Read the labels on dressings and gauze products for contents such as latex or silicone. Ascertain if facility linens are washed in bleach or other harsh chemicals as many patients are sensitive to such products. Recommend the purchase and use of latex-free resistive bands and other equipment to ensure a safer and more skin-friendly environment.

Physical therapists should be aware of other cutaneous disorders that may complicate a patient's treatment course. Insect bites, sexually transmitted diseases, self-induced skin injuries, travel-related illnesses, and rare genetic disorders and disease states can often mimic more common wound etiologies and presentations. When standard interventions fail, clinicians should consider other potential etiologies and discuss the situation with the referring or primary care physician.

Physical therapists need to be cognizant about the use of modalities with patients who have suspicious lesions or dermatological conditions. Most physical agents and mechanical modalities are contraindicated in the presence of cancer or suspected cancer, as the modality may cause mitogenic activity of the cancer cells. Rashes and skin infections could spread to other body parts, tissues, or segments with the application of a modality on the involved area. The parameters of the physical agent or modality may be blunted or exacerbated by the dermatological condition due to the disruption of the skin battery potential, or by alterations in the thickness and structure of the epidermis and dermis. Sound clinical judgment and communication with the referring physician can help to ensure the safety and effectiveness of all physical therapy interventions.

Normal and Abnormal Variations in Non-Caucasian Skin

It is important for wound care clinicians, as well as other health care practitioners, to be able to recognize normal and abnormal variations in darker-pigmented individuals. Pigmentary factors often mask the cutaneous reactions that are normally anticipated with a dermatological condition. For example, cyanosis, erythema, and pallor are more difficult to detect in deeply pigmented skin. Therefore, the early stages of certain diseases where these clinical findings may provide important clues are readily missed.[24] There are several dermatological conditions that occur in black skin that are normal integumentary variations.[10, 24] Table 17–9 describes the more common variations observed in black skin.

TABLE 17–9   Normal Variations in Black Skin

Variation	Clinical Presentation
Futcher's (Voigt's) line	• Sharp, bilateral, pigmentary demarcation lines usually on the extremities • Correspond to underlying spinal nerves innervating a dermatome • A reported incidence of 25% in heavily pigmented black persons • Benign condition
Midline hypopigmentation	• Line of hypopigmentation over the sternum • Black males primarily affected; becomes less noticeable with age • Unknown etiology; may be inherited in an autosomal dominant pattern • Incidence approximately 30–40% in black persons
Nail pigmentation	• Diffuse nail pigmentation or linear dark bands on the nail • May appear brown, blue, or blue-black • Linear hyperpigmented nail streaks represent a normal variant in over 50% of black people • Melanin is deposited in nail plate/matrix, possibly due to trauma or UV light • Positive correlation with advancing age • Thumb and index nails most commonly involved; often bilaterally distributed • Drugs such as antimalarials, bleomycin, doxorubicin, and zidovudine may cause nail pigmentation • Associated with systemic diseases such as Addison's disease and Peutz Jegher's syndrome • An irregular nail pigment or history of changing lesion warrants biopsy, as 20% of melanomas in black people are found in the nails

(Continued)

TABLE 17–9   Continued

Variation	Clinical Presentation
Oral pigmentation	• Oral mucosa appears blue to blue-gray • Symmetrical discoloration usually of anterior gingiva • Certain drugs (antimalarials, phenothiazine) and heavy metals can cause oral pigmentation • Addison's disease, Peutz Jegher's syndrome, and hemochromatosis should also be considered • Benign condition
Palmar changes	• Creases may be hyperpigmented due to localized hypermelanosis • May contain hyperkeratotic papules or pits in the creases
Plantar changes	• Hyperpigmented macules may vary in color and distribution • May present with irregular borders
Idiopathic Guttate Hypomelanosis aka Disseminate Lenticular Leucoderma	• Small, white, irregularly shaped macules primarily on the anterior lower extremities • Unknown etiology; benign • Macules range in size from 2 to 6 mm • More common in women over the age of 40 • Histologically, there is a decrease in the number of melanocytes
Dermatosis Papulosa Nigra	• Dark brown papules ranging in size from 1 to 5 mm • Usually located on the malar region • May affect 35–77% of black individuals • Lesions are histologically indistinguishable from seborrheic keratosis • Begnign condition sometimes referred to as "flesh moles"

Source: Porth C. *Pathophysiology: Concepts of Altered Health States.* 7th ed. Philadelphia: Lippincott, Williams & Wilkins; 2005; Connoly C, Bikowski J. *Dermatological Atlas of Black Skin.* Surrey, UK: Merit Publishing; 2006.

Roughly 80% of the world's population consists of individuals with pigmented skin. In the United States, approximately 29% of the population is non-Caucasian. It is projected that by the year 2050, 48% of the United States population will be non-Caucasian. The problem for clinicians when assessing patients with pigmented skin is the lack of guidance and/or evidence. Lyder et al. (1998) carried out a pilot study to examine the validity of the Braden Scale in black and Latino/Hispanic older adults. Statistical analysis revealed that the Braden score significantly underpredicted those participants at risk for pressure ulcers.[25] U.S. prevalence surveys found dark-skinned African American patients had the most severe category/stage IV pressure ulcers,[26–28] which was probably due to the fact that early nonblanching erythema was not detected and deep tissue injury occurred before corrective action took place.[29]

The total amount of melanin is the principle determinant of skin color. This is determined by the combined effects of two variables: constitutive and faculative skin color. *Constitutive* skin color designates a genetically determined level of cutaneous melanin, in the absence of exogenous or endogenous influences, whereas *faculative* skin color designates an induced level of increased epidermal melanin content due to solar radiation, hormones, and other environmental factors.[30]

The cutaneous pigment melanin is produced by melanocytes. The biosynthesis of melanin occurs within the metabolic unit of the melanocyte, the *melanosome*. The melanocyte, an exocrine cell, resides in the basal layer (or stratum germanitivum) of the epidermis and in the matrix portion of the hair bulb. Studies of human skin revealed *no* significant differences in the actual number of melanocytes,[31] however, racial differences in skin color are attributed to differences in the *rate* at which melanosomes are produced and melanized in melanocytes and then transferred, distributed, and degraded in keratinocytes.

Heredity plays a major role in determining the pigmentation of a person. In addition, other intrinsic and extrinsic factors contribute to the tendency of black individuals to develop specific response patterns to common dermatological conditions. Annular, fibromatous, follicular, granulomatous, keloidal, and ulcerative integumentary responses are all consistently more common in black individuals.[24]

A thorough history is an important part of the examination of black skin to determine a patient's normal skin tone and variations. Hypo- and hyperpigmentation may be indicative of a pathological condition.[10] Palpation, localized tissue discoloration known as *dyschromia* (darker than surrounding tissue and/or blue to purple hues), and temperature discrepancies should be assessed to augment the visual observation of skin color changes. As with all integument disorders, an appropriate diagnosis must be made for optimal treatment to ensue.

CHAPTER SUMMARY

This chapter provides an introduction to identification of dermatological conditions that are commonly seen within the physical therapy setting. However, dermatology is a vast field that deals with a plethora of cutaneous manifestations and diseases. For additional information, consult one of several dermatology texts available.[9, 16]

Physical therapists and physical therapist assistants play an important role in dermatology by early recognition and identification of cutaneous pathologies that warrant referral to other health care providers. When cutaneous lesions do not respond to conventional therapies or a patient's history is suspect, other etiologies and diagnoses should be considered. This is when collaboration with other health care team members becomes imperative. Any suspicious findings should be succinctly documented and discussed with the patient's physician or other specialist. The combined efforts of all team members can facilitate optimal care for the patient and ensure appropriate diagnosis.

REVIEW QUESTIONS

1. A 78-year-old woman has been referred to physical therapy for left shoulder pain of unknown etiology. During your examination, you notice a brown, well-demarcated lesion with an uneven surface on her left scapula. Subjectively, the patient does not know how long the tumor has been present, yet she reports the area surrounding the tumor is tender.

   a. The clinical presentation of this lesion is suggestive of what type of lesions?

   b. How would you describe this lesion to the referring physician?

   c. As a physical therapist, how would you manage this patient?

2. You have been treating a 26-year-old woman who was recently diagnosed with lupus erythematosus. During the treatment session, the patient reports that she developed a rash on her face and upper extremities over the weekend.

   a. Clinically, what do you think could have caused this rash?

   b. What specific questions should you ask the patient?

   c. Given the objective and subjective information from your history, what would you discuss with the referring physician?

Use this address to access the Companion Website created for this textbook. Simply select "Physical Therapy" from the choice of disciplines. Find this book and log in using your username and password to access images, video clips, and additional learning tools.

APPENDIX

Basic Dermatology Terminology

Abscess   Localized collection of purulent material in a cavity formed by necrosis or disintegration of tissues.

Alopecia   Absence of hair in normally hairy areas of the skin.

Aphtha   Small ulcers of the mucous membranes.

Bulla   A rounded or irregularly shaped blister greater than 0.5 cm in diameter, containing serous or seropurulent material.

Burrow   Small and short (as in scabies) or long and tortuous tunnels in the epidermis.

Carbuncle   Necrotizing infection of the skin and subcutaneous tissues composed of a group of furuncles (boils).

Cellulitis (erysipelas)   Inflammation of cellular tissue; purulent inflammation of the dermis, subcutaneous tissue, and soft tissues.

Comedo/Comedones   Plug of keratin and sebum in an orifice; blackhead.

Crusts   Dried blood, serum, or pus mixed with epithelial and bacterial debris.

Cutaneous Horn   Localized spike-shaped area of marked overgrowth of keratin; can stick out above the skin a half an inch or more.

Denude   Loss of epidermis.

Ecchymosis   A macular red or purplish-blue hemorrhage in the skin or mucous membrane more than 2 cm in diameter.

Erosion   Loss of all or portions of the epidermis; heals without scar tissue.

Erythroderma   A generalized redness of the skin.

Excoriation   Linear or punctate abrasion produced by mechanical trauma.

Fibrosis   Formation of excessive fibrous collagen in the tissues.

Fissure   Linear crack or cleft through the epidermis and often into the dermis.

Follicular Plugs   Keratin plugs in the hair follicle 1–3 mm in size.

Furuncle   A localized pyogenic infection originating in a hair follicle.

Granuloma   Chronic inflammatory tissue composed of macrophages, fibroblasts, and granulation tissue.

Keratoderma   Hyperplasia of the stratum corneum.

Keratosis   Horny thickening of the skin.

Kerion   Nodular inflammatory, pustular lesion due to a fungal infection.

Lesion   Pathological or traumatic loss of normal tissue continuity, structure, or function.

Lichenification   Chronic thickening of the epidermis with exaggeration of its normal markings; often from excessive rubbing or scratching.

Macule   Small, circumscribed change in skin color, nonpalpable, present with various shapes.

Malperforans Ulcer   Seen in diabetics and Hansen's disease; associated neuropathy so the ulcers are painless yet deep and destructive.

Milia/Milium   Whitish papules, 1–2 mm in diameter with no visible opening onto skin surface.

Necrobiosis   Describes partial degeneration of tissue.

Nodule   Papule greater than 1 cm in diameter; deeper and firmer than a papule; centered in the dermis or subcutaneous adipose.

Papilloma   Benign tumor projecting from the skin.

Papule   Circumscribed, solid elevations up to 0.5 cm in diameter; present with various shapes.

Patch   Macule greater than 1 cm in diameter.

Petechia   Punctate hemorrhage spot 1–2 mm in diameter.

Plaque   Papule greater than 0.5 cm in diameter; often formed by coalescence of papules; generally flat but may have central depression.

Poikiloderma   Dermatosis characterized by variegated cutaneous pigmentation, atrophy, and telangiectasia.

Primary lesion   Lesion that appears first.

Pruritus   Irritating skin sensation that elicits the scratch response; itch.

Purpura   Discoloration of the skin or mucosa due to extravasation of blood.

Pustule   Small elevations of the skin containing purulent material.

Rash   Temporary eruptions of the skin.

Scales   Dry or greasy laminated masses of keratin.

Scar   Collagen and connective tissue that replaces lost dermis.

Sclerosis   Hardening or induration of the skin; often due to fibrosis.

Secondary lesion   Primary lesion that has been modified by trauma, regression, or other extraneous factors.

Sinus   Cavity or channel in the tissue.

Stria Cutis Distensae   A band or streak of linear, atrophic, pink, white, or purple lesions of the skin due to changes in the connective tissue.

Sycosis   Chronic pustular folliculitis and perifolliculitis involving the beard area.

Telangiectasia   Visible vascular lesion formed by dilation of small cutaneous blood vessels.

Tumor   Soft or firm, movable or fixed mass of various shape, larger than 2 cm.

Vegetation   A growth of pathological tissue consisting of multiple closely set papillary masses.

Verruca   Epidermal tumor caused by a papillary virus; describes lesion with a warty surface.

Vesicle   Circumscribed, fluid-containing, epidermal elevation 1–10 mm in size.

Vibex   A narrow linear mark; usually hemorrhage from scratching.

Wheal   Localized skin edema of irregular shape and variable size that is transient and superficial.

Xerosis   Dryness of the skin; usually presents with scaling, superficial fissures, and pruritus.

PEARSON
myhealthprofessionskit™

Use this address to access the Companion Website created for this textbook. Simply select "Physical Therapy" from the choice of disciplines. Find this book and log in using your username and password to access images, video clips, and additional learning tools.

REFERENCES

Go to myhealthprofessionskit.com to view this chapter's references.

APPENDIX A
Glossary

Abrasion   Wound caused by scraping or friction to the skin's surface.

Abscess   Localized collection of pus within body tissues.

Acute wound   A wound induced by surgery or trauma in an otherwise healthy individual.

Adherence   Patient choosing to follow guidelines suggested by a health care provider. An adherent patient is defined as one who follows at least 80% of suggested guidelines.

Adipose tissue   Vascular, loose connective tissue that stores fat and provides energy, cushioning, and insulation.

Aerobes   Bacteria that require oxygen to survive.

Air-fluidized pressure-relieving device   Dynamic pressure-relieving support surface.

Albumin   Plasma protein. Normal levels are at least 3.5 mg/dL.

Alginate   Absorptive wound dressing made from brown seaweed.

Alternating pressure-relieving device   Dynamic pressure-relieving support surface.

Anaerobes   Bacteria that cannot survive in an oxygen-rich environment.

Anastomoses   Connections between vessels.

Angioblast   Endothelial cell that lines vessel walls.

Angiogenesis   Formation of new blood vessels.

Ankle-brachial index (ABI)   Indirect measure of peripheral perfusion, calculated as the systolic pressure of the ankle divided by the systolic pressure of the brachium. Normally 0.9–1.1.

Antibacterial   Type of antimicrobial that is effective against bacteria.

Antibiotic   Oral or intravenously delivered substance that destroys or inhibits the growth of microorganisms.

Antifungal   Type of antimicrobial that destroys yeasts and molds.

Antimicrobial   Substance that destroys or inhibits the growth of microorganisms.

Antiseptic   Antimicrobial designed to reduce bacterial contamination on intact skin.

Arterial insufficiency   Decreased arterial blood supply, most commonly due to arteriosclerosis.

Arteriography   Invasive procedure in which radioactive dye is used to assess blood flow.

Arteriosclerosis   General term for thickening and hardening of arterial walls.

Atherosclerosis   Systemic, degenerative process in which the arterial lumen is gradually encroached upon by plaque formation.

Autolytic debridement   Form of debridement that uses endogenously produced enzymes to digest necrotic tissue.

Autonomic neuropathy   Dysfunction of the autonomic nervous system that may result from uncontrolled diabetes.

Bactericidal   Antimicrobial agent that is capable of killing bacteria.

Bacteriostatic   Antimicrobial agent that inhibits bacterial cell growth.

Basement membrane   Thin, acellular layer separating the epidermis from the dermis.

Biofilms   Communities of microorganisms that are attached to a wound surface and encased with a glycocalyx.

Biologic debridement   The use of sterile maggots to debride a wound.

Biologic dressings   Wound dressings derived from natural tissues.

Biosynthetic dressings   Wound dressings derived from natural tissues.

Blister   Collection of fluid at the junction between the dermis and epidermis due to friction.

Bottoming out   Occurs when there is less than $3/4$ to 1 inch of support material between the patient and support surface.

Burn shock   Complex clinical syndrome that occurs when perfusion is unable to meet tissue demands after a burn injury.

Calf muscle pump Pressure changes within the venous system in which muscle contraction forces blood proximally.

Callus Localized buildup of stratum corneum cells due to pressure or friction.

Capillary closing pressure Amount of external pressure that must be applied to prohibit capillary blood flow, generally 13–32 mm Hg.

Capillary refill Indicator of surface blood flow. Normally less than 3 seconds.

Cellulitis Inflammation of connective tissue; infection in, or close to, the skin.

Charcot foot Neuropathic fracture/dislocation found in patients with diabetes, most commonly resulting in a "rocker-bottom" foot deformity.

Chemotactic agent Substance that attracts cells.

Chemotaxis Movement along a chemical gradient.

Chronic wound A wound, induced by various causes, whose progression through the phases of wound healing is prolonged or arrested due to underlying conditions.

Clean technique Infection control procedure designed to reduce the number of microbes present and decrease the risk of infection.

Closed wound A wound in which the epithelial integrity has been restored.

Collagen dressings Class of dressings that contain collagen from various animal or human sources that may promote wound healing by providing a scaffolding for the proliferative phase of wound healing, stimulating cell growth and migration, and absorbing wound exudate.

Collagenase Enzyme that breaks down collagen.

Colonization Normal presence of a small number of microbes (i.e., $\leq 10^3$ organisms/gram of tissue).

Complement system A cascade of proteins produced by the body that enhance the body's defense against pathogens.

Composite dressings Multilayer dressings made from a combination of wound dressing categories.

Compression garments Custom or off-the-shelf compression sleeve for venous insufficiency, lymphedema, or burn scar management.

Contamination Presence or anticipated presence of blood, wound fluid, or other potentially infectious waste.

Contracture Pathological shortening of scar tissue resulting in a deformity.

Conversion Process of widening and deepening of a burn injury.

Creatinine Measure of body's protein status; normally 0.7–1.5 mg/dL.

Critical colonization Point at which increasing wound bioburden begins to adversely affect wound healing.

Current of injury Local change of polarity at the site of integumentary injury.

Cytokine Signaling protein during the inflammatory phase of wound healing.

Cytotoxic agent Substance that is poisonous to human cells.

Debridement The removal of necrotic tissue, foreign material, and/or debris from a wound bed.

Deep partial-thickness burn Also called *deep second-degree burn;* involves the epidermis and dermis.

Deep veins Located within muscles, roughly parallel arterial system.

Dehiscence Separation of wound margins.

Delayed primary closure A combination of primary and secondary wound healing processes in which the wound is first observed before primary closure.

Dermal papillae The ridges and valleys of the superior surface of the dermis that conforms with the contours of the epidermal stratum basale to help anchor the two layers together.

Dermatitis Inflammation of the skin associated with itching, redness, and open lesions.

Dermis Inner, vascular layer of the skin.

Diapedesis The movement of PMNs through capillary walls.

Disinfect To clean a surface with an antimicrobial.

Doppler ultrasound Instrument used to assess arterial or venous flow.

Duplex scanning Noninvasive medical test to assess peripheral blood flow, velocity, and turbulence.

Dynamic insufficiency When lymph transport is unable to accommodate for an increase in lymphatic load. Term can also be applied to the venous system.

Dynamic support surface Electric device that uses currents of air or fluid to redistribute pressure across the body.

Elephantiasis Severe disfiguring form of lymphedema caused by filariasis.

Enzymatic debridement Form of debridement using topically applied exogenous enzymes to remove devitalized tissue; requires a physician's prescription.

Epibole Keratinocyte migration over the lip or margin of the dermis.

Epidermis Outer, avascular layer of the skin.

Epithelialization Process by which keratinocytes resurface the wound defect.

Eschar Black necrotic tissue that may be either soft or hard.

Escharotomy   Surgical incision through burn eschar to relieve pressure and restore perfusion.

Exudate   Mixture of fluid, high levels of protein, and cells.

Fascia   Fibrous connective tissue that separates and surrounds structures and facilitates movement between adjacent structures.

Fasciotomy   Surgical incision through fascia to release pressure and restore perfusion.

Fibrin cuff theory   Theory that venous insufficiency ulcers are due to the development of fibrin cuffs around the capillaries.

Fibroblast   Dermal cell that produces collagen, elastin, granulation tissue, and growth factors.

Filariasis   Form of secondary lymphedema caused by the bite of an infected mosquito.

Fistula   A sinus tract connecting two epithelial surfaces.

Fluid aspiration   Method of identifying wound infection in which a physician uses a needle to remove 1.0 mL of fluid from the wound area for analysis.

Fluid-filled pressure-reducing device   Static pressure-reducing support surface made of air, water, or gel.

Foam pressure-reducing device   Static pressure-reducing support surface appropriate for patients with low risk for ulcer development.

Friction   When two surfaces move across one another.

Full-thickness burn   Also called *third-degree burn*; involves damage of the epidermis and dermis to the subcutaneous tissues.

Full-thickness skin graft   Durable and cosmetic skin graft consisting of epidermis and dermis.

Full-thickness wound   Wound that extends through the epidermis and dermis and into or through the subcutaneous tissue.

Galvanotaxis   Stimulation of cells to move along an electrical gradient.

Gangrene   Dead tissue that is dry, dark, cold, and contracted; must be surgically removed.

Gauze   Traditional wound dressing, woven or nonwoven, available in sheets, rolls, and packing strips.

Gram-negative   Method of identifying microorganisms; gram-negative organisms are not stained by crystal violet but are stained by safranin.

Gram-positive   Method of identifying microorganisms; gram-positive organisms are stained by crystal violet.

Granulation tissue   Temporary structure composed of vascularized connective tissue that fills the wound void.

Granuloma   Chronic inflammation around a foreign body.

Growth factor   Growth-promoting substance that increases or enhances cell size, proliferation, or activity.

Hair   Epidermal appendages located within the dermis that are made of soft keratin.

Hand check   Method to assess for bottoming out by placing outstretched hand palm up between the support surface and patient.

Healed wound   A closed wound with tissue strength approaching normal.

Hemosiderin deposition   Occurs when the byproduct of the breakdown of red blood cells is forced into the interstitium by venous hypertension.

Histamine   Chemical mediator released by mast cells that causes vasodilation, increases vessel wall permeability, and attracts other cells to the area.

Homans' sign   Assessment technique historically used to identify a deep vein thrombosis that has since been found to be inaccurate.

Hydrocolloid   Moisture-retentive occlusive wound dressing consisting of gelatin, pectin, and carboxymethylcellulose hydrophilic particles with an adhesive backing.

Hydrogel   Moisture-retentive wound dressing that is 80–99% water or glycerin based, available in sheets and as an amorphous gel.

Hyperbaric oxygen   Modality used to enhance wound healing by having patient breathe 100% oxygen at 2.0–2.5 Atm.

Hypergranular   Error of the proliferative phase in which too much granulation tissue is formed and epithelialization is delayed.

Hypertrophic scarring   Overproduction of collagen that stays within the confines of the original wound.

Hypogranular   A pothole-type wound that fails to build a sufficient granulation tissue matrix.

Impregnated gauze   Mesh gauze with a topical agent such as an amorphous hydrogel or petrolatum incorporated into it.

Incision and drainage   Procedure in which an abscess is surgically opened and thoroughly irrigated.

Induration   Firm edema.

Infection   Invasion and multiplication of microorganisms within body tissues; wound culture reveals greater than 10^5 microbes per gram of tissue.

Inflammation   First phase of wound healing, characterized by rubor, calor, tumor, dolor, and functio laesa; vascular and cellular response to injury of living tissue.

Integrins   Cell surface receptors that allow cells to reversibly bind to the extracellular matrix.

Intermittent claudication   Activity-specific discomfort due to local ischemia.

International NPUAP/EPUAP Pressure Ulcer Classification System   Classification system for pressure ulcers updated in 2009.

Intimal layer   Inner layer of arteries and veins composed of a single endothelial cell layer.

Ischemia reperfusion injury   Repeated bouts of localized tissue ischemia from pressure or peripheral arterial disease and reperfusion that may cause gradual, progressive tissue damage.

Ischemic rest pain   Burning pain due to arterial insufficiency that occurs at rest.

Ischemic ulcer   Arterial insufficiency ulcer.

Keloid   Scar due to the overproduction of collagen that extends beyond the confines of the original wound.

Keratin   A protein produced by keratinocytes. Nails are made of hard keratin; hair is made of soft keratin.

Keratinocyte   Epidermal cell that resurfaces a wound and produces keratin.

Langerhans' cells   Epidermal cells that assist with infection control.

Laplace's law   Formula describing the determinants of the amount of compression exerted by a bandage.

Ligation   Tying off; perforating veins may be ligated to reduce hypertension in the superficial veins.

Lipedema   Bilateral, symmetrical increase in adipose tissue deposition in the abdomen, buttocks, and lower extremities with sparing of the feet.

Lipodermatosclerosis   Hyperpigmentation and accompanying erythema, induration, and plaque-like structural changes due to long-standing venous insufficiency.

Lipolymphedema   Form of lymphedema caused by lipedema, which usually has very limited improvement with interventions.

Low-air-loss pressure-relieving device   Dynamic pressure-relieving support surface.

Low-intensity laser therapy   Light amplification by stimulated emission of radiation; modality that may enhance healing in chronic wounds.

Lund–Browder classification   Alternate method to the rule of nines for estimating burn size as a percent of total body surface area. This method takes into consideration age-related changes in body proportions.

Lymph   Fluid consisting of water, protein, dead or dying cells, cellular components, fatty acids, foreign material, and debris.

Lymph capillaries   The smallest vessels within the lymphatic system, highly permeable.

Lymph collectors   Larger vessels within the lymphatic system with muscular walls and valves to assist with lymph flow.

Lymphatic territories   Areas of the skin made up of several adjacent lymph collectors that drain to the same lymph nodes.

Lymphangiomotoricity   The strength and frequency of lymphangion contraction.

Lymphangions   Functional units of the lymphatic system.

Lymphatic load   Material that is transported within the lymphatic system.

Lymphedema   Accumulation of protein-rich fluid due to congenital malformation of the lymphatics or impaired lymph transport.

Lymphorrhea   The weeping of lymph through small pores in the skin surface with no overt measureable wound.

Maceration   Skin that is white, friable, overhydrated, and sometimes wrinkled.

Macrophage   Cell that directs the repair process, secretes growth factors and enzymes, and destroys bacteria and debris.

Margination   When PMNs are pushed to the sides of a vessel wall.

Mast cell   Cell that helps initiate inflammation; secretes histamine, enzymes, and chemical mediators.

Matrix metalloproteases (MMPs)   Proteases that degrade the extracellular matrix.

Maturation and remodeling   Final phase of wound healing during which collagen matures and reorients along the lines of stress.

Mechanical debridement   Form of debridement using force to remove devitalized tissue, foreign material, and debris from a wound bed.

Mechanical insufficiency   When the lymphatic system is unable to transport the normal amount of lymph due to a functional failure of the system. Term is also be applied to the venous system.

Melanin   Pigment produced by melanocytes that helps protect the body from ultraviolet radiation and is a major determinant of skin color.

Melanocytes   Pigment-producing cells within the epidermis.

Merkel cell   Sensory receptor within the epidermis providing information on light touch.

Moisture barrier   Substance used to protect the periwound and intact skin from excessive moisture. Some moisture barriers are also safe for use on rashes and broken skin.

Moisture-retentive dressing   Specialized synthetic or organic wound dressing.

Moisture-vapor transmission rate The rate at which gas is able to escape through a moisture-retentive dressing.

Moisturizer Substance used to relieve and prevent dry skin.

Motor neuropathy Dysfunction of motor nerves leading to atrophy, weakness, and/or paralysis.

MRSA Methicillin-resistant *Staphylococcus aureus*.

Multilayer compression bandage Compression bandage composed of many layers used for the treatment of venous insufficiency ulcers and/or lymphedema.

Musculocutaneous flap closure Surgical procedure used to close category/stage III and IV pressure ulcers by rotating a muscle and overlying tissue along with the blood supply to fill the wound defect.

Myofibroblast Cell possessing properties of fibroblasts and smooth muscle cells that cause wound contraction.

Nails Epidermal appendage made of hard keratin and located at the dorsal tips of digits.

Necrotic tissue Dead, devitalized tissue adhered to the wound bed.

Negative nitrogen balance Nutritional state that occurs when the body excretes more nitrogen than is ingested; sign of malnutrition.

Negative pressure wound therapy (NPWT) Modality that uses negative pressure to enhance wound healing. Sometimes referred to as vacuum-assisted closure (VAC).

Neuropathic ulcer Ulcer due to insensitivity; previously referred to as a diabetic ulcer.

Nonselective debridement The removal of nonspecific areas of devitalized tissue. May include mechanical or surgical debridement.

Nosocomial infection An infection that is acquired while hospitalized.

Occlusion The ability of a dressing to prevent transmission of moisture vapor and gases from the wound bed.

Open wound Damage to the skin resulting in a loss of skin integrity.

Padded ankle-foot orthosis Method of treating neuropathic ulcers; removable brace that reduces plantar pressure and immobilizes the ankle and foot.

Papillary dermis Thin superficial dermal layer consisting of loosely arranged connective tissue.

Papillomas Cauliflower-like projects of the epithelium caused by distended and dilated superficial lymphatics.

Papillomatosis Cobblestone appearance of the epithelium seen in stage three lymphedema.

Partial-thickness wound Wound involving the epidermis and part of the dermis.

Paste bandage Nonelastic compression bandage, such as Unna's boot.

Percutaneous ablation of perforators (PAPS) Endoscopic surgery for chronic venous insufficiency.

Perforating veins Veins that pierce the fascia to connect the deep and superficial venous systems.

Phagocytizing Process of engulfing and destroying bacteria and/or debris.

Pitting edema Swelling in which a depression remains within the involved tissues after the application of digital pressure.

Platelet Cell that helps control bleeding; releases growth factors and chemotactic agents.

Plethysmography Noninvasive medical test to assess peripheral blood flow.

PMN (Polymorphonuclear neutrophil) Cell that cleans the wound; secretes enzymes and inflammatory mediators.

Positive nitrogen balance Nutritional state that occurs when more nitrogen is ingested than excreted; desired for most efficient wound healing.

Prealbumin Transport protein used as an indicator of nutritional status. Normal levels are 16–40 mg/dL.

Pressure-reducing device Support surface that reduces interface pressures more than a standard hospital mattress or chair surface but not below 23–32 mm Hg.

Pressure-relieving device Support surface that consistently reduces tissue interface pressures below 23 mm Hg.

Pressure ulcer Wound caused by unrelieved pressure, or combination of pressure and shear.

Pressure ulcer assessment instrument Tool to describe various aspects of pressure ulcers and to identify changes in wound status.

Pressure ulcer risk assessment tool Screening device to help predict individuals at risk for pressure ulcers.

Primary closure Process by which wounds heal if the wound margins can be approximated.

Primary dressing Wound covering that comes into direct contact with the wound bed.

Primary lymphedema Congenital malformation or impairment of the lymphatic system resulting in an accumulation of protein-rich fluid.

Proliferation Second phase of wound healing; building and regenerating phase consisting of angiogenesis, granulation tissue formation, wound contraction, and epithelialization.

Prostaglandins   Substances released by injured cells that cause vasodilation.

Pruritus   Severe itching.

Pulsed lavage   Interrupted delivery of wound irrigant under pressure by an electrically powered device.

Pyoderma gangrenosum   Noninfectious, progressive necrotizing skin condition associated with systemic inflammatory conditions.

Radiation fibrosis   Chronic changes in which the skin appears discolored, dry, hairless, atrophied, fibrotic, and inelastic due to increased collagen deposition and vascular damage.

Reactive hyperemia   Localized area of blanchable erythema.

Resistant   A bacteria that cannot be killed by a certain antimicrobial.

Respiratory pump   Pressure changes within the venous system in which inspiration and expiration force blood toward the heart.

Rete pegs   Protrusions of the epidermal stratum basale that extend into the papillary dermis to help anchor the two layers together.

Reticular dermis   Thick, deep dermal layer consisting of dense, irregularly arranged connective tissue.

Rubor of dependency   Test to assess arterial blood flow.

Rule of nines   Method of estimating burn size as a percent of total body surface area by dividing the body into sections roughly equal to 9% of total body surface area.

Scab   Collection of necrotic cells, fibrin, collagen, and platelets that covers a superficial wound.

Sclerotherapy   Injection of an agent to fibrose dysfunctional veins.

Sebaceous gland   Oil gland; epidermal appendage located within the dermis.

Sebum   Oily substance that lubricates the skin and hair.

Secondary closure   Wound healing process in which granulation tissue is formed to fill the wound defect.

Secondary dressing   Wound dressing placed over the primary dressing that provides increased protection, cushioning, absorption, and/or occlusion.

Secondary lymphedema   Disruption or damage to the lymphatic system resulting in an accumulation of protein-rich fluid.

Segmental pressure   Serial blood pressure measurements used to localize an area of decreased arterial blood flow.

Selective debridement   Removal of specific areas of devitalized tissue; may include sharp, enzymatic, or autolytic debridement.

Selective sharp debridement   Form of sharp debridement using scissors or scalpel to cut along the lines of demarcation between viable and nonviable tissue.

Semipermeable film   Moisture-retentive wound dressing consisting of a transparent polyurethane sheet with an adhesive backing; impermeable to bacteria and water.

Semipermeable foam   Moisture-retentive wound dressing consisting of a polyurethane foam with or without an adhesive backing.

Semmes–Weinstein monofilaments   Tools used to assess sensory integrity.

Sensitive   If a bacteria can be killed by a certain antimicrobial.

Sensory neuropathy   Dysfunction of sensory nerves leading to altered or decreased sensation.

Sentinel lymph node   The first lymph node receiving lymph from a given area, usual a tumor.

SEPS procedure   Endoscopic surgery for chronic venous insufficiency.

Serial instrumental debridement   Form of sharp debridement using forceps and scissors to remove loosely adherent devitalized tissue. Usually occurs over a number of visits and may require prior tissue preparation.

Seroma   The accumulation of serum within the tissue, generally localized into a pocket created by surgery.

Serum transferrin   Indicator of nutritional status; normal levels are greater than 170 mg/dL.

Sharp debridement   Selective debridement using forceps, scissors, or a scalpel.

Shear   Force parallel to the body surface.

Short-stretch compression bandage   Compression wrap with low resting pressure and little distensibility.

Silver nitrate   Topical agent applied to decrease hypergranular tissue or stop local bleeding.

Sinus tract   An elongated cavity or abscess that drains to the body surface; may be associated with category/stage IV pressure ulcers.

Skin sealant   Product used on intact periwound to protect the skin from excessive moisture and/or adhesives.

Skin substitutes   Products used for temporary or extended skin coverage.

Slough   Necrotic tissue that is yellow or tan in color and has a stringy or mucinous consistency.

Split-thickness skin graft   Meshed or sheet graft involving the epidermis and a portion of the dermis.

Staging system   Classification system for pressure ulcers that was revised in 2009.

Standard precautions Type of infection control that includes universal precautions, hand washing, and personal protective equipment.

Static support surface Nonmoving pressure-reducing device that provides cushioning and pressure distribution.

Stemmer's sign Inability to pinch a skin fold on the dorsal aspect of a digit. Presence confirms lymphedema in this area.

Sterile technique Method of infection control that uses only sterile equipments.

Sterilization Procedure that destroys all microbes from the area of interest.

Stratum basale Deepest epithelial cell layer; contains continuously dividing cells.

Stratum corneum Outermost epithelial cell layer; consists of dead keratinocytes.

Stratum granulosum Epithelial cell layer located between the stratum spinosum and stratum lucidum.

Stratum lucidum Epithelial cell layer located between the stratum granulosum and stratum corneum.

Stratum spinosum Epithelial cell layer located between the stratum basale and stratum granulosum.

Subcutaneous tissue Composed of adipose tissue and fascia; located beneath the dermis; helps support the skin.

Subdermal burn Also called *fourth-degree burn*; results in destruction beyond the dermis down to fat, muscle, tendon, and/or bone.

Sudoriferous gland Sweat gland; epidermal appendage located within the dermis.

Superficial burn Also called *first-degree burn*; involves only the epidermis.

Superficial partial-thickness burn Also called *superficial second-degree burn*; involves the epidermis and papillary dermis.

Superficial veins Veins located within the subcutaneous tissues; assist with temperature regulation.

Superficial wound Wound involving only the epidermis.

Surfactants Cytotoxic substances within wound cleansers that lower surface tension of loose particulate matter on a wound bed.

Surgical debridement The use of scalpels, scissors, or lasers in a sterile environment by a physician or podiatrist to remove necrotic tissue, foreign material, and debris from the wound bed.

Swab cultures Methods to identify and quantify microbes present in a wound.

Thoracic duct Largest lymphatic vessel, drains into the left venous angle.

Tissue adhesives Also known as skin glue, over-the-counter alternative to sutures and staples for primary wound closure.

Tissue biopsy Procedure in which a physician removes a sample of living tissue from the wound to identify infection.

Tissue inhibitors of matrix metalloproteases (TIMPS) Proteases that regulate the activity of MMPs.

Tissue interface pressure The amount of pressure between a body part and support surface.

Toe pressure Test to assess digit perfusion.

Total contact cast Modified short leg cast used to treat uninfected grade 1 or 2 plantar neuropathic ulcers.

Total lymphocyte count (TLC) Indirect measure of nutritional status and immune function. Normal values are $\geq 1,800/mm^3$.

Transcutaneous oxygen monitoring (TCOM or TcPO$_2$) Test measuring tissue oxygen content.

Transport capacity The ability of the lymphatic system to move fluid.

Transudate Low-protein collection of fluid caused by increased vascular permeability.

Trendelenburg test Test to identify vein incompetence.

Tubular bandage Off-the-shelf sleeves to provide compression.

Tunica externa Protective outer layer of arteries and veins, formerly called the adventitia

Tunica media Middle layer of arteries and veins composed of smooth muscle along with some collagen and elastin fibers.

Tunneling A narrow passageway within a wound bed.

Ulcer Open wound or lesion.

Undermining Area of tissue under the wound edges that becomes eroded, resulting in a large wound with a small opening.

Universal precautions Type of infection control in which all blood and body fluids are considered to be contaminated.

Urea Indicator of malnutrition; normal BUN is 5–25 mg/dL.

Vacuum-Assisted Closure (VAC) More formally known as negative-pressure wound therapy (NPWT), modality that uses negative pressure to enhance wound healing.

Varicose vein, varicosity Dilated vein. In addition to increased lumen size, varicosities typically entail increased vessel length and tortuosity.

Vasopneumatic compression device Pneumatic device consisting of a bilayered sleeve to provide compression.

Vein stripping Surgical resection of veins.

Venography   Invasive procedure in which radioactive dye is used to assess venous blood flow.

Venous filling time   Test to assess peripheral blood flow.

Venous hypertension   Increased backward pressure within the venous system.

Venous stasis ulcer   Ulcer caused by venous insufficiency.

VRE   Vancomycin-resistant *Enterococci*.

Wagner classification   Classification system for neuropathic ulcers.

Walking splint   Bivalved total contact cast used to treat neuropathic ulcers.

Watershed   A natural boundary that separates lymph territories

White blood cell   Cell that helps fight infection.

White blood cell trapping theory   Theory that venous insufficiency ulcers are due to activated white blood cells within the interstitium.

Wound cleanser   Commercially available antiseptic containing surfactants. Not regulated by the FDA.

Wound cleansing   The delivery of a wound cleanser to the wound surface using mechanical force to remove lightly adhered necrotic tissue, debris, and bacteria.

Wound contraction   Process by which myofibroblasts pull wound margins closer together, thereby decreasing the size of the defect.

Wound scrubbing   Mechanical debridement using a sponge, brush, or gauze along with a fluid to break the adherence of devitalized tissue and debris from the wound bed.

Zone of coagulation   Central portion of a burn injury that sustains irreparable damage.

Zone of hyperemia   Outer edge of a burn injury. Generally heals within 7 to 10 days.

Zone of stasis   Area of a burn injury surrounding the zone of coagulation that consists of cellular injury and compromised tissue perfusion.

APPENDIX B
Case Studies

CASE STUDY 1

Refer to color image 24 to answer the following questions.

1. Describe the wound and periwound as you would in the patient's chart.
2. What is the probable etiology of this patient's wound?
3. Does the patient require debridement? Defend your answer.
4. How would you bandage this wound?
5. What additional interventions might be appropriate at this time?

CASE STUDY 2

Refer to color image 25 to answer the following questions.

Your patient is a 44-year-old woman who reports her anterior shin wound began after bumping into a coffee table 2 months ago and has slowly increased in size and pain. She has been bandaging the wound with Dakin's-soaked gauze twice a day. Her past medical history is positive for hypertension and cataracts. The patient reports no history of falls, but acknowledges that she sometimes holds onto furniture or the walls to steady herself. The patient's wound measures 3.7×6.2 cm with slight serosanguinous drainage. Pedal and popliteal pulses are 1+, ABI is 0.77, periwound skin temperature appears normal, and there is no odor present. Range of motion and strength are unremarkable. Transfers are independent. The patient walks with a wide base of support with occasional crossover steps.

1. Describe the wound and periwound as you would in the patient's chart.
2. What is the probable etiology of this patient's wound?
3. Is the patient's current bandaging procedure appropriate at this time?
4. Describe your local wound care for this patient's wound.
5. What additional interventions may be appropriate?
6. What referrals are indicated for this patient?

CASE STUDY 3

Refer to color image 22 to answer the following questions.

Your patient is a 62-year-old woman who reports that the wound on the bottom of her foot has worsened despite home health nursing for bandage changes three times per week for the last month. The patient reports the wound began insidiously 2 months ago. Her past medical history is positive for diabetes mellitus (DM), obesity, and right below-knee amputation (R BKA) 4 months ago secondary to a nonhealing neuropathic ulcer. She lives alone, has been nonambulatory for the past 4 weeks, and uses a manual wheelchair for mobility. She is independent with stand-pivot transfers.

1. Document your objective findings as you would in the patient's chart.
2. What additional tests and measures would you perform on this patient during your examination?
3. What do you hypothesize is the etiology of this patient's wound?
4. Does the wound appear to be infected?

5. Is the patient a candidate for total contact casting? Why or why not?
6. Describe your local wound care.
7. What additional physical therapy interventions would be appropriate at this time? Explain your rationale.
8. What referral may be indicated for this patient?
9. It is now 3 weeks later and the patient's wound presents as in color image 23. Describe the wound presentation.
10. Describe how your intervention strategy would change at this point.

ANSWERS TO CASE STUDIES

Case Study 1

1. Patient presents with a deep partial-thickness burn wound injury to the dorsal hand, wrist, and distal forearm. The wound measures l × w. Alternatively, you could estimate the wound to be approximately 1.5% total body surface area. However, given the wound's small size, direct wound measurement may be a more reliable method to assess and document change in wound status over time. There is no slough present and there is significant angiogenesis throughout the wound bed.
2. Patient history would likely confirm that the wound is due to a burn injury.
3. Because the wound is 100% granular, debridement is not indicated at this time.
4. The wound may be bandaged with a topical antimicrobial, impregnated gauze, gauze square, and two-ply roll gauze. Elastic netting or a self-adherent elastic wrap may assist with keeping the bandage in place.
5. The patient should be instructed in active and active-assistive range of motion exercises for the involved wrist and hand. In addition, the patient should be educated in the use of elevation to control edema. If the patient's motion is severely limited or there is significant pain complaint prohibiting motion, the patient may benefit from pain medications prescribed by a physician and/or a splint to prevent deformities.

Case Study 2

1. Wound bed contains approximately 50% granular tissue, 15% yellow slough, and 35% viable sheath of the tibialis anterior tendon. Wound edges are attached and there is evidence of epithelialization at all edges. A mild erythema extends approximately 0.5 cm from the wound edge. There is minimal hair growth and the skin on the lower leg is mildly anhydrous. A small wound lateral to the main wound is also evident.
2. The wound is likely due to arterial insufficiency with a traumatic onset.
3. The Dakin's solution is not appropriate at this time. The wound does not demonstrate signs of infection and this solution is known to be cytotoxic and may delay wound healing.
4. You should protect the surrounding tissue with a moisturizing ointment and the periwound with a skin sealant. To prevent tendon sheath dehydration, you should apply an amorphous hydrogel to the wound bed and adjust bandage frequency to ensure proper wound hydration. A hydrocolloid was the dressing chosen initially, but the patient's skin proved too fragile as noted by the skin tear upon its removal. A nonadherent semipermeable foam dressing secured with roll gauze would be appropriate as would a nonadherent bismuth-impregnated gauze and a bulky gauze dressing. The patient would benefit from a posterior leaf splint with the involved ankle in slight dorsiflexion to prevent excessive motion of the tendon sheath within the wound bed and promote granulation tissue development over same.
5. The patient may benefit from gait training with an assistive device because she has an unsteady gait and a history of bumping into objects, and is now required to wear a posterior leaf splint.
6. The patient may benefit from a referral to an ophthalmologist to assess and address her visual acuity and cataracts as a potential source of future injury.

Case Study 3

1. Patient presents with full-thickness ulcers on the plantar surface of the forefoot, digits, and lateral foot. Wound size: see wound tracing, measures l × w × d (depth measurements are limited because of the presence of eschar). Wound beds are 100% black eschar covered with the exception of the plantar midfoot, which contains ~15% yellow slough and ~35% healthy granular tissue. Midfoot also demonstrates fragile new epithelium as noted by light pink skin at the base of the third and fourth metatarsophalangeal (MTP) joints.

2. You should test sensation using monofilaments, pulses, and capillary refill. Given the patient's previous amputation and history of diabetes, you should also perform an ABI.

3. The results of your tests and measures should identify neuropathic and circulatory dysfunctions, if present. Although the wound appears similar to a full-thickness burn wound, it is actually the result of a combination of neuropathy and excessive shear forces from walking and transferring solely on her left limb after her right below-knee amputation (R BKA).

4. Although it is possible the patient's circulation is so poor that she is unable to create a sufficient inflammatory response, the wound does not appear to be infected.

5. The patient is not a candidate for total contact casting because of the unknown depth of the wound and the excessive amounts of necrotic tissue.

6. Local wound care should consist of sharp debridement of plantar foot ulcers, protection of epithelial tissue with moisturizing ointment or a skin sealant, a bulky gauze dressing to protect the foot ensuring toes are separated by gauze or cotton, and appropriate temporary footwear. An amorphous hydrogel or enzymatic debrider (with a physician's order) are topical agents of choice.

7. Patient education should include safe transfer techniques to decrease shear to her foot (sliding board or lateral transfers), care for her residual limb, as well as proper foot and wound care guidelines. Whirlpool therapy may be appropriate initially to soften the eschar and assist with debridement. Electrical stimulation may be appropriate to enhance wound healing. A strengthening program should be developed for bilateral upper extremities to improve the patient's transfers now and to prepare for gait with an assistive device after wound closure. Lower extremity strengthening exercises will help the patient prepare for prosthetic gait training. Right gastrocnemius stretching to decrease forefoot shear and pressure are also indicated. An aerobic exercise program to assist with weight loss and glycemic control are also appropriate.

8. To maximize patient nutrition and assist with glycemic control, the patient may need to be referred to a diabetic educator, dietitian, and/or endocrinologist.

9. The patient now presents with a significant amount of fragile healthy epithelial tissue to the plantar aspect of her foot. Three open areas remain. Wound borders are slightly callous, especially at wound 1, which also shows signs of maceration.

Location	Wound Bed Description
1. Plantar second/third web space just distal to the MTP joints	• 40% granular and 60% yellow slough
2. Lateral fifth MTP joint	• 80% granular, 10% fascia and connective tissue, and 10% yellow slough
3. Lateral proximal heel	• 70% granular, 20% fascia and connective tissue, and 10% yellow slough

10. The wound is improving with your current plan of care. Important local wound care would include callus debridement and the use of an amorphous hydrogel along with a bulky gauze dressing to maintain a moist wound healing environment. A moisture barrier and a moisturizing ointment should also be used to protect the intact and macerated skin. The patient is appropriate for total contact casting, although given the wound's current rate of improvement, this is probably not necessary. You should continue to monitor and limit pressure and shear forces. Since the "slowest" area of wound healing is at the lateral border of the foot and the metatarsophalangeal joints, you should assess the patient's dorsiflexion range of motion as a source of increased stress to these areas during transfers. Any limitations noted should then be addressed.

APPENDIX C
Answers to Checkpoint and Chapter Review Questions

CHAPTER 1

Answers to Checkpoint Questions

1. No, the epidermis does not have a blood supply of its own; rather, it relies on diffusion from the underlying dermis.
2. Blisters occur at the junction between the epidermis and the dermis. Therefore, the epidermis and the superficial (papillary) dermis are involved.
3. The epidermis ranges in depth from 0.06 to 0.60 mm, while the dermis ranges in depth from 2.0 to 4.0 mm. Therefore, the wound likely involves at least the epidermis, dermis, and subcutaneous tissue.

Answers to Review Questions

1. See Figure 1–1.
2. A is an example of a superficial wound. B is an example of a partial-thickness wound. C is an example of a full-thickness wound.
3. If the body is cold, the superficial vasculature within the dermis constricts to divert more blood to the body core. Conversely, if the body is hot, dermal vessels dilate, allowing heat to be dissipated into the environment.
4. The skin serves as a physical and chemical barrier; therefore, the patient is at risk for infection. The epidermis helps regulate fluid levels. The loss of such a large amount of skin will cause the patient to become dehydrated if the fluid loss is not replaced with intravenous fluids. The skin helps regulate body temperature. With the loss of such a large amount of skin, the patient may complain of being

cold and require blankets or warmer air temperature. The patient's sense of light touch will be impaired in the affected area, making him unaware of excess pressure from bandages or splints. The patient's self-image may be altered as a result of the current wounds and the fear of future scarring.
5. This is an example of a full-thickness wound.
6. This is an example of a partial-thickness wound.

CHAPTER 2

Answers to Checkpoint Questions

1. A partial-thickness wound involves the epidermis and part of the dermis. Therefore, epithelialization can occur from the wound margins and from the epidermal appendages located within the dermis.
2. This scenario describes delayed primary closure, also known as healing by tertiary intention.
3. a. The wound is now hypergranular.
   b. Physical therapy treatment options include applying pressure or silver nitrate to the hypergranular tissue. In addition, if a hydrocolloid dressing is being used, a different type of dressing should be selected.

Answers to Review Questions

1. Transudate is a collection of fluid caused by increased vascular permeability. Exudate is a mixture of transudate and cells.
2. Polymorphonuclear neutrophils (PMNs) marginate and then pave vessel walls. PMNs force their way

through small openings within the vessel walls produced during the vascular response and into the interstitial space. Once in the interstitium, PMNs migrate to the zone of injury along chemical gradients.

3. Angioblasts, endothelial cells adjacent to a wound, bud and grow into the injured area. Eventually these buds connect, forming functioning capillary loops. Vascular endothelial growth factor (VEGF) is a powerful stimulant for angiogenesis.

4. Granulation tissue is a temporary scaffolding created by fibroblasts consisting of water, proteoglycans, and fibers.

5. Dermal myofibroblasts decrease the size of a wound by pulling the wound margins closer together.

6. Both hypertrophic and keloid scarring result from the overproduction of immature collagen and are more common in individuals with darker skin. Hypertrophic scarring remains within the confines of the original wound, whereas keloids extend beyond the original wound.

7. A wound may become chronically inflamed if a foreign body or debris is in the wound bed, if there is repeated trauma to the wound bed, or if cytotoxic agents such as povidone–iodine are used.

8. a. You should be concerned that the patient may develop a cervical flexion contracture.

   b. There are many correct ways you might prevent a cervical flexion contracture. Two suggestions include (1) encouraging the patient to perform cervical active range of motion exercises, especially into a more extended position; and (2) limiting the patient's use of pillows while in bed to allow gravity to position the patient's neck in a more extended position.

9. Because full-thickness wounds involve the epidermis, dermis, and subcutaneous tissue, this wound should pass through the three phases of wound healing: inflammation, proliferation (consisting of angiogenesis, granulation tissue formation, wound contraction, and epithelialization), and maturation and remodeling.

CHAPTER 3

Answers to Checkpoint Questions

1. First, wounds heal faster in a moist wound environment. Second, chronic wounds are not self-limiting and require aggressive interventions if wound closure is to be achieved.

2. No. A patient may have a severe, life-threatening wound that is painless because of sensory nerve dysfunction.

3. Yes. The patient is at risk for delayed wound healing and, therefore, requires aggressive interventions if this is consistent with the patient's overall plan of care.

Answers to Review Questions

1. Colonization is the presence of microbes. Colonization is normal; therefore, no medical interventions are required. A wound is considered infected if a wound culture contains more than 10^5 microbes per gram of tissue. Infections impair wound healing and are usually treated with antibiotics or topical antimicrobials.

2. No, age-related changes are highly variable from individual to individual. However, it is probably safe to say that most 80-year-old individuals will heal slower than, say, a 40-year-old person with the same medical history.

3. Although Patient X's wound is slightly larger (5.6 cm^2 vs. 5.0 cm^2) and has some debris in it, it is likely to heal faster for three reasons. First, Patient X's wound is in a highly vascular location, the face. Second, Patient X is younger and healthy, while Patient Y has diabetes; therefore, Patient X is likely to be able to handle the small amount of debris present in the wound bed without becoming infected. Third, Patient X's wound is acute and is likely to follow the normal phases of wound healing, while Patient Y's wound has become chronic.

4. Although the wound is closed (there are no open areas), it is not yet healed. The pink scar color means the scar tissue has yet to be remodeled. The running and cutting of basketball-playing at this time would likely be too much stress on this fragile new scar tissue, especially if the wound required 3 months of non-weight-bearing treatment to reach closure. You should suggest the patient begin non-weight-bearing training, such as swimming, at this time.

CHAPTER 4

Answers to Checkpoint Questions

1. a. You should not document wound odor at this time. The wound must first be rinsed and debrided, if necessary, before assessing wound odor. Additionally, old dressings should never be used to assess wound odor.

b. It is not possible to determine the presence of infection from the information given.

2. The patient has a chronic wound. Her macrocirculation is diminished in the lower extremity. She has decreased sensation, although she does have protective sensation. The type, color, and amount of drainage suggest a *Pseudomonas* infection.

3. Sample goal revisions include:
   a. Wound will be completely resurfaced with epithelium in 1 month.
   b. Wound bed will contain at least 80% granular tissue in four visits.
   c. In 1 week, the wound will progress to the proliferative phase of wound healing as evidenced by the presence of granular buds within the wound bed.
   d. Wound will be clinically free of the signs and symptoms of infection in 2 weeks.
   e. Patient will demonstrate proper wound bandaging independently in two visits.

Answers to Review Questions

1. Wound location: anterior right knee

Wound Characteristics

Wound size	A. Superior wound: length × width × depth B. Middle wound: length × width × depth C. Inferior wound: length × width × depth
Tunneling/ under-mining	Unable to assess from photo.
Wound bed	Wound A and wound B are hypogranular, with 97% and 98% granular beds and 3% and 2% yellow slough, respectively. A and B granulation tissue is covered with a fibrous coating. Wound C is 100% covered with yellow slough.
Wound edges	Wound A edges are not attached to the base and appear rolled under from the 6-o'clock position to the 12-o'clock position. Wound B edges are not attached to the base and appear rolled under circumferentially. Wound C edges are attached to the wound base.
Wound drainage	Unable to assess from photo.
Wound odor	Unable to assess from photo.

Characteristics of the Periwound and Associated Skin

Structure and quality	Healed incision noted medial right knee, medial to current wounds. Wounds A–C involve a portion of the incision on the anterior aspect of the right knee.
Color	Mild hyperpigmentation lateral to wound B, medial to wound C, and inferior to wound C.
Epithelial appendages	Minimal leg hair growth noted (compared to contralateral side).
Edema	Right knee edema noted when compared to left, but no distinct periwound edema noted.
Temperature	Unable to assess from photo.

2. The wound fits into Pattern C: Impaired Integumentary Integrity Associated with Partial-Thickness Skin Involvement and Scar Formation.

3. The goals must be specific, measurable, objective, and time-dependent. Sample goals include:
   a. Wound C will be 100% granular in 1 week.
   b. Wound A depth will decrease by 0.2 cm in 2 weeks.

CHAPTER 5

Answers to Checkpoint Questions

1. You should debride the necrotic tissue, absorb exudate, and protect the surrounding tissue.
2. No. The patient's restlessness and agitation would make the use of sharp instruments potentially hazardous for both the patient and the clinician.

Answers to Review Questions

1. a. Autolytic debridement is a possibility and is the treatment of choice if the ulcer is not infected. The benefits of this method include the minimal pain involved with this procedure and the ability to leave the dressing in place for several days, therefore minimizing the time needed for wound care.
   b. Enzymatic debridement is a possibility and is the treatment of choice if the wound is infected.

The benefits of this method are that it causes only minimal pain, is faster than autolytic debridement, and can be used regardless of whether the ulcer is infected. The drawback is the need to change the dressing more frequently (at least daily pending the enzyme chosen).

c. Mechanical debridement is not the best choice for this patient. If the examination itself irritated the patient, any type of mechanical debridement is likely to further increase the patient's distress.

2. The referral is appropriate. The wound has failed to heal on its own and is 90% slough covered so an enzyme is appropriate. The use of an antimicrobial and antibiotic appears to be judicious as the patient presents with the signs and symptoms of an infection (moderate amount of thick yellow drainage, erythema, and fever).

3. Sharp debridement should be performed to hasten the resolution of infection and removal of the necrotic tissue. Some sort of mechanical debridement may be useful because of the high percentage of necrotic tissue, but this is not required.

4. There are many possible answers. The best answers are measurable, objective, and time-dependent. In addition, it is unlikely that a change in wound size would occur in 1 week given the amount of necrotic tissue, active infection, and increase in size since the original injury. Two sample goals include:
   a. In 1 week the wound will be free of yellow slough.
   b. In 1 week there will be no purulent or malodorous drainage.

5. You should consult with the referring physician to change your interventions for two reasons. First, the use of an enzyme in a wound with exposed tendon is contraindicated. Second, the patient no longer shows signs of infection, so the topical antimicrobial is no longer warranted.

6. Sharp debridement continues to be indicated to remove the remaining slough. Autolytic debridement would maintain a warm, moist wound environment and protect the tendons from dehydrating. However, the infection is just recently showing signs of resolution; therefore, there is a risk that autolytic debridement would allow any remaining bacteria to proliferate unchecked. Wet-to-dry dressings are contraindicated because of the exposed tendons. Therefore, you should suggest changing to only sharp debridement.

CHAPTER 6

Answers to Checkpoint Questions

1. The wound is probably infected. The significant amount of thick, blue-green drainage is characteristic of an infection.
2. a. Because there are no other subjective and objective changes, it is unlikely that this response is due to infection. The patient may have an allergy to sulfa.
   b. You should describe your findings to the referring physician and suggest changing to a sulfa-free antimicrobial, such as bacitracin.
3. a. Clean gloves.
   b. Gloves (forearm length or longer if necessary), water-impermeable gown, protective eyewear, and surgical mask or face shield.
   c. Sterile gloves.
   d. Clean gloves.
   e. Clean gloves.

Answers to Review Questions

1. a. The wound's chronicity despite adequate macrocirculation may be an indicator of an infection.
   b. The proportional amount of erythema, the slight local temperature increase, the amount and type of drainage, and the gross lack of edema are consistent with inflammation. The yellow-brown discoloration of the old bandages is due to the povidone–iodine.
   c. The wound appears to be chronically inflamed.
   d. The povidone–iodine should be discontinued. Rather, a moisture-retentive dressing should be chosen (see Chapter 7).
   e. Clean technique is appropriate.
2. a. Induration, purulent drainage, excessive erythema, and increasing pain despite appropriate care are suggestive of infection. Additionally, the patient's history of rheumatoid arthritis increases her risk for infection.
   b. The wound should be irrigated and debrided as much as possible. You should contact the patient's physician and request an order for both an aerobic and an anaerobic swab culture. You should also ask the physician if topical or systemic antimicrobial treatment should be initiated at this time.
   c. Sterile technique should be used when filling the wound tunnel.

CHAPTER 7

Answers to Checkpoint Questions

1. a. Wounds should remain covered, even at night. Keeping the wound bandaged helps retain wound fluids, enzymes, and growth factors; provides thermal insulation; prevents scab formation; helps remove and soften eschar; expedites wound healing; and decreases wound pain.

   b. It is normal for wounds to drain because the barrier function of the skin is lost. If drainage is excessive, is disproportionate to the size of the wound, or has an abnormal color or consistency, an infection should be suspected. In this case, the dressing should be changed at least daily and most moisture-retentive dressings would not be the most cost-effective option.

2. a. You could decrease the frequency of dressing changes to once a week or change to a less absorptive dressing. Appropriate dressing choices might include a sheet hydrogel secured with a roll gauze or an amorphous hydrogel with a nonadherent gauze and gauze square secured with a roll gauze.

   b. You could increase the frequency of dressing changes to three times per week. Alternatively, you could change to a more absorptive type of dressing such as a semipermeable foam or an alginate. You should also use a skin sealant to protect the periwound.

3. A growth factor is not appropriate at this time. The patient's wound is acute and caused by trauma without underlying factors that might deter healing. A growth factor should be reserved for chronic wounds that are recalcitrant to standard interventions.

4. A and C are not appropriate at this time. Because the wound is already very moist, the addition of an amorphous hydrogel will only increase this problem and is, therefore, not indicated. Because the wound exhibits signs of infection (heavy drainage that is milky white as well as warmth and erythema that are disproportionate to the size of the wound), a hydrocolloid is contraindicated at this time.

Answers to Review Questions

1. a. The wound should be irrigated to remove as much foreign debris as possible. A broad-spectrum antimicrobial may be applied to the wound prophylactically. A petrolatum-impregnated gauze is placed over the wound and covered by a sheet gauze. This should be secured with a self-adherent elastic wrap. The self-adherent elastic wrap should extend up to just above where the thigh begins to taper to prevent the dressing from sliding down as the player returns to the game. The advantage of this dressing is that it can be changed and the wound can be irrigated to remove any remaining foreign debris. The disadvantage is that, even with the self-adherent elastic wrap, the dressing is likely to slide during physical activity. This may cause further trauma to the wound bed, require the player to rewrap the wound during play, and be distracting to the player.

   b. The wound should be irrigated to remove as much foreign debris as possible. A broad-spectrum antimicrobial may be applied to the wound prophylactically. The periwound is thoroughly dried and a skin sealant is applied. An appropriately sized semipermeable film is placed over the wound ensuring no wrinkles and covering at least a 1- to 2-cm border of intact skin around the wound. The advantage of this dressing is that it allows visual inspection of the wound and periwound without removing the dressing. The film is also somewhat elastic and highly conformable. Therefore, it is more likely to stay in place and be less distracting to the player. Because this dressing maintains a moist environment better than gauze, it will likely be more comfortable than gauze as well. The only disadvantage of this dressing is that if the wound is bleeding more than minimally, the dressing will be unable to accommodate for this amount of fluid. There is little danger of infection if the majority of debris has been removed through irrigation and the patient is young and otherwise healthy.

2. A skin sealant should be applied to the wound perimeter. A moisturizer should be applied to the patient's foot, but not between the toes. Because of the recent bone infection and the implanted antimicrobial beads, the wound dressing should be changed at least daily. This, and the wound location, lends itself to a gauze dressing. The wound appears slightly dry and may benefit from an amorphous hydrogel to maintain a moist wound environment. A piece of petrolatum-impregnated

gauze should be placed over the wound, covered with a thin sheet of gauze, and secured with a two-ply roll gauze. The fourth toe should be wrapped individually. Alternatively, a small piece of cut gauze may be woven between the toes to provide padding and absorb wound exudate and perspiration, then the entire foot can be enclosed within a bulky (six-ply) roll gauze. Additionally, a temporary shoe should be prescribed for the patient to allow room for the bandages. The patient should be taught how to use an assistive device to unload the foot wound.

3. The dressing may be left on for 5–7 days. However, the dressing should be changed sooner if its integrity is compromised (if the dressing begins to roll up providing a channel into the wound area, if there is strike-through, or if the drainage is within a half inch of the dressing's border) or if the clinician suspects the onset of a wound infection (as indicated by a sudden change in patient status and the cardinal signs of infection).

4. a. The wound is necrotic and nondraining. It requires debridement, establishment of a moist wound environment, and protection of the surrounding tissue. Since the wound is of recent onset and previous treatment (left open to the air) has not been ideal, an enzyme and surgical debridement are not warranted at this time. There are no signs of infection. The patient's skin quality is decreased and the prolonged use of steroids makes her at risk for trauma if adhesive dressings are applied. Sharp debridement should be performed and any remaining eschar should be cross-hatched with a scalpel. The periwound should be protected with a skin sealant. An amorphous hydrogel can be applied to moisten the wound bed, followed by a sheet hydrogel secured with a roll gauze or self-adherent elastic wrap. The dressing can be changed in 3–5 days.

   b. The tunneling present at this time requires the use of gauze packing strips. To prevent further trauma when lightly packing this wound, it would be wise to use either a saline-moistened strip or a hydrogel-impregnated strip. To protect the surrounding tissue, a skin sealant is again applied. A petrolatum-impregnated gauze may be placed over the wound, followed by a gauze sheet. The dressing can then be secured with a roll gauze or a self-adherent elastic wrap.

CHAPTER 8

Answers to Checkpoint Questions

1. a. Whirlpool would be the most appropriate intervention as this would allow the removal of any topical agent, facilitate debridement of eschar, decrease pain, and allow for range of motion exercises.
   b. Pulsed lavage with suction would be most appropriate as this would help remove the thick drainage and allow thorough irrigation of the tunnel.
   c. Normal saline irrigation would be most appropriate as this would allow the wound to be irrigated with minimal wound bed trauma, low cost, and little clinician time.

2. The most appropriate parameters would be to use high-voltage pulsed current with a frequency of 100 Hz (80–125 Hz) and an intensity of 75–200 volts that produces a comfortable paresthesia. Positive polarity (anodal stimulation) should be used to promote granulation tissue formation and epithelialization. Treatment should be 45 minutes, 3 days per week, although other options may also be appropriate.

Answers to Review Questions

1. The following alternative interventions may be indicated for this patient: whirlpool, pulsed lavage with suction, electrical stimulation, ultrasound, and hyperbaric oxygen.

2. Whirlpool is not indicated because the patient is incontinent and does not have a catheter. Pulsed lavage with suction should not be your first choice because the patient is taking anticoagulants, which may result in bleeding at the treatment site and delay wound healing. Although you could use pulsed lavage without suction, the previous treatment included wound irrigation with normal saline twice daily without improvement so this also is unlikely to enhance wound healing.

3. Ultrasound is not indicated because of the wound size and amount of necrosis. Although hyperbaric oxygen may be indicated, the high cost of this intervention and need to transport the patient to a facility for a TCOM assessment and a hyperbaric oxygen chamber make it a less appealing first line of treatment. Therefore, electrical stimulation

would be the most appropriate adjunctive intervention for this patient.

4. Specific electrical stimulation parameters that may be appropriate include high-voltage pulsed current with a frequency of 100 Hz. Intensity may produce a comfortable paresthesia; however, due to the patient's stroke, this sensory response cannot be relied upon, and the intensity should be set at a submotor level that is less than 200 volts. Cathodal stimulation should be used at this time because of the presence of necrotic tissue and infection. Treatment should be 45 minutes daily, although other options may also be appropriate.

5. The wound should be irrigated with normal saline and debrided as much as possible with each session. A skin sealant should be applied to the periwound and an absorptive dressing, such as an alginate and gauze, should be applied after electrical stimulation. A moisture-retentive dressing, such as a hydrocolloid, is not appropriate because of the need for frequent dressing changes and current/recent infection.

6. Additional physical therapy interventions may include therapeutic exercise and mobility training to improve the patient's ability to unweight the affected area to allow healing and prevent additional pressure ulcers from forming. A pressure-relieving mattress and a nutritional assessment (if not already performed) should be ordered. Refer to Chapter 12 for additional information on the examination and treatment of pressure ulcers.

CHAPTER 9

Answers to Checkpoint Questions

1. Although weight loss will enhance wound healing in a patient who is obese, the patient must maintain a positive nitrogen balance to have the energy and materials required for tissue repair and regeneration. Therefore, while a diet that is very low in calories may assist with more rapid weight loss, it will also adversely affect wound healing.

2. A patient with type 2 diabetes may have difficulty following the recommended diet because it involves a major change in lifestyle, because he or she does not know what this diet would consist of, or because he or she does not understand how following this diet will affect wound healing.

3. While performing wound management techniques, you could ask Mr. B about his blood sugar control, including how well he is adhering to his diet and what his most recent blood sugar test results were. You could also ask Mr. B why glycemic control is important.

Answers to Review Questions

1. Miss W is at risk for malnutrition. Because her burns are extensive, she will lose a significant amount of fluid and protein due to wound drainage, placing her at risk for dehydration, hypovolemic shock, and a negative nitrogen balance. Her metabolic rate will increase in response to the injury, resulting in increased energy expenditure that must be counteracted by a high-protein, high-calorie, high-carbohydrate diet. This diet will also provide Miss W with the nutrients required for wound healing. In addition, pain, fear, and significant upper extremity involvement will likely reduce Miss W's ability to eat independently.

2. You should request a dietary consult and ensure someone is present to assist Miss W during mealtimes. You should encourage the patient to drink water during your session. You should also ensure the patient's intravenous line does not become compromised during treatment.

3. Although there are myriad ways these issues might be addressed, the following provides some potential methods to increase patient participation. First, you should ensure adequate pain control prior to therapy sessions, requesting a bolus of medication just prior to treatment, if needed. Second, using terms Miss W can understand, you should briefly explain the purpose of debridement and range of motion exercises as well as the sensations to be expected during treatment. Third, you can enlist the support of Miss W's parents and family to decrease patient fear.

4. The clinician should provide encouragement and praise for participation.

5. Although there are myriad ways this issue might be addressed, the following provides some potential methods to increase patient participation. First, you should define limits for each therapy session. For example, debridement will be stopped after 15 minutes or the patient must perform five repetitions of range of motion exercises in each affected joint. Second, by performing range of motion exercises in the whirlpool, the patient's

pain and anxiety may be decreased. Third, you could distract the patient by playing games or having toys in the whirlpool to encourage movement or allow debridement.

6. Again, there are many potential methods that can be initiated to reinforce occupational therapy goals. For example, you could have the patient assist with removing the bandages or use a gauze square to help remove residual topical agents and loose debris.

CHAPTER 10

Answers to Checkpoint Questions

1. a. The patient's advanced age is a nonmodifiable risk factor.
   b. The following risk factors may be modified or controlled: high cholesterol, hypertension (HTN), high blood sugar, increased body weight, and smoking.
   c. The patient may benefit from:
      1) Closer medical supervision for pharmacological management of hypertension, diabetes mellitus, and cholesterol.
      2) A referral to a registered dietitian to assist with the management of his blood pressure, blood sugar, cholesterol, and weight.
      3) A referral to a smoking cessation program.
      4) In addition to local wound care, physical therapy should provide a graded exercise program to assist with blood pressure and blood sugar regulation and weight control.

2. a. $\text{ABI} = \dfrac{\text{systolic pressure of the lower extremity}}{\text{systolic pressure of the upper extremity}}$

   $= \dfrac{70}{120}$

   $= 0.58$

   b. The patient has moderate arterial insufficiency and likely complains of intermittent claudication. In addition to the low calculated ABI, systolic ankle pressures less than 80 mm Hg are associated with poor healing potential. A trial of conservative interventions may be performed, but the patient should have a vascular consult. Referral is mandatory if the wound worsens or fails to progress with appropriate conservative interventions.

3. a. Performing the ABI is painful because inflation of the cuff further occludes the patient's circulation, causing ischemic pain.
   b. A Doppler ultrasound should be performed to assess distal pulses. The rubor of dependency test and venous filling time would provide additional information regarding the patient's arterial circulation without causing undue discomfort.

4. a. The patient's presentation is consistent with arterial insufficiency in position, presentation, and periwound condition.
   b. The examiner should perform a pulse examination, palpate the affected area for temperature differences, and question the patient about pain at rest and in varying positions. Additional information that would help to clarify the wound's etiology includes the patient's past medical history as well as some additional tests and measures, such as an ABI and sensation.

5. Direct heat to arterial insufficient limbs can cause significant tissue damage. You should tell the patient not to use a heating pad or soak her feet in warm water. Alternatively, you should advise her to wear warm socks.

6. The use of a moisture-retentive dressing is appropriate. However, compression is contraindicated with low ABIs, as the elastic compression wrap will further compromise the patient's circulation.

Answers to Review Questions

1. First, you should reassess the physical therapy plan of care and the follow-through of this plan both within therapy and by the patient/caregiver. If both are deemed appropriate, the patient should be referred to a physician or vascular surgeon immediately. The physical therapy tests and measures performed indicate moderate to severe arterial insufficiency and a potentially limb-threatening situation. An increase in wound size despite appropriate conservative interventions mandates a referral.

2. a. Debridement should be included within the physical therapy plan of care for two reasons. First, the patient has sufficient circulation for debridement in a physical therapy setting. Second, removal of devitalized tissue should facilitate wound healing by decreasing the amount of energy required for autolytic debridement alone.

b. Method 1: Apply an amorphous hydrogel to moisten the wound bed. Method 2 (with physician's prescription): Apply an enzyme to assist with debridement.

c. Using either topical agent described above, Method 1: gauze square, secure with a light gauze wrap, cotton padding between toes as needed. Method 2: cover wounds with toe caps.

d. The ulcer locations are typical for either spontaneous arterial ulceration or ulceration as a result of excessive pressure from a shoe on a foot with compromised circulation. Regardless, the addition of bandages within the patient's current footwear will likely exacerbate the situation. The patient should be fitted for temporary footwear, such as a postoperative or Darco shoe, that allows room for bandages and does not put pressure on any non-weight-bearing areas of the patient's foot.

3. a. You should assess Mrs. Y's pulses (using a Doppler ultrasound if needed) and sensation. You should perform an ABI and, if abnormal, perform segmental pressure measurements.

b. Arterial insufficiency ulcer, left medial malleolus, measuring ($l \times w \times d$), unable to ascertain depth of tissue destruction secondary to necrotic tissue, wound bed is 90% covered with necrotic tissue, 5% granulation tissue at the anterior wound border (from approximately 2-o'clock to 5-o'clock positions, with the head being the 12-o'clock position), 5% of bed centrally contains exposed deltoid ligament, which appears intact. Periwound erythema extending X cm from wound edge. Periwound temperature appears Z compared to ipsilateral calf and thigh. Surrounding tissue exhibits loss of hair growth and is anhydrous.

c. The wound contains necrotic tissue that should be debrided. If the ABI is $>0.3 \geq 0.5$, this may be done within the physical therapy setting.

d. A moisturizer should be applied to the intact skin. A skin sealant should be applied to the wound perimeter. An acceptable wound dressing might include an amorphous hydrogel, an impregnated gauze contact layer, and a layer of gauze padding to protect the wound from further trauma. Secure with a roll gauze without compression.

e. The patient and caregiver should be educated in proper foot/leg care guidelines as well as how to care for the wound. Transfer training and possibly bed mobility training will assist with patient mobility and independence, thereby decreasing the risk of pressure ulcers and deconditioning. Upper extremity aerobic exercise, such as wheelchair mobility or upper body ergometry, may be prescribed to assist with blood sugar control without unduly taxing circulation to the foot. Electrical stimulation may be used as an adjunct to wound healing.

CHAPTER 11

Answers to Checkpoint Questions

1. Inspiratory spirometry or diaphragmatic breathing exercises will enhance the effect of the respiratory pump on venous return. Repeated active ankle dorsiflexion and plantar flexion and walking will enhance the effect of the calf muscle pump on venous return.

2. The periwound is too moist, causing maceration and increasing the size of the wound. You should discontinue the amorphous hydrogel and apply a skin sealant to the periwound. In addition, you should consider either using a more absorptive dressing, such as a semipermeable foam, hydrocolloid, or alginate, or increasing the frequency of dressing changes to twice weekly to better control the wound drainage.

3. Based on Laplace's law, assuming all other variables are equal, the smaller the bandage width, the more compression it will provide. Therefore, the 8-cm bandage will provide the greatest amount of compression.

4. The patient seems to have developed a sensitization to the paste bandage. You should initiate another form of compression therapy that is less likely to cause a reaction, such as a multilayer compression bandage system or CircAid. You should also contact the physician about the use of a topical glucocorticoid ointment to decrease erythema and pruritus.

Answers to Review Questions

1. a. Given the copious, foul-smelling, and neon green color of the drainage, you should request an order for a culture and sensitivity and appropriate topical and/or systemic antimicrobial interventions.

b. The patient does not appear to have arterial insufficiency. His ABI is normal, and his pulses are likely diminished due to peripheral edema.

c. The patient should be treated with compression after appropriate antimicrobial treatment has been initiated.

d. Given that infection is suspected and there is significant wound drainage, the bandage should be changed daily. Appropriate choices for compression include a short-stretch compression wrap, CircAid, or a tubular bandage. An UlcerCare garment should not be used at this time because the swelling will decrease and the garment will no longer fit properly.

2. a. You should assess Mr. V's pulses and perform an ABI and assess for the possibility of a deep vein thrombosis. You may also choose to perform a Trendelenburg's test and a Doppler examination.

b. Venous insufficiency ulcer, medial malleolus, measuring ($l \times w \times d$). Wound bed contains approximately 5% necrotic tissue primarily at wound margins. Periwound maceration extending X cm from wound edge. Periwound temperature appears X compared to ipsilateral calf. Surrounding tissue exhibits hemosiderin deposition and lipodermatosclerosis with discoloration extending X cm from the wound edge.

c. Whirlpool would be contraindicated for this patient because the dependent positioning and warm water would exacerbate Mr. V's edema, venous hypertension, excessive wound drainage, and maceration.

d. A moisturizer should be applied to the intact skin. A skin sealant should be applied to the wound perimeter. An acceptable wound dressing might include an alginate, a nonadhesive semipermeable foam, and a multilayer compression bandage system.

e. The patient should be educated in proper leg care guidelines as well as how to care for the wound. Therapeutic exercise, such as ambulation, repeated ankle pumps, and aerobic exercise, should also be included in the plan of care.

f. As a cashier, the patient stands statically for extended periods of time, which contributes to venous hypertension. If possible, the patient should try to use a chair and prop his leg up on a stool. You should encourage the patient to perform ankle pumps and calf raises, or ambulate when able during his shift.

3. There are no signs of infection. The patient's ABI of 0.8 is within the suggested guidelines for the use of compression. His pulses may be decreased due to edema. However, the wound is increasing in size with compression therapy and the wound bed is pale. The patient likely has concomitant arterial insufficiency. It is possible that he has calcific arterial disease due to his diabetes, making his ABI artificially elevated. Therefore, you should discontinue compression therapy. Either a moisture-retentive dressing or a traditional gauze dressing with an amorphous hydrogel may be used instead. Negative pressure wound therapy may be considered as an adjunct to wound healing if this change in treatment plan does not enhance wound healing. If improvements are not noted during the 2 weeks following this change in the plan of care, you should consult with the patient's physician.

CHAPTER 12

Answers to Checkpoint Questions

1. Patients have less contact with the support surface when seated than when supine. Because pressure is defined as force per unit area, contact pressures are higher when patients are seated. The inverse relationship between pressure and time means that patients may develop pressure ulcers in less time if subjected to higher pressures. Therefore, patients must reposition more often when seated than supine to reduce the risk of pressure ulcer formation.

2. Due to the increased time spent sitting in a wheelchair and impaired sensation below the level of injury, the most common location for pressure ulcers in patients with spinal cord injuries is over the ischium.

3. Although the lighter weight of foam would make wheelchair mobility and lifting her cushion in and out of the car easier, Ms. B is likely to bottom out on foam due to her increased body weight, and the foam cushion would be soiled by incontinence. An air-filled cushion would make transfers more difficult for Ms. B. A gel-filled cushion would be most likely to prevent bottoming out, withstand repeated episodes of incontinence, and allow ease of transfers.

Answers to Review Questions

1. a. No, wound care is not a priority with this patient at this time. Aggressive debridement

would cause the patient undue pain and is not consistent with a palliative care plan. Enzymatic debridement is also not indicated.

b. No, Mrs. K is not a surgical candidate as this is not consistent with a palliative care plan.

c. No, electrical stimulation is not consistent with a palliative care plan.

d. In this situation, clinicians would be wise to choose dressings that minimize patient discomfort as well as the frequency and time needed for dressing changes. A synthetic dressing, such as a hydrocolloid, would be appropriate.

2. a. Pressure ulcer, left greater trochanter, measuring (l × w × d). Wound bed contains 75% granulation tissue or healthy muscle, 15% desiccated adipose tissue posteriorly, 10% necrotic tissue superiorly. Periwound not assessed at this time as it is covered with a hydrocolloid. Erythema right buttock. Skin temperature is comparable to surrounding areas.

b. The wound has about 10% necrotic tissue superiorly that may be debrided in physical therapy to decrease the risk of repeat infection and enhance wound healing.

c. Gauze packing strips covered with bulky gauze pads, such as ABD pads, may be used to take up dead space and absorb drainage. Montgomery straps can be attached to the hydrocolloid on either side of the wound and tied to help approximate the wound edges. A moisture barrier should be applied to Miss T's perineum to protect intact skin.

d. The patient should be placed on a pressure-reducing mattress. She should not be positioned on her right side. To prevent additional pressure ulcers, her heels should be kept off the bed using pillows or wedges, she should not be positioned directly on her right side, and the head of the bed should be kept below 30 degrees except when eating. Miss T should be assisted, if needed, with position changes at least every 2 hours, more often if there is erythema lasting more than 10 minutes on the recently unweighted area.

e. Miss T may benefit from electrical stimulation as an adjunct to wound healing. If she is able to follow directions, she may also benefit from physical therapy for therapeutic exercise to assist with mobility.

f. If not already performed, you should request a dietary consult because of the association of

malnutrition with pressure ulcer development and slow wound healing. If the patient is incontinent, you should also request a urology consult to assess for physical reasons for incontinence, such as a urinary tract infection.

3. a. Because of the exposed bone, the wound should be classified as a category/stage IV pressure ulcer and would fit into Integumentary Preferred Practice Pattern E: Impaired Integumentary Integrity Associated with Skin Involvement Extending into Fascia, Muscle, or Bone and Scar Formation.

b. The wound is improving. Although there is an increase in wound size, the wound is now free of eschar. The eschar present on initial examination did not allow an accurate picture of the true extent of the wound. The undermining is typical for pressure ulcers and is likely a result of previous deep tissue ischemia.

c. No, there are no signs of infection noted. The amount and type of drainage are normal, and there is no odor present.

CHAPTER 13

Answers to Checkpoint Questions

1. Diabetes also adversely affects the eyes, kidneys, blood vessels, immune system, and nerves.
2. Patient Y's ulcer is deep with exposed tendon, capsule, or bone. A grade 2 ulcer would fit into Integumentary Preferred Practice Pattern E.
3. Patients with diabetes have autonomic neuropathy, which leads to dry, cracked skin and increased callus formation. Skin cracks provide a means for microbes to enter the body. Calluses cause localized areas of pressure, which can lead to ulceration. Moisturizing lotion can prevent anhydrous skin and decrease callus formation.
4. A grade 3 ulcer is not appropriate for total contact casting but may be unloaded by having the patient use a padded ankle-foot orthosis, a walker and partial weight-bearing gait pattern, or a wheelchair.

Answers to Review Questions

1. Yes. Improved glycemic control can reduce the development and progression of the long-term complications of diabetes, including neuropathy, retinopathy, vascular disease, and immune response.

2. Patient X may have dry and cracked skin, thick calluses, or foot deformities.

3. Patient D may be nonadherent because (1) he does not understand the importance of using the walker, (2) he has difficulty maintaining non-weight bearing due to lack of balance or fatigue, or (3) his ulcer is not painful. Alternative methods might include allowing Patient D to use a partial weight-bearing gait pattern, obtaining a wheelchair, or using a total contact cast or padded ankle-foot orthosis as indicated. In addition, you should reemphasize the importance of limiting mechanical stress to the ulcer.

4. The tissue is likely the first metatarsophalangeal joint capsule. If you are a physical therapist assistant, you should inform the primary physical therapist. If you are the physical therapist, you should inform the physician because of the risk of osteomyelitis.

5. a. You should perform the following tests and measures related to the patient's wounds: pedal pulses, sensory integrity, wound size, wound depth, and assess for tunneling or undermining. Local temperature may be assessed. An ABI should be performed if pulses are not normal or if there is a history of peripheral vascular disease.

   b. Mr. W presents with a full-thickness neuropathic ulceration on the plantar aspect of his first metatarsal head. (Note the medial first metatarsal wound is not clearly visible in this photo and, therefore, is not described here.) The wound bed is 100% granular; however, the quality of this tissue is suspect, given the deep red color and rough texture. The wound appears hypogranular, and the edges are not attached to the wound base. The wound has a ring of macerated callus surrounding it. The wound is classified as a grade 2 ulcer and would fit into Integumentary Preferred Practice Pattern E.

   c. The callus should be debrided to enhance wound closure.

   d. From this photo alone, the wound does not appear to be infected. However, the quality of the granulation tissue and the significant amount of maceration might lead one to suspect that a subclinical infection may be present.

   e. A moisturizing lotion should be applied to the intact skin. A skin sealant should be applied to the periwound. If a wound infection is suspected, the wound may be wrapped with a calcium alginate contact layer, thick gauze pad, and a roll gauze, secured with tape. A padded ankle-foot orthosis is used to unweight the ulcer. If an infection is not suspected a total contact cast may be used.

   f. Other interventions may include the use of an assistive device, temporary shoe inserts, or a walking shoe to unweight the ulcer. Assuming the ulcer is not infected, the patient may benefit from stretching and/or joint mobilization if dorsiflexion, great toe extension, and gastrocnemius length are not within normal limits. Aerobic exercise such as cycling with relief at the forefoot or upper body ergometry may be prescribed if there is a need to improve glycemic control.

   g. The patient may benefit from a consult with a registered dietitian and the physician attending to his diabetes in order to attain/maintain maximum glycemic control. If Mr. W's blood sugars are not satisfactorily controlled, you should request a consult with the physician attending to his diabetes (primary care physician or endocrinologist). In addition, a consult with a registered dietitian for medical nutrition therapy may be warranted.

CHAPTER 14

Answers to Checkpoint Questions

1. The wound appears to be a superficial partial-thickness burn injury. However, because chemical burns may take 24–72 hours to fully develop, you should reserve making a definitive diagnosis at this time.

2. a. The patient is at high risk for burn shock due to the depth and size (27% TBSA) of the burn wound injury. The clinician should monitor the patient's heart rate during therapy to ensure it stays between 100 and 120 beats per minute to avoid overstressing the patient's system. Intravenous lines should be monitored for signs of compromise to ensure adequate fluid resuscitation. Because the patient's burns are circumferential, there is a risk of compartment syndrome. Therefore, the clinician should closely monitor peripheral pulses. A Doppler ultrasound may be needed. Any decline in status should be reported to the physician immediately. The affected limbs should be elevated to help reduce edema.

b. Because the patient has a history of a closed space injury, there may be pulmonary involvement from smoke inhalation. The clinician should carefully monitor the patient for signs of respiratory distress, such as dyspnea or stridor. Any decline in status should be reported to the physician immediately. To help minimize any pulmonary damage, the clinician should encourage aggressive pulmonary hygiene, including deep breathing.

3. a. Yes. The burns are suspicious as they may have resulted from an intentional submersion in hot water. In cases of accidental scald injuries during bathing, the infant is more likely to present with burns to the posterior trunk, buttocks, and posterior lower extremities.

   b. You should report your findings to a social worker. In addition, you should follow any state laws and facility policies regarding the reporting of suspected abuse of a minor.

Answers to Review Questions

1. The wound appears to be a deep partial-thickness burn injury.
2. Using the rule of nines, the burn covers approximately one-half of the anterior surface of each lower extremity, or $1/2(9\%) \times 2$ legs $= 9\%$ of total body surface area. When using the Lund–Browder classification, the burn covers approximately $[2.75\% (1/2 \text{ of one leg}) + 1.75\% (\text{dorsal foot})] \times 2$ legs $= 9\%$.
3. The wound will reepithelialize from the periphery and from the spared epidermal appendages within the wound area and will require at least 3 weeks to heal. Surgical interventions may be required because of the large size and depth of tissue involvement.
4. Local wound care should consist of whirlpool followed by saline irrigation, debridement, and bandaging with a topical antimicrobial, such as silver sulfadiazine, a nonadherent gauze, gauze pad, and gauze wrap. You may choose to use sterile technique initially because of the depth and extent of injury. A low-stretch compression bandage should be applied to help control edema when the patient is out of bed. Bandages should be changed two times per day to ensure silver sulfadiazine antimicrobial effectiveness.
5. The wound locations may lead to bilateral plantar flexion contractures.

6. These may be prevented or lessened by having the patient perform active dorsiflexion repeatedly throughout the day. If necessary, the patient's caregivers can assist with this exercise. The patient can be positioned in neutral or slight dorsiflexion using posterior leaf splints or a foot board. When the patient is sitting or in bed, her legs should be elevated to decrease edema, which may further restrict range of motion.
7. The patient will likely have difficulty with transfers and gait. To encourage mobility, you should ensure adequate pain control. An assistive device such as a walker may be beneficial.

CHAPTER 15

Answers to Checkpoint Questions

1. a. This scenario describes a low-risk individual partaking in a low-force, high-repetition activity. Taken in context, this individual has a low risk for developing lymphedema.
   b. This scenario describes a high-risk individual partaking in a high-load, high-frequency task. Taken in context, this individual has a significant risk for developing lymphedema.
2. The following anastamoses can be used to move fluid from the left lower extremity to the uncongested neighboring quadrants: the anterior inguino–inguinal pathway, the posterior inguino–inguinal pathway, and the left inguinal–axillary pathway.
3. LaPlace's law is an equation used to determine the amount of compression exerted by a compression wrap.

   Bandage compression
   $$= \frac{(\text{tension}) (\text{layers applied}) (\text{constant})}{(\text{limb girth}) (\text{bandage width})}$$

Answers to Review Questions

1. You should discuss the patient's lymphedema with the hand surgeon and request that the tourniquet time during surgery be a little as possible and with as little compression as is medically necessary to perform the procedure. You should have the patient don her compression sleeve and glove or gauntlet as soon after the procedure as possible. Alternatively, if the patient or caregiver has learned how to perform multilayer compression bandaging, you should have

the patient be bandaged as soon after surgery as possible. The bandage should be rewrapped daily until the post-operative follow-up with the surgeon about a week after surgery. The patient should remeasure her limb at this time. If her arm is swollen at that time, she should continue to wrap and contact you for further more intensive treatment options. If her limb is not swollen, she may return to wearing her compression garment.

2. a. No. Because your arm swelling has resolved at this time you only need to wear your compression garment if you are performing high-risk activities, such as repeated movements or lifting.

b. Yes. This is a lifetime precaution. Because there is less air pressure in the cabin of an airplane while flying, your arm may swell again if you fly without the extra compression provided by wearing your garment.

c. Yes. This is a lifetime precaution. Your lymph system has been permanently changed as a result of your surgery and radiation. The tourniquet-like effect of a blood pressure cuff may further damage your lymphatic system in your left arm and exacerbate your lymphedema.

d. No. This is a lifetime precaution. Being in a jacuzzi or hot tub causes a systemic increase in body temperature. To control your body temperature, blood is shunted to your skin and this extra fluid must be reabsorbed by your lymphatic system. Since the lymph system draining your left arm has been permanently altered, it is possible that this increase in fluid will exacerbate your lymphedema.

e. Yes. It is possible for lymphedema to recur. By regularly self-measuring your arm, you can identify subtle changes in your arm size indicating an exacerbation of your lymphedema rather than waiting for more overt changes, such as tight jewelry or shirt sleeves.

3. a. You would want to assess for a possible deep vein thrombosis by following the Clinical Assessment Guidelines for Deep Vein Thrombosis discussed in Chapter 11. If this is negative, you should perform an ABI. You should also assess Mr. Gerard's sensation using monofilaments.

b. 1. These interventions will assist with post-operative edema control and should be a part of his treatment.

2. These interventions will assist with restoring Mr. Gerard's knee motion after surgery as well as assist in decreasing lower extremity edema by enhancing his calf and leg muscle pumps.

3. A bike will assist with restoring Mr. Gerard's knee motion after surgery as well as assist in decreasing lower extremity edema. If he is able to perform full revolutions at a pace, this may also assist with enhancing Mr. Gerard's respiratory pump, thereby decreasing edema.

4. A below knee compression garment is not indicated at this time because his leg is still swollen. There is no evidence that the garment will reduce his swelling and when his swelling does decrease, the garment may not fit properly. In addition, a below-knee garment does not address Mr. Gerard's knee edema.

5. An above-knee garment would address Mr. Gerard's knee and leg edema but, as noted in the previous answer, is not currently indicated.

6. Multilayer compression bandaging from Mr. Gerard's toes to his groin is indicated to assist with edema control.

7. Manual lymph drainage may be performed, but is not as high a priority as compression wrapping and exercise.

CHAPTER 16

Answers to Checkpoint Questions

1. Abrasions are either superficial or partial-thickness wounds. Therefore, abrasions affect only the epidermis and the dermis.

2. a. A broad-spectrum topical antimicrobial would be beneficial given the overt wound contamination and the potential for infection.

b. No, you should not choose a semipermeable foam dressing. Because the patient's wound is at high risk for infection, the dressing should be changed at least daily. Therefore, a gauze dressing may be preferred.

3. a. Soft tissue mobilization is contraindicated to irradiated tissue because the mechanical forces may damage this fragile tissue, potentially creating an open wound.

b. Thermal interventions, such as ultrasound or hotpacks, are contraindicated because they will increase local tissue perfusion. Since the patient has had trauma to her lymphatic system (surgical node removal, postoperative scarring, and radiation damage), this added blood flow may exceed her lymphatic capacity, creating lymphedema. Second, irradiated tissue is hypovascular and the patient may not be able to dissipate the thermal forces leading to tissue damage.

Answers to Review Questions

1. a. The wound should be irrigated with saline or tap water. Any large pieces of debris should be removed with forceps. If the wound is not very tender, the wound bed may be gently scrubbed with a high-porosity sponge to further remove more embedded debris. A topical antimicrobial should be applied and the wound should be covered with a gauze dressing. A self-adherent elastic wrap, such as Coban, can be applied to help maintain wound coverage while the patient returns to playing.

   b. The patient should be instructed to wash the wound with soap and water once or twice a day and repeat the same bandaging procedure. The patient and his guardian should also be instructed in the signs and symptoms of wound infection and to contact his family physician if these are observed.

2. The wound may be irrigated. Then you should elevate the wound slightly and provide gentle compression to control the bleeding. If there are any areas of devitalized tissue, you should remove them with scissors (a physician's order may be required by law). If the wound edges can be approximated, they should be. The wound should then be covered with a nonadherent dressing secured with a roll gauze. A foam dressing may also be used. However, if the patient's skin integrity is in doubt, a nonadhesive foam should be chosen.

3. First, the patient's wound may be infected. A wound culture or a physician-performed tissue biopsy could be used to determine infection. If positive, the physician should use the results of the sensitivity testing to determine the appropriate antibiotic. Second, the patient may have pyoderma gangrenosum, and the repeated debridement is exacerbating the inflammatory destructive process. A negative wound culture or tissue biopsy would provide further support for

this theory, however, there is no definitive test for pyoderma. If pyoderma is suspected, the physical therapist should perform only minimal debridement of loose slough and the physician will manage the patient pharmacologically.

4. a. Pitting edema at the end of the day that resolves after recumbency is suggestive of venous insufficiency or lymphedema.

   b. After performing an ABI to rule out arterial insufficiency, you should initiate compression using either a multilayer compression bandage or a short-stretch compression bandage. The patient should also be instructed in ankle pumping exercises and proper positioning to assist with edema control.

5. a. The patient may have pyoderma gangrenosum.

   b. Discuss the clinical findings of your examination with the referring physician. Include the physical findings of the wound, the patient's history of ulcerative colitis, and the fact that the wound has not responded to conventional interventions for venous ulcer management. You may recommend a biopsy or referral to a dermatologist for further assessment.

   c. For individuals with dark pigmentation it is important to assess the skin for other clues beyond erythema. Inflammation may be more readily determined by tissue temperature discrepancies. In addition, inflammation may present as a blue to purple discoloration. It is also important to establish the normal color variations of a patient's skin to determine what is normal versus abnormal. You should compare the affected side with the patient's contralateral side and ask the patient about his or her normal skin color variations to determine what may be abnormal.

CHAPTER 17

Answers to Checkpoint Questions

1. a. These lesions may represent dermatitis or eczema.

   b. You should ask Ms. G when the rash occurred, if the skin is itchy, and if she has had a similar rash previously. You should also ask the patient if she has come into contact with any potential irritants, such as a new detergent, soap, or moisturizing lotion.

c. You should instruct the patient to avoid any potential irritants and refrain from scratching the affected areas. In addition, you may suggest Ms. G contact her physician, especially if the condition gets worse or if she requires medication to help control the pruritus.

d. Ultrasound should not be performed over broken skin. Given the extent of the affected area, even if the specific area to be treated does not have any open areas, it would be wise to withhold ultrasound, at least for this day, to reduce the potential for complications.

2. a. Erythema and scaling on the plantar aspect of the feet may represent tinea pedis.

b. You should instruct the patient to wash his feet daily, dry all aspects of his feet thoroughly, and wear clean, dry socks and shoes. The patient should be instructed to use shower shoes rather than walk barefoot through locker rooms and showers. In addition, you should suggest that the patient discuss the use of topical antifungals with his physician.

c. A hydrocolloid dressing is contraindicated for use with tinea pedis as the occlusiveness of this product would exacerbate the infection.

Answers to Review Questions

1. a. Physical therapists do not diagnose specific disease entities. They can, however, formulate a clinical diagnosis and discuss significant findings with other health care providers. The tumor present on this patient may be suggestive of a melanocytic nevi, seborrheic keratosis, malignant melanoma, or dermatofibroma. The patient should be referred back to her referring physician or to a dermatologist to examine the tumor.

b. When discussing the lesion with her physician, it is important to provide objective and subjective findings. You should discuss your clinical findings with the physician and recommend further examination of the tumor because of its suspicious presentation.

c. After examining this patient, a treatment plan should be formulated, based on the objective and subjective findings. However, the use of modalities should be postponed until a physician has examined the tumor. If the lesion is benign, you may continue your therapeutic interventions, including the use of modalities. If the lesion is malignant, the patient should undergo treatment to manage the tumor and resume therapy only after being cleared by her physician.

2. a. This rash may be related to the patient's lupus, as it is common for patients to have cutaneous involvement. However, the rash may also be related to a new medication the patient is taking to manage her condition.

b. Specific questions to ask the patient include:
   • When did you first notice the symptoms?
   • Are you taking any new medications, and if so, when did you start the medication?
   • Have you been in the sun lately?

c. The patient's referring physician should be notified of the rash, and the objective and subjective findings should be discussed. The physician may want to see the patient to determine if the rash is related to the lupus or to a new medication. The physician will also determine if therapy should be continued or deferred.

APPENDIX D
Wound Care Billing and Coding

by *Dr. Lam Le*, MD, CWSP, FACHM, FAPWCA

This Appendix consists of the following basic information needed for wound management billing and coding.

1. Commonly used wound care ICD-9 codes
2. Modifier codes for wound management
3. CPT codes for wound management
4. Reimbursement and documentation for debridement
5. Evaluation and Management CPT codes and descriptions (to be used by physicians in an outpatient setting)

WOUND CARE ICD-9 CODES

Wound care billing and coding can be extremely overwhelming for the clinician. However, there are only a few common CPT and ICD-9 codes that are used in Wound and Hyperbaric Medicine. The following tables provide short lists to help the clinician navigate through wound care billing and coding.

TABLE D–1   Commonly Used Wound Care ICD-9 Codes

ICD-9	Diagnosis
250.8	Diabetes with other specified manifestations
440.21	Atherosclerosis of the extremities with intermittent claudication
440.22	Atherosclerosis of the extremities with rest pain
440.23	Atherosclerosis of the extremities with ulceration
440.24	Atherosclerosis of the extremities with gangrene
444.21	Arterial embolism and thrombosis of arteries of the upper extremities
444.22	Arterial embolism and thrombosis of arteries of the lower extremities
451.2	Phlebitis and thrombophlebitis of lower extremities, unspecified
454.0	Varicose veins of lower extremities with ulcer
454.1	Varicose veins of lower extremities with inflammation
454.2	Varicose veins of lower extremities with ulcer and inflammation
454.8	Varicose veins of lower extremities with other complications
457.1	Lymphedema, chronic
681.0	Cellulitis and abscess of finger

(*continued*)

TABLE D–1   Continued

ICD-9	Diagnosis
681.1	Cellulitis and abscess of toe
682.0	Cellulitis and abscess of face
682.1	Cellulitis and abscess of neck
682.2	Cellulitis and abscess of trunk
682.3	Cellulitis and abscess of upper arm and forearm
682.4	Cellulitis and abscess of hand, except finger
683.5	Cellulitis and abscess of buttock
683.6	Cellulitis and abscess of leg, except foot
683.7	Cellulitis and abscess of foot, except toes
683.8	Cellulitis and abscess of other specified sites
683.9	Cellulitis and abscess of unspecified sites
707.00	Pressure ulcer of unspecified site
707.01	Pressure ulcer of elbow
707.02	Pressure ulcer of upper back
707.03	Pressure ulcer of lower back
707.04	Pressure ulcer of hip
707.05	Pressure ulcer of buttock
707.06	Pressure ulcer of ankle
707.07	Pressure ulcer of heel
707.09	Pressure ulcer of other
707.10	Ulcer of lower limbs, unspecified
707.11	Ulcer of lower limbs, thigh
707.12	Ulcer of lower limbs, calf
707.13	Ulcer of lower limbs, ankle
707.14	Ulcer of lower limbs, heel and midfoot
707.15	Ulcer of lower limbs, other part of foot
707.19	Ulcer of lower limbs, other part of lower limb
707.20	Pressure ulcer, unspecified stage
707.21	Pressure ulcer, stage 1
707.22	Pressure ulcer, stage 2
707.23	Pressure ulcer, stage 3
707.24	Pressure ulcer, stage 4
707.25	Pressure ulcer, unstageable
707.8	Chronic ulcer of other specified sites

TABLE D–1   Continued

ICD-9	Diagnosis
707.9	Chronic ulcer of unspecified sites
730.0	Acute osteomyelitis
730.1	Chronic osteomyelitis
958.3	Posttraumatic wound infection, not elsewhere classified
997.60	Amputation stump with unspecified complication
997.62	Amputation stump with infection
998.3	Disruption of operation wound
998.5	Postoperative infection

TABLE D–2   Modifier Codes for Wound Management

Modifier	Description
25	Significantly, separately identifiable evaluation and management service by the same physician on the same of day of procedure or other service
27	Multiple outpatient hospital E/M encounters on the same date
50	Bilateral procedure
51	Multiple procedures
52	Reduced services
58	Staged procedure
59	Distinct procedural service

TABLE D–3   CPT Codes for Wound Management

CPT	Description
10060	Incision and drainage of abscess; single or simple
10061	Incision and drainage of abscess; complicated or multiple
11040	Debridement; skin, partial thickness
11041	Debridement; skin, full thickness
11042	Debridement; skin, and subcutaneous tissue
11043	Debridement; skin, subcutaneous tissue, and muscle (10-day global)
11044	Debridement; skin, subcutaneous tissue, muscle, and bone (10-day global)
11055	Paring or cutting of benign hyperkeratotic lesion: single lesion
11056	Paring or cutting of benign hyperkeratotic lesion: 2–4 lesions
11057	Paring or cutting of benign hyperkeratotic lesion: >4 lesions
11100	Biopsy of skin, subcutaneous tissue: single lesion

(continued)

TABLE D–3   Continued

CPT	Description
11101	Biopsy of skin, subcutaneous tissue: each separate/additional lesion *Use in conjunction with 11100
11720	Debridement of nails; one to five
11721	Debridement of nails; six or more
15340	Tissue cultured allogenic skin substitute, first 25 square cm
15341	Tissue cultured allogenic skin substitute, each additional 25 square cm *Use in conjunction with 15340
15430	Acellular xenograft implant; first 100 square cm or less
15431	Acellular xenograft implant; each additional 100 square cm *Use in conjunction with 15430
16020	Dressings or debridement of partial-thickness burns; small <5%
16025	Dressings or debridement of partial-thickness burns; medium 5–10%
16030	Dressings or debridement of partial-thickness burns; large >10%
17250	Chemical cauterization of granulation tissue
29580	Unna boot application
29581	Multilayer compression application
97597	Removal of devitalized tissue from wounds, selective debridement without anesthesia; wound surface <20 square cm
97598	Removal of devitalized tissue from wounds, selective debridement without anesthesia; wound surface >20 square cm
97602	Removal of devitalized tissue from wounds, nonselective debridement without anesthesia
97014	Electrical stimulation (unattended)
97032	Electrical stimulation, each 15 minutes (attended)
97022	Whirlpool (unattended)
97026	Infrared (unattended)
97028	Ultraviolet (unattended)
97035	Ultrasound (attended)
97039	Unlisted modality (attended) *specify type and time
97605	Negative pressure wound therapy, wound surface <50 square cm
97606	Negative pressure wound therapy, wound surface >50 square cm
99183	Physician attendance and supervision of hyperbaric oxygen therapy

REIMBURSEMENT AND DOCUMENTATION FOR DEBRIDEMENT

Debridement is the process of removing devitalized tissue and foreign matter from a wound bed. Wound debridement is a vital element of chronic wound treatment. Nonviable tissue within a chronic wound has been shown to impede wound healing and promote bacterial growth. Therefore, the clinician often must debride a wound bed as part of the wound treatment plan.

CPT codes 11040–11044 are used to report surgical removal of devitalized tissue from wounds. They are payable to physicians and qualified nonphysician practitioners licensed by the state to perform the services. CPT codes 97597–97598 are used to report selective debridement of devitalized tissue and are payable to physicians and qualified nonphysician practitioners, licensed

physical therapists, and licensed occupational therapists. CPT code 97602 is used to report nonselective debridement but is separately payable for Medicare Part A only. Removal of nontissue integrated fibrin exudates, crust, biofilms, or other materials from a wound without removal of tissue does not meet the definition of any debridement code and may not be reported and billed as a debridement. When the service provided is only a nonsurgical cleansing of a wound without debridement, the appropriate Evaluation and Management service code should be used and not the debridement codes.

CPT guidelines do not restrict the number of times debridement codes can be reported. However, medical documentation must support medical necessity for performing debridement. Documentation must show the extent of the debridement performed matches the CPT code reported and there must be progressive improvement in the wound with debridement.

TABLE D–4   Debridement Documentation Requirements

1. Describe the medical condition and relevant medical diagnosis.
2. Describe the wound to document medical necessity; size, condition, the presence and extent or absence of infection and nonviable tissue, depth of wound, before and after debridement.
3. Document the type of tissue that was removed and the depth of the excision.
4. Document the method of debridement (excisional/nonexcisional) and instrument used (scalpel/curette).
5. Selective debridement requires the total area of all wounds to be documented.
6. Document all dressings and treatments used.
7. Document the progress of the wound with each treatment.

TABLE D–5   Evaluation and Management CPT Codes and Descriptions*

E/M CPT	Description
99201	Outpatient visit for evaluation and management of a new patient with three key components: • Problem-focused history • Problem-focused examination • Straightforward medical decision making
99202	Outpatient visit for evaluation and management of a new patient with three key components: • Expanded problem-focused history • Expanded problem-focused examination • Straightforward medical decision making
99203	Outpatient visit for evaluation and management of a new patient with three key components: • Detailed history • Detailed examination • Medical decision making of low complexity

(continued)

TABLE D–5   Continued

E/M CPT	Description
99204	Outpatient visit for evaluation and management of a new patient with three key components: • Comprehensive history • Comprehensive examination • Medical decision making of moderate complexity
99205	Outpatient visit for evaluation and management of a new patient with three key components: • Comprehensive history • Comprehensive examination • Medical decision making of high complexity
99211	Outpatient visit for evaluation and management of an established patient with two of three key components: • Does not require the presence of a physician • Presenting problem is minimal • Less than 5 minutes spent performing services
99212	Outpatient visit for evaluation and management of an established patient with two of three key components: • Problem-focused history • Problem-focused examination • Straightforward medical decision making
99213	Outpatient visit for evaluation and management of an established patient with two of three key components: • Expanded problem-focused history • Expanded problem-focused examination • Medical decision making of low complexity
99214	Outpatient visit for evaluation and management of an established patient with two of three key components: • Detailed history • Detailed examination • Medical decision making of moderate complexity
99215	Outpatient visit for evaluation and management of an established patient with two of three key components: • Comprehensive history • Comprehensive examination • Medical decision making of high complexity

*The codes listed above are used to report evaluation and management services provided by a physician in an outpatient setting.

APPENDIX E
Total Contact Casting Procedure and Patient Instructions

TOTAL CONTACT CASTING PROCEDURE

1. **Preparation**
   a. Irrigate and debride wound of devitalized tissue as able.
   b. Pare callus if present with scalpel to remove entirely or at least level with surrounding tissue to eliminate local pressure point.
   c. Document wound size.
   d. Ensure toenails are adequately trimmed.
   e. Apply skin sealant to periwound as needed.
   f. Apply appropriate thin dressing over wound surface.
   g. Apply moisturizing ointment to foot and lower leg (except between toes).

2. **Gather necessary supplies**
   a. Cast padding
   b. Stockinette
   c. Scifoam
   d. Beveled felt padding
   e. Fiberglass casting rolls
   f. Short- or long-stretch compression bandage
   g. Scissors
   h. Paper tape
   i. Basin of water
   j. Gloves

3. **Application**
   a. Position patient prone with knee flexed 90° and ankle in neutral.
   b. Place cotton padding between toes.
   c. Apply stockinette.
      1) Fold distal end over dorsum of foot and secure with paper tape.
      2) Proximal end will be folded over fiberglass.
      3) Ensure stockinette is smooth and wrinkle-free.
   d. Pad the extremity.
      1) Place Scifoam over toes, trim dog-ears.
      2) Place beveled felt pads over malleoli and navicular tuberosity; secure with paper tape.
      3) Place felt strip along tibial crest; secure with paper tape.
      4) Apply cast padding over extremity.
   e. Apply fiberglass casting rolls.
      1) Aide maintains patient position—ankle in neutral and toes turned slightly upward.
      2) Clinician applies initial layer of fiberglass to extremity while clinician and aide contour fiberglass over bony prominences and into plantar arch.
      3) Initial layer is further molded until mostly set by wrapping with a moistened compression bandage.
      4) Clinician applies second layer of fiberglass—first fill the plantar arch with layered fiberglass to provide a level plantar surface, then reinforce the initial layer and roll the proximal end of stockinette back to ensure a soft proximal cast edge.
      5) Compression wrap is repeated.
      6) Use additional fiberglass rolls if needed to reinforce the cast, repeating molding and compression wrap with each roll.

4. **Check cast for proper fit**
   a. Check for positioning by gently grasping the cast and trying to slide it up and down on the patient's leg. If there is more than $\frac{1}{2}$-inch of movement, the cast is too loose.
   b. Once cast is fully set, don cast shoe and gait train with appropriate assistive device as needed to ensure safe mobility.

5. **Instruct patient in follow-up procedure**
   a. Educate patient in proper cast care and provide written instructions to increase adherence.
   b. Arrange for follow-up appointment.
      1) Initial cast usually changed after ~3 days.
      2) Second cast usually changed after ~1 week.
      3) Third cast usually changed every 1–2 weeks.

6. **Cast removal on follow-up visit**
   a. Position patient comfortably in sitting or supine position.
   b. Use cast saw to cut cast medially, distally over Scifoam, and laterally.
   c. Use blunted scissors and cast pliers to remove cast.
   d. Inspect lower leg, foot, and wound.
   e. Clean lower leg and foot as needed.

Modified from McCulloch J. Total contact casting: A management option for diabetics with plantar ulcerations. Course presented at: Bloomington Hospital; April 12–13, 1999; Bloomington, IN.

TOTAL CONTACT CAST PATIENT INSTRUCTIONS

You have had a total contact cast applied to your leg to assist with healing the ulcer (sore) on your foot. This cast is specially made to decrease the amount of pressure and shear (friction) over your entire foot. By decreasing these forces, the cast allows your ulcer to heal. For the cast to be effective, you must know how to take care of it and your leg.

DO NOT

- DO NOT use your cast to strike or hit objects, or damage your cast in any way.
- DO NOT stick objects in the cast or scratch your skin.
- DO NOT remove your cast yourself.

DO

- **Use your cast shoe** whenever you are walking or standing.
- **Limit your walking distance and standing time** as much as possible. Try to decrease the amount you walk by at least one-third.
- **Use an assistive device, such as a cane, crutches, or a walker** as instructed by your clinician. This will help your balance and further decrease the amount of pressure and shear on your foot.
- **Take shorter steps.** This will help your balance and further decrease the amount of pressure and shear on your foot.
- **Keep your cast dry.** Water softens your cast and will increase the risk of infection. Sponge bathing is recommended. When bathing, cover your cast with two layers of plastic bags secured above the cast.
- **Wear a full-length sock on your uncasted leg when sleeping.** This will help protect your other leg from being rubbed by the cast.
- **Inspect your cast daily** for signs of damage to the cast or drainage. If you are unable to do so, have a significant other do this for you.
- **Contact your clinician immediately if any of the following signs or symptoms occur:**
  - Excessive swelling causes the cast to become too tight.
  - The cast becomes too loose and your leg is able to slip more than $\frac{1}{2}$-inch inside the cast.
  - The cast becomes damaged.
  - You notice any drainage on the outside of the cast.
  - You notice a foul odor coming from the cast.
  - You experience leg pain or pressure in the ankle or foot that does not go away after resting.
  - You notice any sudden onset of fever or an unusual increase in your blood sugar.

1. **Call:** _____
2. **Do not walk on your cast.**
3. **Keep your leg elevated.**

APPENDIX F
Internet Wound Care Resources

The following Websites provide a plethora of information on wound management, wound care products, wound guidelines, and wound research. These sites, and the links they contain, can assist clinicians active in wound management to enhance their knowledge, expand their practice, and improve the quality of care they provide. Many of these sites allow clinicians to post clinical practice questions for experienced clinicians to respond to, and many of them provide search engines and access to journal articles on wound management. Although in no way complete, these resources provide a starting point for both novice and master wound management clinicians.

- **http://dermatlas.med.jhmi.edu/derm**

The Derm Atlas Website is sponsored by Johns Hopkins University. The site's purpose is to "enable health care professionals, parents, and patients to access high quality dermatology images for teaching purposes." There are images of over 11,600 pediatric dermatological diagnoses available for review online, with new images added regularly. Site visitors can search the site by word, body site, category, or diagnosis.

- **http://telemedicine.org/stamfor1.htm**

The Electronic Textbook of Dermatology Website is published by the Internet Dermatology Society. This free site contains an anatomical review of the integument and a vast array of dermatological resources and images including common skin pathologies and cutaneous drug reactions.

- **http://aad.org**

This is the website for the American Academy of Dermatology.

- **http://www.aawconline.org**

This is the official Website for the Association for the Advancement of Wound Care (AAWC). Based in the United States, the AAWC is a nonprofit organization of health care workers, manufacturers, caregivers, and patients. The AAWC's mission is to "promote excellence in education, clinical practice, research, and public policy." Of particular interest to clinicians new to wound management, the association offers a wound slide guide that can be purchased. Association membership includes free copies of official association journals: *Ostomy/Wound Management* and *Wounds: A Compendium of Clinical Research and Practice*.

- **http://www.aawm.org**

This is the Website for the American Academy of Wound Management (AAWM). The AAWM is a not-for-profit interdisciplinary organization created to promote education, research, and knowledge of patients with acute and chronic wounds. The AAWM has established standards for credentialing clinicians in wound management as certified wound specialists (CWS)®. Links provide information on upcoming continuing education and conferences in the area of wound management.

- **http://www.ameriburn.org**

This is the official Website of the American Burn Association (ABA). The ABA is committed to education in acute care, rehabilitation, and prevention of burn wound injuries. The ABA is a multidisciplinary organization that encourages national and international research within the burn care field. The ABA's official publication is the *Journal of Burn Care and Research*.

- **http://www.apma.org**

The Website for the American Podiatric Medical Association provides information on diabetic foot ulcers along with links to the *Journal of the American Podiatric Medical Association.*

- **http://www.apta.org**

The official Website of the American Physical Therapy Association provides APTA members with access to PubMed, professional and continuing education opportunities, APTA publications, and practice updates.

- **http://www.apwca.org**

This is the website for the American Professional Wound Care Association. Members receive a free subscription to *Advances in Skin and Wound Care* as well as discounted conference rates.

- **http://www.aswcjournal.com**

This is the Website for the print journal *Advances in Skin and Wound Care.*

- **http://www.cms.gov**

The website for Centers for Medicare and Medicaid Services includes information on national and regional coverage decisions.

- **http://www.cochrane.org**

The Website for the Cochrane Collaboration, a United Kingdom–based, international not-for-profit organization devoted to the prevention of open wounds and interventions for patients with open wounds. The site includes links to the Cochrane Library and over 4,000 completed reviews.

- **http://www.dermnet.com**

This Website provides over 23,000 images of skin diseases as well as links to various dermatological and integumentary resources.

- **http://www.diabetes.org**

The American Diabetes Association Website provides links to journals, articles, and research on diabetes and neuropathic ulcers for clinicians and laypersons.

- **http://www.epuap.org**

This is the website for the European Pressure Ulcer Advisory Panel, which, in conjunction with the National Pressure Ulcer Advisory Panel, compiled the updated pressure ulcer guidelines.

- **http://www.etrs.org**

This is the website for the European Tissue Repair Society with links to its official journal, *Wound Repair and Regeneration.*

- **http://www.fda.gov**

This is the website for the U.S. Food and Drug Administration. Links provided can be used to find updates on medications, medical devices, and nutrition guidelines.

- **http://www.freemedicaljournals.com**

This Website provides free links to full text articles from many medical and scientific journals.

- **http://www.guideline.gov**

The National Clearing House™ is a public resource created by a partnership between the Agency for Healthcare Research and Quality and the American Medical Association.

- **http://www.lymphnet.org**

This is the website for the National Lymphedema Network with links on education, resources, position statements, and certification in the management of lymphedema.

- **http://www.medscape.com/medscapetoday**

The Medscape Website provides registered users with free access to a wide array of medical information as well as a weekly e-mail with links to recent articles of interest. Highlights of this site include a clinical management series, clinical practice guidelines, treatment updates, an editor-conducted journal scan of current medical literature within each specialty area, Medline access, and a drug search program.

- **http://www.ncbi.nlm.nih.gov/PubMed/ medline.html**

This free, government-sponsored Website allows visitors to perform Medline searches. In addition, the site provides links to the National Institutes of Health, the National Library of Medicine, the National Center for Biotechnology, and PubMed Central—a free and unrestricted digital archive of print journals.

- **http://www.npuap.org**

This is the official Website for the National Pressure Ulcer Advisory Panel (NPUAP). The site's goal is to provide multidisciplinary guidance for improved patient outcomes in pressure ulcer prevention and management through education, public policy, and research. This site contains the newest pressure ulcer staging system guidelines, position statements and information on the PUSH Tool, conferences, and a newsletter. Site visitors new to wound management may wish to order one of the educational wound slide sets with accompanying slide guide.

- **http://www.o-wm.com**

This is the *Ostomy/Wound Management* Website. This site includes abstracts and key points of journal articles, a discussion forum, and continuing education unit (CEU) information. In addition, a complete buyer's guide provides links to a vast array of wound product manufacturers.

- **http://www.wocn.org**

This is the official Website for the Wound Ostomy Continence Nursing Society (WOCN). The WOCN's mission is to "promote educational, clinical, and research opportunities; to advance the practice and guide the delivery of expert health care to individuals with wounds, ostomies, and incontinence." The site provides links to full text articles in the *Journal of WOCN*.

- **http://www.worldwidewounds.com**

The mission of *World Wide Wounds* is to be the premier online resource for peer-reviewed information on dressing materials. It also strives to provide health professionals with clinical guidance on all aspects of wound management.

- **http://www.woundsresearch.com**

This is the Website for the peer-reviewed journal *Wounds*.

INDEX

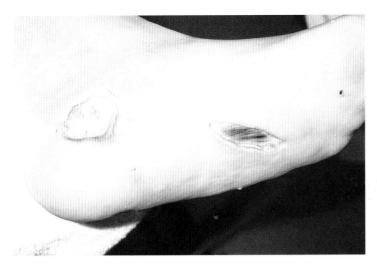

PHOTO C–1   The plantar fascia is exposed on the plantar aspect of this patient's foot. The fascia can be identified by the regular arrangement of the fibers. Note the dark color of the fascia, indicating that, although it is intact, it is no longer viable tissue.

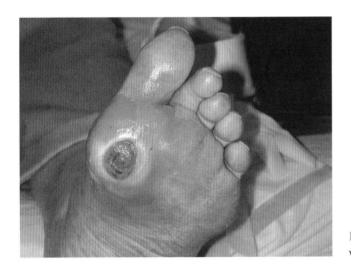

PHOTO C–2   Patient with a plantar first metatarsal wound.

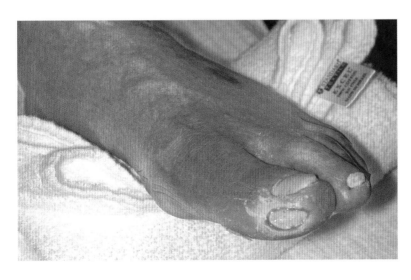

PHOTO C–3   Patient with a wound in the inflammatory phase of wound healing. Notice the edema of the great toe as well as the erythema extending from the wound dorsally down to the area of the metatarsophalangeal joint. The wound bed is covered with a thin layer of yellow slough. The great toe feels slightly warm to the touch. Additionally, the patient reports the toe is tender to the touch.

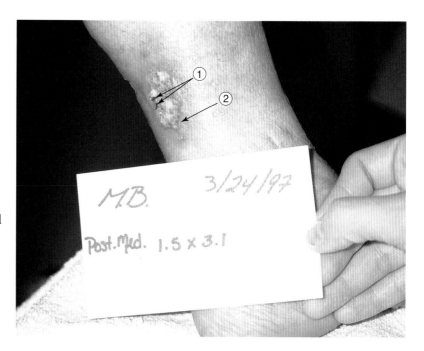

PHOTO C–4   Patient with a wound in the proliferative phase of wound healing. The small endothelial buds (1), which can be seen within the wound bed, indicate angiogenesis. The pale pink epithelial cells at the wound edge (2) are evidence of epithelialization.

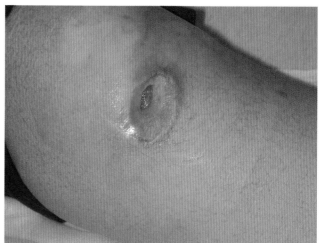

PHOTO C–5   Wound contraction during the proliferative phase of wound healing. This wound, located anteriorly inferior to the patella, is actively contracting toward the center while the perimeter is remodeling. Note the changes in tissue quality. Near the wound edge, less granulation tissue has been formed and the scar is less mature and more pink in color. Farther out, the scar is closer to the patient's natural skin color and flush with the surrounding skin.

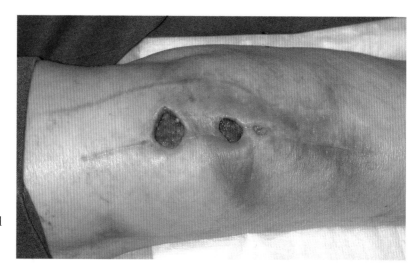

PHOTO C–6   Patient with a total knee replacement with tunneling wound.

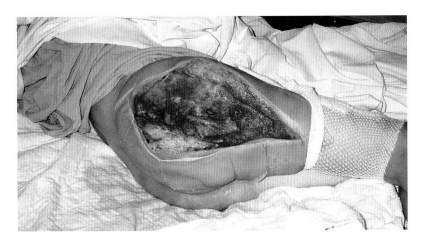

PHOTO C–7   Patient with a lateral thigh pressure ulcer.

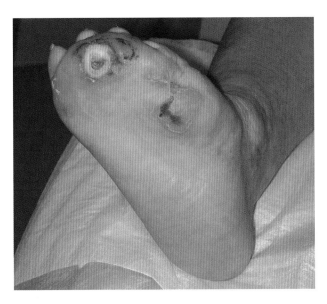

PHOTO C–8   Patient with a neuropathic ulcer prior to debridement. Notice the ring of callus around the wound at the plantar aspect of the metatarsal heads that is typical of neuropathic ulcerations. The pressure point caused by the Charcot deformity is callused and there is evidence of subdermal hemorrhaging. Previous amputations and surgical incisions are also evident.

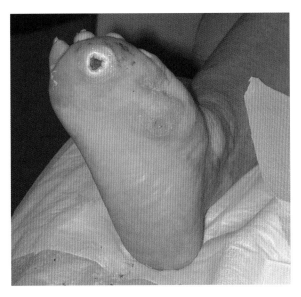

PHOTO C–9   Color image 8 after debridement and application of moisturizing lotion to the intact skin. This would be classified as a Wagner grade 1 ulcer and fit pattern D: Impaired Integumentary Integrity Secondary to Full-Thickness Involvement and Scar Formation.

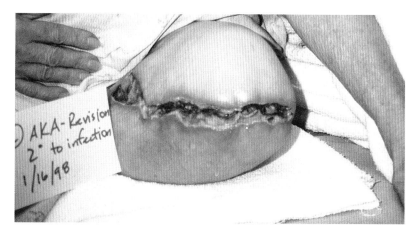

PHOTO C–10   Patient presents with history of peripheral vascular disease, diabetes, and an ulceration that failed to heal secondary to osteomyelitis. Five days after an initial above-knee amputation, infection persisted and a revision of the amputation was performed. Note that the amputation site was not surgically closed. The wound bed contains approximately 98% necrotic tissue, and probing will find several tunnels in the lateral/inferior wound bed. Periwound is mildly erythematous compared to the extent of the wound, which would be consistent with inflammation rather than current infection. However, with a history of peripheral vascular disease and diabetes mellitus, the patient may not be able to build up a significant cellular response to bacterial infection.

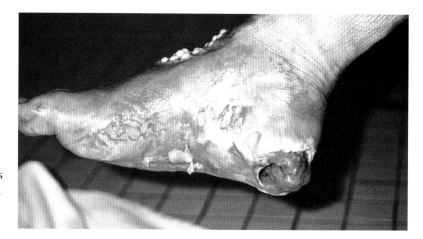

PHOTO C–11   Patient presenting with grossly infected foot wounds. Significant erythema and copious amounts of purulent drainage are evident. The calcaneal wound has very poor quality hypergranular tissue with severe periwound maceration. Also note the presence of antimicrobial beads on the dorsum of the foot. These were placed 2 weeks prior to this photograph in an attempt to control the patient's infection after he refused an amputation.

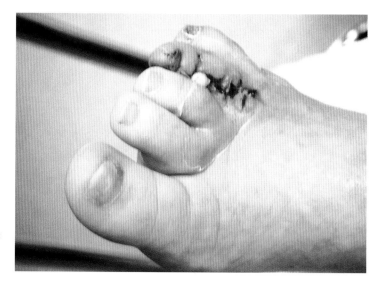

PHOTO C–12   Patient with ulcer of the fourth digit after surgical debridement and implantation of antimicrobial beads.

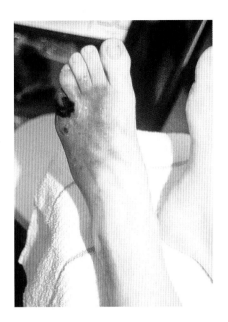

PHOTO C–13   Patient with
a gangrenous toe.

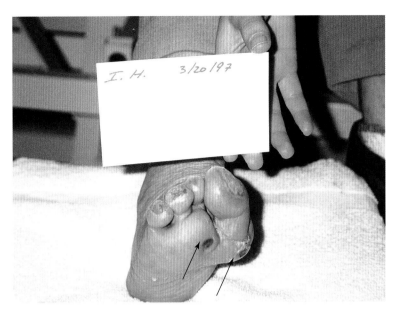

PHOTO C–14   Patient with arterial insufficiency ulcers. Note the
wounds on the distal toes with adherent yellow slough-covered
bases. The wound beds appear to be slightly dry, rather than wet or
moist. The patient presents with a previous amputation of the second
digit and metatarsal due to a previous nonhealing neuropathic ulcer.
This amputation allowed the hallux valgus deformity and a dorsal
migration of the third digit. These deformities caused pressure points
(arrows) at the plantar aspect at the first and third metatarsal heads.

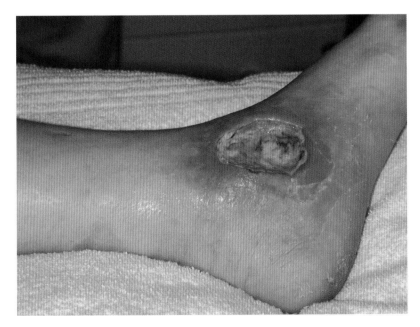

PHOTO C–15   Patient with an
ulcer near the left medial malleolus.

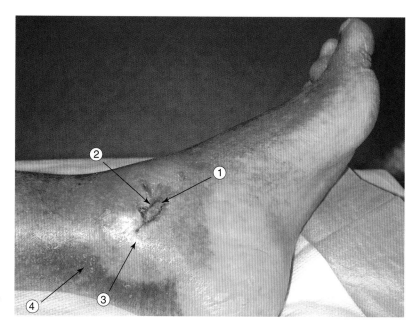

PHOTO C–16 Patient with a typical venous insufficiency ulcer. The wound is located near the medial malleolus. The wound bed is approximately 85% adherent yellow slough (1), with approximately 15% granulation tissue at the wound margins (2). There is scar tissue surrounding the ulcer (3), indicating the wound was once significantly larger than in the current photograph. There is extensive hemosiderin deposition posterior, superior, and anterior to the ulcer (4).

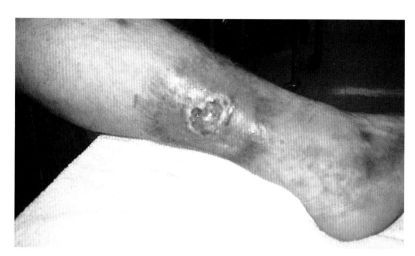

PHOTO C–17 Patient with a medial calf ulcer with hemosiderin deposition.

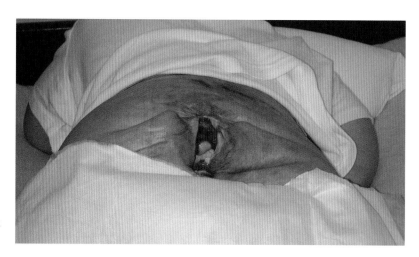

PHOTO C–18 Patient with a stage IV sacral pressure ulcer.

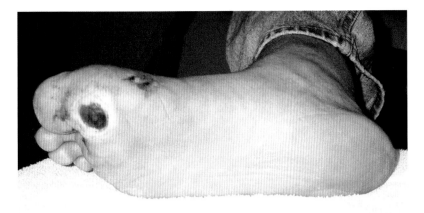

PHOTO C–19   Patient with a plantar first metatarsal ulcer.

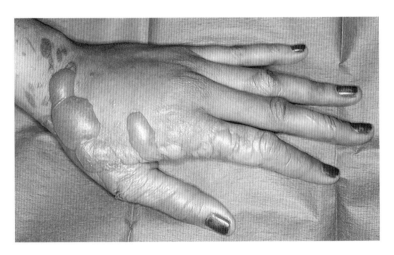

PHOTO C–20   Patient with a superficial partial-thickness burn.

Source: Paramedic care: Principles and Practice— Trauma Emergencies by Bledsoe/Porter/Cherry, © reprinted by permission of Pearson Education, Inc., Upper Saddle River, NJ.

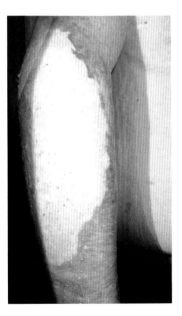

PHOTO C–21   Patient with a deep partial-thickness burn of the right lateral forearm.

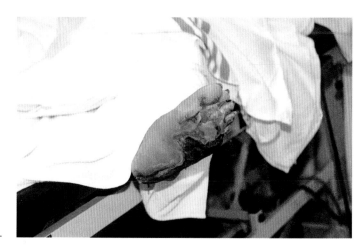

PHOTO C–22   Case Study 3: plantar foot
wound on a patient with below-knee amputation.

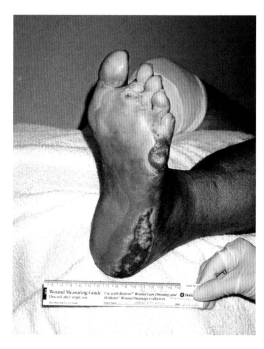

PHOTO C–23   Color image 22 three weeks after initiating
physical therapy.

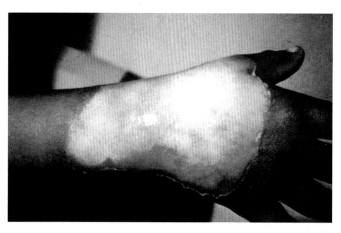

PHOTO C–24   Case Study 1: patient with a dorsal hard,
wrist, and distal forearm wound.

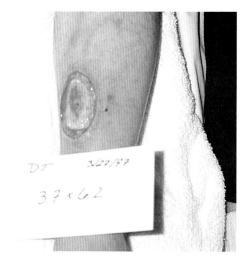

PHOTO C–25   Case Study 2: patient with
an anterior shin wound.